369 0246375

Paediatric Dentistry

Paediatric Dentistry

Fourth edition

Edited by

Richard Welbury

Professor of Paediatric Dentistry
University of Glasgow;
Visiting Professor
University of Zagreb

Monty S. Duggal

Professor of Child Dental Health
Leeds Dental Institute

Marie Thérèse Hosey

Professor of Paediatric Dentistry
King's College London

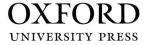

OXFORD

UNIVERSITY PRESS

Great Clarendon Street, Oxford OX2 6DP,
United Kingdom

Oxford University Press is a department of the University of Oxford.
It furthers the University's objective of excellence in research, scholarship,
and education by publishing worldwide. Oxford is a registered trade mark of
Oxford University Press in the UK and in certain other countries

British Library Cataloguing in Publication Data

Data available

Library of Congress Cataloging in Publication

Library of Congress Control Number: 2012939874

ISBN 978-0-19-957491-9

Printed and bound by
Bell & Bain Ltd, Glasgow

Contents

Contributors

M.J. Aldred
Department of Dentistry
Royal Childrens' Hospital, Melbourne

A.S. Blinkhorn
Faculty of Dentistry
University of Sydney

L.A.L. Burbridge
Department of Child Dental Health
Newcastle upon Tyne Dental Hospital
and School

P.J.M. Crawford
Department of Child Dental Health
University of Bristol

P.F. Day
Department of Child Dental Health
Leeds Dental Institute

C. Deery
Professor of Paediatric Dentistry
University of Sheffield

M.S. Duggal
Professor of Child Dental Health
Leeds Dental Institute

S.A. Fayle
Department of Child Dental Health
Leeds Dental Institute

T.J. Gillgrass
Department of Orthodontics
Glasgow Dental Hospital and School

J.C. Harris
Department of Paediatric Dentistry
Sheffield Teaching Hospitals Trust

P.A. Heasman
Professor of Periodontology
University of Newcastle upon Tyne

M.T. Hosey
Professor of Paediatric Dentistry
King's College London

M.L. Hunter
Professor of Paediatric Dentistry
University of Cardiff

N.M. Kilpatrick
Professor of Paediatric Dentistry
Murdoch Children's Research Institute,
Melbourne

L. Lourenço-Matharu
Department of Paediatric Dentistry
King's College London

J.G. Meechan
Department of Oral Surgery
University of Newcastle upon Tyne

J.H. Nunn
Professor of Special Care Dentistry
University of Dublin

G.J. Roberts
Professor of Paediatric Dentistry
King's College London

H.D. Rodd
Professor of Paediatric Dentistry
University of Sheffield

J.A. Smallridge
Department of Child Dental Health
King's College London

K.J. Toumba
Professor of Paediatric Dentistry
University of Leeds

P.J. Waterhouse
Department of Child Dental Health
University of Newcastle upon Tyne

R. Welbury
Professor of Paediatric Dentistry
University of Glasgow

J.M. Whitworth
Department of Restorative Dentistry
University of Newcastle upon Tyne

Preface to the first edition

The child and adolescent deserves the best of care in all the different disciplines of dentistry. I was delighted to be given the opportunity of trying to draw together all the different aspects of paediatric dentistry and am most grateful to my colleagues for agreeing to contribute the various chapters which make up the book. We have tried to cover as much ground as possible within the obvious publishing restrictions and the finished product will inevitably reflect the editor's perceptions of where current needs and deficiencies exist. The sudden increase in both erosive tooth surface loss and cosmetic awareness in our younger patients made their inclusion in Chapter 8 important, where previously they have not achieved such prominence in paediatric texts. Similarly, periodontal disease (Chapter 10), oral pathology and oral surgery (Chapter 14), and disability (Chapter 16) are as deserving of detailed inclusion in a 'paediatric' as much as in any 'general' text.

The book was written with undergraduate dental students in mind, but we hope it will also be useful to those engaged in postgraduate studies and to general dental practitioners. Exhaustive references are deliberately not given but suggested 'further reading' lists are included to help expedite Further enquiry and learning.

I hope we have shown in *Paediatric dentistry* that the early years of life are the time to get it right for the child and adolescent and there is no reason why our young patients should be denied correct and appropriate care.

R. R. W.
Newcastle upon Tyne
April 1996

Preface to the second edition

I am delighted to be given the opportunity to edit the second edition of this popular textbook and am grateful to my colleagues for their continuing contribution. The reviews of the first edition indentified the need for a chapter on the treatment of caries in the preschool child and I am grateful to Stephen Fayle for undertaking this task.

There have been small modifications and updates to most chapters, which should keep the reader abreast with current theory and practice. Greater use has also been made of 'Key points' for revision purposes.

I hope the second edition will continue to help both undergraduates, postgraduates, and general dental practitioners in their practice of paediatric dentistry.

R. R. W.
Newcastle upon Tyne
January *2001*

Preface to the third edition

I was very pleased when my younger colleagues Marie Thérèse Hosey and Monty Duggal accepted my offer to join me in editing this third edition. Our book has now sold four and a half thousand copies since its launch in 1997 and it is essential that we maintain a contemporary outlook and publish changes in techniques and philosophies as soon as they have an evidence base.

Since 2001 and the second edition, there have been a significant number of changes of authorship, as well as a change of chapters for some existing authors.

Gerry Winter died in December 2002. He was a wise colleague and friend who was a mentor to many of us. I continue to miss his expertise and availability for consultation, by post or telephone, which he freely gave even after his retirement.

John Murray, Andrew Rugg-Gunn, and Linda Shaw have now retired from clinical practice. I am indebted to them all for their support, both in my own personal career and in the production of out textbook. I am grateful to them for allowing the new chapter authors to use their texts and figures.

The restorative section of the book has been remodelled. The endodontics chapter in the previous editions has now been incorporated into either chapters 8 or 12, and there are separate chapters relating to the operative care of the primary and the permanent dentitions. Without the help and friendship of Jim Page the original 'Operative care of dental caries' chapter would not have been possible. I am grateful to Jim for allowing us to continue to use his original illustrations from that chapter.

Although designed for the undergraduate we hope the new edition will continue to be used by undergraduate, postgraduate, and general dental practitioner alike, and that their practice of paediatric dentistry will be both fulfilling and enjoyable.

R. R. W
Glasgow
January 2005

Preface to the fourth edition

It is difficult to believe that 17 years have passed since work began on the first edition. Our Portuguese edition was marketed in 2007 and this has broadened our market significantly in Brazil.

This edition contains some new contributors, Liege Lourenço-Matharu, Lucy Burbridge, Jenny Harris, and Toby Gillgrass, and their enthusiasm and insight have been invaluable. We are grateful to the comments from reviewers and OUP staff which have resulted in revision of a number of chapters, and so we hope that the end product will be as well received as previous editions.

The excitement of a new edition is tinged with sadness at the loss of Nigel Carter at such a young age. Nigel always gave very generously of his time to paediatric colleagues. On a happier note, Peter Gordon is now enjoying a well-earned retirement and we would all like to thank him for his contribution to the three previous editions.

In looking at the author list for the fourth edition we are struck by the number of contributors who have gained promotion to professorial positions since they originally contributed to *Paediatric Dentistry*. We must be doing something right!

Richard Welbury
Marie Thérèse Hosey
Monty Duggal

Acknowledgements

Fig. 1.2, *Ten Cate's Oral Histology*, 6th edn, Antonio Nanci, © Elsevier 2011;

Figs 1.3, 1.5, 1.8, 1.14, reproduced from Mitchell, *An Introduction to Orthodontics*, 2007, with permission of Oxford University Press;

Figs 1.6, 1.11, 14.48, reproduced from Johnson and Moore, *Anatomy for Dental Students*, 1997, with permission of Oxford University Press;

Fig. 1.7, redrawn from Proffit, W.R. (2000). *Contemporary Orthodontics*, 3rd edn, Mosby;

Fig. 1.10, courtesy of Professor Steve Richmond;

all figures in Chapter 2 courtesy of David Myers and Eden Bianchi Press;

Fig. 3.14 Green and Vermillion (1964);

Figs 5.2, 5.3, 5.4, 5.9, 5.10, 5.11, 5.12, 5.13, 5.19, 15.1, 15.2, 15.10, 15.16, 15.23, 15.24, 15.25, 15.28, 15.30, 15.31, 15.32, reproduced from *Dental Update* (ISSN 0305-5000), by permission of George Warman Publications (UK) Ltd;

Fig. 6.1, reproduced with permission from Jenkins 1978;

Figs 6.4, 6.5, reproduced from Soames and Southam, *Oral Pathology*, by permission of Oxford University Press;

Fig. 6.7, reproduced from von der Fehr (1994) with kind permission of the *International Dental Journal*;

Fig. 6.8, reproduced from Spencer *et al.* (1994) with kind permission of the *International Dental Journal*;

Fig. 6.15, reproduced by kind permission of Toothfriendly International, Switzerland. http://www.toothfriendly.org;

Figs 8.24, 8.27, reproduced with the kind permission of Professor H.S. Chawla, PGIMER, India;

Figs 10.25, 10.26, by kind permission of Dr J. Winters;

Fig. 11.6, reproduced by permission from MacMillan Publishers Ltd: *British Journal of Dentistry* © 1994;

Fig. 11.7, Reproduced from Heasman, P.A., Factitious Ginival Ulceration: A Manifestation of Munchausen's Syndrome, *Journal of Periodontology*, 1994. With permission of the American Academy of Periodontology;

Fig. 11.11, reproduced by kind permission of Mr N.E. Carter;

Figs 11.12, 11.18, 11.19, reproduced by kind permission of Professor I.L. Chapple, Birmingham, UK;

Fig. 11.13, reproduced by kind permission of Mr D.G. Smith, Consultant in Restorative Dentistry, Newcastle upon Tyne;

Figs 12.55, 12.56, reproduced from Andreasen and Andreasen, *Textbook and colour atlas of traumatic injuries to the teeth* (3rd edition) with permission from John Wiley & Sons;

Fig. 14.1, R. Evans and W. Shaw (1987). Reproduced with kind permission of the Editor of the *European Journal of Orthodontics*;

Figs 14.7, 14.35, courtesy of Mr T.G. Bennett;

Fig. 14.10, courtesy of Professor J.H. Nunn;

Fig. 14.40, courtesy of Mr I.B. Buchanan;

Figs 15.4, 15.6, 15.12, reproduced by kind permission of Informa Healthcare;

Fig. 15.7, by kind permission of the *Journal of Dentistry for Children*;

Fig. 15.13, by kind permission of Professor C. Scully;

Fig. 15.27, image kindly supplied by Straumann Ltd;

Figs 16.5, 16.6, 16.8, courtesy of Dr Linda Shaw;

Figs 16.10, 16.11, 16.12, courtesy of Dr Alex Keightley;

Fig. 16.13 courtesy of Dr Triona Fahey;

Fig. 17.21, courtesy of Shine, www.shinecharity.org.uk;

Fig. 17.22, courtesy of HSE Dental Services, Dun Laoghaire, Ireland;

Fig. 17.23, courtesy of Dr Bitte Ahlborg, Mun-H-Center, Sweden;

Fig. 18.2 data used with permission of Department for Children, Schools and Families 2010;

Figs 18.3, 18.4, 18.7, by kind permission of COPDEND;

Fig. 18.8, reproduced with kind permission of Munksgaard;

Figs 18.9, 18.11, reproduced from Hobbs and Wynne, *Physical Signs of Child Abuse: A Colour Atlas* © Elsevier (2001);

Fig. 18.10, reproduced with kind permission of Professor G.T. Craig.

Fig. 18.13 Adapted from Harris, J.C. *et al.*, Child protection and the dental team. © COPDEND 2006.

Abbreviations

AAGBI	Association of Anaesthetists of Great Britain and Ireland		**EADT**	extra-alveolar dry time
AC	alveolar crest		**EAPD**	European Academy of Paediatric Dentistry
ADHD	attention-deficit hyperactivity disorder		**EAT**	extra-alveolar time
ADJ	amelodentinal junction		**EC**	ethyl chloride
ALL	acute lymphocytic leukaemia		**ECC**	early childhood caries
ALOSS	attachment loss		**ECG**	electrocardiogram
ALP	alkaline phosphatase		**EIR**	external inflammatory resorption
AP	anteroposterior		**ENT**	ear, nose, and throat
APAGBI	Association of Paediatric Anaesthetists of Great Britain and Ireland		**EPT**	electric pulp tester
APF	acidulated phosphate fluoride		**Er:YAG**	erbium: yttrium aluminium garnet
ASA	American Society of Anaesthesiologists		**F**	fluoride
ASD	atrial septal defect		**FOTI**	fibre-optic transillumination
BASCD	British Association for the Study of Community Dentistry		**G6PD**	glucose-6-phosphate dehydrogenase
BDA	British Dental Association		**GA**	general anaesthetic
BNF	*British National Formulary*		**GABA**	gamma-aminobutyric acid
BoNT-A	botulinum neurotoxin type A		**GDP**	general dental practitioner
BPA	bis-phenol A		**GIC**	glass ionomer cement
BPE	Basic Periodontal Examination		**GMP**	general medical practitioner
BSPD	British Society of Paediatric Dentistry		**GORD**	gastro-oesophageal reflux disease
BW	bitewing		**GP**	gutta percha
CAT	computed axial tomography		**HIV**	human immunodeficiency virus
CEJ	cemento-enamel junction		**HLA**	human leucocyte antigen
CJD	Creutzfeldt–Jakob disease		**HOME**	hand over mouth exercise
CLD	certainly lethal dose		**Ho:YAG**	holmium: yttrium aluminium garnet
CLP	cleft lip and palate		**ICDAS**	International Caries Diagnosis and Assessment System
CNS	central nervous system		**ICON**	Index of Complexity, Outcome, and Need
COP-DEND	Committee of Postgraduate Dental Deans and Directors		**IM**	intramuscular
COSHH	Control of Substances Hazardous to Health		**INR**	international normalized ratio
CP	cleft palate		**IOTN**	Index of Orthodontic Treatment Need
CPP-ACP	casein phosphopeptide-amorphous calcium phosphate		**IPC**	indirect pulp capping
			IRM	intermediate restorative material
CT	computed tomography		**IV**	intravenous
DDAVP®	1-desamino-8-D-arginine vasopressin		**KG**	keratinized gingiva
DMFS	decayed, filled, and missing tooth surfaces		**LA**	local anaesthetic
DMFT	decayed, missing, and filled teeth		**LAD**	leucocyte adhesion deficiency syndrome
DO	distal–occlusal		**LCH**	Langerhans' cell histiocytosis
DPC	direct pulp capping		**MDT**	multidisciplinary team
EACA	epsilon-aminocaproic acid		**MFP**	sodium monofluorophosphate
			MHC	major histocompatibility complex
			MIH	molar incisor hypomineralization
			MMR	measles, mumps, and rubella

MRI	magnetic resonance image/imaging	**ppm**	parts per million
MTA	mineral trioxide aggregate	**PRR**	preventive resin restoration
NAI	non-accidental injury	**psi**	pounds per square inch
Nd:YAG	neodymuim: yttrium aluminium garnet	**PVAC–PE**	polyvinylacetate–polyethylene
NECAT	New England Children's Amalgam Trial	**RCOA**	Royal College of Anaesthetists
NICE	National Institute for Health and Clinical Excellence	**RCT**	root canal treatment
		RET	regenerative endodontic technique
NSAID	non-steroidal anti-inflammatory drug	**RMGIC**	resin-modified glass ionomer cement
NUG	necrotizing ulcerative gingivitis	**SBE**	subacute bacterial endocarditis
OCA	operative care advised	**SCAP**	stem cells of the apical papilla
OFG	orofacial granulomatosis	**SDCEP**	Scottish Dental Clinical Effectiveness Programme
OME	otis media	**SIGN**	Scottish Intercollegiate Guidelines Network
OPT	orthopantomogram (also abbreviated to OPG)	**STD**	safely tolerated dose
PAR	Peer Assessment Rating	**TAB**	transient apical breakdown
PCA	preventive care advised	**TENS**	transcutaneous electrical nerve stimulation
PCS	patient-controlled sedation	**TMD**	temporomandibular joint disorder
PDL	periodontal ligament	**TSL**	tooth surface loss
PJC	porcelain jacket crown	**TTP**	tender to percussion
PL	periodontal ligament	**TWA**	time-weighted average
PLD	potentially lethal dose	**TWI**	tooth wear index
PLS	Papillon–Lefèvre syndrome	**VSD**	ventral septal defect
PMC	preformed metal crown	**WHO**	World Health Organization

1
Craniofacial growth and development

T.J. Gillgrass and R. Welbury

Chapter contents

1.1 Introduction

This chapter describes, in general terms, the prenatal development and postnatal growth of the craniofacial skeleton, and the occlusal development of the primary and permanent dentitions.

1.2 Prenatal development

Understanding of embryological development is essential for the dental practitioner who may frequently face patients with the common craniofacial anomalies such as cleft lip and/or palate. For routine care, an understanding of their development and aetiology will bring insight to their likely presenting signs and symptoms.

This section will include a brief summary of the development of the face including the neural crest and pharyngeal arches. It is not the intention of this summary to be in any way a complete or thorough description but simply to describe some of the key cells/interactions and structures.

1.2.1 Neural crest

Neural crest cells are derived from the neural fold, and are highly migratory and specialized cells capable of predetermined differentiation. The differentiation occurs after their migration and is essential for the normal development of face and teeth (Fig. 1.1).

1.2.2 Branchial arches

By week 4 the primitive mouth or stomatodeum is bordered laterally and from the developing heart inferiorly by the pharyngeal or branchial arches (Fig. 1.2). These are six bilateral cylindrical thickenings (although the fifth and sixth are small) which form in the pharyngeal wall and into which the neural crest cells migrate. They are separated externally by the branchial grooves and internally by the pharyngeal pouches. The first groove and pouches are involved in the formation of the auditory apparatus and the Eustachian tube.

Each arch has a derived cartilage rod, muscular, nervous, and vascular component. The first two arches and their associated components are central to the development of the facial structures.

This period is also characterized by the development of the organs for hearing, sight, and smell, namely the otic, optic, and nasal placodes.

1.2.3 Facial development

By the end of week 4, thickenings start to develop in the frontal process. The medial and lateral frontonasal processes develop from these, together with the nasal placodes.

The maxillary process develops from the first pharyngeal arch and grows forward to meet the medial and nasal processes, from which it is separated by distinct grooves at week 7 (Fig. 1.3). Its eventual fusion with them creates the upper lip and, from the two medial nasal processes, the incisor teeth and the primary palate. Where this fusion is disturbed a cleft of the lip may form (Fig. 1.4).

The lower lip is formed by fusion of the mandibular process from the first arch.

By week 8 the odontogenic epithelium, which will differentiate into tooth-forming cells, can be determined on the inferior border of the maxillary process, the lateral aspect of the medial process, and the superior border of the mandibular processes.

1.2.4 Secondary palate

Development of the secondary palate starts around week 7. It is formed from three processes: the nasal septum develops in the midline from the frontonasal process and the two palatine shelves develop from the maxillary processes. At this stage the palatal shelves are directed downwards on either side of the tongue. Between weeks 7 and 8 they elevate to meet the primary palate and nasal septum, to which they fuse (Fig. 1.5).

The trigger for this elevation is still unclear, although high concentrations of glycosaminoglycans which attract water and increase turgidity in the shelves, contractile fibroblasts, and the position of the tongue have all been implicated. Once in contact, the epithelial covering of the shelves must disappear to allow the fusion. Various methods including cell death ('apoptosis') and cell transformation have been suggested as methods by which this epithelial covering is lost.

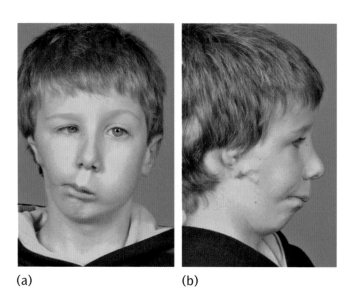

(a)   (b)

Figure 1.1 A child with the hemifacial microsomia part of the oculo-auricular-vertebral spectrum. The unilateral inhibition of neural crest migration and bronchial arch development results in (a) marked asymmetry and (b) ear defects.

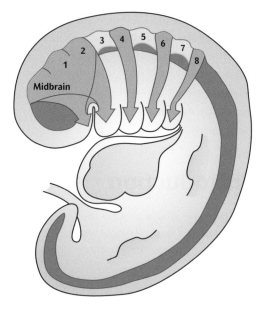

Figure 1.2 Week 6–7 embryo showing branchial arches and migration of neural crest cells into the branchial arch system. (This figure was published in *Ten Cate's Oral Histology*, 6th edition, Antonio Nanci, © Elsevier 2011.)

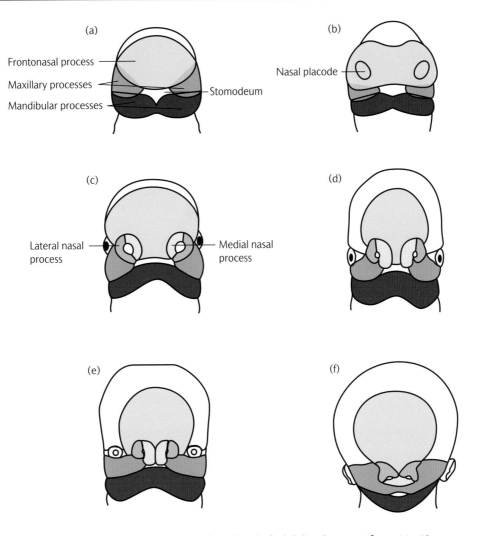

(a)

Frontonasal process

Maxillary processes

Mandibular processes

Stomodeum

(b)

Nasal placode

(c)

Lateral nasal process

Medial nasal process

(d)

(e)

(f)

Figure 1.3 Diagrammatic representation of early facial development from 4 to 10 weeks i.u. (a) 4th week i.u. (b) 28 days i.u. (c) 32 days i.u. (d) 35 days i.u. (e) 48 days i.u. (f) 10 weeks i.u. (Reproduced from Mitchell, *An Introduction to Orthodontics*, 2007, with permission of Oxford University Press.)

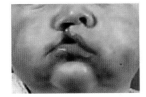

Figure 1.4 Failure of fusion resulting in cleft lip and primary palate.

If the shelve fusion fails, this is likely to result in clefts of the palate. The extent of these clefts varies clinically from submucous clefts affecting the bony structure of the palate and underlying muscular attachment and clefts of the soft palate which may or may not have significant effects on speech to those including the hard palate producing communication between the nasal and oral cavities (Fig. 1.6).

There appear to be distinctive differences between clefts of the palate and those of the lip and palate within different geographical and sexual distributions. This also suggests different disruptive mechanisms and timings as lip closure occurs earlier in development than palatal fusion. However, as clefts of the palate alone and lip with palate can occur in certain families, it suggests the distinction may not be complete.

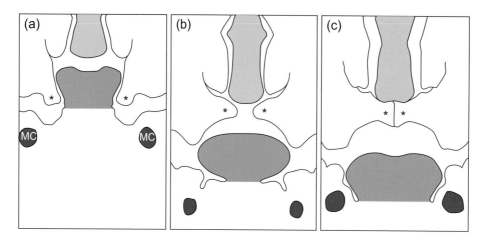

Figure 1.5 Diagrammatic representation of palatal shelf elevation and subsequent fusion. (a) During week 7 *in utero* the palatal shelves begin to develop and lie on either side of the tongue. (b) During week 8 *in utero* the palatine shelves elevate rapidly owing to the internal shelf-elevating force and developmental changes in the face. (c) During week 9 *in utero* the shelves fuse with each other, the primary palate, and the nasal septum. MC, Meckel's cartilage; asterisks, palatal shelves. (Reproduced from Mitchell, *An Introduction to Orthodontics*, 2007, with permission of Oxford University Press.)

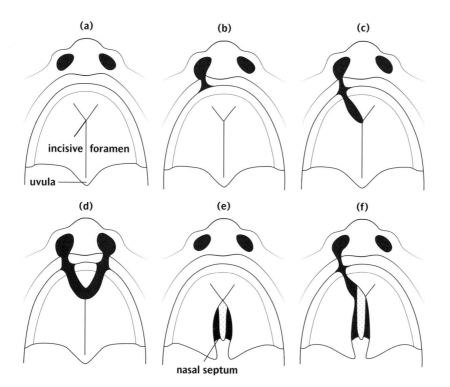

Figure 1.6 Diagrammatic representations of some of the different types of clefts of the lip and palate: (a) Normal; (b) unilateral cleft lip; (c) unilateral cleft lip and anterior palate; (d) bilateral cleft lip and anterior alveolus; (e) cleft of posterior palate (hard and soft); (f) unilateral cleft of the lip and anterior and posterior palate. (Reproduced from Johnson and Moore, *Anatomy for Dental Students*, 1997, with permission of Oxford University Press.)

1.3 Postnatal craniofacial growth

There is a great deal of individual variation in the process of postnatal growth and in the final form of the craniofacial structures. This section presents a simplified and rather idealized account of bone growth in general and as part of craniofacial growth. Occlusal development is then described, before going on to discuss the effect of individual variation in producing departures from this idealized pattern.

An individual's stature can be charted on standard growth charts during growth. This will present an overall view of the process of growth and will help to detect instances where growth is not proceeding in the usual manner. However, it disguises the fact that the various tissues of the body grow at different rates at different ages (Fig. 1.7).

In order to maintain harmonious facial growth, bone growth must synchronize with that of other tissues. For example, growth of the calvarium is linked to growth of the brain. The cranial vault initially grows much more rapidly than the facial bones in order to keep pace with the developing brain, 90% of which is complete by 5 years of age.

1.3.1 Assessment of postnatal craniofacial growth

One way of assessing the changes that take place during craniofacial growth is to superimpose tracings of two lateral skull radiographs taken of the same person at different ages. The two radiographs can be compared, as shown in Fig. 1.8, and the changes that have taken place during growth can be examined. A potential difficulty with this approach is that the various bones of the skull grow at different rates at different ages, and there is no single central point about which growth occurs in a radial fashion, i.e. there is no valid fixed radiographic landmark on which to superimpose the films. One convention is to superimpose the tracings of the radiographs on the outline of the sella turcica, using the line from the sella to the frontonasal suture to orientate the films. If this method of superimposition is used, it appears that the cranium expands in a more or less radial fashion to accommodate the brain and the facial skeleton then grows downwards and forwards, away from the cranial base.

Another difficulty is that radiographs only produce a two-dimensional representation of what is a three-dimensional structure. Newer methods of radiological assessment using computed tomography or lower-radiation-dose cone-beam computed tomography (Fig. 1.9) are capable of producing three-dimensional volumetric images of the facial skeleton.

Soft tissue growth and facial changes are also important for understanding the effects of underlying bony changes. Although computed

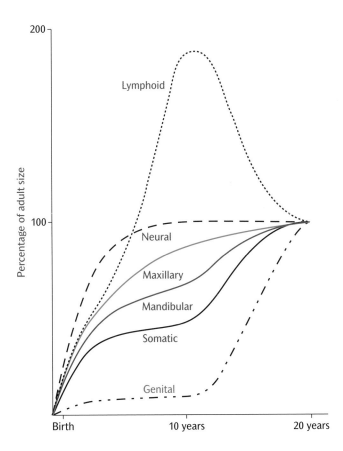

Figure 1.7 Postnatal growth patterns for neural, lymphoid, somatic, and genital tissues shown as percentages of the total increase. The patterns for the maxilla and mandible are shown in blue. (This was originally redrawn from Proffit, W.R. (2000). *Contemporary Orthodontics*, 3rd edn, Mosby.)

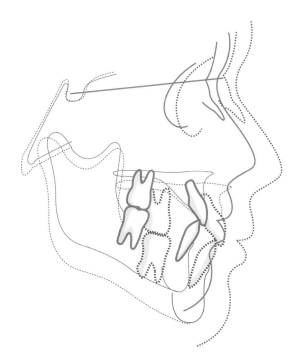

Figure 1.8 Superimpositions on the cranial base showing overall downward and forward direction of facial growth: solid line, 8 years of age; broken line, 18 years of age. (Reproduced from Mitchell, *An Introduction to Orthodontics*, 2007, with permission of Oxford University Press.)

tomography will capture the soft tissue, it does not accurately depict the colour and texture and, particularly in the case of conventional computed tomography, produces a significantly higher radiation dose than plain radiographs.

Non-invasive laser scanning or stereophotogrammetry is capable of producing photo-realistic topography of the facial soft tissues without exposure to radiation. Sequential capture is being used for longitudinal growth studies where colour mapping can help illustrate areas of maximum growth (Fig. 1.10) over a substantial time period.

1.3.2 Bone growth

Mineralized bone is formed through a process known as 'ossification'. This occurs in two ways, **intramembranous ossification** and **endochondral ossification**. Intramembranous ossification occurs by membrane activity and is seen in the bones of the calvarium, the facial bones, and

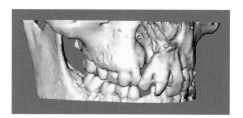

Figure 1.9 Cone-beam computed tomography of a child with a cleft of the alveolus, manipulated to produce a three-dimensional image.

the mandible. **Endochondral ossification** occurs by replacement of a cartilage framework. Classically, endochondral ossification is described in long bones but it also occurs in the craniofacial region, most notably in the cranial base.

Growth in bones formed by endochondral ossification occurs at growth centres known as epiphyseal plates in long bones and synchondroses in the cranial base. These are primary growth centres within which the chondroblasts are aligned and clear zones of cell division, hypertrophy, and calcification occur. The most notable of the three synchondroses within the cranial base is the spheno-occipital synchondrosis. The condylar cartilage has a different histological appearance to that of the epiphyseal plates and synchondroses. Although capable of producing bone, its stimuli appear more reactionary to growth around it rather than the primary growth sites which react to both internal and external stimuli.

The apparent growth of the facial bones is a function of **remodelling** and **displacement** or **translation**. Remodelling results in an alteration in the size and shape of bones by deposition and resorption of material on the external and internal surfaces of the bone and suture systems. It is a function of the 'periosteum' or 'osteogenic membrane'. Deposition and resorption go hand in hand; one seldom occurs without the other. Deposition of bone on one aspect of a cortical plate of bone is accompanied by resorption on the other aspect. Displacement or translation occurs when one bone is moved relative to another, primarily due to another area of growth; for example, the maxilla is translated downwards and forwards by growth of the spheno-occipital synchondroses and nasal septum. Such translation will be accompanied by a degree of remodelling.

The suture systems form bone when subjected to traction. In the case of the calvarial bones, the suture systems form new bone and

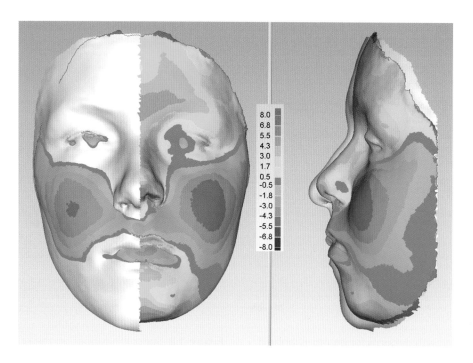

Figure 1.10 Colour mapping after sequential laser scanning showing facial growth in a forward direction (red) and a negative direction (blue) in the AP plane. (Courtesy of Professor Steve Richmond.)

enable the bones to stay in contact with each other when the expansion of the growing brain would otherwise move them apart.

The suture systems allow the bones to respond to growth in neighbouring soft tissue. The suture systems lying between the maxilla and the cranial base allow the downward and forward translation of the maxilla in response to the growth of the soft tissues of the face. It is not proliferation of the vascular connective tissue in the sutures that pushes the bones apart; the whole arrangement of the connective tissue in a suture seems to be designed to enable the suture to respond to a tensile force.

1.3.3 Soft tissue growth

The effects of bony growth can be masked or accentuated by the overlying soft tissues. Notably, this is shown intra-orally in the positions of the dental arches in the so-called neutral zone between the effects of the tongue, lips, and cheeks. The soft tissues are also responsible for dento-alveolar compensation where the position of the teeth attempts to compensate for skeletal jaw discrepancies.

The growth of the soft tissues, particularly the nose and the length and thickness of the lips, has a profound effect on the appearance of the face. Soft tissue growth shows sexual dimorphism, with changes occurring later and for longer in boys. Changes in the the nose continue into adulthood.

1.3.4 Mechanisms of growth

The mechanisms controlling the process of facial growth are not completely understood. In the post-genomic era it is becoming apparent that genetically encoded factors have a major effect on craniofacial growth; after all, children tend to resemble their parents in facial appearance. This may be particularly noted in class III parents and those with a class II division 2 malocclusion. The alternative school of thought is that the growth is only loosely under genetic control; rather, the final shape is under the control of its soft tissue environment. This is known as the 'functional matrix theory'. This is best shown in the cranial vault where the bone growth is reactionary to neural expansion. However, it fails to explain mid-facial growth through the synchondroses.

Therefore it is likely that both come into play, The genetically encoded factors can be affected by factors outwith the DNA 'epigenetic' that are able to switch them off or on. If this is the case, it should be theoretically possible to influence them (e.g. the use of functional appliances to encourage mandibular growth). At present, however, although a positive response is possible, it appears extremely variable and unpredictable between indviduals.

1.3.5 Cranial growth

At birth, the cranium is some 60–65% of its adult longitudinal dimensions, and this increases to about 90% by the age of 5 years. The calvarial bones are carried away from each other by the expanding brain and respond by forming new bone in the sutures that separate the bones of the vault of the skull (Fig. 1.11). The six fontanelles that are present at birth reduce in size. The largest (the anterior fontanelle) closes at about 1 year of age and the last to close (the posterolateral fontanelle) closes at about 18 months. The calvarial bones undergo a process of remodelling, with areas of bone deposition and resorption altering the contour of the bones as the volume of the brain cavity increases.

Early fusion of the cranial sutures, or 'craniostenosis', results in compensatory growth from the other sutures. This can result in unusual head shapes, and may produce detrimental effects on brain growth and development as it may be accompanied by increased intracranial pressure. The most common craniostenosis involves the sagittal suture. Compensatory growth results in a head shape that is increased in anteroposterior direction and narrow laterally—'dolichocephaly'. If the suture fusion is asymmetric, the deformation is also asymmetric—'plagiocephaly' (Fig. 1.12).

The cranial base also grows to accommodate the changes in the size and shape of the brain, but the process is different to that seen in the calvarial bones. There is considerable lateral growth of the cranial base as the cerebral hemispheres expand, but less increase in the anteroposterior dimension. No sutures are present to allow for expansion of the deeper compartments of the cranial base, a process that takes place by surface deposition and extensive remodelling. In addition, the three synchondroses, (spheno-occipital, intersphenoid, and spheno-ethmoidal) in the mid-ventral floor of the cranial base allow for increases in the anteroposterior dimension by endochondral ossification. Growth in the spheno-occipital synchondrosis does not cease until about the age of 15 years in boys, rather earlier in girls, and it closes fully at about the age of 20. The spheno-occipital synchondrosis has a significant influence on the growth of the facial region as the condylar fossa is posterior to it, but the anterior cranial base, and therefore the nasomaxillary complex to which it is attached by a suture system, sits anteriorly. As a consequence, as it grows it has an effect on how the maxilla and mandible relate to each other (Fig. 1.13).

The pattern and the timing of growth in the cranial base is intermediate between the neural type of growth that characterizes the growth of the calvarial bones and the musculoskeletal pattern of growth exhibited by the facial skeleton.

The shape of the cranial fossae is much more complex than the relatively smooth form of the bones of the vault of the skull. Surface deposition and subsequent remodelling occurs, with the final size and shape of the compartments being determined by the size of the lobes of the brain forming the partitions which separate the cranial fossae.

1.3.6 Nasomaxillary growth

The nasomaxillary region, which makes up the middle third of the face, is a complex area comprising a number of bones joined to each other and to the anterior cranial base by a suture system. The nasomaxillary complex grows downwards and forwards relative to the cranial base. This is accomplished through cranial base growth and deposition within the suture system as it is carried forward; there is also deposition in the region of the tuberosity, lengthening the alveolus in this region. The anterior surface is remodelled not by apposition, as might be expected in a bone that is growing forward, but by resorption.

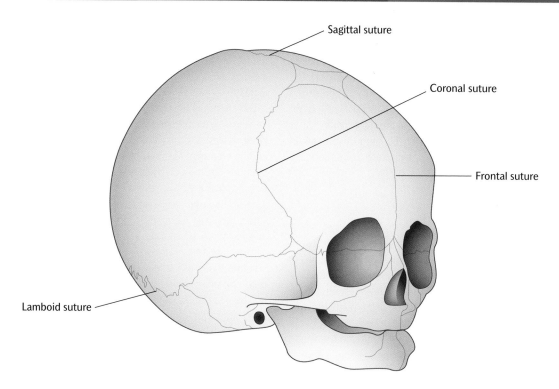

Figure 1.11 The skull at birth showing the sagittal, coronal, frontal, and lamboid sutures. (Reproduced from Johnson and Moore, *Anatomy for Dental Students*, 1997, with permission of Oxford University Press.)

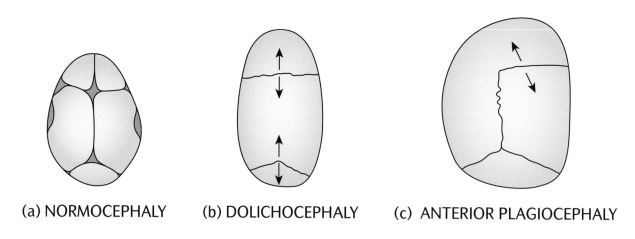

(a) NORMOCEPHALY   (b) DOLICHOCEPHALY   (c) ANTERIOR PLAGIOCEPHALY

Figure 1.12 Skull morphology: (a) normal; (b), (c) abnormal due to early fusion of cranial sutures.

Failure of the cranial base to lengthen, as seen in achondroplasia and a number of other syndromes (Fig. 1.13), results in characteristic faces with lack of mid-face prominence.

Unlike the growth of the cranium, which occurs in conjunction with the growth of the brain, the nasomaxillary complex grows fastest at about the time of the pubertal growth spurt, in conjunction with the general growth of the musculoskeletal system.

As bone is deposited on the external aspect of the maxilla in the region of the tuberosity, and vertically with the development of the alveolus through tooth eruption, it is also resorbed from the internal aspect of the bone in this area, thereby enlarging the maxillary sinus. As the

bone is translated downwards, the nasal cavities and the maxillary sinus expand by a process of bone resorption at the floor of the nose and the sinus, together with bone deposition on the palatal aspect of the maxilla.

1.3.7 Mandibular growth

Growth of the mandible, like that of the maxilla, is coordinated with the pattern of general musculoskeletal growth, growing at its fastest rate at about the time of the pubertal growth spurt. Growth of the mandible has to be coordinated with the downward and forward growth of the maxilla.

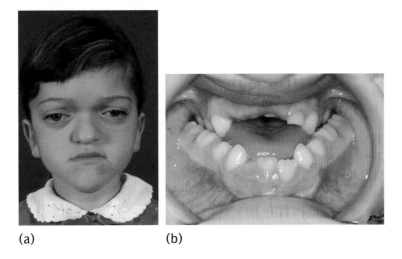

(a)   (b)

Figure 1.13 (a) A facial photograph of a child with Crouzon's syndrome with typical lack of mid-facial growth resulting in (b) a significant class III incisor relationship. Coronal synostosis results in a short wide head (brachycephaly), and early fusion of the sutures surrounding the eye sockets results in shallow orbits and bulging eyes.

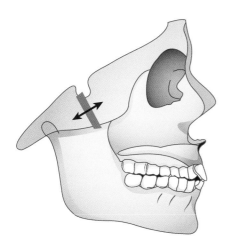

Figure 1.14 Anteroposterior growth at the spheno-occipital synchondrosis affects the anteroposterior relationship of the jaws. (Reproduced from Mitchell, *An Introduction to Orthodontics*, 2007, with permission of Oxford University Press.)

This task is made more complicated by the fact that the mandibular condyles articulate in the glenoid fossa, which lies behind the spheno-occipital synchondrosis, while the maxilla lies in front of it; therefore, growth of the mandible has to keep pace not just with the translation of the maxilla, but also with growth in the cranial base (see Fig. 1.14).

Taking the anterior cranial fossa as a stable reference area, it appears that the mandible, like the maxilla, grows downwards and forwards. As is the case with the maxilla, this downward and forward growth is not achieved by deposition of bone on the anterior aspect of the mandible, but by translation of the bone, accompanied by growth in the region of the ramus and the mandibular condyle. Bone is deposited on the posterior aspects of the ramus and the coronoid processes

and resorbed from the anterior aspect of the ramus. At the same time the condylar cartilage contributes to growth of the mandibular condyle, although its growth appears more reactionary than a primary growth cartilage. That is, it is not proliferation of the condylar cartilage that pushes the mandible downwards and forwards, but the condyle essentially 'fills in' as the mandible is translated.

As the ramus of the mandible grows upwards and backwards, its anterior aspect undergoes resorption and becomes remodelled into the body of the mandible. This process involves resorption on the lateral aspect of the bone and deposition on the lingual aspect, which forms new bone in correct alignment with the body of the mandible and helps maintain an appropriate intercondylar width. Growth of the mandibular ramus and condyle has to keep pace with changes in the position of the maxilla, in both vertical and horizontal directions, and with growth in the middle cranial fossa. Until puberty the mandible will grow at approximately 1–2mm per year, but after puberty this may double. It is easy for a small discrepancy to arise, for example, in the amount of vertical growth of the mandibular ramus, resulting in a rotation of the body of the mandible and a corresponding tilt of the occlusal plane. These rotations have been demonstrated using implant studies. The rotations may be partially masked by resorption but are capable of a significant effect on the vertical dimension of the face and on skeletal relationships.

1.3.8 Normal variation

There is always variation between individuals. Variation in the pattern of facial growth is only to be expected, and there are a number of compensatory mechanisms which operate to minimize the impact of such variation. Variation in the position or size of one structure is often compensated by corresponding change in another. The process of growth is constantly creating imbalances, as related structures grow and develop at different rates, but the overall direction of growth is towards some position of overall balance or harmony.

Anteroposterior discrepancies can arise during facial growth because of the position of a bone, or an imbalance in the sizes of bones, or a mixture of both. A class II skeletal pattern can be caused by insufficient growth of the ramus of the mandible in a backward direction; alternatively, a class II skeletal pattern can be the result of a backward tilt of the middle cranial fossa. This change in angulation results in the maxilla having a more anterior position, relative to the glenoid fossa, than would otherwise have been the case. The normal-sized mandible, occluding in the glenoid fossa, now has a class II relationship with the normal-sized maxilla. In a similar way, a converse alteration in the pattern of growth—excessive backward growth of the ramus of the mandible or a more vertical tilt of the middle cranial fossa—can produce a class III skeletal relationship, with the accompanying dental malocclusion.

Vertical growth in the nasomaxillary region has to be combined with vertical growth of the mandibular ramus. Maxillary growth that is not matched by mandibular growth will result in mandibular rotation. If there is an excess of vertical maxillary growth that is not matched by vertical growth of the ramus, the effect will be to produce a downward and backward rotation of the mandible. This downward and backward rotation will, in turn, produce an anteroposterior discrepancy, with a tendency towards a class II relationship.

Horizontal and vertical discrepancies tend to be accompanied by **dento-alveolar compensations**. In the case of a class III skeletal pattern, the upper incisor teeth are frequently proclined and the lower incisor teeth retroclined, as illustrated in Fig. 1.15.

These compensations are almost certainly brought about by muscular activity in the soft tissue integument affecting the position of the teeth, and they minimize what might otherwise have been a large reversed incisor overjet. In the case of class II skeletal patterns, the dento-alveolar compensation can take two forms. If the lips function in front of the upper incisor teeth, these teeth are generally retroclined, with the effect that the incisor overjet is virtually normal. However, if the lower lip functions behind the upper incisors, these teeth are usually proclined and the lower incisors are retroclined to make way for the lip. This results in an increased incisor overjet (Fig. 1.16).

Downward and backward mandibular rotations tend to be accompanied by a vertical drifting of the premolar, canine, and incisor teeth to compensate for an arrangement that would otherwise have produced an anterior open bite. This vertical drifting should be distinguished from over-eruption, which would produce a lengthening of the clinical crowns of the teeth.

1.3.9 Modification of the pattern of facial growth

Attempts to modify the pattern of facial growth have met with a certain amount of success. Orthodontic appliances have been designed which hold the mandible postured downwards and forwards. This moves the condyle out of the glenoid fossa and encourages upward and backward growth of the mandibular ramus. At the same time, the stretched muscles of mastication exert an upward and backward force (through the appliance) to the maxilla, which tends to inhibit its downward and forward growth. The effect on the growing face is to help correct a developing class II skeletal pattern. If this pattern is being caused not so much by underdevelopment of the mandible (which seems to be the most common cause) but by excessive forward growth of the maxilla, an appliance may be used simply to exert an upward and backward force on the maxilla without involving the mandible, thus helping to influence the course of facial growth.

These appliances apply forces to the developing maxilla and mandible via the teeth—the appliances are attached to the teeth—and work partly by inducing a dento-alveolar compensation for the underlying skeletal discrepancy. This process is sometimes referred to as 'orthodontic camouflage'. There is likely to be some restraint of the downward and forward growth of the maxilla, but the appliances seem to have only a minimal effect on the eventual size of the mandible. The so-called myofunctional appliances, which derive their impetus from

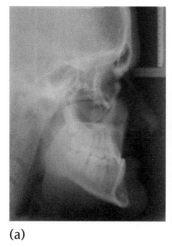
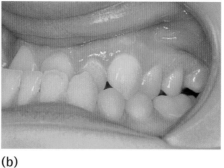

(a)   (b)

Figure 1.15 Dento-alveolar compensation: (a) cephalometric radiograph; (b) clinical photograph.

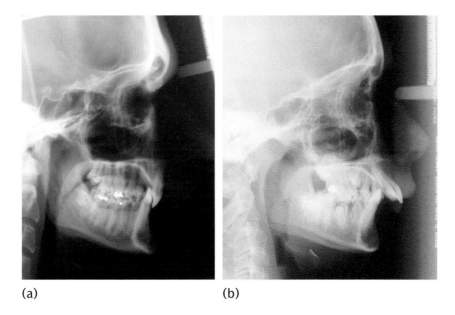

(a)   (b)

Figure 1.16 Cephalometric radiographs of two different patients with a class II skeletal pattern: (a) the upper incisor is within the upper lip, producing retroclination; (b) the upper incisor is outside the upper lip, showing upper incisor proclination.

the muscles of mastication, are used most often to help correct class II malocclusions. The appliances work by maintaining a forward and downward posturing of the mandible. However, while it is possible to use myofunctional–functional appliances to correct a developing class

III malocclusion, they are less often used in this context as it is difficult to obtain the necessary backward posturing of the mandible. In addition, the dento-alveolar compensations that these appliances tend to produce are often already present in untreated class III occlusions.

1.4 Tooth development

Teeth start to form during week 5 of embryonic life, and the process of tooth formation continues until the roots of the third permanent molars are completed at about 20 years of age. The stages of tooth formation are the same whether the tooth is of the primary or the permanent dentition, although obviously the teeth develop at different times. The tooth-germs develop from the dental lamina, a sheet of epithelial cells which itself develops from the primary epithelial band. This is a layer of thickened epithelium which forms around the mouth in the area soon to be occupied by the upper and lower jaws. The primary epithelial band quickly organizes into two discrete epithelial ingrowths—the vestibular lamina and the dental lamina. The vestibular lamina grows down into the underlying ectomesenchyme, and the epithelial cells enlarge and then break down, thereby forming the cleft which becomes the sulcus between the cheeks and the alveolar processes.

The dental lamina forms a series of epithelial buds that grow outwards into the surrounding connective tissue. These buds represent the first stage in the development of the tooth-germs of the primary dentition. The epithelial bud continues to grow and becomes associated with a condensation of mesenchymal cells to form a tooth-germ at the cap stage of development. The epithelial bud develops into the enamel organ, and the condensation of mesenchymal cells constitutes the dental papilla

and extends around the enamel organ to form the dental follicle. The cells at the margin of the epithelial bud continue to proliferate and grow to enfold the mesenchymal cells of the dental follicle, producing a tooth-germ at the bell stage of development. Around this time—the transition from cap stage to bell stage—a process of histodifferentiation produces the recognizable structures of the enamel organ, with its external and internal enamel epithelia, stratum intermedium, and stellate reticulum.

Further proliferation of the cells of the dental lamina at a point adjacent to each primary tooth-germ, but on its lingual aspect, produces the tooth-germ of the permanent successor. The tooth-germs of the permanent molar teeth which have no primary precursors are formed by distal extension of the dental lamina which tunnels backwards as the jaws lengthen posteriorly.

The cells of the inner enamel epithelium lengthen to a columnar shape, with the cell nuclei occupying the portion of the cell beside the stratum intermedium, away from the dental papilla. The cells of the dental papilla adjacent to the internal enamel epithelium also elongate to a columnar form, with their nuclei aligned away from the enamel organ and towards the centre of the dental papilla. These columnar cells of the dental papilla differentiate into odontoblasts, the cells which form dentine. Dentine formation, which is induced by the cells of the internal

Table 1.1 The chronology of the development of the primary dentition

Stage of development	Central incisor		Lateral incisor		Canine		First molar		Second molar		Time
	Max	**Mand**	**Max**	**Mand**	**Max**	**Mand**	**Max**	**Mand**	**Max**	**Mand**	
Hard tissue formation begins	13–16	13–16	14.7–16.5	14.7–16.5	15–18	16–18	14.5–17	14.5–17	16–23.5	17–19.5	Weeks after ovulation
Crown formation complete	1.5	2.5	2.5	3	9	8–9	6	5–6	11	8–11	Months after birth
Beginning of eruption	8–12	6–10	9–13	10–16	16–22	17–23	13–19	14–18	25–33	23–31	Months after birth
Completion of root formation	33	33	33	30	43	43	37	34	47	42	Months after birth

Max, maxilla; Mand, mandible.
Adapted from Schroeder (1991).

enamel epithelium, always precedes enamel formation. Although dentine is formed by the odontoblasts of the dental papilla, the process is initiated by the epithelial cells of the enamel organ. Once dentine formation begins, the cells of the internal enamel epithelium differentiate into ameloblasts and commence the formation of enamel. Dentine and enamel formation initially occurs in the region of the cusp tips and incisal edges of the teeth, and then continues towards the cervical margin of their crowns.

Differentiation of odontoblasts and the formation of dentine is induced by the cells of the internal enamel epithelium. A similar process is involved in the production of dentine to form the roots of teeth. The epithelial cells at the cervical loop of the enamel organ proliferate and migrate in an apical direction to form a tubular epithelial sheath around the dental papilla. These epithelial cells—the root sheath of Hertwig—induce the formation of odontoblasts from the cells of the dental papilla and the production of dentine to form the roots of the teeth, a process which is not complete until 3–5 years after the eruption of the crown of the tooth.

The stages of tooth development are the same for both primary and permanent teeth, although progression through the stages occurs at different times and at varying rates for the different teeth. Tables 1.1 and 1.2 summarize the chronology of tooth development for the two dentitions.

1.5 Tooth eruption

For tooth eruption to occur, a force must be generated to propel the tooth through the bone and gingival tissue. In the case of the secondary dentition the primary tooth roots must also be removed.

The method by which the force is created is open to debate. Some have suggested cellular proliferation at the apex of the tooth; alternatively, a localized change in blood pressure has been implicated. It has also been suggested that the force of eruption causes resorption of bone in the tooth's path, although this has also been questioned. Animal experiments have shown that the resorption process can be uncoupled from the eruption process, i.e. it is not necessary for the tooth to erupt to cause resorption of bone.

The follicle has been shown to play an essential role in active tooth eruption, but it is not fully understood how the coronal part of the follicle is activated to initiate osteoclastic activity in the alveolar bone ahead of the tooth and clear a path for tooth eruption. Once the tooth has broken through the alveolar crestal bone it reaches the supra-alveolar phase of eruption where it is likely that the follicle plays a lesser role.

What causes the tooth to erupt through the opening in the crypt created by the resorption process is also open to question. Suggested theories including root elongation, periodontal ligament, and local changes in vascular pressure have been discounted as major factors, and although bone growth at the base of the crypt is essential for eruption it is possible that this is simply reactive to tooth movement. It is fair to say that this source of eruption remains elusive.

1.6 Occlusal development

1.6.1 The primary dentition

The first tooth to erupt is usually the lower central incisor. Occasionally, this tooth is present at birth, but the average age for its eruption is about 7 or 8 months, although inevitably there is some individual variation. The other incisor teeth follow soon after, with the upper central incisors erupting at about 10 months followed by the upper lateral incisors at about 11 months and the lower lateral incisors at about 13

Table 1.2 The chronology of the development of the permanent dentition

Stage of development	Central incisor		Lateral incisor		Canine		First premolar		Second premolar		Time
	Max	Mand	Max	Mand	Max	Mand	Max	Mand	Max	Mand	
Hard tissue formation begins (histology)	3–4	3–4	10–12	3–4	4–5	4–5	18–24	18–24	24–30	24–30	Months after birth
Hard tissue formation begins (radiology)	–	–	–	–	6	6	19	19	36	36	Months after birth
Crown formation complete	3.3–4.1	3.4–5.4	4.4–4.9	3.1–5.9	4.5–5.8	4.0–4.7	6.3–7.0	5–6	6.6–7.2	6.1–7.1	Years of age (decimal)
Beginning of eruption	6.7–8.1	6.0–6.9	7.0–8.8	6.8–8.1	10.0–12.2	9.2–11.4	9.6–10.9	9.6–11.5	10.2–11.4	10.1–12.1	Years of age (decimal)
Completion of root formation	8.6–9.8	7.7–8.6	9.6–10.8	8.5–9.6	11.2–13.3	10.8–13.0	11.2–13.6	11.0–13.4	11.6–14.0	11.7–14.3	Years of age (decimal)

Stage of development	First molar		Second molar		Third molar		Time
	Max	Mand	Max	Mand	Max	Mand	
Hard tissue formation begins (histology)	7–8ao	7–8ao	30–36mo	30–36mo	7–9yr	8–10yr	Months after ovulation (ao) or months (mo) and years (yr) after birth
Hard tissue formation begins (radiology)	2mo	2mo	36–48mo	36–48mo	9–10yr	9–10yr	Months (mo) or years (yr) after birth
Crown formation complete	2.1–3.5	2.1–3.6	6.9–7.4	6.2–7.4	12.8–13.2	12.0–13.7	Years of age with decimal fractions
Beginning of eruption	6.1–6.7	5.9–6.9	11.9–12.8	11.2–12.2	17.0–19.0	17.0–19.0	Years of age with decimal fractions
Completion of root formation	9.3–10.8	7.8–9.8	12.9–16.2	11.0–15.7	19.5–19.6	20.0–20.8	Years of age with decimal fractions

Max, maxilla; Mand, mandible.
Adapted from Schroeder (1991).

months. The first primary molars put in an appearance at about the age of 16 months, followed by the primary canine teeth at about 19 months. The second primary molars erupt at about 27–29 months, with the lower teeth usually erupting before the upper ones. While the eruption sequence—the order in which the teeth erupt—is usually as described above, there is considerable variation in the actual age at which the teeth erupt. In any event, there is an almost continuous process of tooth eruption between the ages of 7 and 29 months.

Some occlusal features occur relatively frequently in the established primary dentition.

1. The incisor teeth tend to be spaced (Fig. 1.17). If the primary teeth are not spaced, the permanent teeth will be crowded because the larger permanent incisor teeth have to fit into the same space as their smaller primary predecessors. Crowding of the permanent incisor teeth is a relatively common occurrence, but it is seldom so severe that there is no spacing of the primary incisors.

2. So-called anthropoid spaces between the upper lateral incisor and the canine and between the lower canine and the first primary molar are particularly common (Fig. 1.18).

3. In the case of a class I occlusion, the mesiobuccal cusp of the primary upper second molar occludes in the mesiobuccal groove of the primary lower second molar, a situation analogous to the class I occlusion of first permanent molars. However, the primary lower second molar is much longer mesiodistally than the upper second molar. Therefore the class I occlusion of the mesiobuccal cusp of the upper molar means that the distal surfaces of the teeth are in the same vertical plane, which is known as the flush terminal plane (Fig. 1.18).

The incisor relationship tends more towards edge-to-edge than is the case with permanent teeth (although with increasing wear of the primary teeth there may be a postural element in this) and the upper incisors tend to be more upright. There is sometimes an anterior open bite associated with a sucking habit, and there may be cross-bites of the buccal segment teeth (Fig. 1.19). However, in general the teeth in the primary dentition tend to be well aligned. While there may be some anteroposterior, lateral, or vertical discrepancy, these deviations are seldom so marked that they give rise to comment.

1.6.2 The mixed dentition

The primary dentition erupts more or less continuously over a 2-year period. However, the permanent dentition erupts in two stages: first, the incisor teeth and the first permanent molars erupt, and then the other teeth in the buccal segments. The lower central incisor and the first permanent molars erupt at about the age of 6 years. The upper central incisor and the lower lateral incisor erupt at about the age of 7 years and the upper lateral incisor at about the age of 8 years. As with the primary teeth, while some variation in the timing of tooth eruption is only to be expected, this eruption sequence should not vary. In particular, the upper central incisor should erupt before the upper lateral incisor. The upper incisors are usually spaced, and the lateral incisors in particular have a distal inclination. During this period of physiological spacing the canine is closely associated with the distal aspect of the lateral incisor (Fig. 1.20) and should be palpated clinically high in the buccal sulcus from the age of 10 years. The resultant spacing will usually close significantly as the canine erupts.

If the upper lateral incisor erupts before the upper central incisor, almost certainly there is something impeding the eruption of the central incisor, for example a supernumerary tooth or a dilaceration of the root of the central incisor (Fig. 1.21).

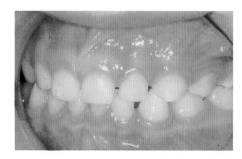

Figure 1.17 Spaced upper arch in the primary dentition of a patient.

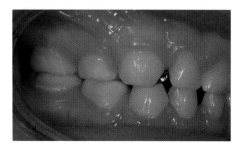

Figure 1.18 Anthropoid spaces and flush terminal plane.

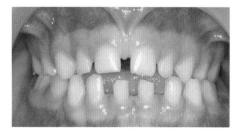

Figure 1.19 The primary dentition with an anterior open bite and unilateral cross-bite consistent with habit.

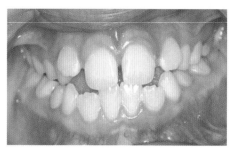

(a)

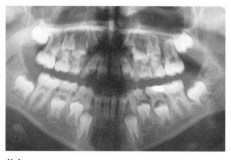

(b)

Figure 1.20 (a) The mixed dentition with spacing between the upper central and lateral incisors. The lateral incisors have a distal inclination. (b) The orthopantomogram (OPT) radiograph of the same patient showing the unerupted canine teeth closely associated with the apex of the lateral incisors.

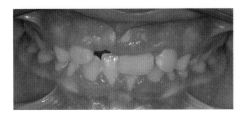

Figure 1.21 Early mixed dentition where the upper left central incisor and both lateral incisors have erupted out of sequence with the upper right central incisor.

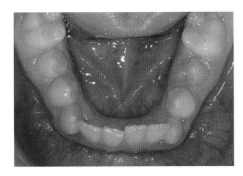

Figure 1.22 Early permanent dentition where a lower left second primary molar has recently been exfoliated and the lower left second premolar is erupting. Note the space mesial and distal to the erupting tooth which is due to the discrepancy in size between the primary molar and premolar.

The lower canine and the first premolar teeth are the next to erupt at about 10 years of age, followed by the upper canine and the second premolar teeth at about the age of 11 and the second molar teeth at about the age of 12. Third molar teeth start to erupt from about the age of 16 onwards, but the eruption of third molars is very variable; not uncommonly, these teeth are impacted against their neighbours and fail to erupt at all.

The upper central incisors are more proclined than their primary counterparts. This allows some forward repositioning of the mandible when the first permanent molars erupt in a cusp-to-cusp relationship with their opponents. The distal surfaces of the second primary molars tend to be in the same vertical plane, so the first permanent molars erupting behind them tend to adopt a class II occlusal relationship. The forward repositioning of the mandible allows the establishment of a class I intercuspal position. The primary teeth in the buccal segments have a larger combined mesiodistal width than the permanent teeth which replace them. Thus, provided that the primary teeth are shed in

the ordinary way, there should be no problem with a lack of space for the permanent teeth in the buccal segments of the dental arch. The 'leeway space' as it is sometimes called—the amount by which the combined size of the primary canine and primary molar teeth exceeds the combined mesiodistal widths of the permanent canine and permanent premolar teeth—amounts to 1.5mm in the upper arch and 2.5mm in the lower with its large second primary molar (Fig. 1.22).

The size and shape of the anterior segments of the dento-alveolar arches do not change much following the eruption of the permanent incisor teeth. There is not much growth by deposition of bone on the labial aspect of the maxilla or mandible—these bones grow by forward and downward translation, with deposition of new bone on their posterior surfaces. If there is insufficient space to accommodate the teeth in the dental arches when the teeth erupt, it is unlikely that the situation will improve as growth proceeds. There is a small expansion in the width of the dental arch, with deposition of bone on the lateral aspect of the maxilla and the mandible, most of which occurs as the lateral incisors are erupting. While most of the 'leeway space' is taken up by mesial movement of the posterior teeth, the mesial molar movement may be restrained using orthodontic appliances to allow some improvement in the alignment of crowded incisors.

1.6.3 The permanent dentition

As with the primary dentition, it is possible to identify occlusal features of the established permanent dentition that occur consistently in ideal dental arches.

1. The mesiobuccal cusp of the upper first permanent molar occludes in the mesiobuccal groove of the lower first permanent molar, with the distal aspect of the upper first molar contacting the mesial aspect of the lower second molar.

2. The teeth should have a normal labiolingual inclination. In the case of the anterior teeth, the crown inclination must be sufficient to prevent over-eruption of the teeth and an increased incisor overbite. In the case of the posterior teeth, the upper teeth should have a lingual inclination, which remains constant in the premolar and molar regions, while the lower teeth have a lingual inclination which becomes more pronounced towards the back of the arch.

3. The teeth should have a normal mesiodistal angulation, with the crowns of the teeth more mesially positioned than their roots.

4. There should be no rotated teeth.

5. There should be no spacing or crowding of the teeth.

6. The occlusal plane should be flat or have only a mild curve of Spee.

Not all these features are necessary for dental health, but taken together they provide a definition of the ideal class I occlusion.

1.7 Summary

The aim of this chapter has been to outline the pattern of normal craniofacial growth.

1 While normal variation of this pattern will produce the differences that occur between individuals, the underlying patterns of growth should not be radically different from those described here, i.e. if development is to proceed in a normal fashion.

2 The growth of the brain and the cranium is almost complete by the age of 5 years.

3 The facial skeleton grows downwards and forwards relative to the cranial base, starting to grow rapidly at about the time of the pubertal growth spurt and with facial growth virtually complete by the age of about 15.5 years in girls, and slightly later in boys.

4 With regard to occlusal development, while the exact age at which structures form will vary from person to person, the overall pattern of tooth development and the process by which the dental occlusion becomes established is largely as described in this chapter.

5 The eruption sequence—the order in which the teeth erupt—is more important than the age at which the teeth erupt. Therefore if there is a local problem with regard to the establishment of a normal occlusion, it is likely to become apparent in the first instance as a disturbance of the eruption sequence.

1.8 Further reading

Enlow, D.H. (1990). *Facial growth* (3rd edn). W.B. Saunders, Philadelphia. *(This is a widely recommended textbook, which deals with the subject of facial growth, very much from a clinical point of view.)*

Nanci, A. (2007). *Ten Cate's Oral Histology—development, structure and function* (7th edn). Mosby, St Louis, MO. (*A popular, complete, and well-illustrated text, which presents the subject clearly and in a modular, well-organized format.*)

1.9 Reference

Schroeder, H.E. (1991). *Oral structural biology*. Georg Thieme Verlag, Stuttgart. (*A pocket-sized book which presents a concise review of the subject, this text is best used as a reference rather than as an introduction to the subject. The points raised in the text are well documented by references to the academic literature.*)

2

Introduction to the dental surgery

A.S. Blinkhorn

Chapter contents

2.1 Introduction

It is a common belief among many individuals that being 'good with people' is an inborn art and owes little to science or training. It is true that some individuals have a more open disposition and can relate well to others (Fig. 2.1). However, there is no logical reason why all of us shouldn't be able to put young patients at their ease and show that we are interested in their problems.

It is particularly important for dentists to learn how to help people relax, as failure to empathize and communicate will result in disappointed patients and an unsuccessful practising career. Communicating effectively with children is of great value, as 'being good with younger patients' is a practice-builder and can reduce the stress involved when offering clinical care.

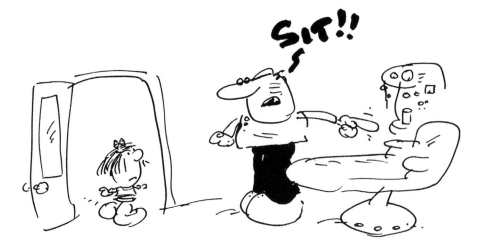

Figure 2.1 Being good with patients is not necessarily an inborn art! (With thanks to David Myers and kind permission of Eden Bianchi Press.)

All undergraduate and postgraduate dental training should include a thorough understanding of how children relate to an adult world, how the dental visit should be structured, and what strategies are available to help children cope with their apprehension about dental procedures. This chapter will consider these items, beginning with a discussion on the theories of psychological development and following this up with sections on parents and their influence on dental treatment, dentist–patient relationships, anxious and uncooperative children, and helping anxious patients to cope with dental care.

2.2 Psychology of child development

At one time the psychological development of children was split into a series of well-defined phases, but more recently this division has been criticized and development should now be seen as a continuum. The phases of development may well differ from child to child, so a rigidly applied definition will be artificial. Nevertheless, for clarity when describing a child's psychological development from infancy to adulthood, certain developmental milestones should be considered.

Academic considerations about psychological development have been dominated by a number of internationally known authorities who have, for the most part, concentrated on different aspects of the systematic progression from child to adult. However, the most important theoretical perspective now influencing thinking about child development is that of attachment theory—a theory developed by the psychoanalyst John Bowlby. In a series of writings over three decades, Bowlby developed his theory that child development could best be understood within the framework of patterns of interaction between the infant and the primary caregiver. If there were problems in this interaction, the child was likely to develop insecure and/or anxious patterns that would affect the ability to form stable relationships with others, to develop a sense of self-worth, and to move towards independence. The other important concept to note is that development is a lifelong process—we do not switch off at 18—nor is it an even process. Development is uneven, influenced by periods of rapid bodily change.

The psychological literature contains many accounts of the changes accompanying development. Therefore a general outline of the major 'psychological signposts' of which the dental team should be aware is presented in this section. As the newborn child is not a 'common' visitor to the dental surgery, no specific description of newborn behaviour will be offered; instead, general accounts of motor, cognitive, perceptual, and social development from birth to adolescence will be included. It is important to understand that the thinking about child development has become less certain and simplistic in its approach; hence dentists who make hard and fast rules about the way they offer care to children will cause stress to both their patients and themselves.

2.2.1 Motor development

A newborn child does not have an extensive range of movements, but these develop rapidly and by the age of 2 years the majority of children are capable of walking on their own. The 'motor milestones' occur in a predictable order, and many of the tests used by paediatricians assess normal development in infancy in terms of motor skills. The predictability of early motor development suggests that it must be genetically programmed. Although this is true to some extent, there is evidence that the environment can influence motor development. This has led to a greater interest in the early diagnosis of motor problems so that remedial intervention can be offered. A good example of intervention is the help offered to Down syndrome babies, who have slow motor development. Specific programmes which focus on practising sensorimotor tasks can greatly accelerate motor development to almost normal levels.

Motor development is really completed in infancy; the changes which follow the walking milestone are refinements rather than the development of new skills. Eye–hand coordination gradually becomes more precise and elaborate with increasing experience. The dominance of one hand emerges at an early age and is usually linked to hemisphere dominance for language processing. The left hemisphere controls the right hand and the right hemisphere controls the left. However, whereas the majority of right-handed people appear to be strongly left-hemisphere dominant for language processing, only 20% of left-handed people have right hemisphere dominance for language processing. Some children with motor retardation may fail to show specific right or left manual dominance and will lack good coordination between the hands.

Children aged 6–7 years usually have sufficient coordination to brush their teeth reasonably well. Below that age many areas of the mouth will be missed and there is a tendency to swallow relatively large amounts of toothpaste; hence parental supervision of brushing is important.

2.2.2 Cognitive development

The cognitive capability of children changes radically from birth through to adulthood, and the process is divided into a number of stages for ease of description. A Swiss psychologist called Piaget formulated the 'stages view' of cognitive development on the basis of detailed observations of his own children, and suggested that children pass through four broad stages of cognitive development (Table 2.1).

Dogma bites the dust

These stages have been highlighted because of the importance of Piaget's early work on cognitive development. However, an over-reliance on 'dogma' may well limit the development of a subject, and this was the case with cognitive development. Few scientists challenged Piaget's findings and the field of infant perception became a rather sterile area for a number of years, but this changed with the work of Bowlby. Enormous developments in research since then have led to many doubts being raised about Piaget's original interpretation of his data. He underestimated the thinking abilities of younger children, and there is evidence to show that not all preschool thinking is totally egocentric. (See Key Point 2.1.)

> **Key Point 2.1**
>
> Babies and children are not unfinished adults. They are able to create, learn, and explore.

2.2.3 Are adults sensible?

Of just as much interest is the modern view that not all adult thinking is logical; many of us are biased and illogical. This is a self-evident truth when one considers the arguments raised against water fluoridation!

Table 2.1 Piaget's stages

Sensorimotor	This stage lasts until about 2 years of age. The prime achievement is 'object permanence'. The infant can think of things as permanent—which continue to exist when out of sight—and can think of objects without having to see them directly.
Preoperational thought	This runs from 2 to 7 years of age. The sensorimotor stage is further developed, allowing the child to predict outcomes of behaviour. Language development facilitates these changes. Thought patterns are not well developed, being egocentric, unable to encompass another person's point of view, single-tracked, and inflexible (sums up most politicians, some dental professors, and hospital administrators). Typically, children in this age band are unable to understand that areas and volumes remain the same despite changes in position or shape.
Concrete operations	This is the stage of thinking that occurs from about 7 to 11 years of age. Children are able to apply logical reasoning, consider another person's point of view, and assess more than one aspect of a particular situation (Fig. 2.2). Thinking is rooted in concrete objects, abstract thought is not well developed.
Formal operations	This is the last stage in the transition to adult thinking ability. It begins at about 11 years of age and results in the development of logical abstract thinking so that different possibilities for action can be considered.

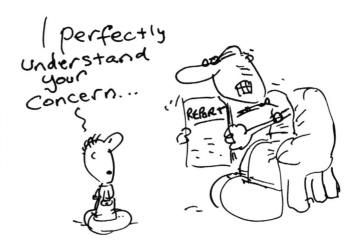

Figure 2.2 Children aged 7–11 years are able to consider another person's point of view. (With thanks to David Myers and kind permission of Eden Bianchi Press.)

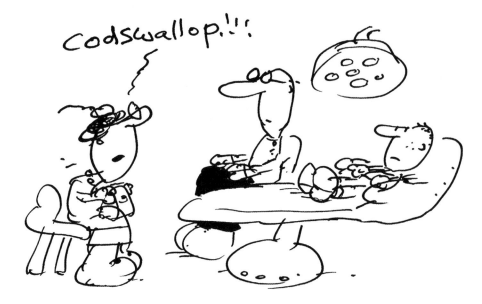

Figure 2.3 Be prepared for parents who don't agree. (With thanks to David Myers and kind permission of Eden Bianchi Press.)

However, there is a serious point to this observation on adult illogicality. We must be prepared for parents who do not agree with our perceived wisdom (Fig. 2.3) or do not understand the basic tenets of specific programmes. Dentists will lead less stressful practising lives if they remember that not all their patients will always agree with or follow oral health advice.

So Piaget should be seen as a pioneer who really set in motion work on cognitive development, but it is now recognized that the developmental stages are not as clear-cut and many kids are smarter than we think!

2.2.4 Perceptual development

Clearly, it is very difficult to discover what babies and infants are experiencing perceptually; so much research has concentrated on eye movements. These types of studies have shown that with increasing age, scanning becomes broader and larger amounts of information are sought. Compared with adults, 6-year-old children cover less of the object, fixate on details, and gain less information. However, children do develop their selective attention, and by the age of 7 years can determine which messages merit attention and which can be ignored. Concentration skills also improve. Some dental advice can be offered to children of this age but, given the importance of the home environment, parents should be the main focus of any information given on oral healthcare.

With increasing age children become more efficient at discriminating between different visual patterns and reach adult proficiency by about 9 years of age.

The majority of perceptual development is a function of the growth of knowledge about the environment in which a child lives, hence the necessity to spend time explaining aspects of dental care to new child patients (Fig. 2.4).

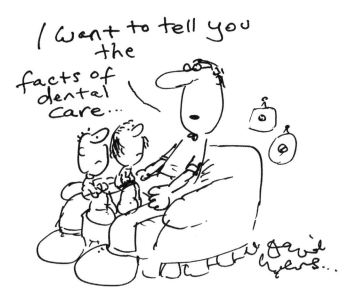

Figure 2.4 Spend time explaining the facts about dental care. (With thanks to David Myers and kind permission of Eden Bianchi Press.)

2.2.5 Language development

A lack of appropriate stimulation will retard a child's learning, particularly language. A child of 5 who can only speak in monosyllables and has no sensible sentence structure will not only be unable to communicate with others but also be unable to think about the things he/she sees and hears. Stimulation is important, as language development is such a rapid process in childhood that any delay can seriously handicap a child. Newborn children show a remarkable ability to distinguish speech sounds, and by the age of 5 years most children can use 2000 or more words. Language and thought are tied together and are important in cognitive development, but the complexities of the relationship between the two are not well understood.

Dentistry has a highly specialized vocabulary and it is unlikely that many children, or even adolescents, will understand our meaning if we rely on jargon. The key to successful communication is to pitch your advice and instructions at just the right level for different age groups of children. There is a risk of being patronizing if every child patient is told that 'little pixies are eating away tiny bits of your tooth and I am going to run my little engine to frighten them away to fairyland'. A streetwise 10-year-old who is a computer games afficionado would probably call the police if you used such language! There is no universal approach to patients, so careful treatment planning and assessment are required before children or their parents are given specific written or verbal advice. (See Key Point 2.2.)

> ### Key Point 2.2
>
> Members of the dental team must assess children's linguistic ability before offering advice. Tailor advice to individual families.

2.2.6 Social development

Until fairly recently it was believed that newborn infants were individuals who spent most of their time sleeping. However, recent research reveals that babies interact quite markedly with their environment, often initiating interactions with other humans by movement of their eyes or limbs.

Separation anxiety

Babies tend to form specific attachments to people and are prone to separation anxiety. At about 8 months infants show a definite fear of strangers. This potential for anxiety separation remains high until about 5 years of age, when separation anxiety declines quite markedly. This is consistent with studies of children in hospital, which show that after the age of 5 there is less distress on entering hospital. Separation anxiety should also be considered by dentists who insist that all young children must enter the dental surgery alone. Clearly, this will cause severe anxiety to patients under 5 years of age. (See Key Point 2.3.)

> ### Key Point 2.3
>
> Parents in the dental surgery cannot be governed by a rule. Each child and parent has different needs. A caring health professional should adopt some flexibility in his/her approach to offering clinical care with or without parents present.

It has been reported that a loving early parental attachment is associated with better social adjustment in later childhood and is a good basis for engendering trust and friendship with peers. This is important, as a successful transition from home to school depends on the ability to interact with other individuals apart from parents. The home environment will play a major part in social development, but the effects of community expectations should not be underestimated. We are all products of our broad social environment, mediated to some extent by parental influences.

2.2.7 Adolescence

The waning of parental influence can be seen in the final stage of child development—adolescence. This is the end of childhood and the beginning of adulthood. It is conceptualized as a period of emotional turmoil and a time of identity formation. This view is a Western creation and is culturally biased. In many societies 'terrible teenagers' do not exist; childhood ends and adult responsibilities are offered at a relatively early age.

It is interesting to note that even in Western industrialized societies there is little real evidence to support the idea that the majority of adolescents are rebellious and non-conformist. The main change is the evolution of a different sort of parental relationship. There is increasing independence and self-sufficiency. The research does show that young people tend to be moody, are oversensitive to criticism, and feel miserable for no apparent reason, but on the whole they do not rebel against their parental role models.

There are some clear messages to dentists who wish to retain their adolescent patients. Don't criticize them excessively as this may compromise their future oral health. These patients are looking for support and reassurance. Many health professionals need to rethink their assumptions about young people, as personal behaviour patterns are not really related to health issues at all. Until there are acute problems 'health *per se*' is of little relevance to adolescents, being a rather abstract concept. Their major issues of concern are finding employment, exploring their sexuality, and having the friendship and support of their peers.

2.3 Parents and their influence on dental treatment

Children learn the basic aspects of everyday life from their parents. This process is termed socialization, and is ongoing and gradual. By the age of 4 years children know many of the conventions current in their culture, such as male and female roles. The process of transmitting cultural information early in life is called primary socialization. In industrialized countries, obtaining information on many aspects of life is gained formally in schools and colleges rather than from the family. This is termed secondary socialization.

2.3.1 Socialization

Interestingly, primary socialization can have a profound and lasting effect. For example, fear of dental treatment and when we first begin to clean our teeth can often be traced back to family influence, so parents can shape a child's expectations and attitudes about oral health. Thus every attempt should be made to involve them when attempting to offer dental care or change a child's health habits. (See Key Point 2.4.)

Key Point 2.4

Maintaining a healthy mouth begins in early childhood as the teeth erupt. It is far simpler to encourage healthy habits than to change ingrained behaviour.

2.3.2 Avoid victim blaming

Involving parents means that the dentist must look to positive reinforcement rather than 'victim blaming'. Parents who are accused of oral neglect may well feel aggrieved or threatened. All too often children's oral health is compromised by a lack of parental knowledge, so programmes have to be carefully designed to reduce any chances of making people feel guilty. Guilt often results in parents spending more time seeking excuses for problems than trying to implement solutions.

Parents who are convinced that their child has an oral health problem which can be solved tend to react in a positive way both to their dental advisor and to the preventive programme itself. It is especially helpful if the preventive strategy can include a system of positive reinforcement for the child (Fig. 2.5). Features such as brushing charts, diet sheets, gold stars for brushing well, and extra pocket money for curtailing thumb-sucking are all useful tips to help parents maintain a child's enthusiasm for a particular dental project.

It must be emphasized that preventive programmes must be carefully planned to include only one major goal at a time. Parents will be unable to cope if too much is expected of them at any one time. Programmes that involve families have much higher success rates than those which concentrate solely on the patient. Interestingly, families also have a profound influence on levels of dental anxiety among their children. Dentally anxious mothers have children who exhibit negative behaviour at the dentist. Hence, dentists need to look 'beyond' the child when assessing the reasons for dental anxiety.

2.3.3 Should parents join children in the surgery?

One of the great debates in paediatric dentistry centres on whether parents should be allowed in the dental surgery while their child is receiving treatment. A child's family, it could be argued, can offer emotional support during treatment. There is no doubt that within the medical field there is great support for the concept of a parent actually 'living in' while a child is hospitalized. However, the issue is not so clear cut in dentistry (Fig. 2.6).

The first issue that must be raised is whether dentists have the ethical/moral right to bar parents from sitting in with their children when dental care is being undertaken. Clearly, parents have views and anxiety levels may be raised if parents feel that their familial rights are being threatened, and a child may be stressed by tension between his/her parents and the operator.

In their comprehensive book on child management, Wright *et al.* (1987) summarize the advantages of keeping parents out of the surgery as follows.

1. The parent often repeats orders, annoying both the dentist and the child patient (Fig. 2.7).

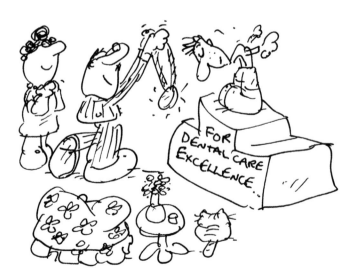

Figure 2.5 Positive reinforcement is important. (With thanks to David Myers and kind permission of Eden Bianchi Press.)

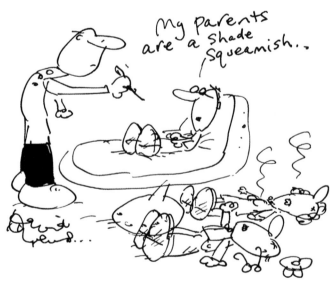

Figure 2.6 Should we allow parents into the surgery? (With thanks to David Myers and kind permission of Eden Bianchi Press.)

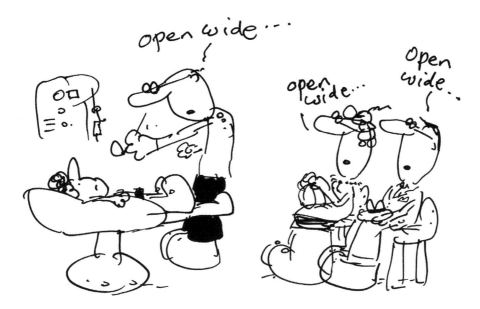

Figure 2.7 Some parents can be very irritating by repeating all your requests. (With thanks to David Myers and kind permission of Eden Bianchi Press.)

2. The parent intercepts orders, becoming a barrier to the development of rapport between the dentist and the child.

3. The dentist is unable to use voice intonation in the presence of the parent because he/she is offended.

4. The child divides his/her attention between the parent and the dentist.

5. The dentist divides his/her attention between the parent and the child.

6. Dentists are probably more relaxed and comfortable when parents remain in the reception area.

These suggestions have merit but they do have a rather authoritarian feel to them, stressing the ordering and voice intonation rather than sympathetic communication. Practical research to support parents in or out of the surgery is not available to suggest whether there is a right or wrong way to handle this particular question. In the end it is a personal decision taken by the dentist in the light of parental concerns and clinical experience. As in any branch of medicine there can be no hard and fast rules for dealing with the general public; an adherence to any type of dogma, come what may, is a recipe for confrontation and stress. Therefore allowing parents to sit in with children should be a decision taken for each individual rather than implementing a 'keep parents out' policy.

2.3.4 Each patient is a unique individual

Patients with special needs require a high degree of parental involvement in oral healthcare, particularly those children with educational, behavioural, and physical difficulties. For example, toothbrushing is a complex cognitive and motor task which will tax the skills of many handicapped children. A parent will have to be taught how to monitor the efficiency of the plaque removal and intervene when necessary to ensure that the mouth is cleaned adequately. Diet is also important, so clear advice must be offered and reinforcement planned at regular intervals.

2.4 Dentist–patient relationship

The way a dentist interacts with patients will have a major influence on the success of any clinical or preventive care. Clearly, only broad guidelines can be presented on how to maintain an effective relationship with a patient, as all of us are unique individuals with different needs and aspirations. This is especially so in paediatric dentistry where a clinician may have to treat a frightened 3-year-old child at one appointment and an hour and a half later be faced with the problem of offering preventive advice on oral health to a recalcitrant 15-year-old. However, there are common research findings which highlight the key issues that will cause a dentist–patient consultation to founder or progress satisfactorily.

2.4.1 People like friendly dentists

The first question that must be considered is 'Why me—what factors did the parents take into account before making an appointment at my practice?'

The obvious answers are that your practice is closest to the bus stop, has good parking, and you are the only one open after 6.00p.m. Surprisingly, the choice is not so simple. Most people try to find out details about different dental practices from friends and colleagues. While the technical skill of the dentist is of some concern, the most important features people look for are that he/she has a gentle friendly manner, explains treatment procedures, and tries to keep any pain to a minimum. (See Key Point 2.5.)

Key Point 2.5

Patients seek out friendly, kind dentists. Taking time to talk and interact with individuals can build a practice.

As with any health issue the social class background of the respondents influences attitudes and beliefs. For example, parents of high socio-economic status are more interested in professional competence and gaining information, whereas parents from poorer areas want a dentist to reassure and be friendly to their child.

So which dentist parents choose to offer care to their child will depend to some extent on reports about technical skill from family and friends, but the major driving force is well-developed interpersonal skills. A major point to emphasize is that technical skill is usually judged in terms of caring and sympathy, a finding which adds further weight to the importance of dentists developing a good 'chair-side manner'.

Explanation, 'taking the time to talk us through what our child's treatment will entail', is another factor which rates highly, and may actually influence the rate of attendance for follow-up appointments.

2.4.2 Structure of the dental consultation

To help students and new graduates improve their dentist–patient interaction skills it is possible to give an outline structure for a successful dental consultation. The proposed model consists of six stages, and is based on the work of Wanless and Holloway (1994). (See Key Point 2.6.)

Key Point 2.6

Most consultation visits should have a set plan. Focus on communication before intervention.

1. *Greeting.* The dentist greets the child by name. Avoid using generalized terms such as 'Hi, sonny' or 'Hello, sunshine', which are general rather than specific to the patient (Fig. 2.8). If parents are present, include them in the conversation but do not forget that the child should be central to the developing relationship. A greeting can be spoilt by proceeding too quickly to an instruction rather than an invitation. For example, 'Hello, Sarah, jump in the chair' is rather abrupt and may prejudice an interactive relationship. The greeting should be used to put the child and parents at ease before proceeding to the next stage.

2. *Preliminary chat.* This phase has three objectives: to assess whether the patient or parents have any particular worries or concerns, to settle the patient into the clinical environment, and to assess the patient's emotional state. The following sequence represents one way of maximizing the effect of the 'preliminary chat'.

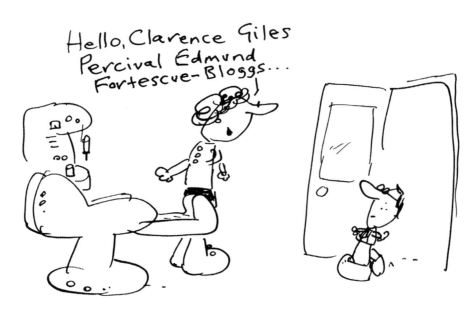

Figure 2.8 Always greet your patient by name. (With thanks to David Myers and kind permission of Eden Bianchi Press.)

(a) Begin with non-dental topics. For children who have been before it is helpful to record useful information such as the names of brothers/sisters, school, pets, and hobbies.

(b) Ask an open question such as 'How are you?/Are you having any problems with your teeth?' Listen to the answer and probe further if necessary. All too often dentists ask questions and then ignore the answer!

By talking generally and taking note of what the child is saying you are offering a degree of control and reducing anxiety.

3. *Preliminary explanation*. In this stage the aim is to explain what the clinical or preventive objectives are in terms that parents and children will understand. This is a vital part of any visit as it establishes the credibility of the dentist as someone who knows what the ultimate goal of the treatment is, and is prepared to take the time and trouble to discuss it in non-technical language. (See Key Point 2.7.)

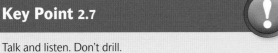

Key Point 2.7

Talk and listen. Don't drill.

While not wishing to labour the point, it must be stressed that sensible information cannot be offered to the patient or parents until the clinician has a full history and a treatment plan based on adequate information. This requires a broad view of the patient and should not be totally tooth-centred. It is all too easy to lose the confidence of parents and children if you find yourself making excuses for clinical decisions taken in a hurried and unscientific manner. Thus the preliminary chat sets the scene prior to actual clinical activity.

4. *Business*. The patient is now in danger of becoming a passive object who is worked on rather than being involved in the treatment. Many jokes are made about dentists who ask questions of patients who are unable to reply because of a mouthful of instruments (Fig. 2.9)! This does not mean that the visit should enter a silent phase. It is important to remain in verbal contact. Check that the patient is not in pain, discuss what you are doing, use the patient's name to show a 'personal' interest, and clarify any misunderstandings.

At the end of the business stage it is helpful to summarize what has been done and offer aftercare advice. If the parent is not present in the surgery, the treatment summary is particularly important as it is a useful way of maintaining contact with the parents.

5. *Health education*. Oral health is, to a large extent, dependent upon personal behaviour and as such it would be unethical for dentists not to include advice on maintaining a healthy mouth. Although offering advice to parents and patients is useful, in many instances the profession treats health education in a 'throw-away' manner. This results in both patients and dentists being disappointed. (See Key Point 2.8.)

Key Point 2.8

Dental health education is a key part of our professional activity. It requires time and commitment.

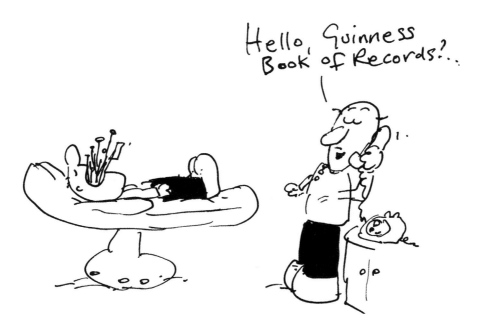

Figure 2.9 Is your patient just a mouthful of instruments? (With thanks to David Myers and kind permission of Eden Bianchi Press.)

The key ways to improve the value of advice sessions are as follows.

(a) Make the advice specific; give a child a personal problem to solve.

(b) Give simple and precise information.

(c) Do not suggest goals of behaviour change which are beyond a patient's capacity to achieve.

(d) Check that the message has been understood and not misinterpreted.

(e) Offer advice in such a way that the child and parents are not threatened or blamed.

(f) If you are trying to improve oral hygiene avoid theoretical discussions; offer a practical demonstration.

(g) At follow-up visits reinforce the advice and offer positive reinforcement.

(See Key Point 2.9.)

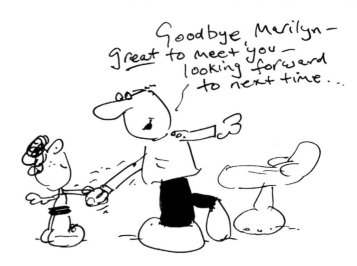

Figure 2.10 Make sure that you offer your patient a definite farewell. (With thanks to David Myers and kind permission of Eden Bianchi Press.)

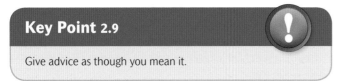

Key Point 2.9

Give advice as though you mean it.

The final part of the health education activity is goal-setting. The dentist sets out in simple terms what the patient should try to achieve by the next visit. It implies a form of contract and as such helps both children and parents to gain a clearer insight into how they can all help to improve the child's oral health. Goal-setting must be used sensibly. If goals are manifestly impossible, parents and child patients become disillusioned. Parents feel that the dentist does not understand their problems and complain that they are being blamed for any dental shortcomings, so always ensure that you plan goal-setting carefully in a positive and friendly manner.

6. *Dismissal.* This is the final part of the visit and should be clearly signposted so that everyone knows that the appointment is over. The patient should be addressed by name and a definite farewell offered (Fig. 2.10). The objective should be to ensure that wherever possible the patient and parents leave with a sense of goodwill.

Clearly, not all appointment sessions can be dissected into these six stages. However, the basic element of according the patient the maximum attention and personalizing your comments should never be forgotten.

In addition it is important to remember that the ability to understand both written and verbal information is highly variable. The majority of the dental team offer their patients oral health education advice, supplemented by written material in an effort to shape behaviours such as diet and toothbrushing. However, we often do not appreciate that literacy is an important contributor to health behaviour, and has far-reaching consequences on our everyday lives (Blinkhorn and Gittani 2009). If compromised, it will affect our ability to gain employment, understand health risks, gain entry into higher education, and participate in screening programmes (Ratzan 2001). (See Key Point 2.10.)

Key Point 2.10

Health literacy is of vital importance, and the dental team should avoid all-purpose advice leaflets!

It is only in recent years that the importance of health literacy has been fully realized (Kickbusch 2001; Powers *et al.* 2010). In 2007 the International Adult Literacy Survey reported that 20% of Americans and 17% of Canadians had difficulty in reading straightforward English prose. The importance of this finding is given increased relevance by Kelly and Haidet (2006) who reported that healthcare professionals overestimate patients' literary ability and erroneously believe that their written and verbal instructions are understood. The problem is compounded by the fact that people with low literacy skills are reluctant to admit their shortcomings (Wolf *et al.* 2005).

Therefore the dental team must take on another role when planning care for children—the ability to enable parents and carers to grasp either what we are 'talking about' or offering them to read! Clearly, experienced staff will be able to assess parents, taking account of social background and their general temperament. The main point to bear in mind is that because literacy skills vary there can be no one way of giving information, nor is it possible to have one advice leaflet for everyone—we are all too different! Such an approach is grounded in common sense, but all too often we as a profession 'hone our clinical skills' but give little attention to how we communicate. To be a successful healthcare professional we must put the same effort and commitment into being an effective advisor as we do into our clinical care. Hence profiling our patients and their families in terms of their ability to understand our advice is an essential requirement for any health professional seeking to improve health knowledge and change behaviour.

2.5 Anxious and uncooperative children

Dental anxiety should concern us as a profession because it not only prevents many potential patients from seeking care but also causes stress to the dentists undertaking dental treatment. Indeed, one of the major sources of stress for general dental practitioners is 'coping with difficult patients' (Fig. 2.11). Dentists do not want to be considered as people who inflict unnecessary anxiety on the general public. However, anxiety and dental care seem to be locked in the general folklore of many countries. In order to understand why, it is helpful to consider 'what is the nature of anxiety'.

2.5.1 Anxiety

Many definitions of anxiety have been suggested and it is a somewhat daunting task to reconcile them. However, it would seem sensible to consider the comments of Kent (see Kent and Blinkhorn 1991) who reported that anxiety is 'a vague unpleasant feeling accompanied by a premonition that something undesirable is going to happen'. In other words it relates to how people feel—a subjective definition. Another point of view is that anxiety manifests itself in behaviour. For example, if a person is anxious, he/she will act in a particular manner. A person will avoid visiting the dentist. Thus anxiety should be seen as a multifactorial problem made up of a number of different components, all of which can exert an effect. (See Key Point 2.11.)

Key Point 2.11

Anxiety is an issue in dental care. Do not get bogged down in definitions but take steps to reduce patient stress. Focus on preventive advice before trying to initiate clinical interventions.

Anxiety must also be seen as a continuum with fear—it is almost impossible to separate the two in much of the research undertaken in the field of dentistry, where the two words are used interchangeably. One could consider that anxiety is more a general feeling of discomfort, while fear is a strong reaction to a specific event. Nevertheless, it is counterproductive to search for elusive definitions as both fear and anxiety are associated with dental visiting and treatment.

From a common-sense point of view it is clear that some situations will arouse more anxiety than others. For example, a fear of heights is relatively common, but it is galling to note that in a US study (Agras *et al.* 1969) it was found that visiting the dentist ranked fourth behind snakes, heights, and storms. Clearly, anxiety about dental care is a problem that we as a profession must take seriously, especially as children remember pain and stress suffered at the dentist and carry the emotional scars into adult life. Some people may develop such a fear of dentistry that they are termed phobics. A phobia is an intense fear which is out of all proportion to the actual threat.

Research in this area suggests that the extent of anxiety that a person experiences does not relate directly to dental knowledge, but is an amalgamation of personal experiences, family concerns, disease levels, and general personality traits. Such a complex situation means that it is no easy task to measure dental anxiety and pinpoint aetiological agents.

Measuring dental anxiety is problematic because it relies on subjective measures. In addition, the influence of the parents, the dentist's behaviour, and the reason for a visit may all exert some effect on a child's anxiety levels.

Questionnaires and rating scales are the most commonly used means by which anxiety has been quantified, although there has been some interest in physiological data such as heart rate. Some questionnaires that have been used to measure anxiety can be applied to a whole variety of

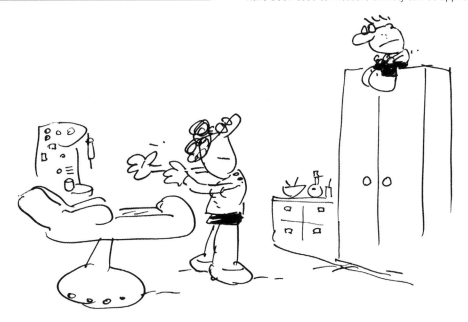

Figure 2.11 Difficult patients can be a source of stress! (With thanks to David Myers and kind permission of Eden Bianchi Press.)

situations, such as recording 'exam nerves' or fear of spiders, while others are specific to the dental situation. The most widely used dental anxiety measure is the Dental Anxiety Scale, which takes the form of a questionnaire. Patients are asked to choose an answer which best sums up their feelings. The answers are scored from 1 to 5 so that a total score can be computed. A high score should alert the dental team that a particular patient is very anxious.

However, patient-administered questionnaires have a limited value in evaluating a young child's anxiety because of their poorly developed vocabulary and understanding. Therefore there has been great interest in measuring anxiety by observing behaviour. One such scale was developed by Frankl to assess the effect of a parent remaining with a child in the surgery (see Kent and Blinkhorn 1991). It consists of four ratings from definitely negative to definitely positive. It is still commonly used in paediatric dental research. Another scale which is popular with researchers is one used by Houpt, which monitors behaviour by allocating a numerical score to items such as body movement and crying (see Kent and Blinkhorn 1991).

Recent studies have used the Frankl scale to select subjects, and then more detailed behaviour evaluation systems have been utilized to monitor compliance with treatment. Behavioural observation research can be problematic as the presence of an observer in the surgery may upset the patient. In addition, it is difficult to be totally objective when different coping strategies are being used, and some bias will occur. The development of cheap lightweight digital video cameras has greatly helped observational research, as the patient's behaviour can be scored by a number of raters away from the surgery. Rescoring the videos allows the researchers to check the reliability of the index used.

Physiological measurements such as a higher pulse rate, perspiration, and peripheral blood flow have been used to quantify children's dental anxiety. However, few physiological signs are specific to one particular emotion and the measuring techniques often provoke anxiety in the child patient, so they are rarely used.

As yet, there is no standard measure of dental anxiety for children, as the reproducibility and reliability of most questionnaires have not been demonstrated, and observational and physiological indices are not well developed. This is a serious problem as the assessment of strategies to reduce anxiety are somewhat compromised by a lack of universally accepted measuring techniques.

2.6 Helping anxious patients to cope with dental care

A number of theories have been suggested in an effort to explain the development of anxiety. Uncertainty about what is to happen is certainly a factor, a poor past experience with a dentist could upset a patient, and others may learn anxiety responses from parents, relations, or friends. (See Key Point 2.12.)

Key Point 2.12

Listening to a child's concerns about dental care is an important skill and may help to reduce anxiety.

A dentist who can alleviate anxiety or prevent it happening in the first place will always be popular with patients. Clearly, the easiest way to control anxiety is to establish an effective preventive programme so that children do not require any treatment. In addition to an effective preventive regimen, it is important to establish a trusting relationship, listening to a child's specific worries and concerns. Every effort must be made to ensure that any treatment is pain free. All too often we forget that local analgesia requires time and patience. With the use of a topical anaesthetic paste and slow release of the anaesthetic solution most 'injections' should be painless. There is no excuse for the 'stab and squirt' method (Fig. 2.12).

Children are not 'little adults'; they are vulnerable and afraid of new surroundings, so effective time management is important. Try to see young patients on time and do not stress yourself or the child by expecting to complete a clinical task in a short time on an apprehensive patient.

Despite the dental team's best efforts anxiety may persist and routine dental care is compromised. Other options to help the child will then have to be considered. An increasingly popular choice is the use of pharmacological agents; these will be discussed in Chapter 4. The alternatives to the pharmacological approach are:

1. reducing uncertainty
2. modelling
3. cognitive approaches
4. relaxation
5. systematic desensitization

These are discussed in more detail in this section.

2.6.1 Reducing uncertainty

The majority of young children have very little idea of what dental treatment involves and this will raise anxiety levels. Most children will cope if given friendly reassurance from the dentist, but some patients will need a more structured programme.

Tell–show–do

One such structured method is the tell–show–do technique. As its name implies it centres on three phases.

1. *Tell:* explanation of procedures at the right age/educational level.
2. *Show:* demonstrate the procedure.
3. *Do:* following on to undertake the task. Praise is an essential part of the exercise (Fig. 2.13).

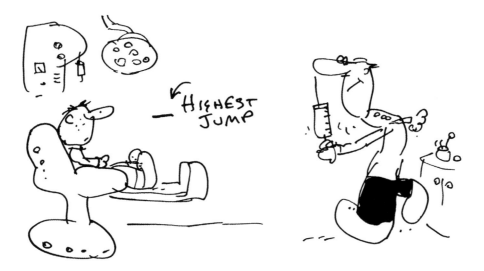

Figure 2.12 Stab and squirt has no place in our anaesthetic technique. (With thanks to David Myers and kind permission of Eden Bianchi Press.)

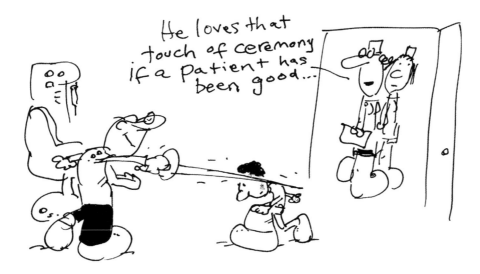

Figure 2.13 Praise costs little, but does show you to be a caring person. (With thanks to David Myers and kind permission of Eden Bianchi Press.)

Although it is a popular technique, there is little experimental work to support its use.

More information for parents

Another technique for reducing anxiety in very worried children is to send a letter home explaining all the details of the proposed first visit so that uncertainty will be reduced. The evidence for this approach is not clear cut as parental anxiety, rather than the child's anxiety, is changed by pre-information.

Acclimatization programmes which gradually introduce the child to dental care over a number of visits have been shown to be of value.

However, this approach is rather time consuming and does little for the really nervous child.

2.6.2 Modelling

Modelling makes use of the fact that individuals learn much about their environment from observing the consequences of other people's behaviour. You or I might repeat an action if we see others being rewarded, or if someone is punished we might well decide not to follow that behaviour. Modelling could be used to alleviate anxiety. If a child could be shown that it is possible to visit the dentist, have treatment,

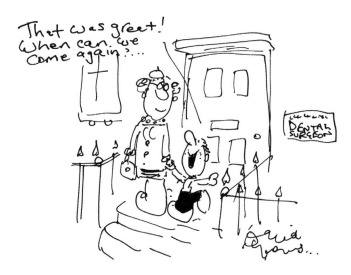

Figure 2.14 We want our patients to leave us in a happy frame of mind. (With thanks to David Myers and kind permission of Eden Bianchi Press.)

and then leave in a happy frame of mind (Fig. 2.14), this could reduce anxiety due to 'fear of the unknown'. A child would see behind that forbidding surgery door!

It is not necessary to use a live model; videos of cooperative patients are of value. However, the following points should be taken into consideration when setting up a programme.

1. Ensure that the model is close in age to the nervous child or children involved.

2. The model should be shown entering and leaving the surgery to prove that treatment has no lasting effect.

3. The dentist should be shown to be a caring person who praises the patient.

2.6.3 Cognitive approaches

Modelling helps people learn about dental treatment from watching others, but it does not take account of an individual's 'cognitions' or thoughts. People may heighten their anxiety by worrying more and more about a dental problem, thus creating a vicious reinforcing circle. Therefore there has been great interest in trying to get individuals to identify and then alter their dysfunctional beliefs. A number of cognitive modification techniques have been suggested, the most common of which are:

1. asking patients to identify and make a record of their negative thoughts;

2. helping patients to recognize their negative thoughts and suggesting more positive alternatives—'reality based';

3. working with a therapist to identify and change the more deep-seated negative beliefs.

Cognitive therapy is useful for focused types of anxiety—hence its value in combating dental anxiety.

Another approach that could be considered a cognitive approach is distraction. This technique attempts to shift attention from the dental setting towards some other kind of situation. Distracters such as videotaped cartoons and stories have been used to help children cope with dental treatment. The results have been somewhat equivocal, and the threat to switch off the video was needed to maintain cooperation.

2.6.4 Relaxation

Relaxation training is of value where patients report high levels of tension, and consists of bringing about deep muscular relaxation. It has also been used in conjunction with biofeedback training. As the techniques require the presence of a trained therapist, the potential value in general paediatric dentistry has still to be assessed.

2.6.5 Systematic desensitization

The basic principle of this treatment consists of allowing the patient to come to terms gradually with a particular fear or set of fears by working through various levels of the feared situation, from the 'mildest' to the 'most anxiety' programme. This technique relies on the use of a trained therapist and in most instances a simple dentally based acclimatization programme should be tried first.

2.6.6 Hand over mouth exercise (HOME)

The physical restraint of children in order to undertake clinical dental care has prompted much debate. Hosey (2002) and Manley (2004) note that in the UK the use of such physical restraint is currently unacceptable. However, some authors (Connick *et al.* 2000; Kupietsky 2004) have suggested that restraint in combination with inhalation sedation may be a helpful procedure if general anaesthesia is not readily available. (See Key Point 2.13.)

> **Key Point 2.13**
>
> HOME is a contentious topic which provokes strong emotions. It is culturally unacceptable in the UK.

In this section alternative options to restraint have been suggested which, although time consuming, are likely to provoke less of a nervous reaction and avoid associating dental care with an unpleasant experience. For those readers who wish to study the topic in more detail, comprehensive clinical guidelines collated by the British Society of Paediatric Dentistry's policy document on consent and the use of physical interventions and also the guideline on behaviour management.

2.7 Summary

1 To prevent the development of anxiety it is more important to maintain trust than to concentrate on finishing a clinical task.

2 The reduction in dental caries means that children with special psychological, medical, and physical needs can be offered the oral healthcare they require.

3 The care of children who are very anxious can be improved by using the techniques described in this chapter.

4 Preventing dental disease should always be given the same status as clinical intervention. However, it is important to ensure that preventive care is appropriate and relevant. The key messages are outlined by Levine and Stillman-Lowe (2009).

(See Key Point 2.14.)

> **Key Point 2.14**
>
> A recurring theme is to ensure that dental caries is prevented by offering parents advice and maximizing the use of fluoride therapy.

2.8 Further reading

Blinkhorn, A.S. and Mackie, I.C. (1992). *Treatment planning for the paedodontic patient*. Quintessence, London. (*There is a comprehensive question and answer section in this book which will help you check up on your treatment planning knowledge.*)

Chadwick, B. (2002). Non-pharmacological behaviour management. Available online at: **http://www.bspd.co.uk**

Clarke, W., Periam, C., and Zoitopoulos, L. (2009). Oral health promotion for linguistically and culturally diverse populations: understanding the local non-English speaking population. *Health Education Journal*, **68**, 119–29. (*A useful discussion on how to promote oral health in non-English speakers.*)

Freeman, R. (1999). The determinants of dental health attitudes and behaviours. *British Dental Journal*, **187**, 15–18. (*This paper examines the role of psychosocial factors on health behaviour, and case-based examples highlight the psychology of patient care in a practical way.*)

Friedman, D.B. and Hoffman-Goetz, L. (2008). Literacy and health literacy as defined in cancer education research: a systematic review. *Health Education Journal*, **67**, 285–304. (*Explains the importance of health literacy.*)

Humphris, G.M., Milsom, K., Tickle, M., Holbrook, H., and Blinkhorn, A.S. (2002). A new dental anxiety scale for 5 year old children (DA5): description and concurrent validity. *Health Education Journal*, **61**, 5–19. (*This paper describes the development of a new dental anxiety scale for children and highlights the key elements associated with measuring anxiety.*)

Rutter, M. and Rutter, M. (1993). *Developing minds*. Penguin Books, London. (*A fascinating insight into how we develop throughout life.*)

Weinman, J. (1987). *An outline of psychology as applied to medicine* (2nd edn), pp.132–4. Butterworth–Heinemann, London. (*This book is for those students who want to take a broader view on the subject of psychology and medicine.*)

2.9 References

Agras, S., Sylvester, D., and Oliveau, D. (1969). The epidemiology of common fears and phobias. *Comprehensive Psychiatry*, **10**, 151–6. (*This paper will show you that fear of dentistry is a problem the dental profession must take seriously.*)

Blinkhorn, A.S. and Gittani, J. (2009). A qualitative evaluation of the views of community workers on the dental health education material available in New South Wales for culturally and linguistically diverse communities. *Health Education Journal*, **68**, 314–19. (*How the way leaflets are presented will affect their potential value.*)

Connick, C., Palat, M., and Pugliese, S. (2000). The appropriate use of physical restraints: considerations. *ASDC Journal of Dentistry for Children*, **67**, 256–62. (*A useful discussion on the role of restraint in clinical paediatric dental practice.*)

Hosey, M.T. (2002). Managing anxious children: the use of conscious sedation in paediatric dentistry. *International Journal of Paediatric Dentistry*, **12**, 359–72. (*A useful guide to managing anxious children.*)

Kelly, P. and Haidet, P. (2006). Physician overestimation of patient literacy: a potential source of healthcare disparities. *Patient Education and Counselling*, **66**, 225–9. (*Doctors often forget that they are talking to real people!*)

Kent, G.G. and Blinkhorn, A.S. (1991). *The psychology of dental care* (2nd edn). John Wright, Bristol. (*This short book highlights the important psychological aspects of providing clinical care, as well as giving details of the Houpt, Frankl, and Corah dental anxiety scales.*)

Kickbusch, I.S. (2001). Health literacy: addressing the health and education divide. *Health Promotion International*, **16**, 289–97.

Kupietzky, A. (2004). Strap him down or knock him out. Is conscious sedation with restraint an alternative to general anaesthesia? *British Dental Journal*, **196**, 133–8. (*A discussion of the role of conscious sedation allied to the use of restraint in paediatric dentistry.*)

Levine, R.S. and Stillman-Lowe, C. (2009). *The scientific basis of oral health education*. BDJ Books, London. (*A comprehensive guide to dental health education and promotion, including the key preventive messages.*)

Manley, M.C.G. (2004). A UK perspective. *British Dental Journal*, **196**, 138–9. (*A view on the use of HOME in the UK.*)

Nunn, J., Foster, M., Master, S., and Greening, S. (2008). Consent and the use of physical intervention in the dental care of children. *International Journal of Paediatric Dentistry*, **18** (Suppl. 1): 39–46.

Powers, B.J., Trinh, J.V., and Bosworth, H.B. (2010). Can this patient read and understand written health information? *Journal of the American Medical Association*, **304**, 76–84.

Ratzan, S. (2001). Health literacy: communication for the public good. *Health Promotion International*, **16**, 207–14. (*Raises the issue of health literacy.*)

Wanless, M.B. and Holloway, P.J. (1994). An analysis of audio-recordings of general dental practitioners' consultations with adolescent patients. *British Dental Journal*, **177**, 94–8. (*Gives advice on how to improve communication skills in the surgery and reminds clinicians that our livelihood depends on effective communication.*)

Wolf, M.S., Bennet, C.L., Davis, T.C., Marin, E., and Arnold, C. (2005). A qualitative study of literacy and patient response to HIV medication adherence questionnaires. *Journal of Health Communication*, **10**, 509–11. (*Makes a case for spending more time and thought on how we give information.*)

Wright, G., Starkey, P.E., Gardener, D.E., and Curzon, M.E.J. (1987). *Child management in dentistry*. John Wright, Bristol. (*A detailed account of child management, including advice on how to introduce different clinical techniques.*)

3

History, examination, risk assessment, and treatment planning

M.L. Hunter and H.D. Rodd

Chapter contents

3.1 Introduction

The provision of dental care for children presents some of the greatest challenges (and rewards) in clinical dental practice. High on the list of challenges is the need to devise a comprehensive yet realistic treatment plan for these young patients. Successful outcomes are very unlikely in the absence of thorough short- and long-term treatment planning. Furthermore, decision-making for children has to take into account many more factors than is the case for adults. This chapter aims to highlight how history-taking, examination, and risk assessment are all critical stages in the treatment planning process. Principles of good treatment planning will also be outlined.

3.2 Ethics and consent

When making decisions about children's dental care, the clinician's foremost ethical responsibility is to do no harm, to act in the child's best interests, and to respect the child's right to refuse treatment. However, reconciling this last principle with the preceding two might well present a dilemma, in which case the clinician should ask him/herself the following questions:

- Is what is being proposed really in the child's best interest?
- Is the child happy to go ahead? If not, is there an alternative?
- If there is no alternative, what will really be the outcome if treatment does not proceed?

In most cases, failure to provide dental care for a child at a specific moment in time will not be life-threatening and a delay will be acceptable. However, there are circumstances in which failure to provide treatment may cause a child pain and distress. On these occasions, the clinician may feel that he/she has no alternative other than to proceed with treatment. Having weighed up the ethical considerations, he/she must then seek valid consent for what is proposed.

Valid consent to examination, investigation, or treatment is fundamental to the provision of dental care. The most important element of the consent process is ensuring that the patient/parent understands the nature and purpose of the proposed treatment, together with any alternatives available, and the potential benefits and risks. In this context, where clinician and patient/parent do not share a common language, the assistance of an interpreter is essential. (See Key Point 3.1.)

Who is permitted to give consent for a child patient is dependent upon:

- the child's age;
- the child's level of understanding relative to the complexity of the proposed treatment;
- who else with an interest in the child is available in the circumstances to take part in the decision-making process;
- the relevant legislation in the country of residence.

The legal position surrounding consent for the treatment of children in the constituent countries of the UK is presented in detail in the British Society of Paediatric Dentistry's policy document on consent and the use of physical intervention in the dental care of children (Nunn *et al.* 2008).

During most of childhood, the adult(s) with responsibility for the child will be required to make decisions about, and give consent for, the child's dental treatment. In the majority of cases, it will be the child's parents who have this role, thus giving rise to the legal concept of 'parental responsibility'. However, parental responsibility is not given solely to parents, nor do all parents have 'parental responsibility' in the legal sense.

Adults acting *in loco parentis* (e.g. childminders, grandparents, and other relatives) have limited rights to consent on a child's behalf. Treatment in the absence of a clear indication of parental wishes should only proceed if the child's life is in danger or if the condition would deteriorate irretrievably as a result of failure to treat. Where treatment is not required urgently, the clinician should seek legal advice as to how to proceed. (See Key Point 3.2.)

Key Point 3.1

A signature on a consent form is not valid consent if the patient/parent has not been given and understood the relevant information.

Key Point 3.2

It is essential to establish what relationship exists between the child and the accompanying adult at the outset.

In all cases, the process whereby consent is gained should be clearly documented. The health record should include a note of all discussions and decisions about treatment, including a statement of the available options. Where physical intervention is considered necessary for examination and/or treatment, a discussion of its nature and use should be an integral part of the consent process.

It should be emphasized that parental rights exist for the benefit of the child and not the parent. Those with parental responsibility have no right to insist on treatment that is not in the best interests of the child, neither should they prohibit a necessary intervention. In cases where such conflict occurs, a second opinion should be sought, with immediate treatment being restricted to the provision of emergency care.

Only one parent normally needs to give consent to treatment. However, if the proposed treatment is irreversible and not medically necessary, it is always prudent to seek the agreement of both parents. In the event that one parent agrees to treatment while the other does not, it is for the clinician to attempt to achieve agreement. It is not uncommon to find that, while the clinician may recommend that treatment proceeds in the child's best interests, a dissenting parent may still request that this decision be reversed. In this case, where the treatment is either controversial or elective, the clinician must seek the authority of the courts before proceeding.

Parental responsibility extends to the right to access a child's health records. However, if the child has capacity to consent, he/she must first indicate his/her agreement. Parental access to records must be withheld if it conflicts with the child's best interests or the clinician has previously given the child an undertaking not to disclose specific aspects of their care. An exception to this principle is justifiable where failure to disclose would be contrary to the child's best interests.

3.2.1 Other ethical considerations

Within the broader remit of providing a high-quality dental service for children, audit, service evaluation, and research have an important role to play. There is increasing recognition of the need to involve children actively, as service users, in the planning, monitoring, and development of health services, as well as in decision-making about their own treatment. Specific ethical principles and regulations govern the involvement of children in medical research; these may vary between countries. In the UK, any proposal to involve children in medical research or audit must be sanctioned by the appropriate ethics committee or audit/clinical governance group (Royal College of Paediatrics and Child Health 2000). Legally, valid consent should be obtained from the parent or guardian, and the agreement of school-age children should also be sought.

3.3 History

Taking a comprehensive case history is an essential prelude to clinical examination, diagnosis, and treatment planning. It is also an excellent opportunity for the dentist to establish a relationship with the child and his/her parent. Generally speaking, information is best gathered by way of a relaxed conversation with the child and his/her parent in which the dentist assumes the role of an interested listener rather than an inquisitor. While some clinicians may prefer to employ a pro forma to ensure the completeness of the process, this is less important than adherence to a set routine.

A complete case history should consist of:

- personal details
- presenting complaint(s)

- social history
- medical history
- dental history.

Table 3.1 summarizes the key information that should be included under each heading.

3.3.1 Personal details

A note should be made of the patient's name (including any abbreviated name or nickname), age, address, and telephone number. Where these details have been entered in the case notes prior to the appointment

Table 3.1 History-taking for the paediatric dental patient

1	Personal details	Name	Abbreviated name/nickname
		Contact details	Address, telephone number
		Date of birth	Age
		GMP details	Name and address
2	Presenting complaint	Planned/emergency appointment	
		Pain or swelling	Duration, nature, exacerbating and relieving factors
		Trauma	Detailed history of event
		Particular concerns	Colour, shape, position of teeth
3	Social history	With whom does the child live?	Parental responsibility (consent)
		Parental occupation	Ease of dental attendance
		Siblings	Number and ages
		School	
		Interests	

Table 3.1 Continued

4	Medical history		
	Pregnancy/birth/neonatal	Maternal health	
		Birth details	Delivery, complications, weight
		Neonatal period	Feeding or respiratory problems, neonatal teeth
		Development	Somatic, psychomotor
		Trauma injuries and childhood illnesses	Age, severity
	Systems	Respiratory	Asthma, hayfever
		Cardiovascular	SBE risk factors
		Haematological	Anaemia, bleeding, bruising
		Immunological	Predisposition to infections
		Endocrine	Diabetes
		Gastrointestinal	Abnormal bowel habits
		Neuromuscular	
		Skeletal	
	Hospitalization	Age and cause of admission	
		Operations	
		Experience of GA	
	Medication	Regular prescriptions	Format: tablets, liquid, inhalers
		Recent/current medication allergies	
	Additional information	Learning difficulties	
		Behavioural problems	ADHD, autistic spectrum disorders
	Relevant family medical history	Problems with GA, allergies, bleeding disorders, any siblings with significant medical problems	
5	Dental history		
	Professional care	Attendance pattern	Regular or irregular attender
		Previous treatment	Prevention, restorations, extractions
		LA/GA/sedation	Any problems encountered
		Previous cooperation	
	Home care	Diet	Bottle/breast feeding, snacks, drinks
		Oral hygiene	Frequency, type of brush and paste, assistance
		Fluoride	Fluoridated water, drops, tablets, mouth rinses
	Habits	Sucking/biting	Dummy, digit-sucking, nail-biting
		Parafunction	Bruxism

GMP, general medical practitioner; SBE, subacute bacterial endocarditis; LA, local anaesthetic; GA, general anaesthetic; ADHD, attention-deficit hyperactivity disorder.

they should be verified. Details of the patient's medical practitioner should also be noted.

3.3.2 Presenting complaint(s)

It is important to ascertain from the child and his/her parent why the visit has been made or what they are seeking from treatment. It is good practice to ask this question to the child before involving the parent as this establishes the child's importance in the process, although the dentist should be prepared to receive different answers from these two sources.

Where a child presents in pain or has a particular concern, this should be recorded in the child's own words and, if relevant, the history of the present complaint (e.g. duration, mode of onset, progression) should be documented. It should be recognized that, even where other (perhaps more important) treatment is required, failure to take into consideration the patient's/parent's needs or wishes at this stage may be detrimental to both the development of the dentist–patient–parent relationship and the outcome of care.

3.3.3 Social (family) history

A child is a product of his/her environment. Factors such as whether both parents are alive and well, the number and age of siblings, the parents' occupations, and ease of travel, as well as attendance at school or day-care facilities are all important if a realistic treatment plan is to be arrived at. However, since some parents will consider this kind of information confidential, the dentist may need to exercise considerable tact in order to obtain it.

This stage of history-taking also presents an opportunity to engage the child in conversation. In this way, the dentist gains an insight into the child's interests (e.g. pets, favourite subjects at school, favourite pastimes) and is able to record potential topics of conversation that can act as 'ice-breakers' in future appointments.

3.3.4 Medical history

Various diseases or functional disturbances may directly or indirectly cause or predispose to oral problems. Likewise, they may affect the delivery of oral and dental care. Conditions that will be of significance include allergies, severe asthma, diabetes, cerebral palsy, cardiac conditions, haematological disorders, and oncology.

Wherever possible, a comprehensive medical history should commence with information relating to pregnancy and birth, the neonatal period, and early childhood. Indeed, asking a mother about her child's health since birth will not infrequently stimulate the production of a complete medical history! Previous and current problems associated with each of the major systems should be elicited through careful questioning, and here a pro forma may well be helpful. Details about previous hospitalizations, operations (or planned operations), illnesses, allergies (particularly adverse reactions to drugs), and traumatic injuries should be recorded, as well as those relating to previous and current medical treatment. (See Key Point 3.3.)

> ### Key Point 3.3
>
> If any relevant conditions become apparent, these may need to be investigated in greater detail, contacting the child's general medical practitioner or hospital consultant where necessary.

It is useful to end by asking the parent whether there is anything else that they think the dentist should know about their child. (Sometimes, important details are not volunteered until this point!) This is a particularly useful approach in relation to children who suffer from behavioural or learning problems, such as attention-deficit hyperactivity disorder (ADHD) or autism. (See Key Point 3.4.)

> ### Key Point 3.4
>
> Sensitive questioning is required if the child appears to have a behavioural problem that has not been mentioned by the parent during the formal medical history.

It is important to bear in mind that many children with significant medical problems will have been subjected to multiple hospital admissions/attendances. These experiences may have a negative effect on the attitude of both the child and his/her parents towards dental treatment. In addition, dental care may not be seen as a priority in the context of total care.

Finally, a brief enquiry should also be made regarding the health of siblings and close family. Significant family medical problems, for instance problems in relation to general anaesthesia, may not only alert the practitioner to potential risks for the child, but also be factors to consider when planning treatment. Likewise, if the patient has a sick sibling, it may not be possible for the parents to commit to a prolonged course of dental treatment.

3.3.5 Dental history

A child's previous dental experiences may affect the way in which he/she reacts to further treatment. Evaluation of a child's previous behaviour requires the dentist to obtain information about the kind of dental treatment a child has received (including the method of pain and anxiety control that has been offered) and the way in which he/she has reacted to this. In so doing, specific procedures may emerge as having proved particularly problematic; such prior knowledge will enable the dentist to modify the treatment plan appropriately.

The dental history should also identify factors that have been responsible for existing oral and dental problems as well as those which might have an impact on future health. These include dietary, oral hygiene, dummy/digit sucking, and parafunctional habits. Specific questions should be asked about drinks (particularly the use of a bottle at bedtime in the younger age group), between-meal snacks, frequency of brushing, and type of toothpaste used.

Finally, a thorough dental history is an opportunity to evaluate the attitude of the parent to his/her child's dental treatment. For example, the regularity of previous dental care may be an indicator of the value that the parent places on the child's dental health. (See Key Point 3.5.)

> ### Key Point 3.5
>
> Embarking on a treatment plan that is at significant variance with parental attitudes and expectations without clear explanation and justification invites non-completion.

3.4 Examination

3.4.1 First impressions

An initial impression of the child's overall health and development can be gained as soon as he/she is greeted in the waiting room or enters the surgery. In particular, it is useful to note the following:

- General health—does the child look well?
- Overall physical and mental development—does it seem appropriate for the child's chronological age?
- Weight—is the child grossly under- or overweight?
- Coordination—does the child have an abnormal gait or obvious motor impairment?

While the history is being taken, the clinician should also be making an 'unofficial' assessment of the child's likely level of cooperation in order that the most appropriate approach for the examination can be adopted right from the start (hopefully saving both time and tears). Broadly speaking, prospective young patients may fall into one of the following categories:

- Happy and confident—this child is likely to hop into the chair for a check-up without further coaxing.
- A little anxious or shy but displaying some rapport with the dental team—this child will probably allow an examination after some simple acclimatization and reassurance (if the child is very young, the option of sitting on the parent's knee could be given).
- Very frightened, crying, clutching their parent, avoiding eye contact, or not responding to direct questions—this child is unlikely to accept a conventional examination at this visit (though the child may allow a brief examination while sitting on a non-dental chair, perhaps even in the waiting room). Further acclimatization will be required before a thorough examination can be undertaken.
- Severe behavioural problem or learning disability—in a few cases, this may preclude the child from ever voluntarily accepting an examination. Restraint (with or without pharmacological management) may be indicated to facilitate an intra-oral examination.

(See Key Point 3.6.)

> **Key Point 3.6**
>
> It is not good practice to formulate a definitive treatment plan, especially one involving a general anaesthetic, without first performing a thorough examination.

3.4.2 Physical intervention

In an ideal world, pre-cooperative children (see Section 4.3) would be given the time and opportunity to accept a dental examination voluntarily over a series of desensitizing visits. In reality, if a child presents with a reported problem but remains pre-cooperative after gentle coaxing and normal behaviour management strategies, it may be deemed necessary to carry out an examination in a controlled but restraining manner. This should always be viewed as a last resort in an 'urgent' clinical situation, and the child's rights and best interests should remain paramount.

Physical intervention should only be considered for infants/very young children, or children with severe learning difficulties (provided that they are not too big or strong to make any restraint potentially dangerous or uncontrolled). The issue of informed consent is important here, as it is imperative that the need for the examination and the manner in which it is going to be conducted are clearly understood by all concerned. It is best to:

- explain in advance how the child is to be positioned;
- ask parents for their active help;
- give reassurance that the child is not going to be hurt in any way;
- document the event and outcomes.

In the most controlled approach, the child is laid across the parent's knees with his/her head in the lap of the operator (Fig. 3.1). The parent is able to hold the child's arms, although a dental nurse may need to restrain the child's legs. It may be easier to examine larger children who have special needs while they are held in their own wheelchair, with the dental nurse supporting the child's head during the examination (see also Chapter 17).

3.4.3 Extra-oral examination

General examination

Before carrying out a detailed examination of the craniofacial structures, a more general physical assessment should be undertaken. Valuable information about a child's overall health, development, or even habits can often be determined by noting the following:

- Height—is the child very tall or very small for his/her age? In a few cases, it may be appropriate to take an accurate height measurement (Fig. 3.2) and plot data on a standard growth chart (Fig. 3.3). Children whose height lies below the third centile or above the 97th centile or who exhibit less than 3–5cm growth per year should be referred to a paediatrician for further investigation.

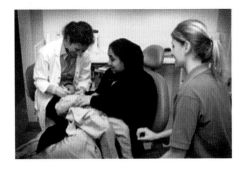

Figure 3.1 Controlled examination of a young boy laid across his mother's knee.

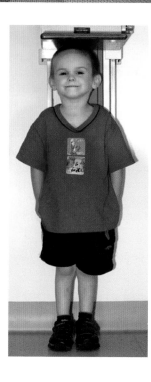

Figure 3.2 Use of a wall-mounted stediometer to take an accurate height measurement (the patient's shoes should be removed!).

- Weight—could there be an underlying eating disorder? Is general anaesthesia contraindicated because of the child's obesity? Is there an underlying endocrine problem?
- Skin—look for any notable bruising or injury on exposed arms or legs (Fig. 3.4).
- Hands—assess for evidence of digit-sucking or nail-biting, warts, finger clubbing, or abnormal nail or finger morphology (Fig. 3.5).

Head and neck

During the examination of the head and neck, the following structures should be briefly assessed:

- head—note size, shape (abnormalities may be seen in certain syndromes), and any facial asymmetry (Fig. 3.6);
- hair—note if sparse (look out for head lice!);
- eyes—is there any visual impairment or abnormality of the sclera?
- ears—record any abnormal morphology or presence of hearing aids;
- skin—document any scars, bruising, lacerations, pallor, and birthmarks (Fig. 3.7), and be aware of contagious infections such as impetigo;

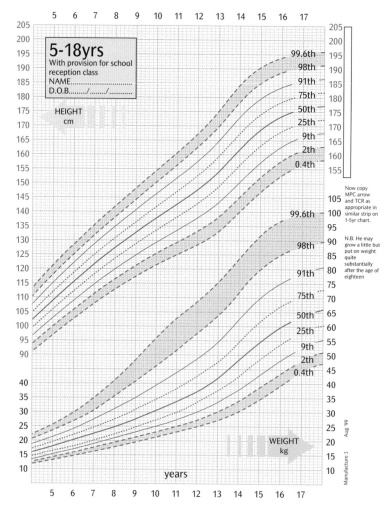

Figure 3.3 Standard growth chart showing plot of height against age for boy who has a severe growth deficiency.

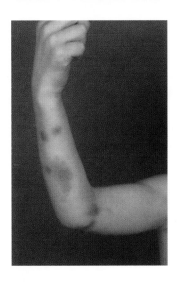

Figure 3.4 Multiple bruises on the arm of a child with a platelet disorder.

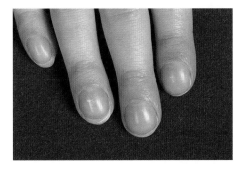

Figure 3.5 Finger clubbing in a child with a congenital heart disorder.

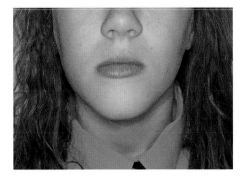

Figure 3.6 Facial asymmetry in a teenage girl.

- temporomandibular joint—is there any pain, crepitus, deviation, or restricted opening?
- lymph nodes—palpate for enlarged submandibular or cervical lymph nodes (bear in mind that lymphadenopathy is not uncommon in children because of frequent viral infections) (Fig. 3.8);
- lips—note the presence of cold sores, swelling, or abnormal colouring (Fig. 3.9).

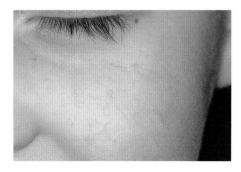

Figure 3.7 Telangiectasia noted on the face of a young boy.

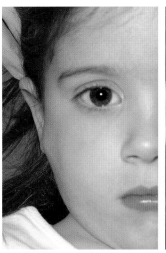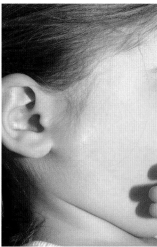

Figure 3.8 Three-year-old girl with swelling possibly in the pre-auricular lymph node or the parotid gland.

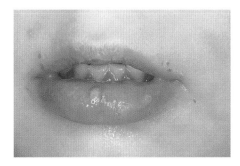

Figure 3.9 Multiple vesicles on the lip of a young patient with acute herpetic gingivostomatitis.

Any positive findings should be recorded carefully. Clinical photographs or annotated sketches (Fig. 3.10) may be very helpful for future reference, particularly with respect to medico-legal purposes, or in cases of suspected child physical abuse (see Chapters 12 and 18). Obviously, when the child presents with a specific problem, such as a facial swelling, a more thorough examination of the presenting condition is needed (see Chapter 15).

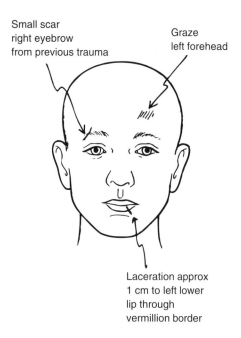

Small scar
right eyebrow
from previous trauma

Graze
left forehead

Laceration approx
1 cm to left lower
lip through
vermillion border

Figure 3.10 Example of an annotated sketch used to record trauma.

3.4.4 Intra-oral examination

A systematic approach should be adopted for the intra-oral examination. The following is a suggested order:

- soft tissues
- gingival and periodontal tissues
- teeth
- occlusion.

Soft tissues

An abnormal appearance of the oral soft tissues may be indicative of an underlying systemic disease or nutritional deficiency. In addition, a variety of oral pathologies may be seen in children (see Chapter 15). Therefore it is important to examine the tongue, palate, throat, and cheeks carefully, noting any colour changes, ulceration, swelling, or other pathology (Fig. 3.11).

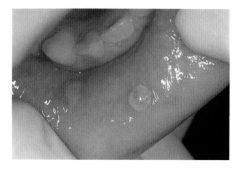

Figure 3.11 Mucocoele of labial mucosa: an incidental finding.

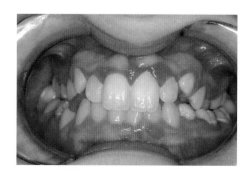

Figure 3.12 Plaque-induced gingival inflammation.

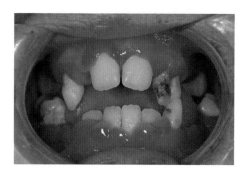

Figure 3.13 Severe gingival inflammation in patient with cyclical neutropenia.

It is also sensible to check for abnormal frenal attachment or tongue-tie, which may have functional implications. If a tongue-tie or abnormal tongue function is observed, some consideration should be given to the child's speech. During examination of the soft tissues, an overall impression of salivary flow rate and consistency should also be gained.

Gingival and periodontal tissues

A visual examination of the gingival tissues is usually all that is indicated for young children, as periodontal disease is very uncommon in this age group. The presence of colour change (redness), swelling, ulceration, spontaneous bleeding, or recession (Figs 3.12 and 3.13) should be carefully noted and the aetiology sought. (See Key Point 3.7.)

Key Point 3.7

The presence of profound gingival inflammation in the absence of gross plaque deposits, lateral periodontal abscesses, prematurely exfoliating teeth, or mobile permanent teeth may indicate a more serious underlying problem, warranting further investigation.

During inspection of the gingival tissues, an assessment of oral cleanliness should also be made and the presence of any plaque or calculus deposits noted. A number of simple oral hygiene indices have been developed to provide an objective record of oral cleanliness. One such index, the oral debris index (Greene and Vermillion 1964), requires

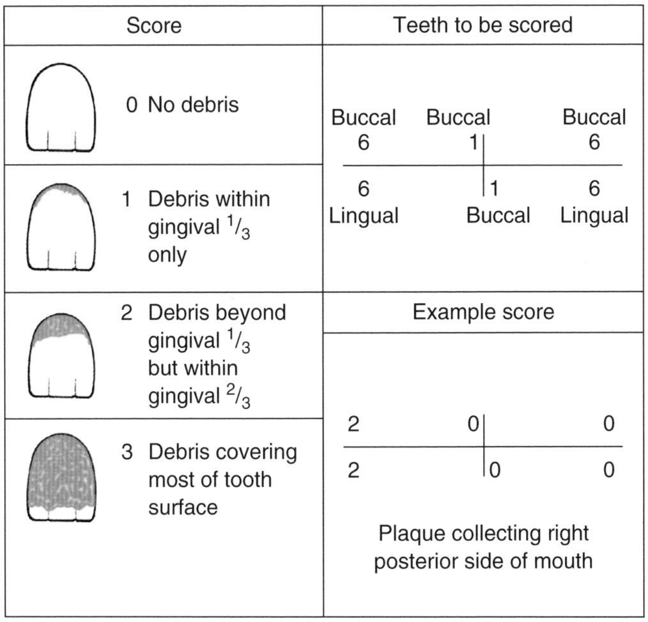

Score		Teeth to be scored	
0 No debris		Buccal 6　Buccal 1　Buccal 6	
1 Debris within gingival $^{1}/_{3}$ only		6　　　1　　6 Lingual　Buccal　Lingual	
2 Debris beyond gingival $^{1}/_{3}$ but within gingival $^{2}/_{3}$		Example score	
3 Debris covering most of tooth surface		2　0｜0 2　　0　0 Plaque collecting right posterior side of mouth	

Figure 3.14 Oral debris index (Greene and Vermillion 1964).

disclosing prior to an evaluation of the amount of plaque on selected teeth (first permanent molars, and upper right and lower left central incisors) as shown in Fig. 3.14.

There are no universally agreed guidelines for the periodontal screening of children and young people, although this is an area that is currently under review and development (Clerehugh 2008). Until such guidelines are published, a simplified periodontal assessment has been advocated for the under-18s which involves examination of all four first permanent molars and the upper right and lower left central incisors. The use of a WHO 621 probe with a 0.5mm ball end and black band at 3.5–5.5mm can be used to determine a Basic Periodontal Examination (BPE) code for each of these six teeth (Table 3.2). It should be borne in mind that children found to have aggressive periodontitis or conditions that predispose them to periodontal destruction should be referred for specialist care (see Chapter 11).

Teeth

Following assessment of the oral soft tissues, a full dental charting should be performed. A thorough knowledge of eruption dates for the primary and permanent dentition is essential, as any delayed or premature eruption may alert the clinician to a potential problem. However, simply recording the presence or absence of a tooth is not adequate: closer scrutiny of each tooth's condition, structure, and shape is also required. Suggested features to note are listed briefly below.

- Caries—is it active/arrested, restorable/unrestorable? Check for the presence of a chronic sinus associated with grossly carious teeth.
- Restorations—are they intact/deficient?
- Fissure sealants—are they intact/deficient?
- Tooth surface loss—note any erosion/attrition, site, extent (Fig. 3.15).
- Trauma—note extent, site, or signs of loss of vitality.

Table 3.2 Codes and clinical criteria for a simplified BPE for use in children.

BPE code	Clinical criteria
0	Healthy periodontal tissues, no bleeding after gentle probing
1	Bleeding after gentle probing, black band remains completely visible above gingival margin, no calculus or defective margins detected
2	Supra-gingival and/or sub-gingival calculus and/or other plaque retention factor, black band remains completely visible above gingival margin
3	Shallow pocket (4–5mm), black band partially visible in the deepest pocket on the index tooth
4	Deep pocked (≥6mm), black band disappears in the pocket
*	Furcation involvement, recession and probing depth ≥7mm

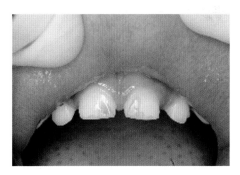

Figure 3.15 Unusual pattern of erosion affecting the labial surface of maxillary primary incisors and attributed to the use of lemon tea in a feeder cup.

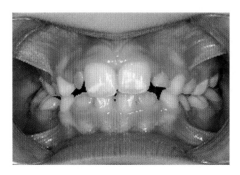

Figure 3.16 Localized white enamel opacities affecting permanent maxillary central incisors.

- Tooth structure—record any enamel opacities/hypoplasia (are defects localized/generalized?) (Figs 3.16–3.18).
- Tooth shape/size—note the presence of double teeth, conical teeth, macro/microdontia, talon cusps, deep cingulum pits (Fig. 3.19).

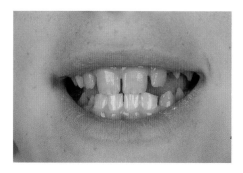

Figure 3.17 Generalized inherited enamel defect (amelogenesis imperfecta).

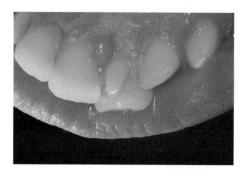

Figure 3.19 Maxillary central incisor with talon cusp.

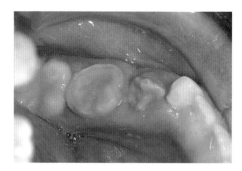

Figure 3.18 Partially erupted mandibular first premolar showing severe enamel hypoplasia.

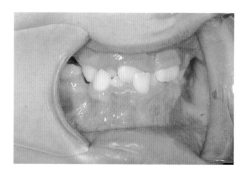

Figure 3.20 Cross-bite in early mixed dentition.

- Tooth number—any missing/extra teeth?
- Tooth mobility—is it physiological or pathological?
- Tooth eruption—are there any impactions, infra-occluded primary molars, or ectopically erupting first permanent molars?

Occlusion

Clearly, a full orthodontic assessment is not indicated every time a child is examined. However, tooth alignment and occlusion should be considered briefly, as these may provide an early prompt as to the need for interceptive orthodontic treatment. It is certainly worth noting:

- severe skeletal abnormalities
- overjet and overbite
- first molar relationships
- presence of crowding/spacing
- deviations/displacements.

There are also two key stages of dental development, when the clinician should be particularly vigilant in checking tooth eruption and position.

1. Age 8–9 years—eruption of upper permanent incisors.
    - Increased overjet—may predispose to trauma.
    - Cross-bite—need for early intervention? (Fig. 3.20)
    - Traumatic bite—associated with localized gingival recession of lower incisor?

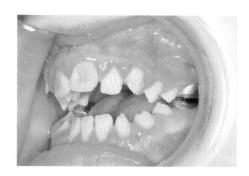

Figure 3.21 Severe anterior open bite (in association with amelogenesis imperfecta).

- Anterior open bite—skeletal problem, digit-sucking habit, or tongue thrust? (Fig. 3.21)
- Failure of eruption—presence of a supernumerary, crown/root dilaceration, retained primary incisor, congenitally missing lateral incisors? (Fig. 3.22)

2. Age ≥10 years—eruption of upper permanent canines.
    - Are the permanent canines palpable buccally? If not, they may be heading in a palatal direction.
    - Are the primary canines becoming mobile? If not, the permanent canines may be ectopic.

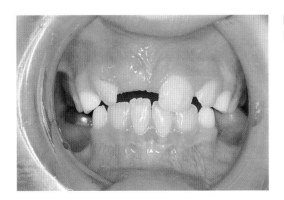

Figure 3.22 Failure of eruption of maxillary left central incisor—time to be concerned!

3.5 Further investigations

Having carried out a thorough extra- and intra-oral examination as described above, the clinician may feel that further investigations are indicated for diagnostic purposes. Table 3.3 highlights the range of dental (and more general) investigations that may be employed to aid diagnosis of the presenting complaint. The use of radiographs is described more fully in the following section.

Table 3.3 Special investigations for the paediatric dental patient

Investigation	Comment
Intra-oral	
Sensibility testing	Use of ethyl chloride or electric pulp tester may be useful for determining pulpal status following trauma; caution should be exercised in interpretation of results
Transillumination	Useful for interproximal caries detection, or trauma-related sequelae such as pulpal haemorrhage or enamel infractions
Mobility	Gentle finger pressure will reveal any pathological or physiological mobility
Percussion	A 'cracked tea-cup' sound on gentle tapping of tooth indicates likely ankylosis
Periodontal probing	Indicated in specific periodontal conditions or to detect the presence of a foreign body
Saliva tests	May be appropriate to test salivary flow rate and buffering capacity in cases of suspected xerostomia
Oral microbial tests	*Streptococcus mutans* or *Lactobacillus* counts may be indicated in children presenting with rampant caries
	Culture and sensitivity of micro-organisms from intra-oral pus sample may aid antibiotic selection
	Cytology of intra-oral swab may confirm suspected candidal infection
Tooth measurement	Space analysis and measurement of tooth size may be necessary for treatment planning
Oral histology/ pathology	Specialist examination of soft or hard tissue specimens may be essential to obtain diagnosis of presenting complaint
Study models	May be useful for treatment planning (± Kesling set-up) or providing record of presenting problems such as erosion, infra-occlusion, orthodontic status
Photographs	Provide record of presenting problem and pre- and post-treatment status
General	
Specialist imaging	Computed axial tomography (CAT), ultrasound, magnetic resonance imaging (MRI), or sialography may be indicated in special cases
Haematology	Full blood picture, electrophoresis (for sickle-cell status), clinical chemistry, or immunological tests may be requested in certain cases
Height and weight	Assessment of height may be indicated where there is an obvious deviation from normal or where detection of pubertal growth spurt is indicated for orthodontic purposes (use of functional appliances)
	Weight assessment may be necessary to determine suitability of patient for out-patient general anaesthesia

Table 3.3 Continued

Investigation	Comment
General	
Dietary assessment	A 3-day dietary record may be analysed to identify potential cariogenic and/or erosive components and provide basis for dietary advice
Temperature	Assessment of any pyrexia is indicated when a child presents with an acute orofacial infection

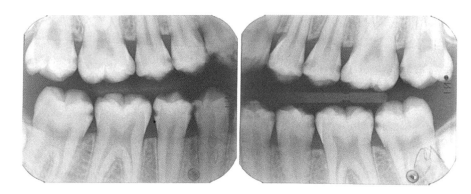

Figure 3.23 Left and right bitewing radiographs showing multiple interproximal carious lesions not evident clinically.

3.5.1 Radiographs

Comprehensive clinical guidelines for the radiographic assessment of children have been proposed by the European Academy of Paediatric Dentistry (Espelid *et al.* 2003). 'Routine' radiographic screening is certainly not indicated for children. However, radiographs may be indicated in order to facilitate:

- caries diagnosis
- trauma assessment
- orthodontic treatment planning
- identification of any abnormalities in dental development
- detection of any bony or dental pathology.

(See Key Point 3.8.)

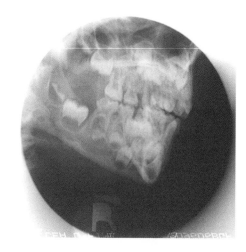

Figure 3.24 Right lateral oblique radiograph showing caries in lower primary molars.

> **Key Point 3.8**
>
> Since patients should not be overexposed to ionizing radiation, every radiographic investigation should be clinically justified and have a clear diagnostic purpose.

Caries diagnosis

Bitewing radiographs are invaluable for the detection of early interproximal carious lesions (Fig. 3.23), or occult occlusal lesions. Indeed, bitewing radiography will increase the identification of interproximal lesions by a factor of between 2 and 8 compared with visual assessment alone. Bitewing radiographs are usually recommended for all new

patients, especially those with a high risk of caries, to provide a baseline caries assessment. However, they may not be necessary for very young patients with open primary molar contacts.

The bitewing radiograph is the view of choice for interproximal caries detection, but it does require a reasonable degree of patient cooperation. The lateral oblique radiograph provides a useful alternative for patients unable to tolerate intra-oral films (Fig. 3.24). This view has the added advantage of including the developing permanent dentition.

Following the initial radiographic investigation of caries, a decision should be made regarding the frequency of any future assessment. The

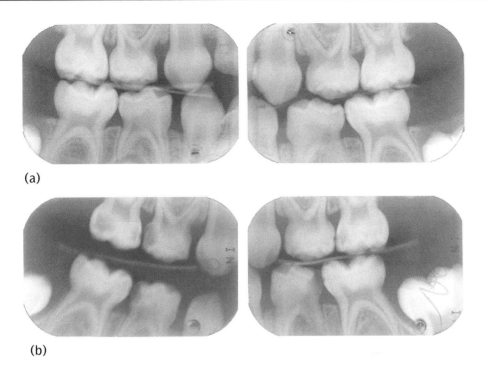

(a)

(b)

Figure 3.25 Left and right bitewing radiographs of a young boy from high-carious-risk family at (a) 3 years 10 months and (b) 4 years 10 months, demonstrating rapid carious development.

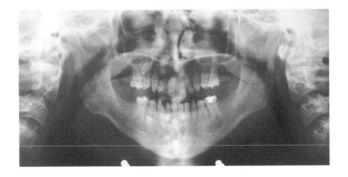

Figure 3.26 Panoral radiograph of a 10-year-old boy with severe hypodontia (only two permanent units are present). Note taurodont mandibular second primary molars.

interval will depend on the patient's individual caries risk (see Section 3.6) as follows:

- high caries risk—repeat bitewings in 12 months (Fig. 3.25);
- low caries risk—repeat bitewings in 24–36 months.

Trauma assessment

Radiographs may be indicated for patients who have sustained facial or dental trauma. This topic will be discussed in more detail in Chapter 12.

Orthodontic treatment planning

A discussion of radiographic views for orthodontic treatment planning is not within the remit of this chapter. However, a panoral radiograph is usually mandatory prior to any orthodontic treatment. The need for other views, such as an upper standard occlusal or lateral cephalometric radiograph, depends on the individual clinical situation (Chapter 14).

Dental development

The need for radiographic assessment of the developing dentition may be prompted by any of the following clinical features:

- delayed/premature dental development;
- suspected missing/extra teeth (Fig. 3.26);
- potential ectopic tooth position (especially upper maxillary canines);
- first permanent molars of poor prognosis—in cases where first permanent molars are to be extracted it is mandatory to check for the radiographic presence of all other permanent teeth, including third molars, and to assess the stage of dental development of the lower second permanent molars in order to determine the optimum time for any first permanent molar extractions (see Chapter 14).

The panoral radiograph provides the optimum view for an overall assessment of normal or abnormal dental development. Furthermore, accurate determination of chronological age can be achieved by calculating dental age using a panoral radiograph and a technique for dental aging, such as that described by Demirjian *et al.* (1973).

A panoral radiograph may be supplemented with an intra-oral radiograph, such as an upper standard occlusal, when an 'abnormality' presents in the anterior maxilla. The combination of these two views provides the opportunity to confirm the exact position of any unerupted maxillary canines or supernumerary teeth using the vertical parallax technique (Fig. 3.27). (See Key Point 3.9.)

Key Point 3.9

The 'SLOB' rule: if the tooth in question moves in the **s**ame direction as the X-ray tube, then the tooth is **l**ingually or palatally positioned (in relation to the reference point). However, if the tooth moves in the **o**pposite direction to the X-ray tube, it is **b**uccally placed.

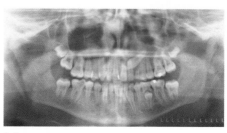

(a)

Detection of pathology

Selected radiographs may be required in cases of suspected pathology. The actual view is obviously dictated by the presenting complaint, but a periapical radiograph is frequently indicated for localized pathologies, such as:

- periapical or inter-radicular infection (primary molars) associated with non-vital teeth;
- periodontal conditions;
- trauma-related sequelae such as root resorption.

A panoral view is particularly valuable where the pathology involves more than one quadrant or has extensive bony involvement. A sectional panoral radiograph may be prescribed in some situations since this approach helps to reduce ionizing exposure.

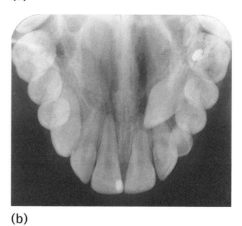

(b)

Figure 3.27 (a) Panoral radiograph and (b) upper standard occlusal radiograph used to confirm the palatal position of the unerupted maxillary left canine by the vertical parallax technique.

3.6 Risk assessment

Having gathered relevant information by taking a history, conducting an examination, and carrying out any special investigations, there is one final consideration to make prior to treatment planning, i.e. risk assessment. (See Key Point 3.10.)

Key Point 3.10

Risk assessment is simply an assessment of the likelihood of a disease or condition developing in an individual patient.

Risk assessment is certainly not a new concept, but it has now become a more recognized step in the decision-making process. When conducting a risk assessment, the clinician needs to consider all factors that may have a negative or positive effect on oral health. Generally, risk assessments are undertaken with respect to caries, but there are other recognized 'risks' to consider for the young dental patient including:

- periodontal disease
- erosion
- orofacial trauma.

The rationale for risk assessment is to target resources to those who most need them. Ideally, any preventive or operative treatment programme should be directed by an appreciation of the patient's risk status, thus ensuring that service delivery is both effective and cost-efficient. Risk assessment is also relevant when determining an optimum recall interval, as not all patients need to be seen with the same frequency. Furthermore, a child's risk status is not static; it may change due to any number of changes in personal circumstances. Therefore it is important to continually reassess risk status at future visits.

3.6.1 Caries

The aim of caries risk assessment is to predict whether the disease is likely to develop in an as-yet caries-free individual, or to determine the rate of disease progression in a patient who already has some caries experience. Ascribing caries risk status to each patient is fundamental to treatment planning as it prompts the clinician to propose the most appropriate preventive strategy. In addition, it should dictate the frequency of radiographic investigation for caries diagnosis and recall visits. However, it should be borne in mind that caries risk status is not static and will have to be reconsidered at subsequent assessments.

Table 3.4 Factors relevant to caries risk assessment

Socio-demographic	Dental	Other
Low-risk status		
Affluent	No previous caries experience	Fluoride exposure (water, milk, toothpaste)
Well-educated mother	Good oral hygiene	No significant medical history
	Low family caries experience	Good dietary control
	Regular brushing with fluoride toothpaste from early age	
High-risk status		
Poverty	Past caries experience (especially in first permanent molars)	Limited/no exposure to fluoride
Poorly educated mother	Current caries experience (especially if involving smooth surfaces, lower incisors)	Use of sweetened drinks in bottles in young children
Immigrant status	Plaque accumulation (especially primary maxillary incisors)	Significant medical history (especially if associated with xerostomia)
	Matrilinear transmission of *Streptococcus mutans* in early childhood	Frequent intake of fermentable carbohydrates
	Low salivary flow	
	Family history of high caries experience	
	Caries-prone sites: deep pits and fissures	
	Hypomineralized/hypoplastic enamel	

Interestingly, research has shown that the experienced clinician can actually achieve a high level of prediction simply on the basis of a socio-demographic history and clinical examination. Thus the need for specific testing, such as microbiological investigation, may not confer significant additional benefit. In particular, past caries experience has proved to be the most useful clinical predictor of caries risk. Additionally, poor oral hygiene (visible plaque on maxillary incisors) in very young children has been found to be a reliable indicator of high caries risk. Table 3.4 highlights the key risk factors that should be taken into consideration when conducting a risk assessment.

Very simply, children can be categorized as low, moderate, or high caries risk according to the following criteria:

- Low risk—intact dentition, good oral hygiene, well-educated affluent family background, good dietary control, and use of fluoride regimens.
- Moderate risk—one or two new lesions per year, poor oral hygiene, and non-optimum fluoride use.
- High risk—three or more new lesions per year, poor oral hygiene and dietary control, significant medical history, immigrant status, poverty, low education, and poor uptake of fluoride regimens.

It is important to bear in mind that the risk of caries development also varies significantly for:

- different age groups—children aged 1–2 years and 5–7 years are considered at high risk;
- individual teeth—first primary molars and first permanent molars are high risk;
- different tooth surfaces: interproximal primary molar surfaces and occlusal surfaces of first permanent molars are high risk.

3.6.2 Periodontal disease

While periodontal disease is not common in children, there are some recognized risk factors associated with increased likelihood of its development. These include:

- smoking;
- diabetes;
- plaque accumulation, although this is not such a reliable indicator at an individual level;
- family history (genetic factors).

Hormonal changes around puberty, low vitamin C or calcium intake, socio-economic status, psychosocial factors, tooth position, and occlusal relationships may also influence periodontal health but are not considered reliable risk indicators.

3.6.3 Erosion

There is no established model for risk prediction in relation to erosion. However, it has been suggested that:

- intake of more than six carbonated drinks weekly is associated with moderate erosion risk;
- intake of more than 14 carbonated drinks weekly is associated with high erosion risk.

In addition, the following risk factors have been reported to have some association with erosion:

- intake of more than two citrus fruits daily;
- frequent sports participation;

- eating disorders;
- gastric reflux, rumination.

3.6.4 Orofacial trauma

Most orofacial trauma cannot be prevented, as it usually results from an unavoidable accident. However, there are some recognized trauma risk factors that warrant consideration and appropriate prevention where possible.

- Increased overjet—children with an overjet >9mm are twice as likely to sustain dental trauma.
- Contact sports—active participation in sports such as rugby, hockey, and martial arts carries an increased risk of sustaining orofacial trauma.

- Previous dental trauma—there is a significant risk of sustaining further trauma.
- Motor disabilities—children with poor coordination are at greater risk of sustaining trauma.
- Neurological disabilities—uncontrolled epileptics are at high risk of trauma.
- Age—peak ages for sustaining orofacial trauma are around 1–2 years and 8–10 years.
- Gender—boys are at greater risk than girls.

3.7 Principles of treatment planning

In planning dental care for child patients, the dentist must satisfy two, sometimes apparently conflicting, objectives. First, it is clearly necessary to ensure that the child reaches adulthood with the optimum achievable dental health. Second, it is essential that the child both learns to trust the dental team and develops a positive attitude towards dental treatment. Therefore, at any point in time, the desirability of 'ideal' care (whatever this might be) must be carefully balanced against:

- the child's potential to cope with the proposed treatment;
- the ability and willingness of the child and parent to attend for care;
- parental preference.

Thus the dentist may be required to exercise a degree of compromise which those more used to treating adults may find unfamiliar and even a little uncomfortable. However, it is important to accept that there will be no winners if, at the outset, a treatment plan is unrealistic or insufficiently flexible to allow modification, should this become necessary, as treatment progresses.

From the foregoing comments, it should be evident that it is not possible to adopt a 'one size fits all' approach to treatment planning; very different treatment plans may be drawn up for children who present with very similar problems. However, basic principles underlie all treatment plans and these are set out in Fig. 3.28. (The reader should note the emphasis that has been placed on repeated assessment and discussion.) Several aspects of this approach are worthy of special comment.

3.7.1 Management of acute dental problems

The management of acute problems present at the time of the child's first visit is undoubtedly a priority. However, it is important that any treatment that is provided sits well in the context of a holistic treatment plan and does not jeopardize its completion. Therefore in most cases pain relief should be provided without recourse to extraction.

3.7.2 Prevention

Any treatment plan relies for its support on a 'spine' of prevention (Chapter 6). Restorations placed in a mouth in which the caries process is still active are prone to failure: repeated restorations may be detrimental to the child's ability to cooperate and to the dentist–parent relationship (as well as frustrating to the dental team). Likewise, managing a child's grossly carious teeth by multiple extractions without ensuring that he/she receives appropriate preventive input does nothing to assist that child in maintaining dental health in the future.

An added advantage of a 'prevention first' approach is its importance in behaviour management, acclimatizing the child to future treatment. Procedures such as fluoride varnish applications or disclosing are good confidence-building steps.

Any preventive strategy should be dictated by an individual's risk assessment; for instance, children at low risk of caries do not routinely require fissure sealants. The delivery of preventive advice and interventions should not be restricted to the commencement of treatment. Rather, prevention should be reinforced as treatment progresses, with modifications being incorporated if they become necessary. (See Key Point 3.11.)

> ### Key Point 3.11
>
> Preventive advice, whether this is in relation to diet, oral hygiene, fluoride supplementation, or even the prevention of dental trauma, should be realistic and specifically tailored to the individual child and parent.

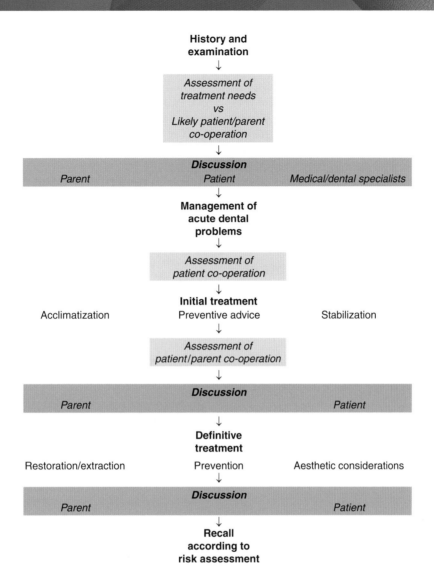

Figure 3.28 Principles of treatment planning for a paediatric dental patient.

Clearly, prevention is not simply a job for the members of the dental team. It demands the creation of a partnership in which both the child and the parent are key players, though the relative role and prominence of each will vary with the age of the child. In the case of young children, parents are (or at least should be) responsible for food choices and oral hygiene, though the latter responsibility is not infrequently abdicated before the child has sufficient manual dexterity to brush adequately alone. As the child approaches the teenage years (and particularly when he/she enters secondary schooling), parental control inevitably decreases. Therefore any discussion of the proposed treatment plan should include an agreement as to what is required of the child and/or parent as well as what will be offered by various members of the dental team (including Dental Care Professionals). It may be helpful to document this agreement in the form of a written 'contract'.

3.7.3 Stabilization

Where a child has open cavities, a phase of stabilization should precede the provision of definitive treatment, whether this is to be entirely restorative in nature or a combination of restorations and extractions. In this process, no attempt is made to render the cavities caries free; rather, minimal tissue is removed without local anaesthesia, allowing placement of an appropriate temporary dressing. The inclusion of such a phase in a holistic treatment plan reduces the overall bacterial load and slows caries progression, renders the child less likely to present with pain and sepsis, and buys time for the implementation of preventive measures and for the child to be acclimatized to treatment.

However, a word of caution is offered: it is essential that the parent understands the purpose of stabilization, and that which has been provided are not permanent restorations. Otherwise, it is possible that they will perceive that treatment is failing to progress.

Following stabilization, the child's response to acclimatization and compliance with the suggested preventive regime should be assessed. This is particularly important before proceeding with definitive treatment. For example, in a scenario in which a child has not responded to acclimatization and has either refused stabilization or accepted this only with extreme difficulty, the dentist may be entirely justified in considering extractions. This will allow the child and his/her family to enjoy a period where no active treatment is required and in which prevention can be established (always provided, of course, that they return for continuing care).

3.7.4 Scheduling operative treatment

In any treatment plan, it is necessary to give careful consideration to the order in which items of operative care are provided. The following are general rules of thumb.

- Small simple restorations should be completed first.
- Maxillary teeth should be treated before mandibular ones (since it is usually easier to administer local anaesthesia in the upper jaw).
- Posterior teeth should be treated before anteriors (this usually ensures that the patient returns for treatment).
- Quadrant dentistry should be practised wherever possible (this reduces the number of visits to a minimum), but only if the time in chair is not excessive for a very young patient.
- Endodontic treatment should follow completion of simple restorative treatment.
- Extractions should be the last items of operative care (at this stage, patient cooperation can be more reliably assured) unless the patient presents with an acute problem mid-treatment.

3.7.5 Recall

Treatment planning (in its broadest sense) clearly does not end with the completion of one treatment journey. The determination of a recall schedule tailored to the needs of the individual child is an essential part of the treatment-planning process.

It is generally accepted that children should receive a dental assessment more frequently than adults since:

- there is evidence that the rate of progression of dental caries can be more rapid in children than in adults;
- the rate of progression of caries and erosive tooth wear is faster in primary than in permanent teeth;
- periodic assessment of orofacial growth and the developing occlusion is required.

In the last context, there is considerable merit in ensuring that recall examinations coincide with particular milestones in dental development, for example around 6, 9, and 12 years. Generally speaking,

recall intervals of no more than 12 months offer the dentist the opportunity to deliver and reinforce preventive advice during the crucial period when a child is establishing the basis for his/her future dental health. However, the exact recall interval (3, 6, 9, or 12 months) should be tailored to meet, and vary with, the child's needs. This requires an assessment of disease levels as well as risk of/from dental disease.

3.7.6 Treatment planning for general anaesthesia

Treatment planning for general anaesthesia is an extremely complex area that merits special mention. However, a full discussion lies outside the scope of this chapter. It is sufficient to emphasize here that, in this context, a comprehensive approach must be taken. Providing treatment under general anaesthesia for a child who has been shown to be unable to cope with operative dental care under local anaesthesia (with or without the support of conscious sedation) will do absolutely nothing to improve his/her future cooperation. Therefore such treatment should include the restoration or extraction (as appropriate) of *all* carious teeth. (See Key Point 3.12.)

Key Point 3.12

The practice of extracting only the most grossly carious or symptomatic teeth (and assuming that other carious teeth can be restored under local anaesthetic at a later stage) predisposes to a high rate of repeat general anaesthesia and should be discouraged.

The orthodontic implications of any proposed treatment should always be considered. This is particularly the case when the loss of one or more permanent units is to be included in the treatment plan. In such cases, the plan should ideally be drawn up in consultation with a specialist in paediatric dentistry and/or orthodontics.

Treatment under general anaesthesia, irrespective of whether this includes restorative treatment or is limited to extractions, should be followed with an appropriate preventive programme. Failure to provide this almost inevitably leads to the child undergoing further treatment (usually extractions) under general anaesthesia.

3.7.7 Treatment planning for complex cases

The clinician should always have a clear long-term 'vision' for the management of the individual patient. In creating this, appropriate specialist paediatric dentistry input to treatment planning should be sought where indicated. In addition, it may be appropriate for the patient to be seen at a multidisciplinary clinic involving a number of other specialties, including orthodontics, restorative dentistry, or oral and maxillofacial surgery. Treatment planning of complex cases, such as those presenting with generalized defects of enamel or dentine formation, hypodontia, or clefts of lip and palate certainly require interdisciplinary specialist input. For example, such input may result in:

- the retention of anterior roots to maintain alveolar bone in preparation for future implants;

- the use of preformed metal crowns to maintain clinical crown height in preparation for definitive crowns;

- the use of direct/laboratory-formed composite veneers in preparation for porcelain veneers when growth (and any orthodontic treatment) is complete.

3.8 Summary

Treatment planning for young patients should not only address current needs but also plan ahead for those of the future, thus ensuring that every child reaches adulthood with a healthy, functional, and aesthetic dentition as well as positive attitudes towards dentistry. Meticulous history-taking, clinical examination, and risk assessment contribute to the decision-making process, but one should never lose sight of what is realistic and practical for the child in the context of his/her environment. To do otherwise not only courts non-compliance but also fails to recognize the most important aspect of all—a child's individuality. (See Key Point 3.13.)

> ### Key Point 3.13
>
> The one overriding consideration is this: management in early adulthood should never be compromised by inappropriate treatment at a young age.

3.9 Further reading

Mascarenhas, A.K. (1998). Oral hygiene as a risk indicator of enamel and dentine caries. *Community Dentistry and Oral Epidemiology*, **26**, 331–9. (*This study reviews the clinical indicators employed in caries risk assessment and highlights the relationship between poor oral hygiene and caries.*)

Powell, L.V. (1988). Caries risk assessment: relevance to the practitioner. *Journal of the American Dental Association*, **129**, 349–53.

(*This comprehensive paper reviews the practical aspects of caries risk assessment.*)

Rodd, H.D. and Wray, A. (2004). *Treatment planning for the developing dentition*. Quintessence, London. (*This practical and easily read book covers all aspects of treatment planning for children.*)

3.10 References

Clerehugh V. (2008). Periodontal diseases in children and adolescents. *British Dental Journal*, **204**, 469–71.

Demirjian, A., Goldstein, H., and Tanner, J.M. (1973). A new system of dental age assessment. *Human Biology*, **45**, 211–27. (*This paper describes how to undertake an accurate dental age assessment for patients using a panoral radiograph.*)

Espelid, I., Mejàre, I., and Weerheijm, K. (2003). EAPD guidelines for the use of radiographs in children. *European Journal of Paediatric Dentistry*, **4**, 40–8. (*This excellent and comprehensive paper describes the appropriate use of dental radiographs for young patients.*)

Greene, J.C. and Vermillion, J.R. (1964). The simplified oral hygiene index. *Journal of the American Dental Association*, **68**, 7–13.

Nunn, J., Foster M., Master, S., and Greening S. (2008). British Society of Paediatric Dentistry: a policy document on consent and the use of physical intervention in the dental care of children. *International Journal of Paediatric Dentistry* **18** (Suppl.1), 39–46. (*This document provides guidance on ethical and legal aspects of the dental care of children in the UK.*)

Royal College of Paediatrics and Child Health: Ethics Advisory Committee (2000). Guidelines for the ethical conduct of medical research involving children. *Archives of Diseases in Childhood*, **82**: 177–82.

4

Management of pain and anxiety

M.T. Hosey, L. Lourenço-Matharu, and G.J. Roberts

Chapter contents

4.1 Introduction

Pain and anxiety are natural physiological and psychological responses. Pain is a direct response to an adverse stimulus that *has* occurred; anxiety is the unpleasant feeling, the worry that something unpleasant *might* occur. Pain and anxiety are often intertwined, especially in the dental setting. The best way to manage child dental anxiety is to avoid its occurrence in the first place through prevention of dental disease, good behaviour management, pain-free operative care, and treatment planning that is tailored to the needs and developmental stage of each individual child. These issues are detailed in the previous chapters. This chapter specifically focuses on pharmacological pain and anxiety control and explores the roles of conscious sedation and general anaesthesia (GA) as adjuncts to behaviour management.

A child's perception of pain is purely subjective and varies widely, particularly with age. Infants up to about 2 years of age are unable to distinguish between pressure and pain. Older children begin to have some understanding of 'hurt' and begin to distinguish it from pressure or 'a heavy push'. It is not always possible to identify which children are amenable to explanation and will respond by being cooperative when challenged with local anaesthesia (LA) and dental treatment in the form of drilling or extractions. Children over 10 years of age are much more likely to be able to think abstractly and participate more actively

in the decision to use LA, sedation, or GA. Indeed, as children enter their teenage years they are rapidly becoming more and more like adults and are able to determine more directly, sometimes aggressively, whether or not a particular method of pain control will be used. The response is further determined by the child's coping ability influenced by family values, level of general anxiety (trait), and intelligence.

There is a strong relationship between the perception of pain experienced and the degree of anxiety perceived by the patient. Painful procedures cause fear and anxiety; fear and anxiety intensify pain. This circle of cause and effect is central to the management of all patients. Good behaviour management reduces anxiety, which in turn reduces the perceived intensity of pain, which further reduces the experience of anxiety. (See Key Point 4.1.)

Key Point 4.1

Children's response to pain is influenced by age, memory of previous negative dental experience, and coping ability.

4.2 The use of analgesics to manage pain in children

A number of oral conditions, such as ulcers, teething, and pulpitis, can lead to children complaining of pain. Studies have shown that almost a quarter of 5-year-old preschool children have had a recent episode of dentally related pain. This can lead to the child being sent home from nursery or school, work time lost by parents, and visits to the dentist or doctor.

The management of the dental pain depends on the cause but usually involves some form of clinical intervention (e.g. a dressing). This operative management of toothache and the management of other dental emergencies are covered elsewhere in this text. However, sometimes the use of oral analgesics to achieve pain relief is required whilst the operative measures are taking effect. Children may need pain control for 'toothache' for a day or two before the removal of carious teeth. Additionally, analgesia is required postoperatively, usually after dento-alveolar surgery, and perioperatively during extractions under GA.

The use of analgesics should be viewed as a temporary solution whilst the causative factors are being brought under control (see

Box 4.1). The most commonly used analgesics for oral pain in children are also the familiar 'over-the-counter' medicines, namely paracetamol and non-steroidal anti-inflammatory drugs (NSAIDs). Therefore a prescription is not required. Most parents are already familiar with these preparations and their brand names.

Box 4.1 The general principles of analgesic management

1. Treat the cause of the pain.
2. Suggest measures to relieve the factors that may be making the situation worse (e.g. anxiety or lack of sleep, dehydration, hunger due to pain on eating).
3. Keep the analgesic simple—'over-the-counter' preparations will suffice.

Table 4.1 Over-the-counter analgesics

Analgesic	Age	Dose	Frequency	Preparations
Paracetamol	1–3 months	30–60mg	Every 8 hours	Dispersible tablets
	3–12 months	60–120mg	Every 4–6 hours	Oral suspension
	1–6 years	120–250mg	Every 4–6 hours	Dispersible tablets
	6–12 years	250–500mg	Every 4–6 hours	Oral suspension
NSAID (e.g. ibuprofen)	Children	1.2–1.8g	Daily in divided doses	Tablets (200, 400, and 600mg)
				Elixir
				Effervescent granules

The most common method of administration is by mouth. Small children and some recalcitrant adolescents refuse to take tablets, so liquid preparations are needed. Sugar-free preparations are readily available.

It should be remembered that the dose for children of different ages needs to be carefully estimated to avoid the risk of an overdose (dangerous) or an underdose (ineffective) (Table 4.1). The parents must be advised that all drugs must be stored in a safe place in a child-proof container. Bathroom cabinets or kitchen cabinets are the safest places as they are out of reach and out of sight of small children. Specific advice on prescribing for children can be obtained from a local pharmacist or the *British National Formulary* (*BNF*).

4.2.1 Paracetamol (Acetaminophen)

Paracetamol is a non-opiod analgesic. For children, it is available as an oral suspension (120/5mL or 250/5mL). It is also available as

tablets, soluble tablets, and suppositories. Overdosage can cause symptoms of nausea and vomiting. Single or repeated dosages totalling as little as 150mg/kg within 24 hours may cause liver damage, so parents should be advised to read instructions on the packet.

4.2.2 Non-steroidal anti-inflammatory drugs (Ibuprofen)

The most commonly prescribed drug in this category is ibuprofen. NSAIDs have the added advantage of being anti-inflammatory and therefore may be of benefit in pulpitis or when a child is pyrexic. Overdosage may cause nausea, vomiting, epigastric pain, and tinnitus. Ibuprofen should be avoided in asthmatics since it has been known to precipitate bronchoconstriction. NSAIDs are known to cause stomach ulceration, and so parents should be advised to avoid prolonged usage.

4.3 Pharmacological management of the anxious child

The different methods of anxiety control vary from simple behaviour management to full intubational GA in a hospital operating theatre. The majority of dental procedures on children can be carried out using a combination of behavioural management and local anaesthesia.

Children's behaviour can be characterized in four ways: (1) cooperative; (2) potentially cooperative; (3) lacking cooperative ability (precooperative); (4) uncooperative. Potentially cooperative children may manage a simple examination, but operative procedures, especially if these are carried out too early in the treatment plan, may be beyond their coping ability. An example of this is a child who readily accepts fissure sealants but who is upset at tooth extraction. Thoughtful treatment planning and good behaviour management will usually suffice for this group, especially if the child is asymptomatic and treatment can progress at an easy pace. However, when invasive treatment is unavoidable (maybe it is all that is required, e.g. orthodontic premolar extractions) or when an emergency situation arises, conscious sedation may be needed.

The pre-cooperative child is the very young child with whom communication cannot yet be established even though they may potentially cooperate later, when they are more mature. The uncooperative child is too anxious to cope with any procedure. Children with specific disabilities with whom cooperation in the usual manner may not ever be achieved also fall into this category. Both of these groups need a different approach, which may include conscious sedation or GA.

Children learn to be anxious by experience, through either a real traumatic event or what they perceive to be a traumatic event. This is why irregular dental attendees who first present with toothache and require an emergency operative intervention can be so traumatized by the event that they become dentally anxious. Although pharmacological management is an adjunct to, rather than a replacement for, the specific behavioural techniques that are employed, its use should be considered in an emergency and in potentially traumatic situations. This is known as 'prophylactic' sedation.

4.3.1 Children are different from adults

Children are different from adults and sedating them can be unpredictable. They are more likely to become hypoxic, i.e. low blood oxygen leading to low brain oxygen. The reason for caution when sedating children is related to child anatomy, physiology, drug response, and emotional development. Anatomically, children have large heads, tongues, tonsils, and adenoids. They also have a U-shaped larynx and narrow pharyx. They have a greater ratio of body surface area to body weight, a higher metabolic rate, and higher oxygen consumption. It is common for children to present with upper respiratory tract infections. Cardiac output in children is 30–50% higher than in adults, and the arterial blood pressure is lower. Children have smaller veins, which are often hidden under subcutaneous fat. They are emotionally and psychologically underdeveloped, which may result in the occurrence of dysphoria during and after sedation. (See Key Point 4.2.)

> **Key Point 4.2**
>
> Children are anatomically and physiologically different from adults. This results in them becoming hypoxic more easily.

4.3.2 Guidelines

According to the National Institute for Health and Clinical Excellence (NICE) guidelines (NICE 2010), sedation may be considered in children and young patients when a procedure is too frightening or too painful, or needs to be carried out in a child or young person who is ill or in pain or who has behavioural problems. Nitrous oxide inhalation sedation is the most common and also the safest sedative agent for use in children's dentistry and is considered to be the 'standard technique'.

In the UK, attitudes related to GA have changed since the Poswillo Report in 1990 (Department of Health 1990). This report included recommendations to discourage GA in favour of sedation. This resulted in a renewed interest in conscious sedation techniques and drugs for behavioural and anxiety control in children. In common with many European countries, 'deep sedation' is not recommended for paediatric

dental practice. These techniques are considered to be a form of GA, and as such further regulations and safeguards apply.

Dental treatment should only be carried out under GA when this is judged to be the most clinically appropriate method of pain and anxiety management. Children undergoing outpatient dental GA receive the same standard of preparation and assessment, including pre-admission, as children admitted for medical procedures. The Association of Paediatric Anaesthetists of Great Britain and Ireland (APAGBI), in collaboration with a wide range of stakeholders, has published guidelines to develop an evidence-based consensus on the care pathway from referral to discharge for children and young people who are considered for outpatient dental extractions under GA (APAGBI 2011).

4.3.3 Evidence

Numerous studies have been carried out worldwide to explore the use of pharmacological agents in paediatric dental management. Despite this, a Cochrane systematic review was unable to conclude which sedative drug is the most effective (Matharu and Ashley 2006). This was because the majority of studies, especially those carried out in the USA, used polypharmacy in conjunction with either 30% or 50% nitrous oxide, and many also used some form of physical restraint. Indeed, 19 different drugs or combinations of drugs and various modes of administration were reported. Therefore the choice of drug and method of sedation is largely determined by the culture, legal framework, professional ethics, and accepted definition of conscious sedation in any given country.

4.3.4 Medical status

The American Society of Anesthesiologists (ASA) classification (Table 4.2) provides an excellent guide to the appropriateness of the pharmacological management and the setting in which the patient should be treated (ASA 2006). In general, ASA I and ASA II patients are suitable for treatment in primary care settings and simple sedatives can be used. There are a wide variety of medical problems and medically compromised children are usually treated in hospital under the care of a team led by a paediatric dentistry consultant so that there is liaison with medical services and access to inpatient facilities if required.

4.4 Clinical decision-making

The decision as to whether a patient should be treated under GA, LA, or LA with sedation depends on a combination of factors, the most important of which are the age of the child, the degree of surgical trauma involved, the perceived anxiety and how the patient may respond (or has responded) to similar levels of surgical trauma, the complexity of the operative procedure, the number of quadrants involved, and the medical status of the child.

There are no hard and fast rules. Every procedure in every child must be assessed individually and the different elements considered

in collaboration with the parent and, where appropriate, the child (Box 4.2). For example, the younger the child, the greater is the likelihood of the need for GA. At the other end of the age range it is unlikely that a 15-year-old will need GA for simple orthodontic extractions, although this might be required for moderately complex surgery such as exposing and bonding an impacted canine. The degree of trauma involved is also another factor; a single extraction is most likely to be carried out under LA, whereas removal of the four first permanent molars is most likely to be carried out under

Table 4.2 ASA physical status classification

I	Normal healthy patient
II	Patient with mild systemic disease
III	Patient with severe systemic disease
IV	Patient with severe systemic disease that is a constant threat to life
V	Moribund patient who is not expected to survive without an operation
VI	Declared brain-dead patient whose organs are being removed for donor purpose

GA. Anxiety perceived as excessive, especially after an attempt at treatment under LA and sedation, might lead to simple treatment such as conservative dentistry being carried out under GA, usually involving endotracheal intubation. Serious medical problems (e.g. cystic fibrosis with its associated respiratory problems) would justify using sedation instead of GA even for more traumatic surgery, such as removal of impacted canines, but it would be appropriate to carry out this sedation in a hospital environment. The degree of intellectual and/or physical impairment in special needs or medically compromised children is also a factor to be considered.

The need for the use of LA is also a factor in determining the best management option. Sedated patients still need to have LA administered. It is important that usage, and especially the dosage, of LA is considered in the decision-making process. Readers are reminded that care must be taken to avoid overdosage in children. Therefore several visits may be needed to complete treatment if sedation is planned.

Box 4.2 Assessing suitability for sedation or GA

A thorough dental and medical assessment is required and should include the following:

- Anticipated dental treatment
- Current medical condition
- Specific surgical problems
- Weight
- Medical problems (associated with previous sedation or anaesthesia)
- Current and previous medication
- Allergies
- Physical status
- Airway patency
- Psychological status
- Developmental status.

4.4.1 The choice of pharmacological management

The choice of the most suitable pharmacological technique should be based on all the following factors:

- invasiveness of the proposed procedure
- level of sedation anticipated
- contraindications
- side-effects
- patient (or parent/carer) preference
- operator preference.

4.5 Conscious sedation: drugs and routes

The routes of administration of sedative drugs used in clinical paediatric dentistry are oral, inhalational, intravenous (IV), and transmucosal (e.g. nasal, rectal, and sublingual). Nitrous oxide inhalation sedation is considered to be the standard conscious sedation technique. Other drugs and routes are seldom used in the UK. Whilst there is considerable recent interest in the use of midazolam, a benzodiazepine, this is generally confined to paediatric dentistry specialist units rather than primary care settings. 'Advanced techniques' such as propofol target-controlled infusion pumps and patient-controlled sedation (PCS) require further research. (See Key Points 4.3.)

4.5.1 A definition of conscious sedation

Conscious sedation is a technique in which the use of a drug or drugs produces a state of depression of the central nervous system (CNS)

enabling treatment to be carried out, but during which verbal contact with the patient is maintained throughout the period of sedation. The drugs and techniques used to provide conscious sedation for dental treatment should carry a margin of safety wide enough to render loss of

Key Points 4.3

- The goal of conscious sedation is to use a pharmacological agent to augment behavioural management and to decrease anxiety levels while maintaining a responsive patient.
- In the UK, the recommendation is to use a single-drug technique for sedating children.
- Nitrous oxide inhalation sedation is the mainstay of paediatric dental sedation.

consciousness unlikely. The level of sedation must be such that the patient remains conscious, retains protective reflexes, and is able to understand and respond to commands.

The ideal qualities of a sedative agent are:

- both sedative and analgesic effects
- easy and acceptable method of administration
- easy titration
- minimal cardiovascular side-effects

- minimal respiratory side-effects
- rapid onset of action
- rapid recovery
- no accumulation in renal/hepatic dysfunction
- inactive metabolites
- inexpensive
- no interactions with other drugs.

4.6 Environment, facilities, and pre- and postoperative instructions

4.6.1 Environment

There should be a suitable child-friendly area where the child can be treated in a calm, peaceful setting without noise or interruption. When oral sedation is planned, a 'quiet room' is needed so that the child can sit quietly before the dental procedure. This is the place where the sedative is administered and the child monitored while sedation is taking effect.

Irrespective of the choice of sedative drug, all equipment must be checked to ensure that it is working correctly before the child enters the surgery. This includes the operating light, dental chair, three-in-one, dental headpieces, dental materials, instruments, and suction.

Sedated patients may hallucinate or misinterpret words and actions, so a chaperone must be present at all times to safeguard the operator–sedationist. Once treatment is complete the child must sit quietly until sufficiently recovered to be accompanied home. (See Key Points 4.4.)

Key Points 4.4

- Sedation needs to be carried out in a calm peaceful environment
- A checklist helps ensure that all facilities are in place before sedation is commenced.
- The dentist must be chaperoned at all times.
- The child must have an adult escort.

4.6.2 Facilities

The use of sedative drugs carries the risk of inadvertent loss of consciousness. Although the techniques are designed to reduce this risk to a minimum, it should always be borne in mind that every time a sedative is given to a patient there is a risk of an idiosyncratic reaction to the drug which may result in hypoxia or unexpected loss of consciousness.

4.6.3 Pre- and postoperative instructions

All instructions should be provided verbally and in writing in advance of the sedation visit and then confirmed at the time of sedation.

Fasting is not required prior to either nitrous oxide inhalation sedation or IV midazolam sedation. The '2–4–6' rule applies for oral sedation and GA. This is 2 hours fast for clear fluids, 4 hours fast for milk, and 6 hours fast for solids.

Preoperative information should also include any possible side-effects and requirements for postoperative care, since families need to plan the return home in advance. Suitable arrangements need to be in place for travel, to ensure that the child plays quietly at home, and that permission to be absent from school has been obtained. Further advice such as control of haemorrhage and avoidance of lip biting, together with instructions for oral hygiene measures, might also need to be included.

Psychologically, the child or young person should be involved in the treatment planning process and taught how to cope with the procedure. Probable sensations, such as pressure or numbness, should be explained. Instructions should also make it clear that a suitable escort must accompany the child home. The escort should be over 18 years old, able-bodied, and capable of ensuring that the postoperative instructions are followed.

4.7 Monitoring the sedated child

4.7.1 Alert clinical monitoring

Sedative drugs are CNS and respiratory depressants. As such, they can cause a variety of effects ranging from hypoxia to oversedation and GA.

For this reason, facilities and emergency training are necessary. It is important that dental surgeons working with children have a very clear

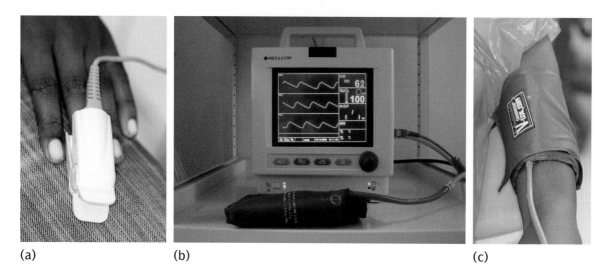

(a)   (b)   (c)

Figure 4.1 (a) Pulse oximeter finger clip. (b) Pulse oximeter and pressure cuff. (c) Blood pressure cuff.

idea of the clinical status of sedated patients so that unintended loss of consciousness can be avoided. Important clinical status indicators are:

- eyes open
- able to respond verbally to questions
- able to maintain an open mouth independently (this should preclude the use of a mouth prop)
- able to maintain a patent airway independently
- able to swallow
- healthy looking, well-perfused skin colour.

All these criteria are evidence of 'normality' in the sedated status. For this reason it is important not to let a child go to sleep in the dental chair while receiving treatment with sedation. Closed eyes may be a sign of sleep, oversedation, loss of consciousness, or cardiovascular collapse. The sedationist must continuously monitor, interpret, and be able to respond to any changes. Monitoring information should be clearly documented in the patient's record, and monitoring should continue until the child is fully recovered. This level of alert clinical monitoring is all that is required for nitrous oxide inhalation sedation.

4.7.2 Pulse oximeter and other monitors

A pulse oximeter is required in all forms of sedation, except when nitrous oxide is used as the single agent. The pulse oximeter is a non-invasive method of measuring arterial oxygen saturation using a sensor probe that is placed on the child's finger or ear lobe. It has a red light source to detect the relative difference in the absorption of light between saturated and desaturated haemoglobin (Figs 4.1(a) and 4.1(b)). The probe is prone to movement artefact, relative hypothermia, ambient light, and abnormal haemoglobinaemias, so false readings may occur. In room air, a child's normal oxygen saturation (Sao_2) is 97%. Adequate oxygenation of the tissues occurs above 95%, while oxygen saturations lower than this are considered hypoxaemic.

Blood pressure monitoring is a requirement for IV sedation (Fig. 4.1(c)). There is a minimal requirement for at least a baseline and postoperative blood pressure check when IV sedation is used. (See Key Points 4.5.)

Key Points 4.5

Monitoring a sedated child involves the following:

- Clinical monitoring—alertness, verbal contact, skin colour, response to stimulus, ability to keep mouth open, ability both to swallow and to maintain an independent airway, normal radial pulse.
- The use of a pulse oximeter (except for nitrous oxide inhalation sedation).

4.7.3 Protocols and checklists

Everyone providing sedation for children should follow national guidelines and recommendations. Each team carrying out sedation should follow a protocol for each technique and develop checklists to ensure that the necessary equipment, drugs, dental materials, and facilities are in place before sedation is commenced. In this way, a high clinical standard is maintained and the safety and security of both the child and the dental team are safeguarded.

4.7.4 Requirements for training

Conscious sedation must only be provided by those who are trained and experienced in both paediatric dental sedation and in the delivery of high-quality operative treatment. The sedationist must be skilled in assessment so that the most effective, safe, and appropriate treatment is planned for each child. Dentists delivering sedation should have documented up-to-date evidence of competency including the following:

- Satisfactory completion of a theoretical training course covering the principles of sedation practice.
- Documented evidence of practical experience in the sedation technique used, including details of:
  - sedation in children and young people performed under supervision
  - successful completion of assessments.

4.7.5 Management of unexpected loss of consciousness

On the rare occasions when the patient becomes unconscious the dentist and his/her staff should proceed according to the following routine:

1. Cease the operative procedure immediately.
2. Ensure that the mouth is cleared of all fluids by using high-volume suction.
3. Turn the patient on to his/her side in the 'recovery position'.
4. Consider the administration of 100% oxygen.
5. If IV sedation is being used, leave the Venflon (cannula) in place so that emergency drugs can be administered through it if required.
6. Consider monitoring pulse, blood pressure, and respiration. Be ready to start resuscitation.
7. The dentist should stay with the patient until full signs of being awake are present (eyes open, independent maintenance of the airways, and verbal contact).
8. Follow up the patient by review within 3 days.
9. Document the incident fully.
10. Inform the patient's general medical practitioner about the incident.

4.8 Nitrous oxide inhalation sedation

Nitrous oxide sedation is the technique of choice for the paediatric dental patient and can be used in primary care settings. It has an excellent safety record, is easy to deliver by titrating the level of nitrous oxide to the patient's needs, and has been shown to have a continued beneficial effect. It involves the inhalation of an oxygen–nitrous oxide gas mixture in relatively low concentrations, usually 20–50% nitrous oxide. The technique has been well described in the literature and was reported as early as 1889 when it was used during cavity preparation in Liverpool Dental School.

The operator is able to titrate the gas to match each individual patient, i.e. the operator gradually increases the concentration to the patient, observes the effect, and increases more (or sometimes decreases) the concentration as appropriate to obtain optimum sedation in the individual patient.

Although nitrous oxide inhalation sedation is very effective, it is important that it is used in combination with behavioural therapy and incorporated into the treatment plan. Failure frequently occurs when nitrous oxide is used as a 'one-off' and not as part of a planned course of treatment that incorporates behavioural management. Although nitrous oxide gas is well noted for its mild analgesic and anaesthetic properties, LA is still required for dental procedures.

Only a dedicated dental nitrous oxide delivery system should be used, since only this will allow titration of the dose. A nitrous oxide scavenging system is also needed to combat chronic environmental exposure to dental staff.

4.8.1 Pen picture of the child undergoing nitrous oxide inhalation sedation

The child has to be capable and willing to collaborate by breathing in and out through his/her nose. There isn't a precise lower age limit; it depends on the child's development and comprehension, but researchers predominantely report usage in school-age children (Fig. 4.2). It is also less successful in pre-cooperative or very anxious children or those who need repeat visits for extractions in multiple quadrants.

4.8.2 Indications and contraindications

- Indications:
  - mildly anxious children
  - unpleasant procedure
  - medically compromised
  - needle phobia
  - gag reflex
  - other sedation methods contraindicated
  - alternative to GA.
- Relative contraindications:
  - acute and chronic nasal obstruction
  - mouth breathers
  - first trimester of pregnancy
  - inability to cooperate or understand.
- Absolute contraindications:
  - inability to breathe nasally with open mouth
  - myasthenia gravis and multiple sclerosis
  - chronic obstructive airways disease
  - nasal or facial deformity
  - severe psychological disorders and nasal hood phobia.

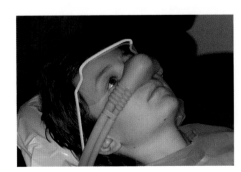

Figure 4.2 Inhalation sedation.

4.8.3 Equipment

Nitrous oxide inhalation sedation equipment is used solely for dentistry and is either wall-mounted or portable. The equipment enables the operator to deliver carefully titrated volumes and concentrations of gases to the child (Fig. 4.3). The dedicated dental equipment is completely different from that used in midwifery where premixed 50:50 gas tanks are common but do not allow titration of the dose.

The safety features of dedicated dental machines are as follows:

- The oxygen cylinder is black (turquoise in the USA).
- The nitrous oxide cylinder is blue.
- A pin index system ensures that the nitrous oxide cylinders cannot be inadvertently fixed to the oxygen delivery side.
- Nitrous oxide is cut out if the oxygen cylinder empties completely.
- No less than 30% oxygen can be given.

Before starting sedation the following checks must be made:

- 'in use' and 'full' gas cylinders correctly identified and labelled;
- oxygen fail-safe system confirmed to be working;
- reservoir bag, tubing, and nasal hoods checked for leakage;
- scavenging and venting system switched on;
- emergency equipment and drugs available;
- other equipment (e.g. radiography equipment and dental instruments) to hand so that the dental nurse does not need to leave the surgery.

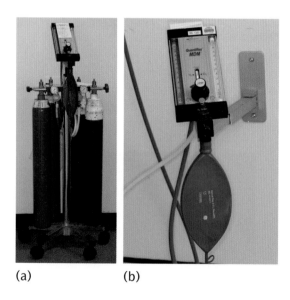

(a) (b)

Figure 4.3 (a) Portable nitrous oxide machine with gas tanks. (b) Wall-mounted nitrous oxide machine.

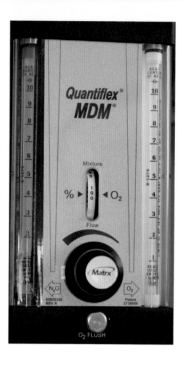

Figure 4.4 Titrating the dose.

4.8.4 The inhalation sedation technique

Inhalation sedation should be carried out with a calm, reassuring voice, using semi-hypnotic suggestion, and accompanied by distraction techniques. The patient should be encouraged to relax.

Steps in the technique

1. Carry out the safety checks.
2. Select the appropriate size of nasal mask.
3. Connect the scavenging pipe.
4. Set the mixture dial to 100% oxygen.
5. Settle the patient in the dental chair.
6. Turn the flow control to approximately 5L/min and allow the reservoir bag to fill with oxygen.
7. With the patient's help, position the nasal mask gently and comfortably but securely enough to avoid any leaks.
8. Begin to tell the child a 'story' that involves hypnotic suggestion.
9. Turn the flow control knob to the left until the flow rate of oxygen matches the patient's tidal volume. This can be monitored by watching the reservoir bag moving slightly inwards and outwards, which may take 15–20 seconds. A flow rate of 5–6L/min is usually comfortable for a child (Fig. 4.4).
10. Simultaneously, reassure the patient about the sensations that will be felt. Encourage the patient to concentrate on breathing gently through the nose. If the reservoir bag appears to be getting too empty, the oxygen flow should be increased until the flow rate matches the patient's respiratory rate.

11. Turn the mixture dial vertically to 90% oxygen (10% nitrous oxide). Wait for 60 seconds, continually encouraging and reassuring the child.

12. Turn the mixture dial to 80% oxygen (20% nitrous oxide). Wait for 60 seconds. Above this level the operator should exercise more caution and consider whether further increments should be only 5%. With experience, operators will be able to judge whether further increments are needed; the authors seldom need to use more than 30% nitrous oxide.

13. At the appropriate level of sedation, dental treatment can be started.

14. To bring about recovery turn the mixture dial to 100% oxygen and oxygenate the patient for 2 minutes before removing the nasal mask.

15. Turn the flow control to zero and switch off the machine.

16. The patient should breathe room air for a further 5 minutes before leaving the dental chair. The patient should be allowed to recover for a total period of 10 minutes before leaving the surgery.

An example of a story that includes hypnotic suggestion to encourage relaxation

I want you to imagine you are lying down on a very fluffy and soft white cloud. The ones that look like cotton. The sky is light blue, the sun is shining, and you feel nice and warm. If you pay attention you can hear the birds singing.

Take a nice breath through your nose and listen. That's good—in and out through your nose.

Can you hear them yet?

Take a nice breath—easy breath—in and out—through your nose, and listen.

The good thing about this lovely cloud is that when the wind blows you can go wherever you want to go. You must be feeling nice and floaty now, and your feet and hands are feeling heavy and sinking into the fluffy cloud.

Take a nice breath through your nose—in and out—can you smell the nice fresh air?

As the gentle wind blows your cloud across the sky your arms and legs are feeling heavy and you feel comfortable and relaxed. Can you count the birds (or stars) in the sky?

Take a nice e-a-s-y breath through your nose—in and out while you count them.

What a great cloud you have! . . . .

Signs of sedation
The overall demeanour of the patient will be relaxed and acquiescent. The signs of a sedated child are:

- reduced body and facial tension
- reduced frequency of blinking
- slowed responses
- laughing/giggling
- glazed eyes
- relaxed feet

- tingling in the fingers and toes (parasthesia)
- visual changes
- auditory changes
- feelings of lightness and/or heaviness
- feelings of temperature change
- floating or melting sensations
- dissociation
- day-dreaming
- change of mood
- engagement with hypnotic suggestion (story-telling).

4.8.5 Environmental pollution

There is concern about the effect of environmental pollution with nitrous oxide on dental staff. This includes potential damage to the reproductive, hepatic, renal, CNS, and haemopoietic systems. Regular use in an unventilated room can cause megaloblastic anaemia, distal renal tubule calcification, neuropathy, and problems with both conception and pregnancy. Control of Substances Hazardous to Health (COSHH) advice is that the exposure should not exceed 100 parts per

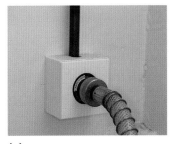

(a)

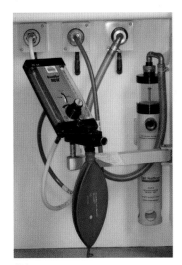

(b)

Figure 4.5 (a) Active scavenging. (b) Active scavenging and piped gases.

million (ppm)over a time-weighted average (TWA) of 8 hours (Health Services Advisory Committee 1995). There are two types of scavenging system for combating environmental exposure: passive and active. Active systems (Fig. 4.5) are best and those that incorporate a scavenging nasal mask (Fig. 4.6) are recommended. The patient should be encouraged to breathe in and out through the nose and not through the mouth. A rubber dam should be used whenever possible. The scavenging nasal mask should remain in place until recovery is complete.

4.8.6 Monitoring during inhalation sedation

Alert clinical monitoring is all that is necessary when using inhalation sedation.

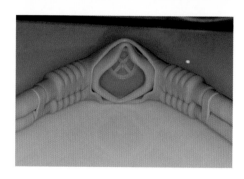

Figure 4.6 Scavenging nose piece.

4.9 Intravenous sedation

IV sedation usually involves the use of midazolam, a benzodiazepine. It intervenes in the mechanism of gamma-aminobutyric acid (GABA), a transmitter substance in the CNS. Midazolam has a variety of effects: it is an anticonvulsant, a muscle relaxant, and an anxiolytic, and has amnesic and sedative–hypnotic qualities. Therefore patients are unlikely to remember the treatment. Usage in adults is well reported, but in children it is confined to 'mature' adolescents.

4.9.1 Pen picture of the child undergoing intravenous midazolam sedation

Most researchers report usage in teenagers, those who are fully engaged with the treatment planning, and those who are willing to allow the placement of a needle. They may need extraction of a grossly carious permanent molar, extensive multiquadrant restorations, or dento-alveolar surgery. Needle phobics will be less likely to choose this option.

4.9.2 Indications and contraindications

- Indications:
  - emotionally mature adolescents
  - an unpleasant or complicated procedure
  - treatment too lengthy for GA
  - ASA I or II.
- Relative contraindications:
  - alcohol or narcotic dependency or known recreational drug use
  - impairment of renal function
  - impairment of hepatic function
  - high blood pressure (very rare in children)
  - lack of escort or presence of other children in addition to the patient.

- Absolute contraindications:
  - allergy to benzodiazepines
  - pregnancy and breastfeeding
  - psychiatric illness.
- Advantages:
  - titrated to patient's response
  - rapid onset
  - amnesia—will not remember the procedure
  - can be reversed by flumazenil in case of emergency.
- Disadvantages:
  - needle phobia—children's thin veins and subcutaneous fat
  - respiratory depression
  - disinhibition effects
  - longer postoperative recovery required
  - becauso of amnesia the patient may not learn to cope with future treatment.

4.9.3 Equipment

A disposable tray (Fig. 4.7) should be prepared with the following:

- midazolam ampoules 5mg/5mL
- cannulas—Y-can and Venflon
- 5/10mL syringes
- alcohol wipes
- midazolam syringe labels
- pulse oximeter
- tourniquet
- blood pressure recorder
- needles
- tape

- oxygen
- flumazenil 500 micrograms/5mL—reversal agent
- flumazenil syringe labels.

4.9.4 Intravenous midazolam technique

The standard regimen is to infuse midazolam slowly until the signs of satisfactory sedation are seen. This usually entails a loading dose followed by further increments as appropriate.

The technique requires the insertion of a Venflon or Y-Can needle that is allowed to remain *in situ* until the treatment for that visit is complete. The two most common sites of access are the antecubital fossa (Fig. 4.8) and the dorsum of the hand.

Record

- batch number and expiry date
- pre-sedation blood pressure
- time of administration
- dosage delivered
- oxygen saturation

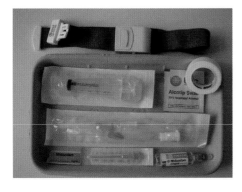

Figure 4.7 IV midazolam tray.

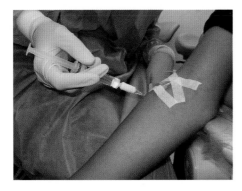

Figure 4.8 Titrating IV midazolam in the antecubital fossa.

- site of cannulation
- overall behaviour
- times that sedation started and finished
- post-sedation blood pressure
- time of discharge.

Steps in the technique

1. Topical skin anaesthetics such as EMLA® cream should be applied 60 minutes before cannulation (lasts 10–20 minutes) or Ametop® gel applied 30 minutes before cannulation (lasts 4–6 hours).
2. After preoperative checks are carried out, the child's blood pressure is taken and noted.
3. An ampule of midazolam 5mg dose in a 5 mL concentration should be carefully opened and withdrawn with a labelled 5mL syringe.
4. A tourniquet is used to reveal the vein, the skin is cleaned with an alcohol wipe, and cannulation is carried out using a Venflon or Y-Can, which should be fixed to the skin with tape. This may need lots of distraction and encouragement.
5. Attach the pulse oximeter clip to the patient's finger.
6. Give 1mL (1mg) of midazolam from the syringe over 30 seconds, always maintaining a conversation with the child.
7. Wait for 90 seconds and observe the effect.
8. Give increments of 0.5mL (0.5 mg) midazolam at 30-second intervals until adequate sedation is achieved.

Signs of sedation

This is best observed while engaging the patient in conversation. Their speech becomes slurred and their responses become slower, and the eyes often lose their focus. They should be responsive to commands at all times. In general, it is inappropriate to use a mouth prop since this makes it difficult to judge the level of sedation, although there are some occasions when an experienced operator may need to do so.

4.9.5 Monitoring during IV sedation

Continual alert clinical monitoring should be carried out by the clinician and sedation nurse. Baseline and postoperative blood pressure readings are recommended. A pulse oximeter must be used throughout.

4.9.6 Flumazenil reversal

In the unlikely event of the patient becoming oversedated, 500 micrograms/5mL flumazenil can be administered intravenously. Flumazenil antagonizes the action of midazolam, reversing the sedative, cardiovascular, and respiratory depressant effects. However, re-sedation can occur because the half-life is shorter than midazolam. Therefore the use of flumazenil is for rescue only and is not a routine part of the procedure.

4.10 Oral sedation

Drugs given orally have a variable absorption from the gastrointestinal tract. They can be affected by the rate of gastric clearance, the amount of food in the stomach, and even by the time of day. Therefore fasting is required. Oral dosages are determined by the body weight; therefore the child needs to be weighed in advance so that the dose of agent can be calculated. Some children spit the drug out, leaving the clinician uncertain about the exact dosage that was administered. To make it more acceptable, a flavoured drink may be added to the sedative (Fig. 4.9). A needleless syringe placed in the buccal pouch can also be helpful. The drug of choice for oral sedation is midazolam, although evidence is still relatively scant.

4.10.1 Oral midazolam conscious sedation

Midazolam is often used for oral sedation although, in common with many drugs used in children, it is not specifically licensed for oral administration. It is unpredictable in children, who can have paradoxical effects; for example, they can become hyperactive and disinhibited rather than sedated. This type of sedation is not usually carried out in primary care settings.

4.10.2 Pen picture of the child undergoing oral sedation using midazolam

This technique is usually used for younger patients, for example a pre-cooperative child who needs one or two primary incisors extracted following trauma. It can also be of value in a child who needs to undergo a simple extraction of an erupted supernumerary. The child is unlikely to remember the episode. Some sedationists confine usage to children under 30kg in weight since those who are heavier than this need such a high dose that the level of sedation becomes less predictable and paradoxical effects are more likely.

4.10.3 Indications and contraindications for oral midazolam

Oral midazolam is indicated in ASA I or II children, usually those under 30kg in weight, and for short procedures such as single tooth extraction. The contraindications are the same as for IV sedation.

4.10.4 Oral midazolam technique

The oral dose ranges from 0.3 to 0.7mg/kg. The maximum recommended dosage for oral midazolam sedation is 20mg (Fig. 4.10).

Record

- batch number and expiry date
- time of administration

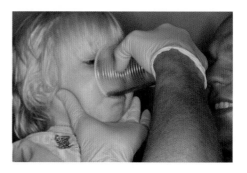

Figure 4.9 Giving a child oral midazolam.

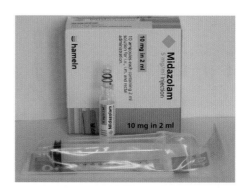

Figure 4.10 Oral midazolam.

- dosage delivered
- oxygen saturation and pulse rate before both commencement and discharge
- overall behaviour
- number of times that the sedative is administered
- time of discharge.

Steps in the technique

1. Encourage the child to go to the toilet before beginning the procedure.
2. Medical history and medication should be checked.
3. Weigh the child and calculate the dose.
4. Mix with flavoured juice.
5. Administer with help from the parent.
6. Place the child and parent in a quiet room while sedation is taking effect and monitor throughout.

Signs of sedation

The child will appear 'floppy' and in a dream-like trance. Speech becomes slurred and responses slower. They should be responsive to commands at all times. The child may move around and might appear upset.

4.10.5 Monitoring during oral sedation

Continual and alert clinical monitoring should be carried out by the clinician and the sedation nurse. This must be augmented by the use of a pulse oximeter.

4.10.6 Other drugs used for oral sedation

A number of different oral drugs are used worldwide. One of these is chloral hydrate, a sedative–hypnotic drug with weak analgesic properties. It is an alcohol and may cause nausea and vomiting due to gastric irritation. It depresses the blood pressure and the respiratory rate; myocardial depression and arrhythmia can also occur. Recently, there has been concern that there is a theoretical risk of carcinogenesis from the breakdown products. Chloral hydrate is often used in combination with hydroxyzine hydrochloride and promethazine hydrochloride since these have an antiemetic effect (helps prevent vomiting), and they are psychosedatives with an antihistaminic and antispasmodic effect. Common side-effects of hydroxyzine hydrochloride and promethazine hydrochloride are dry mouth, fever, and skin rash. They may be used alone or in combination with chloral hydrate. Ketamine is a powerful general anaesthetic agent which, in small dosages, can produce a state of dissociation while maintaining the protective reflexes. Side-effects of ketamine include hypertension, vivid hallucinations, physical movement, increased salivation, and risk of laryngospasm. It carries the additional risk of an increase in blood pressure and heart rate, and a fall in oxygen saturation, when used in combination with other sedatives.

Evidence to support the single use of hydroxyzine hydrochloride, promethazine hydrochloride, or ketamine for paediatric dental sedation is poor, and the 'deep sedation' that ensues is better classified as general anaesthesia.

4.11 General anaesthesia

The concept of 'being put completely to sleep' or having a general anaesthetic is attractive to many parents as they believe that there is no fear and no pain, and the treatment can be completed in one visit. The reality is that, for the vast majority of dental procedures, such a 'quick-fix' approach is inappropriate. The reasons for this are the inherent risk of a complication related to the GA, the limitations on the amount of treatment that can be performed in a constrained operating time, and that procedures are limited to those that can be completed under one general anaesthetic. A plan that involves multiple visits to complete treatment under GA is regarded as unacceptable. Moreover, many parents are unaware of the large number of staff and resources that are needed to carry out dental treatment safely under GA. These include the anaesthetist, the anaesthetic assistant, operating theatre nurses, recovery staff, and the dentist and dental nurse.

GA to enable dental treatment to be provided to children is an important pharmacological means of achieving pain control and behaviour management. As far as is possible, alternative methods should be considered and GA for some children remains an option of 'last resort'. The use of conscious sedation has contributed considerably to a reduction in the demand for GA, especially for extractions only (e.g. premolars for orthodontics) and where extraction is confined to a single quadrant.

4.11.1 What is general anaesthesia?

GA is a state of controlled unconsciousness during which you feel nothing and can be described as 'anaesthetized'. This is essential for some operations and may be used as an alternative to regional anaesthesia for others.

Anaesthetic drugs are injected into a vein, or anaesthetic gases are inhaled into the lungs, and they are then carried to the brain by the blood. They stop the brain recognizing messages coming from the nerves in the body. Anaesthetic unconsciousness is different from unconsciousness due to disease or injury, and is different from sleep. As the anaesthetic drugs wear off, consciousness starts to return. The most common type of GA service for children is known as 'day case'. This means that the child is not kept overnight in hospital, but goes home after normal bodily functions are restored (e.g. they can walk unaided, swallow, and go to the toilet). However, it takes approximately 2 days for cognition to return fully, even after a short general anaesthetic. Therefore postoperative care is needed during this recovery time (e.g. the child may need time away from school).

4.11.2 Risks associated with general anaesthesia

Major risks

Major risks are rare. The real risk of a serious outcome is probably less than one in 400 000, although it is not possible to estimate this properly because of the lack of contemporary, robust data. This figure is based on a joint publication from the Royal College of Anaesthetists and the Association of Anaesthetists of Great Britain and Ireland (RCoA–AAGBI 2008). The main concern of parents is that a child who has been anaesthetized will either not wake up again or wake up with brain damage. This is a real, but vanishingly small, risk that is associated with past times when GA for dental treatment in children was carried out in general dental surgeries. Nowadays, it is mandatory in the UK for all GA to be carried out in a hospital setting with immediate access or transfer to a paediatric critical care unit. The general anaesthetic must be administered by a consultant trained in paediatric aspects of GA. Indeed, the same safeguards, framework, and care pathway apply to children anaesthetized for dental treatment as they do to those undergoing GA for medical procedures. Despite this, dentists are obliged to point out to parents that there is a risk of a major adverse event.

Minor risks

The minor risks are common: approximately two-thirds of families report these the next day and a quarter still have complaints 7 days later. The families of the most anxious children are likely to report the most postoperative complications. Parents must also be alerted to these in advance of the procedure.

Common minor risks:

- pain
- headache
- sore nose
- sore throat
- nausea and vomiting
- upset
- greater anxiety about future dental treatment.

4.11.3 Indications for general anaesthesia

The justification for the choice of GA needs to be carefully thought out and discussed with the parents. This discussion must include (1) the pros and cons of alternative pharmacological measures such as conscious sedation, and (2) the operative dental procedures and how the choice of GA might affect the treatment plan. This is to ensure that the parents fully understand the treatment and the risks that are involved so that they can not only give informed consent but also fully support the child.

There are two indications for a GA for paediatric dentistry:

1. The child needs to be put completely to sleep because there is a belief that he/she is too young, too anxious, or too uncooperative to accept treatment by any other method of pain control. An example of this is a child with early childhood caries, especially when there are painful, unrestorable teeth in multiple quadrants.

2. The dental surgeon needs a guarantee of a completely still patient, usually because the planned dental procedure is complex and requires full 'cooperation' as the operation is surgically challenging. Complete stillness is required to ensure satisfactory operating conditions. An example of this is a child who needs the surgical removal of a supernumerary.

4.11.4 Referral

Once a primary care dentist has determined that dental treatment under GA is considered to be the most clinically appropriate method of management, they will normally refer the child to a local GA service provider. There is usually a local referral process, referral letter template, and guidance. The referral letter should clearly justify the need for the use of GA.

The assessment process at the GA service

The GA service provider is usually located in a hospital remote from the initial primary care clinic. The child patient will undergo two further assessments.

- Dental—to check and confirm the treatment plan. This will probably be undertaken by a specialist in paediatric dentistry.
- Medical—to determine fitness to undergo a general anaesthetic.

These may take place together at the same visit or on different days. Rarely, they may even take place on the same day as the GA. Local guidance and care pathways will vary.

The referring dentist needs to be familiar with the local set-up so that families can be prepared and warned not to fast the child needlessly. Families also need to be alerted to possible changes in the initial treatment plan based on more detailed investigation. Irrespective of the local referral protocol, a dental examination, including radiographs if appropriate, will be performed and options for the dental treatment, including LA, LA supplemented with conscious sedation, or GA, will be explained to the carer and child (where appropriate). The associated benefits and risks of each technique will also have to be discussed. Unless there is an urgent clinical need for treatment, this assessment is undertaken at a separate appointment from the GA visit. In this way, the family has an opportunity to change their mind or to prepare fully.

The role of the dental assessor at the GA service

The assessing dentist will probably be a specialist in paediatric dentistry or should at least be trained and experienced in the behavioural management of children. This expertise will include conscious sedation, particularly inhalational sedation. The dentist will also be conversant with the current evidence and guidelines on the management of caries in the primary and mixed dentition, and have experience of treating these children, especially under GA.

The specialist assessment includes psychological assessment, confirmation of the plan of treatment, preparation for the procedure including information sharing, fasting instructions, discharge planning, and postoperative pain management. This assessment requires time to allow the parent and child to arrive at a considered decision and to give informed consent.

The medical fitness check

This is commonly undertaken by a paediatric nurse or an anaesthetic nurse trained in GA perioperative care and recovery. The opinion of an appropriately trained and experienced anaesthetist is normally available, if required, and relevant medical case records should be provided.

4.11.5 Consent for dental treatment under GA

The primary care dentist makes the initial decision that a general anaesthetic is required and therefore takes the preliminary consent for both the dental treatment and GA. Thus the general dental practitioner (GDP) will be expected to have discussed the need for such a referral, the need for the proposed dental treatment, and the rationale behind the use of GA in favour of other alternatives. The referring dentist should make the family aware of the risks associated with this treatment. Nowadays, the referral will predominantly be to a hospital GA service provider or to a specialist paediatric dentistry unit. At this specialist assessment visit the first stage of the informed consent process will be finalized and documented.

The information leaflet should include:

- preoperative preparation including fasting;
- overview of the proposed treatment including benefits and minor and major risks;
- the general anaesthetic procedure;
- an adult escort should bring the child patient—no other child should accompany them;
- postoperative arrangements including the need for suitable transport home;
- postoperative care and pain control.

4.11.6 The general anaesthesia service, site, and facilities

All children who need a medical procedure, especially if this involves hospital admission, should be managed in a child-friendly setting. In addition, it is necessary to have space, facilities, equipment, and appropriately trained personnel if an emergency arises and resuscitation is required. Agreed protocols and appropriate communication links must be in place, both to summon additional assistance in an emergency situation and to ensure timely transfer to specialist anaesthetic and medical care such as a high-dependency or intensive care unit.

4.11.7 What is day surgery?

The term 'day surgery' is used to describe short-stay ambulatory care which does not involve the use of a hospital bed overnight. Many hospitals now incorporate their paediatric dental service within a day-case surgical service. Whatever the length of stay, children undergoing GA for dental treatment receive the same standard of care and have a similar pathway as those undergoing medical procedures. The facilities and organization of such services vary and can be affected by geographic location; for example, a healthy child from a rural area might have too far to travel and so will need to stay overnight.

4.11.8 The shared airway

The challenge for anaesthetists is that the operating dentist often encroaches upon the airway. In the anaesthetized supine child the head and neck need to be positioned carefully so that they are extended but not over-extended. The anaesthetist attempts to hold the mandible forward to maintain a patent airway. However, during dental treatment, especially extractions in the lower arch, the mandible easily falls backwards and the chin is tipped towards the chest. Therefore this is an area of clinical skill where collaboration is needed to ensure both an optimum airway and sufficient dental operative access.

4.11.9 Induction of GA

The objective is to ensure that sufficient anaesthetic enters the blood stream to enable controlled loss of consciousness. This is commonly achieved by the delivery of a gaseous mix of oxygen and nitrous oxide

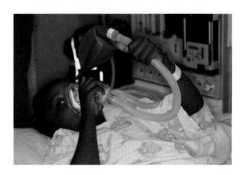

Figure 4.11 Anaesthetic induction.

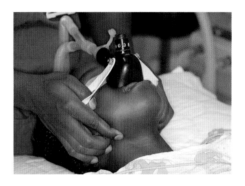

Figure 4.12 Placement of a nasal mask.

which carries an anaesthetic inhalation adjunct such as sevoflurane. The process of induction of GA is completely under the control of the anaesthetist and the operating room assistant. A simple gaseous induction with a nasal mask (Fig. 4.11) or a facial mask enables a relatively quick transition to the anaesthetic state. Another common approach is to use the IV route to administer an anaesthetic drug. This is usually the dorsum of the hand as it is easy to hold still and, once the drug is injected, anaesthesia occurs very quickly.

4.11.10 Types of GA for paediatric dentistry

GA for dentistry is largely broken down into 'short' procedures and 'long' procedures. This is a flexible concept, and variations on these two modes of GA revolve around the way in which the anaesthetist controls and protects the airway.

Short GA

Once the patient is fully asleep, the anaesthetist maintains a patent oro- and nasopharyngeal airway by appropriate elevation of the mandible and placement of a nasal mask in combination with a holding technique that allows the dental surgeon access to the mouth for short procedures (Fig. 4.12). A short procedure can be expected to last for 15 minutes or less. A refinement of this technique is to insert an airway into the nose so there is a patent airway as far back as the nasopharynx. The advantage of this approach is that simpler anaesthetic agents are needed. The disadvantage is the extra care required to maintain the patency of the shared airway.

During the procedure (usually only simple extractions) there is a risk of saliva, blood, or a tooth passing down the throat and into the lungs. To avoid this, the operating dental surgeon places an absorbent gauze pack over the fauces, behind the teeth, to act as a barrier, but care is needed to avoid interference with the airway.

A commonly used alternative to the nasal mask for airway control is a laryngeal mask. This involves a tube with a mask being passed through the mouth to rest over the epiglottis and vocal cords. A small dental pack is placed around it to provide additional protection to the airway. The advantage of this is that there is no need for the additional anaesthetic agents that paralyse the laryngeal muscles to allow insertion of an endotracheal tube.

The type of airway control used is the choice of the anaesthetist. The *single most important feature* of GA is that a satisfactory patent airway can be maintained throughout the whole of the surgical procedure. However, any airway tubes that pass through the mouth reduce the ease of access for operative procedures. Therefore, a joint decision is reached between the operating dentist and the anaesthetist based on the patient's airway anatomy and the planned dental procedure.

Long or extended GA

This is usually reserved for (1) surgical procedures such as the removal of buried and/or malpositioned teeth or the surgical exposure and bonding of an orthodontic bracket, and (2) extensive conservation and extraction. The latter is an effective way of providing care for children with learning disabilities or medical problems.

The dental operative time is approximately 45 minutes and so an endotracheal tube, or at least a laryngeal mask, is needed. The former is passed through either the mouth or the nose. An orotracheal tube has the advantage of a slightly easier intubation process for the anaesthetist and the avoidance of a sore nose for the child, but the disadvantage of taking up a considerable amount of space in the oral cavity making access for treatment more difficult. Whatever the form of airway, the operating dentist usually uses rubber dam if conservation is required, since this not only retracts the soft tissues but also isolates the teeth to improve both access and moisture control.

4.11.11 Monitoring procedures

Once anaesthesia is established, steps are taken to ensure patient safety. In effect, a constant supply of oxygen needs to be delivered to the brain. To this end, the blood needs to maintain good oxygen saturation and needs to be pumped from the lungs to the brain. A pulse oximeter is used to measure blood oxygenation. It is common for anaesthetists to place a blood pressure cuff for continuous recording of systolic and diastolic blood pressure and to use an electrocardiogram (ECG). Many GA machines also have the facility to monitor the carbon

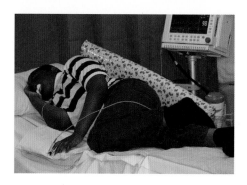

Figure 4.13 Recovery position after general anaesthesia.

dioxide output. Altogether, this array of monitoring helps the anaesthetist to provide safe and effective anaesthesia. In addition, even when an inhalational route is used, many anaesthetists insert an IV cannula for use if further IV drugs or fluids are needed or to deliver perioperative analgesia (e.g. IV NSAID).

4.11.12 Recovery

Once the treatment is complete, the dental surgeon must remove any material such as packs and mouth props placed in the mouth. The child is usually placed in the recovery position (Fig. 4.13) and the recovery is monitored, usually by an anaesthetic recovery nurse. Once the child is awake, the remaining recovery takes place back on the day surgery ward, still under close professional supervision but reunited with the parent. Once the child is fully recovered he/she is discharged home.

4.11.13 Follow-up

Arrangements need to be made for the child to be seen in a few weeks, usually with the GDP. This may be to check that postoperative healing has taken place and that preventive advice is being followed and reinforced. Occasionally, it may be necessary to remove sutures or packs.

4.11.14 Treatment planning for GA

The general principle to be applied is that greater effort needs to be made to ensure that the treatment procedure carried out has a reliable and clear prognostic outcome. This is so that the patient is not faced with the possibility of having a second general anaesthetic to repeat or undo failed dental treatment. The first consideration is to reduce the risk of a repeat general anaesthetic by suitably radical treatment—erring on the side of extractions. Sick children are a special case, where the emphasis on conservative dentistry and extractions varies from one medical problem to another. For example, the high level of extractions in cardiac cases or in an immune compromised child is to ensure that no potential focus of infection remains.

4.12 Summary

Pain and anxiety are often intertwined, especially in the dental setting. The best way to manage child dental anxiety is to avoid its occurrence in the first place through prevention of dental disease, good behaviour management, pain-free operative care, and treatment planning that is tailored to the needs and developmental stage of each individual child. Children's response to pain is influenced by age, memory of previous negative dental experience, and coping ability. The use of analgesics should be viewed as a temporary solution whilst the causative factors are being brought under control. The most commonly used analgesics for oral pain in children are also familiar 'over-the-counter' medicines, namely paracetamol and NSAIDs.

Conscious sedation may be considered in children when a procedure is too frightening, too painful, or needs to be carried out in a child or young person who is ill or in pain, or who has behavioural problems. Nitrous oxide inhalation sedation is the most common and the safest sedative agent for use in children's dentistry and is considered to be the 'standard technique'. The decision as to whether a patient should be treated under GA or LA, or LA with sedation, depends on a combination of factors, the most important of which are the age of the child, the degree of surgical trauma involved, the perceived anxiety and how the patient may (or has) responded to similar levels of surgical trauma, the complexity of the operative procedure, the number of quadrants involved, and the medical status.

When conscious sedation or GA is considered a thorough assessment is required. This includes psychological assessment, confirmation of the plan of treatment, together with preparation for the procedure including information sharing, fasting instructions if required, discharge planning, and postoperative pain management. The parent and child need time and information to consider the treatment options and to give informed consent.

4.13 Further reading

Atan, S., Ashley, P., Gilthorpe, M.S., Scheer, B., Mason, C., and Roberts, G. (2004). Morbidity following dental treatment of children under intubation general anaesthesia in a day-stay unit. *International Journal of Paediatric Dentistry*, **14**, 9–16.

Hosey, M.T. (2002). National Clinical Guideline. Managing anxious children: the use of conscious sedation in paediatric dentistry. *International Journal of Paediatric Dentistry*, **12**, 359–72 (revised 2009).

Hosey, M.T., Macpherson, L.M., Adair, P., Tochel, C., Burnside, G., and Pine, C. (2006). Dental anxiety, distress at induction and postoperative morbidity in children undergoing tooth extraction using general anaesthesia. *British Dental Journal*, **200**, 39–43.

Millar, K., Asbury, A.J., Bowman, A.W., Hosey, M.T., Musiello, A., and Welbury, R.R. (2006). The effects of brief sevoflurane–nitrous oxide anaesthesia upon children's postoperative cognition and behaviour. *Anaesthesia*, **61**, 541–7.

Nunn, J., Foster, M., Master, S., and Greening, S. (2008). British Society of Paediatric Dentistry: a policy document on consent and the use of physical intervention in the dental care of children. *International Journal of Paediatric Dentistry*, **18**, 39–46.

Wilson, K.E., Welbury, R.R., and Girdler, N.M. (2002). A randomized double blind crossover trial of oral midazolam for paediatric dental sedation. *Anaesthesia*, **57**, 860–7.

4.14 References

APAGBI (2011). *Guidelines for the management of children referred for dental extractions under general anaesthesia.* Available online at:
http://www.rcoa.ac.uk

ASA (2006). *Physical status classification system.* Available online at:
http://www.asahq.org/clinical/physicalstatus.htm

Department of Health (1990). *A conscious decision: a review of the use of general anaesthesia and conscious sedation in primary dental care.* Available online at:
http://www.dh.gov.uk/en/Publicationsandstatistics/Publications/PublicationsPolicyAndGuidance/DH_4074702

Health Services Advisory Committee (1995). *Anaesthetic agents: controlling exposure under COSHH.* HMSO, London.

Matharu, L. and Ashley, P.F. (2006). Sedation of anxious children undergoing dental treatment. *Cochrane Database of Systematic Reviews*, **1**, CD003877.

NICE (2010). *Sedation for diagnostic and therapeutic procedures in children and young people.* Available online at:
http://guidance.nice.org.uk/CG112

RCoA–AAGBI (2008). *Your child's general anaesthetic for dental treatment. Information for parents and guardians of children.* Available online at:
http://www.rcoa.ac.uk/system/files/PI_ycgadt.pdf

5

Local anaesthesia
for children

J.G. Meechan

Chapter contents

5.1 Introduction

This chapter considers the use of LA in children and describes methods of injection that should produce minimal discomfort. The complications and contraindications to the use of LA in children are also discussed. The major use of local anaesthetics is in providing operative pain control. However, it should not be forgotten that these drugs can be used as diagnostic tools and in the control of haemorrhage.

5.2 Surface anaesthesia

Surface anaesthesia can be achieved by physical or pharmacological methods (topical anaesthetics). One physical method employed in dentistry is the use of refrigeration. This employs the application of volatile liquids such as ethyl chloride. The latent heat of evaporation of this material reduces the temperature of the surface tissue and this produces anaesthesia. This method is rarely used in children as it is difficult to direct the stream of liquid accurately without contacting associated sensitive structures such as teeth. In addition, the general anaesthetic action of ethyl chloride should not be forgotten.

5.2.1 Intra-oral topical agents

The success of topical anaesthesia depends on the technique. Topical anaesthetic agents can anaesthetize a 2–3mm depth of surface tissue when used properly.

The following points should be noted when using intra-oral topical anaesthetics:

- the area of application should be dried;
- the anaesthetic should be applied over a limited area;
- the anaesthetic should be applied for sufficient time.

A number of different preparations varying in the active agent and in concentration are available for intra-oral use. In the UK the agents most commonly employed are lidocaine (lignocaine) and benzocaine. Topical anaesthetics are provided as sprays, solutions, creams, or ointments. Sprays are the least convenient as they are difficult to direct. Some sprays taste unpleasant and can lead to excess salivation if they inadvertently reach the tongue. In addition, unless a metered dose is delivered, the quantity of anaesthetic used is poorly controlled. It is important to limit the amount of topical anaesthetic used. The active agent is present in greater concentration in topical preparations than in local anaesthetic solutions and uptake from the mucosa is rapid. Systemic uptake is even quicker in damaged tissue. An effective method of application is to spread some cream on the end of a cotton bud (Fig. 5.1). All the conventional intra-oral topical anaesthetics are equally effective when used on reflected mucosa. The length of time of administration is crucial for the success of topical anaesthetics. Applications of around 15

seconds or so are useless. An application time of around 5 minutes is recommended. It is important that topical anaesthetics are given sufficient time to achieve their effect. This is especially important in children as this may be their initial experience of intra-oral pain-control techniques. If the first method encountered is unsuccessful, confidence in the operator and his armamentarium will not be established.

Although the main use of topical anaesthetics is as a pre-injection treatment, these agents have been used as the sole means of anaesthesia for some intra-oral procedures in children including the extraction of mobile primary teeth.

5.2.2 Topical anaesthetics that will anaesthetize skin

EMLA® cream (a 5% Eutectic Mixture of the Local Anaesthetic agents prilocaine and lidocaine) was the first topical anaesthetic to be shown to produce effective surface anaesthesia of intact skin. Therefore it is a useful adjunct to the provision of general anaesthesia in children as it allows pain-free venepuncture.

When used on skin it has to be applied for about an hour so it is only appropriate for elective general anaesthetics. Clinical trials of the intra-oral use of EMLA® have shown it to be more effective than conventional local anaesthetics when applied to attached gingiva such as the hard palate and interdental papillae. It appears to be no more effective than conventional topical agents when applied to reflected mucosa. Intra-oral use of EMLA® is not recommended by its manufacturers. An intra-oral formulation of the combination of prilocaine and lidocaine (Oraqix®) is available as a topical treatment for application to gingival pockets to help reduce the discomfort of dental scaling.

Tetracaine (amethocaine) 4% gel is another topical anaesthetic for skin that may be useful prior to venepuncture. Unlike EMLA,® which consists of amide local anaesthetics, tetracaine is an ester.

5.2.3 Controlled-release devices

The use of topically active agents incorporated into materials that adhere to mucosa and allow the slow release of the agent is a potential growth area in the field of local anaesthetic delivery. Such techniques might prove to be of value in paediatric dentistry. Clinical studies investigating the release of lidocaine from intra-oral patches have shown some promise. The use of anaesthetic agents incorporated into liposomes is also promising in this regard.

5.2.4 Jet injectors

Jet injectors belong in a category somewhere between topical anaesthesia and LA but will be discussed here for completeness. These devices allow anaesthesia of the surface to a depth of over 1cm without the use of a needle. They deliver a jet of solution through the tissue under high pressure (Fig. 5.2).

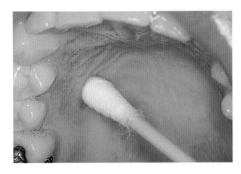

Figure 5.1 Use of a cotton bud to apply a topical anaesthetic over a limited area

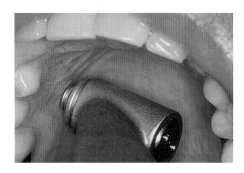

Figure 5.2 The jet injector. (Reproduced from *Dental Update* (ISSN 0305-5000), by permission of George Warman Publications (UK) Ltd.)

Conventional local anaesthetic solutions are used in specialized syringes and have been successful in children with bleeding diatheses where deep injection is contraindicated. Jet injection has been used both as the sole means of achieving LA and prior to conventional techniques. This method of anaesthesia has been used alone and in combination with sedation to allow the pain-free extraction of primary teeth. The use of jet injection is not widespread for a number of reasons. Expensive equipment is required, soft tissue damage can be produced if a careless technique is employed, and the specialized syringes can be frightening to children because of both their appearance and the sound produced during anaesthetic delivery. In addition, the unpleasant taste of the anaesthetic solution, which can accompany the use of this technique, can be off-putting.

Although no needle is employed, the technique is not painless. Indeed, careful use of conventional techniques has been shown to produce similar levels of discomfort to jet injection.

5.3 Non-pharmacological pain control

A number of non-pharmacological methods for reducing the pain of operative dentistry are now available, including the use of electrical stimulation and radio waves. Hypnosis also belongs in this category. There are reports that some lasers have the potential to produce LA as dental hard tissue can be removed painlessly by such devices. The use of refrigeration techniques was mentioned above.

Electroanalgesia or transcutaneous electrical nerve stimulation (TENS) has been shown to be effective in providing anaesthesia for restorative procedures in children aged 3–12 years. The technique has also been used to provide pain control during the extraction of primary teeth and as a 'deep topical agent' to reduce the pain of local anaesthetic injections. In younger children the level of stimulation is controlled by the operator. Children over 10 years of age can understand the method sufficiently well to be able to control the level of stimulus themselves.

TENS blocks transmission of the acute pain of dental operative procedures because large myelinated nerve fibres (such as those responding to touch) have a lower threshold for electrical stimulation than smaller unmyelinated pain fibres. Stimulation of these fibres by the current from the TENS machine closes the 'gate' to central transmission of the signal from the pain fibres. This is quite different from the use of TENS in the treatment of chronic pain, where the release of endogenous painkillers such as β-endorphins is stimulated. In addition, if the patient operates the machine, the feeling of control may help allay anxiety and aid in pain management.

Non-pharmacological methods of pain control offer two advantages. First, systemic toxicity will not occur and, second, the soft tissue anaesthesia resolves at the end of the procedure. This reduces the chances of self-inflicted trauma.

Hypnosis can be used as an adjunct to LA in children by decreasing the pulse rate and the incidence of crying. It appears to be most effective in young children.

5.4 Local anaesthetic solutions

A number of local anaesthetic solutions that can provide anaesthesia lasting from 10 minutes to over 6 hours are now available. There are few, if any, indications for the use of the so-called long-acting agents in children. The gold standard for many years has been lidocaine with adrenaline (epinephrine). Unless there is a true allergy to lidocaine, 2% lidocaine with 1:80 000 adrenaline is the solution of choice in the UK for most techniques. One technique where lidocaine with adrenaline is not the best choice is infiltration anaesthesia in the mandible. A number of studies in adults have shown that 4% articaine with adrenaline is superior for this method in both the molar and incisor regions. 'Short-acting' agents such as plain lidocaine are seldom employed as the sole agent because, although pulpal anaesthesia may be short-lived, soft tissue effects can still last for over an hour or so. More importantly, the efficacy of plain solutions is much less than those containing a vasoconstrictor.

5.5 Techniques of local anaesthesia

There are no techniques of local anaesthetic administration that are unique to children; however, modifications to standard methods are sometimes required. As far as positioning the child is concerned, the upper body should be around 30° to the vertical. Sitting upright can increase the chances of fainting, whilst at the other extreme (fully supine) the child may feel ill at ease. When there is a choice of sites at which to administer the first local anaesthetic injection, the primary maxillary molar area should be chosen. This is the region that is most easily anaesthetized with the least discomfort.

5.5.1 Infiltration anaesthesia

Infiltration anaesthesia is the method of choice in the maxilla. The infiltration of 0.5–1.0mL of local anaesthetic is sufficient for pulpal anaesthesia of most teeth in children. The objective is to deposit local anaesthetic solution as close as possible to the apex of the tooth of interest; however, the presence of bone prevents direct apposition. As the apices of most teeth are closer to the buccal side, a buccal approach is employed and the needle is directed towards the apex after insertion through reflected mucosa. Direct deposition under the periosteum can be painful; therefore a compromise is made and the solution is delivered supra-periosteally. The one area where pulpal anaesthesia can prove troublesome in the child's maxilla is the upper first permanent molar region where the proximity of the zygomatic buttress can inhibit the spread of solution to the apical area (see below).

The use of buccal infiltration anaesthesia in the mandible will often produce pulpal anaesthesia of the primary teeth. However, it may be unreliable when operating on the permanent dentition, with the exception of the lower incisor teeth (Jaber *et al.* 2010). An alternative form of anaesthesia in the posterior mandible is inferior alveolar nerve block anaesthesia.

5.5.2 Regional block anaesthesia

Inferior alveolar and lingual nerve blocks

Administration of the inferior alveolar and lingual nerve block is easier to perform successfully in children than in adults. A common fault in adults is placing the needle too low on the ramus of the mandible with deposition of solution inferior to the mandibular foramen. In children, the mandibular foramen is low relative to the occlusal plane (Fig. 5.3), and it is difficult to place the needle inferior to this site if it is introduced parallel to the occlusal plane. Thus in children it is easier to ensure that the solution is deposited around the nerve before it enters the mandibular canal.

The technique of administration is identical to that used in adults and is best performed with the child's mouth fully open. The direct approach (introducing the needle from the primary molars of the opposite side) is recommended as less needle movement is required after tissue penetration with this method compared with the indirect technique. The operator's non-dominant hand supports the mandible with the thumb intra-orally in the retromolar region of the mandible. The index or middle finger is placed extra-orally at the posterior border of the ramus at the same height as the thumb. The needle is advanced from the primary molar region of the opposite side with the syringe held parallel to the mandibular occlusal plane. The needle is inserted through mucosa in the mandibular retromolar region lateral to the pterygomandibular raphe midway between the raphe and the anterior border of the ascending ramus of the mandible, aiming for a point halfway between the operator's thumb and index finger. The height of

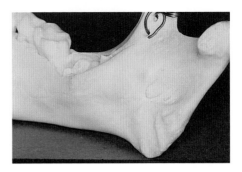

Figure 5.3 The mandibular foramen is below the occlusal plane in children. (Reproduced from *Dental Update* (ISSN 0305-5000), by permission of George Warman Publications (UK) Ltd.)

insertion is about 5mm above the mandibular occlusal plane, although in young children entry at the height of the occlusal plane should also be successful. The needle should be advanced until the medial border of the mandible is reached. In young children bone will be reached after about 15mm and thus a 25mm needle can be used; however, in older children a long (35mm) needle should be employed as penetration up to 25mm may be required. Once bone has been touched, the needle is withdrawn slightly until it is supra-periosteal, aspiration is performed, and 1.5mL of solution is deposited. The lingual nerve is blocked by withdrawing the needle halfway, aspirating again, and depositing most of the remaining solution at this point. The final contents of the cartridge are expelled as the needle is withdrawn through the tissues. A common fault is to contact bone only a few millimetres following insertion. In most children this will lead to unsuccessful anaesthesia. This usually occurs because the angle of entry is too obtuse. If this happens, the needle should not be completely withdrawn but pulled back a couple of millimetres and then advanced parallel to the ramus for about 1cm with the barrel of the syringe over the mandibular teeth of the same side. The body of the syringe is then repositioned across the primary molars or premolars on the opposite side and advanced towards the medial border of the ramus.

Long buccal and mental and incisive nerve blocks

The long buccal injection usually equates to a buccal infiltration in children. The mental and incisive nerve block is readily administered in children as the orientation of the mental foramen is such that it faces forward rather than posteriorly as in adults (Fig. 5.4). Thus it is easier for solution to diffuse through the foramen when approached from an anterior direction. The needle is advanced in the buccal sulcus and directed towards the region between the first and second primary molar apices. Blockade of transmission in the mental nerve provides excellent soft tissue anaesthesia. Flow of solution through the mental foramen to the incisive nerve (which supplies the dental pulps) can produce anaesthesia of the premolar teeth and occasionally the first molar. The efficacy is not as good in the anterior teeth compared with the premolars following mental and incisive nerve block.

The pulps of the lower incisor teeth may not be satisfactorily anaesthetized by inferior alveolar nerve or mental and incisive nerve block

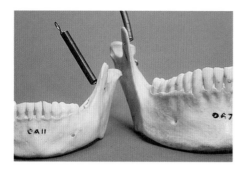

Figure 5.4 The mental foramen faces anteriorly in children (left) compared with posteriorly in adults. (Reproduced from *Dental Update* (ISSN 0305-5000), by permission of George Warman Publications (UK) Ltd.)

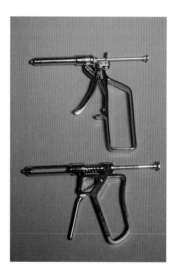

Figure 5.5 Intra-ligamentary injection in a child.

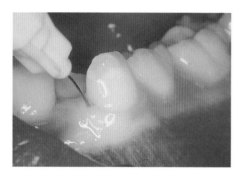

Figure 5.6 Pistol-grip intra-ligamentary syringes.

injections because of cross-over supply from the contralateral inferior alveolar nerve. A buccal infiltration adjacent to the tooth of interest is sufficient to deal with this supply. The method of choice for pulpal anaesthesia in the permanent lower incisors is a combination of buccal and lingual infiltrations.

Maxillary block techniques

Regional block techniques are seldom required in a child's maxilla. Greater palatine and nasopalatine nerve blocks are avoided by infiltrating local anaesthetic solution through already anaesthetized buccal papillae and 'chasing' the anaesthetic through to the palatal mucosa (see below). This technique is equally effective in anaesthetizing lingual gingivae in the lower jaw if infiltration or mental and incisive nerve block techniques have been used (obviously it is not needed if a lingual block has been administered with an inferior alveolar nerve block injection).

The effects of an infra-orbital block are often achieved by infiltration anaesthesia in the canine/maxillary first primary molar region in young children.

5.5.3 Intra-ligamentary anaesthesia

Intra-ligamentary or periodontal ligament (PDL) anaesthesia is a very effective technique in children (Fig. 5.5). This is a method of intra-osseous injection with local anaesthetic reaching the cancellous space in the bone via the periodontal ligament. This method allows the use of small amounts of local anaesthetic solution; the recommended dose per root is 0.2mL. The technique is significantly more successful when a vasoconstrictor-containing solution is employed, although pulpal anaesthesia is not the result of ischaemia. The anaesthetic of choice is 2% lidocaine with 1:80 000 adrenaline. Sensible dose limitations must be used, as entry into the circulation of intra-osseously administered drugs is as rapid as by the IV route.

The technique involves inserting a 30 gauge needle at an angle of approximately 30° to the long axis of the tooth into the gingival sulcus at the mesiobuccal aspect of each root and advancing the needle until firm resistance is met. It would seem sensible to have the bevel facing the bone when the solution is being expelled; however, it has never been demonstrated that the direction in which the bevel faces affects the efficacy of the technique. The needle will not advance far down the ligament as a 30 gauge needle is many times wider than a healthy periodontal ligament. It normally remains wedged at the alveolar crest. The solution is then injected under firm controlled pressure until 0.2mL has been delivered. The application of the appropriate pressure is easier with specialized syringes (Figs 5.6 and 5.7), but the technique is equally effective with conventional dental syringes. Another advantage of specialized syringes is that they deliver a set dose per depression of the trigger (0.06–0.2mL depending on the design). When using conventional syringes for intra-ligamentary injections the recommended dose of 0.2mL for each root can be visualized as it is approximately the volume of the rubber plunger in the cartridge. It is important not to inject too quickly; about 15 seconds per depression of the specialized syringe lever is needed. Also, it is best to wait for about 5 seconds after the injection before withdrawing the needle. This allows the expressed solution to diffuse through the bone; otherwise it escapes via the gingival sulcus into the mouth.

Intra-ligamentary anaesthesia reduces, but does not completely eliminate, the soft tissue anaesthesia that accompanies regional

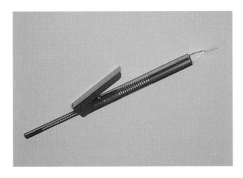

Figure 5.7 A pen-grip intra-ligamentary syringe. This is a less aggressive looking instrument than the pistol-grip type and is preferred for children

block anaesthesia in the mandible. This should help reduce the occurrence of self-mutilation of the lip and tongue. Intra-ligamentary anaesthesia is often mistakenly considered a 'one-tooth' anaesthetic. Adjacent teeth may exhibit anaesthesia, and care must be taken if this method is being used as a diagnostic tool in the location of a painful tooth. There are few indications for the use of the PDL technique in the maxilla because reliable pain-free anaesthesia should be possible in all regions of the upper jaw using infiltration techniques. In the maxilla, intra-ligamentary anaesthesia is best considered as a supplementary method of achieving pain control if conventional techniques have failed. The technique can be invaluable in the posterior mandible and can eliminate the need for uncomfortable regional block injections.

5.6 Pain-free local anaesthesia

The administration of pain-free LA depends on a number of factors that are within the control of the operator. These factors relate to equipment, materials, and techniques.

5.6.1 Equipment

All components of the local anaesthetic delivery system can contribute to the discomfort of the injection. Needles should be sharp. This means that a fresh needle should be used for each penetration as even passage through soft tissue can blunt needles. The gauge of the needles used in dentistry has been shown to have very little impact on injection discomfort, although there is some evidence that the use of the narrowest gauge (30 gauge) may reduce crying in children during inferior alveolar nerve blocks compared with the use of wider needles (Ram *et al.* 2007), and therefore the finest available gauge should be used. A narrow gauge does not interfere with the ability to aspirate blood, but it should be noted that narrow needles are more likely to penetrate blood vessels than their wider counterparts. The choice of syringe used for conventional local anaesthetic injections in children must allow aspiration both before and during injection. There is evidence that inadvertent intravascular injection is more likely to occur in younger patients. Positive aspirate incidences of 20% of inferior alveolar nerve block injections in the 7- to 12-year age group have been reported. One aspect of local anaesthetic delivery that can contribute to discomfort is the speed of injection. The use of computerized delivery systems permits very slow delivery of solution (Fig. 5.8). This is particularly useful when injecting into tissue of low compliance such as the palatal mucosa and periodontal ligament. When using conventional syringes the choice of anaesthetic cartridge can also contribute to the discomfort experienced during injection. The type of cartridge used should allow depression of the rubber bung at a constant rate with a constant force. Cartridges that produce a juddering action should not be employed.

5.6.2 Materials

In the past, heating the contents of local anaesthetic cartridges to body temperature prior to injection has been advised. There is no sound basis for this recommendation. There is ample evidence to suggest that patients cannot differentiate between local anaesthetics at room and body temperature. Indeed, storage of cartridges at higher temperatures can be detrimental to the solution as this can increase the chances of bacterial contamination, decrease the activity of adrenaline in the solution as a result of increased oxidation, and finally decrease the pH of the solution (see below). Cartridges stored in a refrigerator should be allowed to reach room temperature before use. The pH of the injected solution may affect the discomfort of the injection. Local anaesthetic solutions vary in their pHs, with those containing vasoconstrictors having lower values. For example, 2% plain lidocaine has pH 6.8 compared with pH 3.2 for 2% lidocaine with 1:80 000 adrenaline. Thus if minimal sensation is to be produced, it may be worthwhile using a small dose of a plain solution as an initial

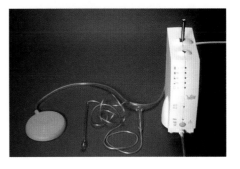

Figure 5.8 The Wand computerized injection system, which permits slow delivery of solution.

injection before using a vasoconstrictor-containing solution as the definitive local anaesthetic.

5.6.3 Techniques

Posterior maxillary buccal infiltrations

Assuming that the proper materials and equipment have been chosen, the following technique can be used to reduce the discomfort of buccal infiltration injections in the maxilla posterior to the canine.

1. Dry the mucosa and apply a topical anaesthetic for 5 minutes.

2. Wipe off excess topical anaesthetic.

3. Stretch the mucosa.

4. Distract the patient (stretching the mucosa and gentle pressure on the lip between finger and thumb can achieve this).

5. Insert the needle—if bone is contacted, withdraw slightly.

6. Aspirate; if positive, reposition the needle without withdrawing from the mucosa and when negative proceed.

7. Inject 0.5–1.0 mL supra-periosteally very slowly (15–30 seconds or via a computerized system).

Anterior maxillary buccal infiltrations

Injection into the anterior aspect of the maxilla can be uncomfortable if some preparatory steps are not taken. Using the method described in steps 1–6 above, deposit about 0.2mL of local anaesthetic painlessly in the first primary molar buccal sulcus on the side to be treated (Fig. 5.9). The next injection is placed anteriorly to this a minute later when soft tissue anaesthesia has spread radially from the initial injection site, and further 0.2mL increments are placed in the anterior aspect of the already anaesthetized area until the tooth of interest is reached. The buccal infiltration of 0.5–1.0mL can now be delivered painlessly through the soft tissue which is already anaesthetized.

Palatal anaesthesia

Injection directly into the palatal mucosa is painful. In some individuals the deposition of the solution close to a cotton-wool bud coated with topical anaesthetic and applied with firm pressure may reduce

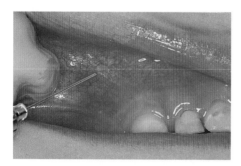

Figure 5.9 Buccal infiltration injection in the upper primary molar region. (Reproduced from *Dental Update* (ISSN 0305-5000), by permission of George Warman Publications (UK) Ltd).

discomfort, especially when the pressure on the bud is increased simultaneously with needle insertion and the child is warned of this pressure increase (Fig. 5.10). As mentioned earlier, conventional topical anaesthetics are not very effective on the attached mucosa of the hard palate and this method is not universally successful. The use of computerized delivery systems may reduce injection pain during palatal injections. A method of reducing the discomfort of palatal injections when using conventional syringes is to approach the palatal mucosa via already anaesthetized buccal interdental papillae. This is most readily achieved using an ultra-short (12mm) 30-gauge needle which is inserted into the base of the interdental papilla at an angle of approximately 90° to the surface. The needle is advanced palatally while injecting local anaesthetic into the papilla. This is performed through both distal and mesial papillae. Blanching should be seen around the palatal gingival margin (Figs 5.11–5.13). With practice this technique can be used without the needle breaching the palatal mucosal surface, which prevents the unpleasant-tasting solution inadvertently appearing in the mouth. This method usually provides sufficient anaesthesia for extractions. However, it can be supplemented by a painless gingival sulcus injection on the palatal side.

Mandibular anaesthesia

Inferior alveolar nerve block injections can be uncomfortable and infiltration anaesthesia may not be successful in the posterior permanent dentition. Alternatively, intra-ligamental (PDL) injections may be employed to anaesthetize the posterior mandibular teeth. This technique is not very successful in the lower permanent incisors. This is the result of a paucity of perforations in the cribriform plate of the lower incisor sockets. As mentioned above, infiltration anaesthesia is the method of choice for the incisor teeth. Lingual anaesthesia can be obtained by chasing through the buccal papillae as described for palatal injections above.

Studies in adults have suggested that PDL techniques are less unpleasant than conventional methods, but many children find delivery of anaesthetic solution via the PDL uncomfortable. The discomfort can be overcome by using the following methods. The mesial buccal papilla can be treated with topical anaesthetic applied with pressure. While pressure is still being applied, a papillary injection is administered followed by the intra-ligamental injection.

As conventional topical local anaesthetics are not very effective on attached gingiva, this method is not successful with all children. Alternatively, a small-dose buccal infiltration is given apical to the tooth (this can be given as one depression of the PDL syringe). This is followed by a papillary injection, which should now be painless, and finally by the intra-ligamental injection (Figs 5.14–5.16).

Lingual gingival anaesthesia is obtained via the PDL by directing the needle through the interdental space (Fig. 5.17).

The techniques described should produce minimal discomfort during local anaesthetic administration in children. When these methods are combined with relative analgesia the production of injection pain is even less likely to arise. When pain-free reliable LA is achieved in children confidence is gained by both the child and the operator, and a sound basis for a satisfactory professional relationship is established. This means that many of the treatments traditionally performed under GA (such as multiple-quadrant extractions and minor oral surgery) can readily be performed in the conscious sedated child.

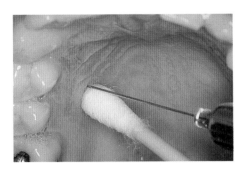

Figure 5.10 Use of pressure and topical anaesthesia to lessen the discomfort of a palatal injection. (Reproduced from *Dental Update* (ISSN 0305-5000), by permission of George Warman Publications (UK) Ltd.)

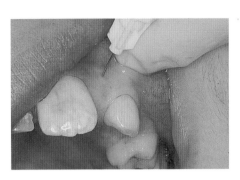

Figure 5.13 It is simple to advance towards the palate when the teeth are spaced (Reproduced from *Dental Update* (ISSN 0305-5000), by permission of George Warman Publications (UK) Ltd.)

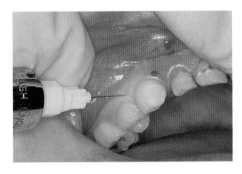

Figure 5.11 Advancing local anaesthetic towards the palate via the buccal papilla. (Reproduced from *Dental Update* (ISSN 0305-5000), by permission of George Warman Publications (UK) Ltd.)

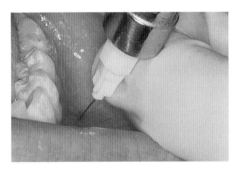

Figure 5.14 Small-dose buccal infiltration in the lower premolar region for removal of a lower second molar.

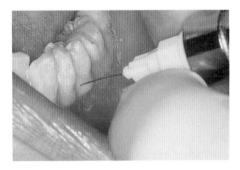

Figure 5.15 Papillary injection after buccal infiltration.

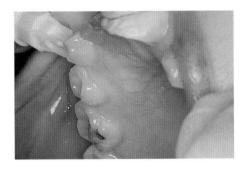

Figure 5.12 Palatal view of Fig. 5.11 showing blanching of the palate. (Reproduced from *Dental Update* (ISSN 0305-5000), by permission of George Warman Publications (UK) Ltd.)

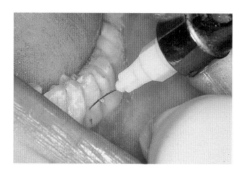

Figure 5.16 Intra-ligamentary injection after papillary injection

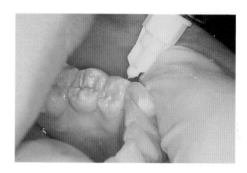

Figure 5.17 Lingual view showing blanching of the lingual gingiva.

5.7 Complications of local anaesthesia

Complications can be classified as generalized and localized, and divided into early and late.

5.7.1 Generalized complications

Psychogenic

The most common psychogenic complication of LA is fainting. The chances of this happening are reduced by sympathetic management and administration of the anaesthetic to children in the semi-supine position.

Allergy

Allergy to local anaesthetics is a very rare occurrence, especially to the amide group to which most of the commonly used dental anaesthetics (such as lidocaine, prilocaine, mepivacaine, and articaine) belong. The only members of the ester group of local anaesthetics routinely used in the UK are benzocaine and tetracaine (amethocaine), which are available as topical anaesthetic preparations.

Allergy can manifest in a variety of forms, ranging from a minor localized reaction to the medical emergency of anaphylactic shock. If there is any suggestion that a child is allergic to a local anaesthetic they should be referred for allergy testing to the local dermatology or clinical pharmacology department. Such testing will confirm or refute the diagnosis, and in addition should determine which alternative local anaesthetic can be used safely on the child. The majority of referrals prove to have no local anaesthetic allergy.

Children who are allergic to latex merit consideration as this material is included in the rubber plungers of some cartridges. When treating such a child it is imperative to use a latex-free cartridge. Details of which cartridges are latex-free can be obtained from the manufacturers.

Toxicity

Overdosage of local anaesthetics leading to toxicity is rarely a problem in adults but can occur in children. Children over 6 months of age absorb local anaesthetics more rapidly than adults; however, this is balanced by the fact that children have a relatively larger volume of distribution and elimination is also rapid because of a relatively large liver. Nevertheless, doses which are well below toxic levels in adults can produce problems in children, and fatalities attributable to dental local anaesthetic overdose have been reported. As with all drugs, dosages should be related to body weight. The maximum dose of lidocaine is 4.4mg/kg. This is an easy dose to remember if one notes that the largest 2% (i.e. 20mg/mL) lidocaine anaesthetic cartridges available in the UK are 2.2mL, which means they contain 44mg of lidocaine. Thus a safe maximum dose is one-tenth of the largest cartridge available per kilogram. If the tenth of a cartridge per kilogram rule is adhered to, overdose will not occur. When it is noted that a typical 5-year-old weighs 20kg it is easy to see that overdose can easily occur unless care is exercised. The use of vasoconstrictor-containing local anaesthetics for definitive LA is recommended in children, as agents such as adrenaline might reduce the entry of local anaesthetic agents into the circulation. In addition, as vasoconstrictor-containing solutions are more effective, the need for multiple repeat injections is reduced.

Cardiovascular effects

Cardiovascular effects caused by the injection of a dental local anaesthetic solution are the result of the combined action of the anaesthetic agent and the vasoconstrictor. Local anaesthetics affect the cardiovascular system by their direct action on cardiac tissue and the peripheral vasculature. They also act indirectly via inhibition of the autonomic nerves that regulate cardiac and peripheral vascular function. Most local anaesthetic agents will decrease cardiac excitability, and indeed lidocaine is used in the treatment of cardiac arrhythmias. Both vasoconstrictors commonly used in the UK, namely adrenaline and felypressin, can influence cardiovascular function. In addition to the beneficial effect of peripheral vasoconstriction on surgical procedures, adrenaline has both direct and indirect effects on the heart. The doses used in clinical dentistry will increase cardiac output, although this is unlikely to be hazardous in healthy children (Meechan *et al.* 2001). Felypressin at high doses causes coronary artery vasoconstriction, but the plasma levels that produce this are unlikely to be achieved during clinical dentistry.

CNS effects

The fact that local anaesthetic agents influence activity in nerves other than peripheral sensory nerves is obvious to any practitioner who has inadvertently paralysed the peripheral branches of the motor facial nerve during an inferior alveolar nerve block injection. Similarly, the CNS is not immune to the effects of local anaesthetic agents. Indeed, plasma concentrations of local anaesthetics that are incapable of influencing peripheral nerve function can profoundly affect the CNS. At low doses the effect is excitatory as CNS inhibitory fibres are blocked; at high doses the effect is depressant and can lead to unconsciousness and respiratory arrest. Fatalities due to local anaesthetic overdose in children are generally the result of central nervous tissue depression.

Methaemoglobinaemia

Some local anaesthetics cause specific adverse reactions when given in overdose. Prilocaine causes cyanosis due to methaemoglobinaemia. In methaemoglobinaemia the ferrous iron of normal haemoglobin is converted to the ferric form, which cannot combine with oxygen.

Treatment of toxicity

The best treatment of toxicity is prevention. Prevention is aided by:

- aspiration
- slow injection
- dose limitation.

When a toxic reaction occurs, the procedure is as follows:

1. Stop the dental treatment.
2. Provide basic life support.
3. Call for medical assistance.
4. Protect the patient from injury.
5. Monitor vital signs.

Drug interactions

Specialist advice from the appropriate physician should be requested in the treatment of children on significant long-term drug therapy. Apparently innocuous drug combinations can interact and cause significant problems in children. For example, an episode of methaemoglobinaemia has been reported in a 3-month-old child following the application of EMLA®. It was concluded in this case that prilocaine (in EMLA®) had interacted with a sulfonamide (which can also produce methaemoglobinaemia) that the child was already receiving.

Infection

The introduction of agents capable of producing a generalized infection, such as human immunodeficiency virus (HIV) infection and hepatitis, is a complication that should not occur when appropriate cross-infection control measures are employed.

5.7.2 Early localized complications

Pain

Pain resulting from local anaesthetic injections can occur at the time of the injection as a result of the needle penetrating the mucosa, too rapid an injection, or injection into an inappropriate site. The sites at which injection may be painful include intra-epithelial, sub-periosteal, into the nerve trunk, and intravascular. An intra-epithelial injection is uncomfortable because at the start of the injection the solution does not disperse and this causes the tissues to balloon out. Sub-periosteal injections may produce pain both at the time of injection and postoperatively. The initial pain is due to injection into a confined space, with the delivery of solution causing the periosteum to be stripped from the bone.

Direct contact of the nerve trunk by the needle produces a sensation similar to an electric shock and immediate anaesthesia. This is most likely to occur in the lingual and inferior alveolar nerves during inferior alveolar nerve blocks. Unfortunately, this complication is more common with experienced operators as it represents good location of the needle. When it does occur the solution should not be injected at that point but delivered after the needle has been moved slightly, thus avoiding an intraneural injection. If the needle does contact the nerve, the patient and parent should be warned that anaesthesia of the nerve may be prolonged. Altered sensation may last up to a few weeks in some cases.

Intravascular injection

Accidental intravascular injections can occur in children if aspiration is not performed. Intravascular injections can cause local pain if the vessel penetrated is an artery and arterial spasm occurs. Intravenous injections can produce systemic effects such as tachycardia and palpitations. Intra-arterial injections are much rarer than intravenous injections; however, the consequences of an intra-arterial injection can be alarming. Such effects range from local pain and cutaneous blanching (Fig. 5.18) to severe intracranial problems. The reported rare cases of hemiplegia following local anaesthetic injections can be accounted for by rapid intra-arterial injection. This can produce sufficient intracranial blood levels of the local anaesthetic to cause central nervous tissue depression.

Failure of local anaesthesia

The inability to complete the prescribed treatment because of failure of the local anaesthetic can be the result of a number of causes, including anatomy, pathology, and operator technique. Anatomical causes of failed LA can result from either bony anatomy or accessory innervation. Bony anatomy can inhibit the diffusion of a solution to the apical region when infiltration techniques are used. This can occur in children in the upper first permanent molar region as the result of a low zygomatic buttress. To overcome this problem the anaesthetic is infiltrated both mesially and distally to the upper first molar/zygomatic buttress region.

Accessory innervation may also produce failed LA. In the upper molar region this may be the consequence of pulpal supply from the

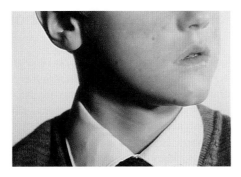

Figure 5.18 Blanching of the cheek after an intra-arterial injection in a child

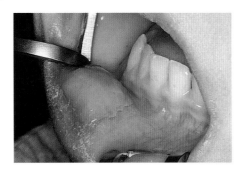

Figure 5.19 Self-inflicted trauma following an inferior dental block injection. (Reproduced from *Dental Update* (ISSN 0305-5000), by permission of George Warman Publications (UK) Ltd.)

greater palatine nerves, which can be blocked by supplementary palatal anaesthesia. In the mandible, accessory supply from the mylohyoid, auriculotemporal, and cervical nerves will not be blocked by inferior alveolar, lingual, and long buccal nerve blocks and may require supplementary injections. The most common area of accessory supply occurs near the midline, where bilateral supply often necessitates supplemental injections when regional block techniques are employed. The presence of acute infection interferes with the action of local anaesthetics. This is partly because the reduction in tissue pH decreases the number of un-ionized local anaesthetic molecules, which in turn inhibits their diffusion through lipid to the site of action (the number of ionized versus un-ionized molecules is governed by the pH and pKa of the agent). More importantly, nerve endings stimulated by the presence of acute infection are hyperalgesic. Regional block and intra-ligamental methods of LA depend on technique, and failure of these forms of LA is often the result of operator error. This cause of failure becomes less common with experience. Infiltration anaesthesia is a very simple method that is readily mastered by novices. When this injection fails, reasons other than operator technique should be sought.

Motor nerve paralysis

Paralysis of the facial nerve can occur following deposition of local anaesthetic solution within the substance of the parotid gland because of

malpositioning of the needle during inferior alveolar nerve block injections. The terminal branches of the facial nerve run through the parotid gland and will be paralysed by the anaesthetic agent. The most dramatic manifestation of this complication is the loss of ability to close the eyelids on the affected side. An eye-patch should be provided until the paralysis wears off. This side-effect is probably more common in adults—the anatomy of the child's mandible is such that inability to palpate the medial aspect of the mandible with the needle successfully is uncommon. Although paralysis of the eyelid is most often due to faulty technique during inferior alveolar nerve block anaesthesia, it can also result from the use of excessive amounts of solution in the maxillary buccal sulcus.

Interference with special senses

There have been reports of interference with vision and hearing after the intra-oral injection of local anaesthetics. Such occurrences most probably result from accidental intra-arterial injections.

Haematoma formation

Penetration of a blood vessel can occur during local anaesthetic administration. However, haematoma formation is rarely a problem unless it occurs in muscle following inferior alveolar nerve block techniques when it may lead to trismus (see below).

5.7.3 Late localized complications

Self-inflicted trauma

Self-inflicted trauma may occur after local anaesthetic injections in children. It may follow regional techniques in the mandible and infiltration anaesthesia in the maxilla. The most common site is the lower lip (Fig. 5.19), but the tongue and upper lip can also be affected. Significant soft tissue loss has been reported in some cases (Akram *et al.* 2008). It can be prevented by adequate explanation to the patient and parent by the clinician. The use of periodontal ligament techniques may reduce the frequency of this complication. However, it must be stressed that soft tissue anaesthesia is not completely avoided with this method in all cases.

Oral ulceration

Occasionally children will develop oral ulceration a few days after local anaesthetic injections. This is usually the result of trauma initiating an aphthous ulcer. On rare occasions, needle trauma may activate a latent form of herpes simplex.

Long-lasting anaesthesia

As mentioned above, long-lasting anaesthesia can result from direct trauma to a nerve trunk from the needle or injection of solution into the nerve. This may occur after regional block techniques, but it is a rare complication.

Trismus

Trismus may follow inferior alveolar nerve block injections and is usually the result of bleeding within muscle following penetration of a blood vessel by the needle. Injection of a solution directly into muscle tissue may also result in trismus. The condition is self-resolving, although it may take a few weeks before normal opening is restored.

Infection

Localized infection due to the introduction of bacteria at the injection site is a complication that is rarely encountered.

Developmental defects

Local anaesthetic agents are cytotoxic to the cells of the enamel organ. It is possible that the incorporation of these agents into the developing tooth-germ could cause developmental defects. There is experimental evidence that such defects can arise following intra-ligamental injections in primary teeth in animal models. Such occurrences in humans have not been reported. In addition to the cytotoxic effects of the anaesthetic agent, it is possible that physical damage caused by the needle to permanent successors could result from the over-enthusiastic use of intra-ligamentary anaesthesia in the primary dentition.

5.8 Contraindications to local anaesthesia

In certain children some local anaesthetic materials will be contraindicated; in others specific techniques are not advised.

5.8.1 General

Immaturity

Very young children are not suited to treatment under LA as they will not provide the degree of cooperation required for completion of treatment. A child who cannot differentiate between painful and non-painful stimuli (such as pressure) is unsuitable for treatment under LA.

Mental or physical handicap

Local anaesthesia is contraindicated where the degree of handicap prevents cooperation.

Treatment factors

Certain factors related to the proposed treatment may contraindicate the use of LA. These factors include duration and access. Prolonged treatment sessions, especially if some discomfort may be produced such as during surgical procedures, cannot satisfactorily be completed under LA. It is unreasonable to expect a child to cooperate for more than 30–40 minutes under such circumstances even when sedated. Similarly, where access proves difficult or uncomfortable (e.g. during biopsies of the posterior part of the tongue or soft palate), satisfactory cooperation may be impossible under LA.

Acute infection

As mentioned above, acute infection reduces the efficacy of local anaesthetic solutions.

5.8.2 Specific agents

Allergy

Allergy to a specific agent or group of agents is an absolute contraindication to the use of that local anaesthetic. Cartridges containing latex must be avoided in those who are allergic to this material.

Medical conditions

Some medical conditions present relative contraindications to the use of some agents. For example, in liver disease the dose of amide local anaesthetics should be reduced. Ester local anaesthetics should be avoided in children who have a deficiency of the enzyme pseudocholinesterase.

Poor blood supply

The use of vasoconstrictor-containing local anaesthetic solutions should be avoided in areas where the blood supply has been compromised, for example after therapeutic irradiation.

5.8.3 Specific techniques

Bleeding diatheses

Injection into deep tissues should be avoided in patients with bleeding diatheses such as haemophilia. Inferior alveolar nerve block techniques should not be used unless appropriate prophylaxis has been provided (e.g. Factor VIII for those with haemophilia). This can be overcome by the use of intra-ligamentary injections in the mandible for restorative dentistry in such patients.

Incomplete root formation

The use of intra-ligamental techniques for restorative procedures on permanent teeth with poorly formed roots could lead to avulsion of the tooth if inappropriate force is applied during the injection.

Trismus

Trismus will preclude the usual direct approach to the inferior alveolar nerve block.

Epilepsy

As seizure disorders can be triggered by pulsing stimuli (such as pulses of light), it is perhaps unwise to use electro-analgesia in children with epilepsy.

5.9 Summary

1 Surface anaesthesia is best achieved with a topical agent on a cotton bud applied to dry mucosa for 5 minutes.

2 Buccal infiltration anaesthesia is successful in the maxilla.

3 Regional block anaesthesia is successful in the mandible.

4 Intra-ligamentary anaesthesia is successful in children. This method may be the first choice in the posterior mandible and a supplementary technique in the maxilla.

5 Pain-free LA in the maxilla is possible with buccal infiltration and by anaesthetizing the palate via the buccal papillae.

6 In the mandible, intra-ligamental techniques can be used to avoid the discomfort of regional block injections.

7 Complications of LA are reduced by careful technique and sensible dose limitations.

8 Contraindications to LA may be related to certain agents or specific techniques.

5.10 Further reading

Malamed, S.F. (2004). *Handbook of local anesthesia* (5th edn). Mosby, St Louis. (*An excellent reference book.*)

Meechan, J.G. (2010). *Practical dental local anaesthesia* (2nd edn). Quintessence, London. (*A practical guide to the administration of local anaesthesia.*)

Moore, P.A. (1992). Preventing local anesthesia toxicity. *Journal of the American Dental Association*, **123**, 60–4. (*A salutary case report of a paediatric local anaesthetic fatality.*)

5.11 References

Akram, A., Kerr, R.M.F., and McLennan, A.S. (2008) Amputation of lower left lip following dental local anaesthetic. *Oral Surgery*, **1**, 111–13.

Jaber, A., Whitworth, J.M., Corbett, I.P., Al-Baqshi, B., Kanaa, M.D., and Meechan, J.G. (2010). The efficacy of infiltration anaesthesia for adult mandibular incisors: a randomized double-blind cross-over trial comparing articaine and lidocaine buccal and buccal plus lingual infiltrations. *British Dental Journal*, **209**, E16.

Meechan, J.G., Cole, B., and Welbury, R.R. (2001). The influence of two different dental local anaesthetic solutions on the haemodynamic responses of children undergoing restorative dentistry: a randomised, single-blind, split-mouth study. *British Dental Journal*, **190**, 502–4.

Ram, D., Hermida, B.L., and Amir, E. (2007). Reaction of children to dental injection with 27- or 30-gauge needles. *International Journal of Paediatric Dentistry*, **17**, 383–7.

6

Diagnosis and prevention of dental caries

C. Deery and K.J. Toumba

Chapter contents

6.1 Development of dental caries *85*

6.2 The epidemiology of dental caries *88*

6.3 Caries detection and diagnosis *90*

6.4 Prevention of dental caries *92*

6.4.1 Plaque control and toothbrushing *92*

6.4.2 Nutrition and diet in caries control *93*

6.1 Development of dental caries

Almost all research on the process of dental caries supports the chemo-parasitic theory proposed by W.D. Miller in 1890. This is now more commonly known as the acidogenic theory of caries aetiology. The main features of the caries process are as follows.

1. Fermentation of carbohydrate to organic acids by micro-organisms in plaque on the tooth surface;

2. Rapid acid formation, which lowers the pH at the enamel surface below the level (the critical pH) at which enamel will dissolve;

3. When carbohydrate is no longer available to the plaque micro-organisms, the pH within plaque will rise because of the outward diffusion of acids and their metabolism and neutralization in plaque, so that remineralization of enamel can occur;

4. Dental caries progresses only when demineralization is greater than remineralization. The realization that demineralization and remineralization are in equilibrium is key to understanding the dynamics of the carious lesion and its prevention.

One of the interesting features of an early carious lesion of the enamel is that the lesion is subsurface, i.e. most of the mineral loss occurs beneath a relatively intact enamel surface. This contrasts strongly with the histological appearance of enamel after a clean tooth surface has been exposed to acid, where the surface is etched and there is no subsurface lesion. This dissolution of the surface of enamel, or etching, is a feature of enamel erosion caused, among other things, by dietary acids. The explanation for the intact surface layer in enamel caries seems to lie in diffusion dynamics: the layer of dental plaque on the tooth surface acts as a partial barrier to diffusion. Further erosion occurs at much lower pH values (pH <4) than caries.

Dental plaque forms on uncleaned tooth surfaces and is readily apparent if toothbrushing is stopped for 2–3 days. Contrary to popular opinion, plaque does not consist of food debris; 70% is comprised of micro-organisms—about 100 million organisms per milligram of plaque. When plaque is young cocci predominate, but as plaque ages the proportions of filamentous organisms and veillonellae increase. Diet influences the composition of the plaque flora considerably, with *Mutans* streptococci much more numerous when the diet is rich in sugar and other carbohydrates. These organisms are particularly good at metabolizing sugars to acids.

Knowledge of the dental caries process increased considerably with the development of pH electrodes, particularly microelectrodes which could be inserted into plaque before, during, and after the ingestion of various foods. The pioneer in this area of research was Robert Stephan, and the plot of plaque pH against time (Fig. 6.1) has become known as the Stephan curve. Within 2–3 minutes of eating sugar or rinsing with a sugar solution, plaque pH falls from an average of about 6.8 to near pH 5, and takes about 40 minutes to return to its original value. Demineralization of the enamel occurs below pH 5.5, which is known as the critical pH.

The clinical appearance of these early lesions is now well recognized (Figs 6.2–6.5). They appear as a white area that coincides with the distribution of plaque. This might be around the gingival margin, as in Fig. 6.2, or between the teeth, as in Fig. 6.3. A histological section through a lesion such as that shown in Fig. 6.3 would look like Fig. 6.4 and a microradiograph would look like Fig. 6.5—the subsurface body of the lesion and surface zone can be seen clearly in both. If the process of dental caries continues, support for the surface layer will become so weak that it will crumble like an eggshell, creating a cavity. Once a cavity is formed, the process of dental caries continues in a more sheltered environment, and the protein matrix of enamel and then dentine is removed by proteolytic enzymes produced by plaque organisms.

The progression of caries is traditionally described as enamel caries progressing through to the amelodentine junction at which the enamel breaks down and a cavity forms. However, it is now understood that the process is not this simple and cavitation can occur at an earlier stage (the enamel cavity) and frequently at a much later stage when the caries has progressed significantly into dentine. Figure 6.6 shows the labial surface of a maxillary canine with a variety of stages of carious lesion ranging from white spot enamel caries to dentine cavity.

The ability of early carious lesions ('pre-cavitation carious lesions') to remineralize is now well understood. Periods of demineralization are interspersed with periods of remineralization, and the outcome—health or disease—is the result of a push in one direction or the other on this

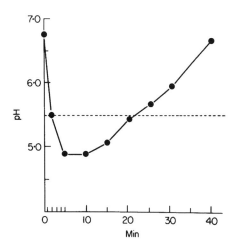

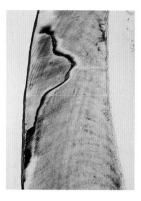

Figure 6.3 Clinical appearance of a pre-cavitation carious lesion on the mesial surface of a maxillary first molar tooth (brown spot lesion).

Figure 6.1 Plot of the pH of dental plaque against time. This is commonly known as a Stephan curve. The curve was produced by rinsing with a 10% glucose solution. The dotted line represents a typical pH value below which enamel will dissolve (the critical pH). (Reproduced with permission from Jenkins 1978.)

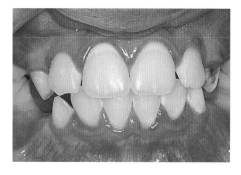

Figure 6.2 Clinical appearance of pre-cavitation carious lesions on the buccal surfaces of maxillary incisor teeth (white spot lesion).

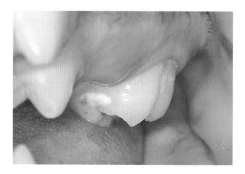

Figure 6.4 Longitudinal ground section through a carious lesion of the type shown in Fig. 6.3 examined in water by polarized light (magnification: 50×). (Reproduced from Soames and Southam, *Oral Pathology*, by permission of Oxford University Press.)

dynamic equilibrium. The shorter the time during which plaque-covered teeth are exposed to acid attack and the longer the time remineralization can occur, the greater is the opportunity for a carious lesion to heal. Satisfactory healing of the carious lesion can only occur if the surface layer is unbroken, and this is why the 'pre-cavitation' stage in the process of dental caries is so relevant to preventive dentistry. Once the surface has been broken and a cavity has formed, it is usually necessary to restore the tooth surface with a filling. The carious process is driven by the plaque on the surface and therefore it is possible to arrest the caries by effective removal of plaque even after cavitation has occurred. However, the lost tissue cannot be replaced.

The first stage of dental caries to be visible is the 'white spot' pre-cavitation lesion stage. This can occur within a few weeks if conditions are favourable for its development. However, in the general population it commonly takes 2–4 years for caries to progress through enamel into dentine at approximal sites.

The most important of the natural defences against dental caries is saliva. If salivary flow is impaired, dental caries can progress very rapidly. Saliva has many functions, which are listed in Table 6.1. The presence of food in the mouth is a powerful stimulus to salivation, with strong-tasting acid foods being the best stimulants. Saliva not only physically removes dietary substrates and acids produced by plaque from the mouth, but also has a most important role in buffering the pH in saliva and within plaque. Fast-flowing saliva is alkaline, reaching pH values of 7.5–8.0, and is vitally important in raising the pH of dental plaque previously lowered by exposure to sugar and carbohydrates. Because teeth consist largely of calcium and phosphate, the concentration of calcium and phosphate in saliva and plaque is thought to be important in determining the progression or regression of caries. Also, it is well known that fluoride aids the remineralization process. Although it may seem sensible to try to maximize the availability of calcium, phosphate, and fluoride in the environs of the tooth, in practice fluoride is much the most important. (See Key Points 6.1.)

Key Points 6.1

- Dental caries occurs in plaque-covered areas frequently exposed to dietary carbohydrates.
- The initial lesion is subsurface before the thin surface layer collapses.
- The initial or pre-cavitation lesion is reversible.
- Saliva plays an essential part in caries prevention.
- If all plaque is removed from the surface the carious process stops.

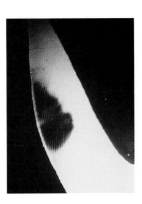

Figure 6.5 Microradiograph of a longitudinal ground section through a lesion of the type shown in Figs 6.3 and 6.4. The body of the lesion shows marked radiolucency (loss of mineral) in contrast with sound enamel and the surface layer (magnification: 70×). (Reproduced from Soames and Southam, *Oral Pathology*, by permission of Oxford University Press.)

Table 6.1 The general functions of saliva

Digestive functions
Assisting the mastication of food
Forming a bolus
Assisting in swallowing a bolus
Taste perception
Metabolism of starch
Protective functions
Ensuring comfort through lubrication
Preventing desiccation of oral mucosa, gingivae, and lips
Antimicrobial
Lavage
Bacteriostatic, bacteriocidal
Inhibiting adhesion of bacteria
Inhibiting aggregation of bacteria
Buffering
Within saliva
Within dental plaque
Removal of toxins (including carcinogens)
Aids speech

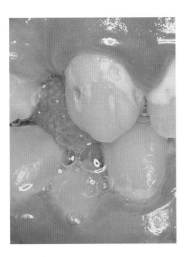

Figure 6.6 Maxillary permanent canine tooth showing a variety of carious lesions ranging from white spot enamel caries to cavitated dentine caries.

6.2 The epidemiology of dental caries

Dental caries is one of our most prevalent diseases and yet there is considerable variation in its occurrence between countries, between regions within countries, between areas within regions, and between social and ethnic groups. One of the tasks of epidemiology is to record the level of disease and the variation between groups. A second task is to record changes in the levels of dental caries in populations over time, and a third task is to try to explain these variations.

The UK has one of the best series of national statistics on dental caries. The dental health of adults and children has been recorded every 10 years, beginning with the Adult Dental Health Survey of 1968 (Table 6.2).

The advantages of this series of surveys are as follows:

1. They are national, using sound sampling methods to obtain representative samples of the populations.

2. They include both clinical and sociological data, giving the interaction between knowledge, attitude, behaviour, and disease.

3. The methods are well described and carefully standardized, resulting in meaningful longitudinal information.

Data on children at the ages of 5, 12, and 14 years are also available through the annual studies conducted under the auspices of the British Association for the Study of Community Dentistry and the UK National Health Service.

The ravages of dental caries were so severe in the past that the extent of disease in a population was measured by the proportion of the population with no natural teeth or edentulousness. A marked decrease in the percentage who were edentulous was recorded between 1968 and 2009, especially in adults aged 35–54 years. For younger people, it is common to record the prevalence (the proportion of people affected) and the severity (number of teeth affected per person) of dental caries and the percentage of carious teeth restored (Care Index). The drastic improvement in these parameters in the UK between 1973 and 2003 is shown in Table 6.3. About half of all children are now clinically 'caries free'. What is of concern is the opinion that the improvement is not continuing in the youngest age groups, and indeed there are signs that caries experience is increasing in some areas. This is compounded by a decline in the Care Index in the UK.

A decline in caries, first noticed during the 1970s, has been recorded in a large number of industrialized countries. The dental health of older children continued to improve in the 1980s, but caries experience in primary teeth, measured at age 5 or 6 years, stayed fairly constant. The Nordic countries used to have very high caries experience and the dramatic improvement in all five Nordic countries can be seen in Fig. 6.7, although it occurred somewhat later in Iceland. One of the most dramatic improvements has been recorded in Switzerland where the mean DMFT (decayed, missing, and filled teeth) in 12-year-olds fell from 8.0 in 1964 to 5.1 in 1972, 3.0 in 1980, and 1.1 in 1992. DMFT in 15-year-olds fell from 13.9 in 1964 to 2.2 in 1992. Caries experience in Australian children has been well recorded and indicates a dramatic improvement in dental health (Fig. 6.8). Reports from North America indicate that caries prevalence and severity in the permanent dentition have continued to decline since 1982 in Canada and the USA, but that

Table 6.2 National surveys of the dental health of children and adults in the UK

Children	
England and Wales	1973
United Kingdom*	1983
United Kingdom*	1993
United Kingdom*	2003
Adults	
England and Wales	1968
Scotland	1972
United Kingdom*	1978
United Kingdom*	1988
United Kingdom*	1998
United Kingdom*	2009

*England, Wales, Scotland, and Northern Ireland.

Table 6.3 Decay experience of 5-year-old children (primary teeth), 12- and 14- to 15-year-old children (permanent teeth) in the UK (1973, England and Wales), as recorded in national surveys

	1973	1983	1993	2003
Five-year-olds				
Percentage affected	72	50	45	43
Mean DMFT	4.0	1.8	1.7	1.6
Filled as a percentage of decay experience	–	28	17	15
12-year-olds				
Percentage affected	93	81	52	34
Mean DMFT	4.8	3.1	1.4	0.8
Filled as a percentage of decay experience	–	70	58	69
14- to 15-year-olds				
Percentage affected	96	93	63	49
Mean DMFT	7.4	5.9	2.5	1.6
Filled as a percentage of decay experience	–	74	57	77

DMFT, decayed, missing, and filled teeth

caries experience in the primary dentition may have stabilized since about 1986–1987.

While dental surveys of schoolchildren have been quite common, there is much less information on the dental health of preschool children mainly because access to them is more difficult (Table 6.4). The prevalence and severity of dental caries in British preschool children were reviewed by Holt (1990) and in preschool children around the world by Holm (1990). In most European countries, North America, and Australia, caries experience has declined in parallel with the increasing use of fluoride toothpastes, although this decline appears to have stopped in the UK. The ChildSmile Programme in Scotland is showing promising results in terms of caries control in preschool children (McMahon *et al.* 2010). This programme provides more up-to-date data drawn from the West of Scotland, a region with high level of caries. In 2007–2008, 25% of 3-year-olds had obvious dental caries, with a much higher level of 32% in children from deprived areas. Caries experience in preschool children in Southeast Asia, Central America, and parts of Africa is high, and there are discernible trends of increasing prevalence in parallel with the rise in availability of sugar-containing snacks and drinks.

While the state of the permanent dentition in children has improved dramatically in many countries, caries in primary teeth is still a considerable problem in preschool and school-aged children. In industrialized countries, caries experience is highest in the more deprived groups of society and often in ethnic minority groups. In developing countries, the reverse social trend is observed, with the well-off urban children having the most caries experience. Most of these variations in children's dental health can be explained in terms of the preventive role of fluoride and the caries-inducing role of sugary snacks. In adults, provision of dental services and patient preference for treatments can have a major effect on the state of the dentition, in addition to the aetiological and preventive roles of sugar, fermentable carbohydrates, and fluoride. (See Key Points 6.2.)

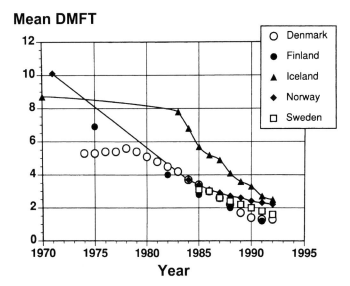

Figure 6.7 Caries experience (DMFT) for 12-year-old children in Nordic countries. (Reproduced from von der Fehr (1994) with kind permission of the *International Dental Journal*.)

Key Points 6.2

- Epidemiology indicates the size of the problem of caries and changes over time.
- Since 1968 there have been surveys of adult and child dental health every 10 years in the UK.
- Prevalence and extent have fallen markedly since the late 1970s in many countries. However, this decline may have ceased.
- Dental caries remains a significant problem for society and the individual.

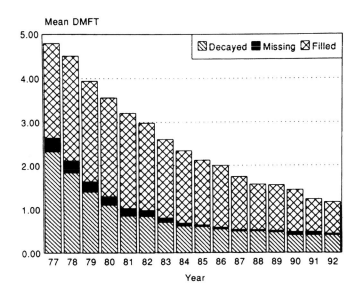

Figure 6.8 Caries experience in Australian 12-year-olds. (Reproduced from Spencer *et al.* (1994) with kind permission of the *International Dental Journal*.)

Table 6.4 Caries prevalence in UK preschool children in 1992–1993

Age (years)	Prevalence (%)
1.5–2.5	4
2.5–3.5	14
3.5–4.5	30

6.3 Caries detection and diagnosis

The presentation of caries has been described as resembling an iceberg with the dentine lesions (those traditionally described as requiring restoration) being above the waterline. Below the waterline lie enamel lesions, the most amenable to preventive intervention. Some form of additional aid is required to detect and diagnose many carious lesions. This can range from radiographs in the clinical situation to histopathology in the *in vitro* setting.

Caries detection and diagnosis is difficult—it is a multistage process. Unfortunately, current training of undergraduate dental students and remuneration systems frequently lead dentists just to think of the diagnostic process as a treatment, i.e. a dentinal carious lesion on the distal surface of a premolar is recorded as a DO (distal–occlusal) amalgam.

The identification of caries depends on a systematic examination of clean dry teeth. The basic equipment consists of adequate lighting, compressed air for drying, a dental mirror, and a blunt or ball-ended probe. The emphasis is on a visual examination, rather than a visual–tactile examination. The sharp probes which were traditionally used to aid diagnoses are contraindicated for a number of reasons.

- The probe does not improve diagnosis—all a 'sticky' fissure means is that the probe fits the fissure.

- Probing a demineralized lesion will break the enamel matrix, making remineralization impossible and thus creating an iatrogenic cavity.

- The probe may transfer cariogenic bacteria from one site to another—in effect inoculate caries-free sites with cariogenic bacteria.

A ball-ended or blunt probe can be used gently to confirm the presence of cavitation, sealants, and restorations.

The first visible sign of caries is the white spot lesion, which at first can only be seen when the surface is dried (Fig. 6.9). This is because when demineralized enamel becomes porous, the pores contain water; if dried, the water in the pores is replaced with air and the lesion becomes more obvious. As the caries progresses the lesion will become obvious even when wet.

Unfortunately, active carious lesions are not the only causes of white areas on teeth. Hypoplasia, fluorosis, and arrested hypermineralized

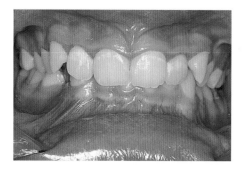

Figure 6.9 Clinical appearance of white spot lesions on the labial and approximal surfaces of the upper permanent incisors.

carious lesions, to name but a few, can all mimic a white spot carious lesion. The decision as to the aetiology depends on factors such as site and surface characteristics. Caries tends to occur at predilection sites; therefore a white area at the gingival margin is much more likely to be caries than one of similar appearance at the incisal edge. Active carious lesions are matt white with a rough surface, while arrested lesions tend to be glossy with a smooth surface. A similar process is conducted for brown spot lesions.

Although large cavities are relatively easily identified, dentine caries presents its own problems. On occlusal surfaces there may be no visible break in the surface, the evidence of caries being shadowing under the enamel. A similar picture is seen for approximal lesions.

Therefore, as even the most thorough visual clinical examination will detect only some of the enamel and dentine carious lesions present, the clinician needs to be helped by diagnostic aids. The most commonly used are radiographs. The views which are of value for caries diagnosis are:

- bitewings
- orthopantomograms (OPTs)
- bimolars
- periapicals.

Bitewings are the first choice view for caries diagnosis. These provide information on both occlusal dentine caries and approximal enamel and dentine caries. OPTs can detect the presence of an occlusal dentine carious lesion with a high degree of accuracy. OPTs and bitewings taken in OPT machines are of much less value in the detection of approximal lesions.

Bimolars are not as useful a view as bitewings because there is often overlap of structures. However, they are of use in the pre-cooperative child who will not cope with bitewings or an OPT. Periapicals are as accurate as bitewings for caries diagnosis, but obviously less information is available on any one film.

As with the visual examination, it is vital that the radiographs are viewed in a systematic way with appropriate illumination and ideal magnification.

Although not all children will tolerate them, bitewing radiographs should be considered for all children from the age of 4 years and above who are at risk of caries. The clinician should ask the question 'Why not take bitewings?' rather than 'Why take bitewings?'

The decision to take radiographs and the frequency of further radiographic examinations need to be based on a thorough carious risk assessment, with the dentist having to balance the benefits of the additional diagnostic yield with the risks of exposure to ionizing radiation. Current guidelines from the Faculty of General Dental Practice UK (2004) suggest radiographic examinations every 6 months for the carious-active child and views every 12–18 months for the child with controlled caries in primary or mixed dentitions (Table 6.5).

An interesting clinical phenomenon which may help the clinician decide whether radiographs are warranted is the presence of a bleeding papilla, which suggests the presence of an approximal cavity (Ekstrand *et al.* 1998).

This occurs because the cavity is full of plaque which, together with driving the carious process, will cause gingivitis and thus the bleeding papilla.

Other diagnostic aids which may assist with approximal caries diagnosis include fibre-optic transillumination (FOTI) and temporary tooth separation. FOTI consists of the placement of a 0.5mm light source in the embrasure (Fig. 6.10). If a carious lesion is present, it will show as a dark shadow. Some studies have suggested that FOTI is as accurate as radiographs, but the situation is confused by other studies which question its benefit. Certainly, if it is used, FOTI provides the clinician with more information on which to base a decision. Temporary tooth separation consists of the placement of an orthodontic elastomeric separator between the teeth (Fig. 6.11). The patient returns after 3–4 days, the teeth having separated allowing direct access for examination.

Three adjuncts have been developed to assist with the diagnosis of occlusal carious lesions: FOTI as discussed above, laser fluorescence devices, and electronic caries meters.

Laser fluorescence devices measure the fluorescence of the tooth and, of particular importance, the fluorescence of bacterial by-products in the carious lesion (Fig. 6.12). This provides a digital reading indicating the status of the surface. Research on these devices is very promising, but false readings are generated by staining, calculus, and hyperplasia. When used appropriately these devices provide a standardized reproducible measure which not only helps with the diagnostic decision but also allows the possibility of monitoring over time.

Table 6.5 Faculty of General Dental Practice UK (2004) recommendations for the frequency of radiographic examinations in children

Caries risk status	Frequency
High	6 monthly
Moderate	12 monthly
Low	12–18 monthly in the primary and mixed dentition
	24 monthly in the permanent dentition

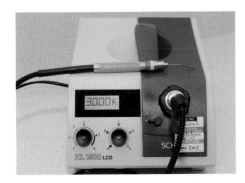

Figure 6.10 A portable FOTI light source with a 0.5mm diameter tip. As dental headpieces contain fibre-optics these are often incorporated into the dental unit.

Electronic caries meters measure the decrease in the resistance of carious lesions compared with sound surfaces. When used meticulously these meters have shown good accuracy in clinical trials. However, the readings of electronic caries meters are confounded by areas of hyperplasia, immature teeth, and particularly moisture.

The research on caries diagnosis has focused on two approaches: developing adjuncts, as discussed above, and improving the information provided by the visual examination. The use of a meticulous visual examination actually dates back to the 1950s. Currently, the International Caries Diagnosis and Assessment System (ICDAS II) delivers a diagnostic method which, with relatively little training, can provide a valid and reproducible examination that permits staging of caries from white spot to pulpal involvement.

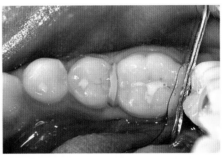

(a)

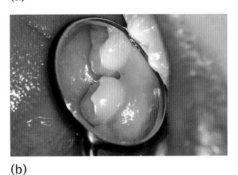

(b)

Figure 6.11 (a) Temporary tooth separation: an elastomeric separator between a lower second premolar and first permanent molar. (b) The appearance after separation, showing access for examination of the approximal surfaces.

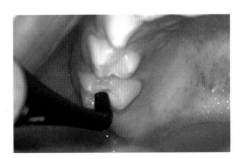

Figure 6.12 The tip of a laser fluorescence device in place on the occlusal surface of a maxillary first permanent molar.

Table 6.6 outlines the ICDAS II codes and criteria, but to gain a full understanding visit the ICDAS website (www.icdas.org) which provides more in-depth information.

At present the highest-quality examination is delivered using a meticulous visual examination supported by appropriate radiographs. (See Key Point 6.3.)

Key Point 6.3

The stages in caries diagnostic process:

- detect
- diagnose
- record.

Table 6.6 The ICDAS II codes and criteria

Code	Criteria
0	Sound
1	First visual change in enamel (seen only after prolonged air drying or restricted to within the confines of a pit or fissure)
2	Distinct visual change in enamel
3	Localized enamel breakdown (without clinical visual signs of dentinal involvement)
4	Underlying dark shadow from dentine
5	Distinct cavity with visible dentine
6	Extensive distinct cavity with visible dentine

6.4 Prevention of dental caries

The dramatic improvement in dental health, especially in children, in many developed countries during the past 20 years is proof that prevention works. Dental caries is not inevitable; the causes are well known, and discouraging caries development and encouraging caries healing are realities to be grasped. Failure to do so is, at least, to provide second-class dental care.

There are four practical pillars to the prevention of dental caries: plaque control/toothbrushing, diet, fluoride, and fissure sealing. Each of these will be considered in turn before being brought together in treatment planning and in relation to caries risk. Prevention of caries is easy in theory but in practice involves many skills. The main reason for this is that control of the aetiological agents—plaque and fermentable carbohydrates—involves a change in behaviour. The value of fluoride is that it can be delivered in a variety of ways, some of which require minimal action by the patient. There is no 'magic bullet' that can be applied to teeth which will render them totally resistant to caries. Fissure sealants come close to this but they are expensive to apply, some fall off, and they only prevent caries of pits and fissures.

In dentistry there is no doubt that prevention is better than cure. Prevention of dental caries underpins all dental care provided to children. All children require preventive input. The type of input depends on the child and their caries risk. Forming a comprehensive treatment strategy, tailored to the needs of each individual child, is an essential component of all paediatric treatment planning.

Despite dental caries being a preventable disease epidemiological surveys in children in many countries have shown that its distribution has become 'bimodal', with 80% of the disease present in only 20% of the child population. Consequently, two approaches are required to improve dental health. This strategy will involve maintaining good dental health in those without dental decay, and targeting resources to those who are at risk of developing decay. This means targeting the 'high-caries-risk' groups comprising:

- the caries prone—especially early childhood caries (nursing bottle caries);
- the handicapped—mental and physical;

- the socially deprived, that is, low socio-economic groups;
- ethnic minority groups usually residing in inner city areas.

Low-caries-risk children are those who are caries free or have well-controlled caries, have good oral and dietary habits, are highly motivated, and attend their dental appointments regularly.

Thus it is important to institute effective preventive measures for children and advice for their patients. This is best achieved at treatment planning prior to commencing any restorative work (other than emergency and stabilizing procedures). It is also important to clarify what constitutes high- and low-caries-risk children (Chapter 3).

The mainstays of preventive measures are:

1. plaque control and regular toothbrushing with a fluoride toothpaste;
2. sensible dietary advice;
3. use of fluorides;
4. fissure sealants;
5. regular dental checks with appropriate radiographs.

All of these measures need to be coordinated and supervised by the dental team and reinforced with good patient and parental motivation.

6.4.1 Plaque control and toothbrushing

A number of plaque disclosing tablets and solutions are available. Children need close supervision when using these agents and appropriate advice should be given to parents and guardians. Plaque charts can be used to monitor progress and to identify areas where cleaning is not ideal. It is customary to report the percentage number of clean surfaces so that patients aim to achieve as close to 100% clean as possible. After demonstrating the plaque disclosing procedure (Fig. 6.13) and performing the charting, it is initially advisable to instruct patients to use

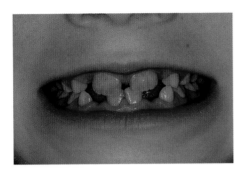

Figure 6.13 Plaque disclosure of upper and lower dentition.

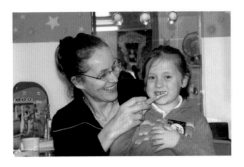

Figure 6.14 Parent assisting toothbrushing of their young child's teeth.

the disclosing agent prior to toothbrushing. After a week it is advisable for patients to brush first and then disclose in order to identify areas that are being missed.

Toothbrushing

Advise regular toothbrushing with an appropriate concentration of fluoride toothpaste. Toothbrushing should become a routine and be performed on at least two occasions every day. Numerous types of brushes (manual and powered) and toothpastes are available. Many brushes and pastes are decorated with cartoon characters, etc., which can be good motivators for many children. Manual brushes (preferably with a small head) and electric brushes are equally effective for plaque removal. However, the cost of brushes and pastes can be prohibitive for some low socio-economic groups where, in reality, toothbrushing has become a low priority. This is where community and school-based programmes are needed to ensure provision of oral health measures. Young children under 5 years need help with toothbrushing (Fig. 6.14). Children do not have the manual dexterity to brush their teeth effectively until they can tie their own shoelaces (about 7 years of age). However, even after this children should still be supervised to establish a regular routine and ensure good oral health practice. Only a small smear of fluoride toothpaste should be used up to 3 years of age; after this age a 'pea-sized' amount should be used Fluoride is cleared so quickly from the oral cavity that many advise swishing the toothpaste saliva slurry around the mouth and not rinsing with water in order to maintain elevated intra-oral fluoride levels for longer periods of time. A simple message for patients is 'Brush your teeth first thing in the morning and last thing at night'.

As dental caries is caused by bacteria in plaque fermenting dietary carbohydrates to acids which dissolve enamel, it is logical to prevent caries by removing plaque from teeth, usually with a toothbrush. Unfortunately, many investigations indicate that caries reduction is not brought about by improved toothbrushing alone. However, it must be said straight away that, first, toothbrushing is a very important way of controlling gingivitis and periodontal disease and, second, toothbrushing with toothpaste is a very important way of conveying fluoride to the tooth surface.

The results of the few studies investigating the effect of flossing on dental caries are mixed. Daily flossing of the teeth of young children reduced caries in one study but no preventive effect was observed in older children who flossed their own teeth. Over 30 years ago, in Kalstaad, Sweden, caries increments were virtually eliminated in children who had fortnightly prophylaxes and intensive preventive advice

by dental hygienists (Axelsson *et al.* 1976). Other workers have tried to reproduce those sensational results (96% caries reduction compared with a control group) but have failed to do so, illustrating the difficulty of extrapolating findings of trials from one country to another.

Plaque growth can be prevented by twice-daily rinsing with chlorhexidine, but because of the intra-oral side-effects of chlorhexidine (changed taste sensation, poor taste, and tooth staining), it is usually recommended for short-term use only to aid periodontal care.

6.4.2 Nutrition and diet in caries control

We are constantly eating and snacking, and it is very important to be able to give sensible practical advice regarding diet and dental caries. Some consider that there are 'good foods' and 'bad foods', while others believe that there are 'good diets' and 'bad diets'. Further, some consider sugar to be the arch villain and enemy of dentistry. Caries has declined despite increased sales and consumption of sugars. However, the literature is controversial, and there are many conflicting views and opinions regarding sugar consumption. The Committee on Medical Aspects of Food Policy (COMA) reports classify sugars as being either intrinsic (sugar within a cell membrane, e.g. fruits) or extrinsic (readily available sugars, e.g. refined sugars). A recent reference can be found at the end of this chapter. Are intrinsic sugars converted to extrinsic sugars on chewing? This is probably irrelevant, as bacteria need a fermentable source of carbohydrate to produce acid. The review by Burt and Pai (2001) summarizes the conflict in opinions on sugar. However, we should concentrate on giving sensible practical everyday advice to our patients as shown in Table 6.7. Advising parents to completely stop their children from eating sugary foods is not achievable! We should aim to ensure that our patients eat sensibly and safely. Baby drinks given in baby bottles led to 'nursing bottle' caries (early childhood caries (ECC)). Plaque pH responses to these drinks showed falls to below the critical pH of apatite (pH <5.5). We should advise that only milk or water is given to children in a baby bottle. Many are not aware that no added-sugar drinks contain natural sugar. We should advise that young children consume drinks from trainer cups or beakers and use straws. 'Safer foods' have been recommended as alternatives for frequent snackers or nibblers. These alternatives include cheeses that have been shown to raise plaque pH. In addition to fruit and vegetables, crisps and peanuts have also been recommended as safer alternatives. However, citrus fruits have been implicated in the aetiology of dental erosion and peanuts are associated with inhalation risk in small children. The development of one 'safer' drink showed that the plaque pH did not fall below the critical pH for enamel (Toumba and Duggal 1999).

Frequency of eating

Frequency of eating has an important effect on teeth. However, is this anecdotal or based on scientific evidence? Eating meals leads to periods of acid attack when tooth mineral is lost. At the end of the meal or snack the acid is buffered by saliva and the mineral loss stops and reverses under favourable conditions. Frequent snackers have predominantly mineral loss and little if any remineralization. Duggal *et al.* (2001) demonstrated the importance of fluoride and frequency of sugar consumption in an *in situ* study using enamel slabs and transverse microradiography. When volunteers did not use a fluoride toothpaste mineral demineralization was observed with the frequency of sugar consumption as low as three times per day. However, when fluoride toothpaste was used twice daily no significant mineral demineralization was observed up to a frequency of sugar consumption of seven

Table 6.7 Practical diet advice

Confectionery and such foods should be used at mealtimes as a dessert rather than consumed between meals
Only milk or water should be given to children in a baby bottle.

For the consumption of soft drinks the following recommendations should be followed:
    Ideally serve only at meal times
    Use a straw whenever possible
    Do not give at bedtime or during the night

Table 6.8 Permitted sweeteners in foods (UK)

Bulk sweeteners
Sorbitol
Mannitol
Hydrogenated glucose syrup*
Isomalt*
Xylitol*
Lactitol†
Maltitol‡
Intense sweeteners
Saccharin
Acesulfame K*
Aspartame*
Thaumatin*

*Permitted 1982.
†Permitted 1988.
‡Permitted 1986.

times per day. Therefore subjects who brush twice daily with a fluoride toothpaste should safely be able to have five mealtimes per day. This is a sensible and achievable dietary message for patients.

Non-sugar sweeteners

Sweeteners allowed for use in food and drink in the UK are listed in Table 6.8. The list is very similar for most countries. There is much evidence that they are non-cariogenic or virtually so. The intense sweeteners and xylitol are non-cariogenic; the other bulk sweeteners can be metabolized by plaque bacteria but the rate is so slow that these sweeteners can be considered safe for teeth. The use of non-sugar sweeteners is growing rapidly, particularly in confectionery and soft drinks. Confectionery products which have passed a well-established acidogenicity test can be labelled with the Mr Happy-Tooth logo (Fig. 6.15), which is a protected trademark informing the purchaser and consumer that these products are dentally safe. Tooth-friendly sweets are available in about 26 countries; in Switzerland about 20% of confectionery sold carries the Toothfriendly (or Mr Happy-Tooth) logo. There is good evidence that sugarless chewing gums not only are non-cariogenic but also positively prevent dental caries by stimulating salivary flow. Indeed, xylitol gums are used in school-based preventive programmes in Finland. In the UK, the British Dental Association (BDA) used to accredit products which benefited oral health. As an example, it accredited dentifrices which had proven effectiveness for many years. Later, foods and drinks were accredited—for example, a fruit-flavoured drink which was demonstrated to have negligible cariogenic and erosive potential. The Toothfriendly and BDA accreditation schemes help the consumer to make better choices. Bulk sweeteners can have a laxative effect and should not be given to children below 3 years of age. People vary in their sensitivity to these polyols, as some adults in the Turku sugar studies were consuming up to 100g of xylitol per day without effect.

Dietary advice for the prevention of dental caries

The basic advice is straightforward—reduce the frequency and amount of intake of fermentable carbohydrates. Dietary advice should be on two levels. First, every patient should receive basic advice. This

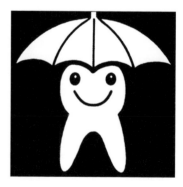

Figure 6.15 Pictogram of Mr Happy-Tooth. This is the protected logo of the International Toothfriendly Association to be seen on products that have passed the internationally accepted toothfriendly test. (Reproduced by kind permission of Toothfriendly International, Switzerland. http://www.toothfriendly.org.)

especially applies to parents of young children who need to be given the correct advice for the appropriate age of the child. Dietary advice is often too negative; energy that has been provided by confectionery has to be replaced and it is very important to emphasize positive eating habits. The variety of foods available has increased enormously in most countries in recent years; we must use this increased choice to assist our patients to make better food choices. The second level of advice is a more thorough analysis of the diet of children with a caries problem. A well-accepted method is the 3-day diary record. One practical drawback of this method is that it requires at least three visits—an introductory visit where the patient is motivated and informed about the procedure and the diet diary is given out, the diary collection visit, and a separate visit for advice and to agree targets. Each of these stages is important. At the first visit it is vital that the patient and parent appreciate that there is a dental problem and that you are offering your expert advice to help them overcome it. Once motivated, they must understand how the diary is to be completed. Any requests by parents for advice at the first visit should be parried and delayed until the third visit. At the third visit, advice must be personal, practical, and positive— all three of these are important (Table 6.7). The food preferences of children, cooking skills, food availability, and financial considerations vary enormously—advice must be personally tailored and practical for each patient. Positive advice has a much greater chance of acceptance than negative advice such as 'avoid this', 'don't eat that'—nagging is a demotivator. Dietary changes are difficult, targets often have to be limited, and constant reinforcement of advice and encouragement is essential. However, health gains can be considerable, to general as well as dental health and often to other members of the family, so that dietary advice is an essential part of care of children.

6.4.3 Fluoride and caries control

The use of fluorides dates back to as early as 1874 when the German Erharde suggested the use of potassium fluoride tablets for expectant mothers and children in order to strengthen teeth. This recommendation was made without any scientific evidence. What we now know to be dental fluorosis (mottling) was noted by dentists long ago who reported on 'Colorado stain' without the aetiology of the tooth defect being established.

Mode of action of fluoride and the caries process

The mineral of tooth tissue exists as a carbonated apatite which contains calcium, phosphate, and hydroxyl ions, making it a hydroxyapatite $[Ca_{10}(PO_4)_6(OH)_2]$. Carbonated portions weaken the structure and render the tissue susceptible to attack. Food remnants and debris mix with saliva and adhere to tooth surfaces as a slimy film known as dental plaque. Oral bacteria, and most importantly certain types of cariogenic bacteria (e.g. *Mutans streptococci* and *Lactobacilli* species), metabolize dental plaque and produce acid which lowers the pH of the oral environment. When the pH is below the critical pH for hydroxyapatite (<5.5), demineralization occurs with a net outward flow of calcium and phosphorus ions from the enamel surface into plaque and saliva. When the pH returns to 7.0, remineralization occurs with a net inward flow of ions into the enamel surface. If fluoride is present during remineralization, it

is incorporated to form fluorapatite $[Ca_{10}(PO_4)_6F_2]$, which is more stable and resistant to further acid attacks. The process of demineralization and remineralization is ongoing and is frequently referred to as 'the ionic seesaw' or 'tug-of-war'. This is now widely believed to be the most important preventive action of fluoride, and a constant post-eruptive supply of ionic fluoride is thought to be most effective.

A number of mechanisms have been proposed to explain the action of fluoride (Table 6.9). The first is that fluoride has an effect during tooth formation by substitution of hydroxyl ions by fluoride ions, thereby reducing the solubility of the tooth tissues. Second, fluoride can inhibit plaque bacterial growth and glycolysis. At pH 7.0, fluoride ions are precluded from entering bacteria. However, at pH 5.0, fluoride exists as hydrofluoric acid, which crosses the bacterial cell membrane and interferes with its metabolism by specifically inhibiting the enzyme enolase in the glycolytic pathway. Third, fluoride inhibits the demineralization of tooth mineral when present in solution at the tooth surface. Fourth, fluoride enhances remineralization by combining with calcium and phosphate to form fluorapatite. Fluoride enhances crystal growth, stabilizes the tissue, and makes it resistant to further acid attack. Enamel apatite demineralizes when the pH drops to 5.5. However, when fluorapatite is formed during remineralization, it is even more resistant to demineralization as the critical pH for fluorapatite is pH 3.5. Therefore it is most important to have an intra-oral source of fluoride when remineralization is taking place. Lastly, fluoride affects the morphology of the crown of the tooth, making the coronal pits and fissures shallower. Such shallow pits and fissures will be less likely to collect food debris, allow stagnation, and become decayed. The most important of these mechanisms is that when fluoride is present in the oral environment at the time of the acid attack it inhibits demineralization and promotes remineralization.

As early as 1890, Miller drew attention to the dissolutive process of dental caries and directed efforts to inhibit dissolution. The clinical findings of the anti-caries activity of drinking water with fluoride caused researchers to seek reasons for this. The finding that fluoride-treated enamel had a lower solubility led many to consider this as a cause-and-effect relationship. The anti-caries action of fluoride was thought to be one of preventing dissolution of enamel, and efforts were made to incorporate increasing amounts of fluoride into surface enamel. The first topical agent used, after water fluoridation, was a 2% sodium fluoride solution, and there was a greater uptake of fluoride into enamel from acidified solutions. Numerous fluoride preparations with varying

Table 6.9 Mechanisms of action of fluoride

1.	It has an effect during tooth formation making the enamel crystals larger and more stable
2.	It inhibits plaque bacteria by blocking the enzyme enolase during glycolysis
3.	It inhibits demineralization when in solution
4.	It enhances remineralization by forming fluorapatite when in solution
5.	It affects the crown morphology making the pits and fissures shallower and hence less likely to create stagnation areas.

concentrations of fluoride were employed for topical application and used as anti-caries agents. It was noted that there was not much difference in the caries reductions reported from the topical fluoride studies despite great variations in the fluoride concentrations used. In addition, the difference in the levels of fluoride in surface enamel of residents of fluoridated and non-fluoridated areas was limited. Therefore it is difficult to explain the 50% reduction of caries observed on the basis of the fluoride level in the surface enamel. Furthermore, there has been no study to show any clear-cut inverse relationship between fluoride content of surface enamel and dental caries.

All the available evidence is that caries results from the presence of an acidogenic plaque on elements of the tooth mineral. The diffusion of acidic components into the tooth mineral is accompanied by the reverse diffusion of components of the mineral. During the carious process there is a preferential loss of calcium, accompanied by dissolution of magnesium and carbonate. The first clinical sign of enamel caries is the so-called white spot lesion, where an apparently sound surface overlies an area of decalcification. The remineralization effect of fluoride has since come into favour. It has been reported that attacked enamel could re-harden on exposure to saliva and that softened enamel could be re-hardened by solutions of calcium phosphates *in vitro*. However, it is now known that it is the presence of fluoride in the oral cavity, and in particular its presence in the liquid phase at the enamel–plaque interface, that is of most importance.

In the past it was thought that the systemic action of fluoride was important for caries prevention. This view has completely changed and it is now known that it is the topical action of fluoride that is essential for caries prevention. It is the presence of fluoride in the liquid phase at the plaque–enamel interface that is of most importance. Studies have shown that even low levels of fluoride (0.10ppm) are effective in preventing the dissolution of enamel. It has been stated that it is the activity of the fluoride ion in the oral fluid that is important in reducing the solubility of the enamel rather than a high content of fluoride in the enamel. Saliva, the fluid that bathes the teeth, has been extensively studied. The level of fluoride in saliva is thought to be important for caries prevention and it has been shown that caries-susceptible subjects have salivary fluoride levels <0.02ppm, whereas caries-resistant subjects have levels >0.04ppm. (See Key Points 6.4.)

Key Points 6.4

Fluorides

- It is the activity of the fluoride ion in the oral fluid that is of most importance in reducing enamel solubility rather than having a high content of fluoride in surface enamel.

- A constant supply of low levels of intra-oral fluoride, particularly at the saliva–plaque–enamel interface, is of most benefit in preventing dental caries.

A vast number of fluoride products are available for systemic and topical use. They can be applied professionally by the dental team or by the patient at home.

Water fluoridation

This is a systemic method of providing fluoride on a community basis. Over 300 million people worldwide receive naturally or artificially fluoridated water. In 1942, Dean showed that 1.0ppm fluoride was the optimum level. This was in the pre-fluoride era, and perhaps the optimum level needs to be reviewed. There have been 113 studies in 23 countries over the last 60 years showing that water fluoridation reduces dental caries by 50%. Water fluoridation has been reviewed recently (Parnell *et al.* 2009), and the York review (McDonagh *et al.* 2000) remains one of the most comprehensive reviews of the topic. It is cheap and cost effective but there are opponents to its use.

Fluoride supplements

These are provided in the form of tablets and drops. Caries reductions vary from 20% to 80%. There is usually very poor patient compliance, especially for high-caries-risk groups. A 'Catch 22' situation exists in that those patients who are compliant do not need supplements whereas those who will benefit will not take them. The doses vary worldwide and are increasingly being held responsible for the rise in fluorosis. The fluoride supplement doses depend on the age of the patient and the level of fluoride in the drinking water. No supplements should be prescribed if the water fluoride level is greater than 0.7ppm. The European view on supplements is that they have no role as a public health measure, and when they are prescribed 0.5mg per day should be the maximum dose. The tablets should be allowed to dissolve slowly in the mouth, thus providing a topical application of fluoride to the teeth.

Other methods for providing systemic fluoride

There are, of course, other systemic methods for providing fluoride to the community:

1. salt—50% caries reduction in Switzerland and Hungary;
2. milk—15–65% caries reduction;
3. mineral water—46% caries reduction in Bulgaria.

Are we receiving more than the optimum daily amount of fluoride and therefore at increased risk of fluorosis? Are there other hidden sources of fluoride? Mineral water is used extensively as the main source of household drinking water. The fluoride levels of bottled water vary considerably, usually in the range 0.0–2.0ppm, but can be as high as 10.0–13.0ppm in some countries. Therefore, before prescribing fluoride supplements, we must first determine the fluoride level of the patient's drinking water, be it tap or bottled water. In addition some baby milk formulas have high amounts of fluoride themselves, and if they are made up with a high-fluoride bottled water the infant may be at increased risk of developing dental fluorosis. The maxillary permanent central incisors are most susceptible to fluorosis at about 2 years of age. In Continental Europe fluoride chewing gum is available, providing 0.25mg fluoride per stick of gum. Some foods (e.g. fish and tea) have high fluoride contents. We also ingest fluoride without realizing it. The 'halo effect' is the term used to describe the ingestion of fluoride from hidden sources. For example, fizzy drinks like Pepsi and Coca-Cola may contain fluoride if the bottling plant is in a fluoridated area and therefore uses fluoridated water. The 'fluoridated' drinks may be transported to non-fluoridated areas. The same applies to foods that are processed and canned or packaged in plants using fluoridated water.

Toothpastes

A dramatic decrease in worldwide caries levels has been seen since the introduction of fluoride-containing toothpastes in the early 1970s. They usually contain 1000 or 1450ppm fluoride. The fluoride is in the form of sodium fluoride, sodium monofluorophosphate (MFP), a combination of both, amine fluoride, or stannous fluoride. Stannous fluoride was the first formulation to be used in toothpastes when they first became available in the late 1960s and early 1970s. However, because of its instability and the undesirable staining observed it was removed from toothpastes until recently. However, stannous fluoride has now been stabilized with sodium hexamataphosphate and has been re-introduced in toothpaste. There are many different brands to suit all tastes. Child formulations contain no more than 750ppm fluoride to limit fluoride ingestion and therefore reduce the risk of fluorosis. There are limited studies on the efficacy of child formulations in preventing caries. A systematic review of low-fluoride toothpastes showed a reduced efficacy of 250ppm fluoride compared with 1000ppm fluoride. Therefore it is advisable to recommend toothpastes for children containing at least 1000ppm fluoride to ensure effective caries prevention. It is sometimes difficult to decide which concentration of fluoride toothpaste should be recommended to parents for their children. There is a balance between caries risk and fluorosis risk. If the child is caries free, low-fluoride (500ppm) children's toothpastes can be recommended to minimize the risk of fluorosis. However, if a young child under 6 years presents with caries, a toothpaste containing at least 1000ppm fluoride is indicated, as these have been proved to be more efficacious for caries prevention. High-concentration fluoride toothpastes containing 2800 and 5000ppm fluoride are now available on prescription only for high-caries-risk patients. These very high fluoride pastes should be used with caution in children, bearing in mind potential fluoride toxicity.

Burt (1998) described toothbrushing with fluoridated toothpaste as being close to an ideal public health method in that its use is convenient, inexpensive, culturally approved, and widespread. The use of fluoride toothpaste in children and adolescents has been subjected to several systematic reviews, and the updated European Academy of Paediatric Dentistry (EAPD) guidelines for the caries-preventive effectiveness of fluoridated toothpastes, expressed as prevented fraction, are summarized in Table 6.10. Evidence-based statements from the EAPD guidelines for the use of fluoridated toothpaste in children are shown in Table 6.11 and the EAPD recommended use of fluoride toothpaste in children is shown in Table 6.12.

Fluoride gels

These can be applied in trays or by brush, and 26% caries reductions have been reported. They are high in fluoride (1.23% = 12 300ppm) for professional use and lower (1000ppm) for home use. There is a risk of

Table 6.10 Factors influencing the caries-preventive effect of fluoride toothpaste as displayed in systematic reviews: prevented fraction (PF %) with confidence intervals (CI)

Intervention	Control	PF (95% CI)
Fluoride toothpaste	Placebo	24 (21–28)
Supervised brushing	Non-supervised brushing	11 (4–18)
Brushing twice per day	Brushing once per day	14 (6–22)
1450–1500ppm F	1000–1100 ppm F	14 (6–22)
F-toothpaste + other fluoride sources*	F-toothpaste	10 (2–17)

*Water fluoridation, fluoride varnish, fluoride gel, or fluoride rinsing.
Reproduced from *European Archives of Paediatric Dentistry* (2009).

Table 6.11 EAPD statements with level of evidence according to the Scottish Intercollegiate Guidelines Network (2000)

Statement	Level of evidence
Brushing with fluoride toothpaste daily prevents caries	1++
Increasing the frequency of brushing with fluoride toothpaste improves caries prevention	1+
Adult assistance/supervision of toothbrushing in children improves caries prevention	2+
Toothpastes containing higher concentrations of fluoride are more effective than those with lower levels of fluoride in preventing caries	1++
Commencement of toothbrushing prior to 1 year of age reduces the probability of developing caries	3
Ingestion of fluoridated toothpaste by young children is associated with an increased risk of dental fluorosis	2–

Reproduced from *European Archives of Paediatric Dentistry* (2009).

Table 6.12 EAPD recommended use of fluoride toothpaste in children

Age group	Fluoride concentration (ppm)	Daily use	Amount to be used
6 months to <2 years	500	Twice	Pea-size
2 to <6 years	1000(+)	Twice	Pea size
6 years and over	1450	Twice	1–2cm

Reproduced from *European Archives of Paediatric Dentistry* (2009).

toxicity with the high-fluoride gels and the following safety recommendations should be followed:

- no more than 2mL per tray;
- sit patient upright with head inclined forward;
- use a saliva ejector;
- instruct the patient to spit out for 30 seconds after the procedure (older gels have to be applied for 4 minutes but newer gels only 1 minute);
- do not use for children under 6 years.

Home-use gels contain 1000–5000ppm fluoride for use by patients at home at bedtime in addition to toothbrushing. Caries reductions of 36% have been reported.

Fluoride mouth rinses

These can be either daily rinses containing 0.05% (225ppm) sodium fluoride or weekly rinses containing 0.20% (900ppm) sodium fluoride. It is best to advise patients to use their fluoride rinses at a different time to toothbrushing so that the number of fluoride exposures increases. Caries reductions of 20–50% have been reported for fluoride rinse studies. The effect of toothbrushing and rinsing with fluoride has been shown to be additive. All orthodontic patients should be using a daily fluoride rinse to minimize the risk of demineralization and white spot lesions. Children under the age of 6 years should not be recommended to use fluoride mouth rinses because of the increased risk of swallowing the product.

Fluoride varnishes

Duraphat® (5wt% fluoride = 22 600ppm fluoride) is the most widely available fluoride varnish. This has a very high fluoride concentration, so again there is the possibility of toxicity with young children. It should be used sparingly with a cotton bud; a small pea-size amount is sufficient for a full mouth application in children up to 6 years. However, the fluoride is released relatively slowly from the varnish and therefore the potential risks of toxicity are less than with gels. Caries reductions of 50–70% have been reported in Scandinavian studies, but a more realistic reduction of 33% was found in a Cochrane review.

Slow-release fluoride devices

Many dental materials such as amalgam, composites, cements, acrylics, and fissure sealants have had fluoride added, but either the fluoride release was short term or the properties of the materials were adversely affected so that they were not of any use as a long-term source of intraoral fluoride. Glass ionomer cements are a group of materials that contain fluoride, but long-term release is debatable. Some researchers

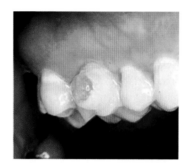

Figure 6.16 A fluoride slow-release glass device attached to the buccal surface of the upper right first permanent molar tooth.

have reported that these materials have a fluoride 'recharging' capacity, i.e. material that has released fluoride later takes up fluoride from other dental products that are used by the patient (e.g. fluoride toothpaste or mouth rinse) and this fluoride is released at a later time. The very latest fluoride research is with slow-release devices. The objective is to develop an intra-oral device that will release a constant supply of fluoride over a period of at least a year. Fluoride glass slow-release devices (Fig. 6.16) developed in Leeds have been shown to release fluoride for at least 2 years (Toumba 2001). Studies in Leeds demonstrated that there were 67% fewer new carious teeth and 76% fewer new carious surfaces in high-caries-risk children after 2 years in a clinical caries trial for children with the fluoride devices compared with a control group with placebo devices. There were 55% fewer new occlusal fissure carious cavities, showing that occlusal surfaces were also protected by the fluoride released from the devices. The fluoride glass devices release low levels of fluoride for at least 2 years and have great potential for use in preventing dental caries in high-caries-risk groups and irregular dental attenders. These devices have been patented and commercial development is now under progress. The provision of fluoride must be tailored for each individual to suit varying social and working circumstances. Slow-release fluoride devices seem to be ideal for targeting the high-caries-risk groups who are notoriously bad dental attenders with very poor oral hygiene and motivation. This is a very promising development with applications in numerous high-risk groups including the medically compromised.

Casein phosphopeptide-amorphous calcium phosphate (CPP-ACP)

Remineralization of dental hard tissue relies on the presence of ionic calcium (Ca^{2+}) and phosphate (PO_4^{3-}) from saliva. The presence of

Table 6.13 Suggestions for fluoride use in various clinical situations

Caries 0–6 years	Caries >6 years
Fluoride toothpaste (>1000ppm fluoride)	Fluoride toothpaste (>1350ppm fluoride)
Fluoride supplements (0.5mg/day)	Fluoride supplements (1.0mg/day)
Fluoride varnish every 3 months	APF gels or fluoride varnish every 6 months or fluoride varnish every 3 months
	Home-use fluoride gels or fluoride daily rinse
Rampant caries 0–6 years	Rampant caries >6 years
Fluoride toothpaste (>1000ppm fluoride)	Fluoride toothpaste (>1350ppm fluoride)
Fluoride supplements (0.5mg/day)	Fluoride supplements (1.0mg/day)
Fluoride varnish every 3 months	APF gels or fluoride varnish every 3 months
	Home-use fluoride gels or fluoride daily rinse
Caries free 0–6 years	Caries free >6 years
Low-fluoride toothpaste (500–1000ppm fluoride)	Fluoride toothpaste (>1350ppm fluoride)
	Home-use fluoride gels or fluoride daily rinse
	Fluoride varnish every 6 months
Orthodontic cases	Erosion cases
Fluoride toothpaste	Fluoride toothpaste
Daily fluoride rinse	Fluoride varnish
	Daily fluoride rinse

APF, Acidulated phosphate fluoride.

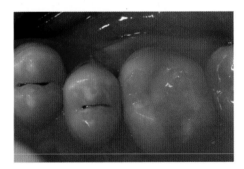

Figure 6.17 Fissure sealant placed on a first permanent molar tooth of a high-caries-risk child.

fluoride increases the speed of the remineralization and favours the formation of the less soluble fluorapatite. However, the remineralizing action of fluoride is limited by the amount of Ca^{2+} and PO_4^{3-} in saliva. Recently, technology related to a milk-based protein complex stabilizing Ca^{2+} and PO_4^{3-} (casein phosphopeptide-amorphous calcium phosphate (CPP-ACP)) has been released commercially, and added to topical creams (Tooth Mousse) and chewing gum. CPP-ACP stabilizes Ca^{2+} and PO_4^{3-} via the action of phosphorylated serine groups, and allows the creation of highly supersaturated solutions of Ca^{2+} and PO_4^{3-}, driving remineralization of enamel via concentration gradients and maintenance of intra-oral supersaturation relative to enamel mineral. (Shen *et al.* 2011). The CPP-ACP is retained in the oral cavity for at least 3 hours, providing a long-lasting source of bio-available Ca^{2+} and PO_4^{3-} and increasing the efficacy of any fluoride present. Products such as Tooth Mousse (MI Paste) should be used in children at risk of dental caries as a preventive agent, and in those with early-stage caries (white spot lesions) to assist remineralization. It is suggested that the cream is used after brushing at night, and also in the morning in high-risk children. A fluoridated CPP-ACP cream (Tooth Mousse plus, 900ppm NaF) improves the remineralization efficacy by approximately 25%. However, it should generally be used in children over 10 years old to decrease the chance of fluorosis from ingestion.

Deciding which fluoride preparation to use for differing clinical situations

This will depend on the following:

- Which groups of children?
- Which fluoride preparation?
- Daily or weekly use?
- Topical or systemic application?

In addition, the expected patient/parent motivation and compliance is very important in deciding what to use. Each patient will require a tailor-made fluoride regime, and the dentist will need to use his/her expertise and knowledge of the patient in formulating individual fluoride regimes and preventive treatment plans. Table 6.13 gives some suggestions for some different clinical situations.

6.4.4 Fissure sealing

Pit and fissure sealants (sealants) have been described as materials which are applied in order to obliterate the fissures and remove the sheltered environment in which caries may thrive (Fig. 6.17). Initially developed to prevent caries, their use has been developed further and they now have a place in the treatment of caries.

The decline in caries observed in industrialized countries over recent decades has affected all tooth surfaces but has been greatest on smooth surfaces. Therefore pitted and fissured surfaces, particularly of the molars, have the greatest disease susceptibility. This means that the potential benefits of effectively used sealants continue to increase.

The placement of sealants is relatively simple but is technique sensitive. Salivary contamination of as little as half a second can affect the bond and therefore the retention of the sealant. (See Key Points 6.5.)

Key Points 6.5

Fissure sealing technique

- Prophylaxis before etching does not enhance retention but is advisable if abundant plaque is present. A dry brush should be used rather than paste as these are retained in the depths of the fissures preventing penetration of the resin.
- Isolate the tooth surface.
- Etch for 20–30 seconds with 37% phosphoric acid.
- Wash and dry the surface, maintaining isolation.
- Apply the resin.
- Cure.
- Check for adequacy.

Several sealant materials are available, but the most effective is bis-GMA resin. Current resin materials are either autopolymerizing or photo-initiated, and most operators prefer the advantages of demand set offered by photo-initiation, although there are theoretical advantages to chemically cured materials in terms of retention as these materials have longer resin tags extending into the etched surface. Filled and unfilled resins are available; the filled materials are produced to provide greater wear resistance. However, this is not clinically relevant and clinical trials demonstrate superior efficacy for unfilled materials. Irrespective of the presence of fillers, some materials are opaque or tinted to aid evaluation. This is an advantage but means that the clinician is unable to view the enamel surface to assist with caries detection and to detect the presence of restorations such as sealant restorations.

Isolation is critical to successful sealant application. Operator and nurse must act as a team as it is impossible for single operators to apply sealant effectively. The vast majority of trials have demonstrated cotton wool and suction to be an effective means of isolation. A rubber dam is advocated by some because of the superior isolation offered by this material. This is probably true, but its use is frequently not possible because of the stage of eruption of the tooth or level of cooperation of the patient. It would be inappropriate to delay sealant application to allow further eruption to permit the application of rubber dam. The

application of sealant is a relatively non-invasive technique, frequently used to acclimatize a patient. On both clinical and economic grounds, it is difficult to justify the use of a rubber dam, with the associated use of local anaesthetic and clamps, for the majority of patients.

Glass ionomers have also been used as sealants; the application technique is less sensitive than that for resins. Unfortunately, glass ionomer sealants have poor retention. It is suggested that the fluoride release from glass ionomers provides additional protection, but the clinical relevance of this remains doubtful. The addition of fluoride to resin sealants has been demonstrated to provide no additional benefit. Glass ionomer sealants only have a place as temporary sealants during tooth eruption, when adequate isolation to permit the application of resin is not possible, or in patients whose level of anxiety or cooperation similarly prevent placement of resin. Glass ionomers have been developed specifically for this role but clinical evidence of their effectiveness is not yet available. (See Key Points 6.6.)

Key Points 6.6

Application of glass ionomer sealants

- Clean the surface.
- Isolate the tooth.
- Run the glass ionomer into the fissusres.
- Protect the material during initial setting.
- Apply unfilled resin, petroleum jelly, or fluoride varnish to protect the material.

For anxious patients application can be done with a gloved finger until the material is set.

Resin fissure sealants are effective; a recent systematic review has demonstrated 60% caries reductions with retention rates of 52% at 4 years (Ahovuo-Saloranta *et al*. 2008). To gain full caries preventive benefit, sealants should be maintained, i.e. sealants with less than optimal coverage should be identified and additional resin applied.

Since the development of sealants there has been a question regarding the consequences of sealing over caries, the concern being that it will progress unidentified under the sealant. Given the difficulty in diagnosing caries this must be a frequent occurrence in daily practice. A number of trials have examined this by actively sealing over caries, and all have shown that sealants arrest or slow the rate of caries progression. We are now at the point where sealing of non-cavited active caries is recommended by most authorities, and the maxim 'If in doubt seal' is good advice. The surface should then be monitored clinically and radiographically at regular intervals until its status is confirmed. One instance where actively sealing over caries is particularly to be recommended is in the pre-cooperative patient where the placement of sealant may help to acclimatize the patient, with the added benefit of controlling the caries, until a definitive restoration can be placed.

Sealants are also effective at preventing pit and fissure caries in primary teeth. Primary teeth have more aprismatic enamel than permanent teeth, and doubt about the effectiveness of etching deciduous enamel led to a belief that they required prolonged etching times. This has been demonstrated not to be the case, and the technique for sealant application to primary teeth is identical to that employed with permanent teeth.

Although the effectiveness of fissure sealants is beyond doubt, to be used cost effectively their use should be targeted. Guidelines for patient selection and tooth selection have been published by the British Society of Paediatric Dentistry, and these are summarized below (British Society of Paediatric Dentistry 2000).

Patient selection

1. Children with special needs. Fissure sealing of all occlusal surfaces of permanent teeth should be considered for those who are medically compromised, physically or mentally disabled, or have learning difficulties, or for those from a disadvantaged social background.
2. Children with extensive caries in their primary teeth should have all permanent molars sealed soon after their eruption.
3. Children with carious-free primary dentitions do not need to have first permanent molars sealed routinely; rather, these teeth should be reviewed at regular intervals.

Tooth selection

1. Fissure sealants have the greatest benefit on the occlusal surfaces of permanent molar teeth. Other surfaces should not be neglected, in particular the cingulum pits of upper incisors, the buccal pits of lower molars, and the palatal pits of upper molars.
2. Sealants should normally be applied as soon as the selected tooth has erupted sufficiently to permit moisture control.

3. Any child with occlusal caries in one first permanent molar should have the fissures of the sound first permanent molars sealed.
4. Occlusal caries affecting one or more first permanent molars indicates a need to seal the second permanent molars as soon as they have erupted sufficiently.

Since the development of sealants in the mid-1960s there have been a number of advances in sealant technology. There is evidence that the use of bonding agents during sealant placement helps reduce the effect on retention of slight salivary contamination; however, this prolongs the procedure, increasing the risk of contamination. Therefore large trials are required to answer this question before changing the standard technique outlined above. Single-stage etch/prime/bonding systems exist, but although they are effective on cut and smooth surfaces, they do not give predictable results on occlusal surfaces because they are not acidic enough to burn off the plaque and etch the enamel surface effectively.

Recently studies have examined the effect of sealing smooth approximal surfaces, not as a preventive measure but to arrest the progression of enamel caries. These studies initially used conventional sealant resin and results suggest that caries progression is prevented in approximately 50% of cases. This technology has been further developed with resins, which do not just coat the surface but act by infiltrating the carious lesion (Fig. 6.18). Success rates of 80%, with only 20% of lesions progressing, are being reported. This technique is more akin to very minimal restorations than sealing as it involves the application of 18% hydrochloric acid to the surface of the carious lesion, which removes the surface layer to allow the resin to penetrate the lesion. Therefore a rubber dam is mandatory to protect the soft tissues and local anaesthetic will normally be necessary.

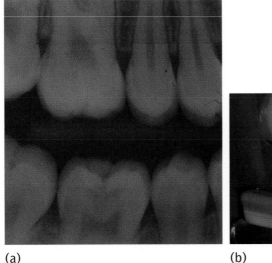
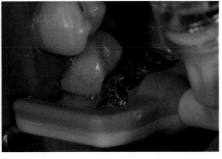

(a)   (b)

Figure 6.18 Approximal sealants. (a) Radiograph showing a number of carious lesions. The lesion on the distal surface of the upper second permanent premolar is amenable to infiltration. (b) Application of the resin infiltrant to a carious lesion on the distal surface of the upper second permanent premolar enamel.

6.5 Treatment planning for caries prevention

The preceding summaries of the various methods of preventing dental caries have highlighted the advantages and disadvantages of the four practical methods of caries prevention: diet, fluoride, fissure sealing, and plaque control. Each is capable of preventing caries, but achieving changes in diet and toothbrushing, undertaking fissure sealing, and applying fluoride in the dental chair are all time-consuming. It is unrealistic to attempt to use each method to its maximum potential and it is necessary to agree an overall philosophy. Everyone should receive some advice on caries prevention, and those perceived to be at greater risk of dental caries should be investigated more thoroughly and given a preventive treatment plan.

Four clear preventive messages are promoted in *The Scientific basis of oral health education* (Levine and Stillman-Lowe 2009) (see Table 6.14). This is the minimum advice. Parents of infants and young children should be advised on sensible eating habits, the abuse of sugar-containing fruit-flavoured drinks, and the need for meals which will reduce the demand for snacks. Toothbrushing should be observed in the surgery, giving an opportunity to discuss the type of toothbrush and toothpaste. Some patients are more likely to develop dental caries than others, and these patients need more aggressive preventive advice and therapy. Effective toothbrushing with an appropriate fluoride toothpaste is an essential first goal. Other forms of fluoride therapy, as outlined above, should be considered: drops/tablets (if the drinking water is fluoride deficient), mouth rinses, and topical applications of solutions, gel, or varnish. Dietary habits should be investigated using a 3-day diet diary and appropriate advice given that is personal, practical, and positive. As toothbrushing, rinsing, and dietary control all require changes in lifestyle, especially at home, continuous encouragement is essential. Fissure sealing in line with the guidelines set out above is likely to be sensible.

The order in which the various carious preventive measures are scheduled in the treatment plan is of some importance. It is sensible to investigate toothbrushing early, as it is a good bridge between the home and the dental surgery and it gives proper emphasis to this vital preventive measure. If done first, it allows you to work on clean teeth. As investigation of diet and dietary advice requires at least three visits, it is sensible to introduce this at an early appointment. Fissure sealing can be commenced early in the treatment plan as a relatively easy procedure, emphasizing prevention rather than restoration, while topical fluoride therapy could be carried out after fissure sealing. If fluoride dietary supplements and/or mouth rinses are going to be recommended, it is sensible to introduce them at the first or second appointment so that continuous encouragement in their use can be given at later appointments. The intensive preventive therapy described above is for patients at risk of developing caries. This begs the question on how to predict future caries development. There has been much work on this topic with many risk factors or markers of caries risk proposed. Overall, the findings are not encouraging. The most successful are past caries experience, saliva properties (flow rate, buffering power, and microbiological content), and social status. These can be used in combination to increase discriminatory power. Despite much work, one large American investigation showed that the best predictor of future caries increment in children was 'intuition of the dentist'.

Table 6.14 Summary of recommendations in *The Scientific basis of oral health education*

1.	Reduce the consumption, and especially the frequency of intake, of sugar-containing food and drink and very acid drinks
2.	Clean the teeth thoroughly every day with a fluoride toothpaste
3.	Request your local water company to supply water with the optimum fluoride level
4.	Have an oral examination every year

Levine and Stillman-Lowe (2009).

6.6 Summary

1 Dental caries is caused by dietary carbohydrates being fermented by plaque bacteria to acid.

2 Caries detection and diagnosis requires a meticulous systematic approach.

3 The pre-cavitation lesion is a danger sign indicating the need for prevention.

4 The four practical pillars to caries prevention are toothbrushing, diet, fluoride, and fissure sealing.

5 Preventive advice must be given to the parent and child and should be appropriate to the age and circumstances of the child.

6 Motivation and continuous encouragement are essential if prevention is to be successful.

6.7 Acknowledgement

Some parts of this text have been reproduced from *Dental Update*, by permission of George Warman Publications.

6.8 Further reading

Bader, J.D., Shugars, D.A., and Bonito, A.J. (2002). A systematic review of the performance of methods for identifying carious lesions. *Journal of Public Health Dentistry*, **62**: 201–213.

Ekstrand, K.R., Ricketts, D.N., and Kidd, E.A. (2001). Occlusal caries: pathology, diagnosis and logical management. *Dental Update*, **28**, 380–7.

Feigal, R.J. (2002). The use of pit and fissure sealants. *Pediatric Dentistry*, **24**, 415–22.

Kidd, E.A.M. and Joyston-Bechal, S. (1996). *Essentials of dental caries* (2nd edn). Oxford University Press, Oxford.

Marinho, V.C.C., Higgins, J.P.T., Sheiham, A., and Logan, S. (2004). Combinations of topical fluoride (toothpastes, mouthrinses, gels, varnishes) versus single topical fluoride for preventing dental caries in children and adolescents. *Cochrane Database of Systematic Reviews*, Issue 1, CD002781.pub2.

Naylor, M.N. (1994). Second International Conference on Declining Caries. *International Dental Journal*, **44** (Suppl. 1), 363–458.

Nyvad, B., ten Cate, J.M., and Robinson, C. (eds.) (2004). Cariology in the 21st Century. *Caries Research*, **38**, 167–329.

Paris, S., Hopfenmuller, W., and Meyer-Lueckel, H. (2010). Resin infiltration of caries lesions: an efficacy randomized trial. *Journal of Dental Research*, **89**, 823–6.

Pitts, N.B. (ed.) (2009). Detection, assessment, diagnosis and monitoring of caries. *Monographs in Oral Science*, Vol 21. Karger, Basel.

Rugg-Gunn, A.J. and Nunn, J.H. (1999). *Nutrition, diet and dental health*. Oxford University Press, Oxford.

Scottish Intercollegiate Guidelines Network. (2005). *Preventing dental caries in the pre-school child. National Guideline*. Royal College of Physicians, Edinburgh.

6.9 References

Ahovuo-Saloranta, A., Hiiri, A., Nordblad, A., Mäkelä, M., and Worthington, H.V. (2008). Pit and fissure sealants for preventing dental decay in the permanent teeth of children and adolescents. *Cochrane Database of Systematic Reviews*, Issue 4, CD001830.

Ashwell, M. (1991). 4: The COMA Report on dietary reference values. *Nutrition Bulletin*, **16**, 132–5.

Axelsson, P., Lindhe, J., and Waseby, J. (1976). The effect of various plaque control measures on gingivitis and caries in schoolchildren. *Community Dentistry and Oral Epidemiology*, **4**, 232–9.

British Society of Paediatric Dentistry. (2000). Guideline for the use of fissure sealants including management of the stained fissure in first permanent molars. *International Journal of Paediatric Dentistry*, **20** (Suppl 1), 3.

Burt, B.A. (1998). Prevention policies in the light of the changed distribution of dental caries. *Acta Odontologica Scandinavica*, **56**, 179–86.

Burt, B.A. and Pai, S. (2001). Sugar consumption and caries risk: a systematic review. *Journal of Dental Education*, **65**, 1017–23.

Duggal, M.S., Toumba, K.J., Amaechi, B.T., Kowash, M.B., and Higham, S.M. (2001). Enamel demineralization *in situ* with various frequencies of carbohydrate consumption with and without fluoride toothpaste. *Journal of Dental Research*, **80**, 1721–4.

Ekstrand, K.R., Bruun, G., and Bruun, M. (1998). Plaque and gingival status as indicators for caries progression on approximal surfaces. *Caries Research*, **32**, 41–5.

European Academy of Paediatric Dentistry (2009). Guidelines on the use of fluoride in children: an EAPD policy document. *European Archives of Paediatric Dentistry*, **10**, 129–35.

Faculty of General Dental Practice (UK) (2004). *Selection criteria for dental radiography* (2nd edn). Faculty of General Dental Practice (UK), London.

Holm, A.K. (1990). Caries in the preschool child: international trends. *Journal of Dentistry*, 18, 291–5.

Holt, R.D. (1990). Caries in the pre-school child: British trends. *Journal of Dentistry*, **18**, 296–9.

Jenkins, G.N. (1978). *The physiology and biochemistry of the mouth* (4th edn). Blackwell, Oxford.

Levine, R. and Stillman-Lowe, C. (2009). *The Scientific Basis of Oral Health Education* (6th edn). British Dental Association, London.

McDonagh, M.S., Whiting, P.F., Wilson, P.M., *et al.* (2000). *A systematic review of public water fluoridation*. NHS Centre for Reviews and Dissemination, York.

McMahon, A.D., Blair, Y., McCall, D.R., and Macpherson, L.M. (2010). The dental health of three-year-old children in Greater Glasgow, Scotland. *British Dental Journal*, **2009**, E5.

Parnell, C., Whelton, H., and O'Mullane, D. (2009). Water fluoridation. *European Archives of Paediatric Dentistry*, **10**, 141–8.

Scottish Intercollegiate Guidelines Network (2000). *Preventing dental caries in high risk children. National Guideline 47. National Guideline*. Royal College of Physicians, Edinburgh.

Shen, P., Manton, D.J., Cochrane, N.J., *et al.* (2011). Effect of added calcium phosphate on enamel remineralization by fluoride in a randomized controlled *in situ* trial. *Journal of Dentistry*, **39**, 518–25.

Soames, J.V. and Southam, J.C. (1998). *Oral pathology* (3rd edn). Oxford University Press, Oxford.

Spencer, A.J., Davies, M., Slade, G., and Brennan, D. (1994). Caries prevalence in Australasia. *International Dental Journal*, **44**, 415–23.

Toumba, K.J. (2001). Slow-release devices for fluoride delivery to high-risk individuals. *Caries Research*, **35** (Suppl. 1), 10–13.

Toumba, K.J. and Duggal, M.S. (1999). Effect on plaque pH of fruit drinks with reduced carbohydrate content. *British Dental Journal*, **186**, 626–9.

von der Fehr, F.R. (1994). Caries prevalence in the Nordic countries. *International Dental Journal*, **44**, 371–8.

7
Treatment of dental caries in the preschool child

S.A. Fayle

Chapter contents

7.1 Introduction

Dental caries is still one of the most prevalent pathological conditions in the child population of most Western countries. A UK study of children aged from 1.5 to 4.5 years demonstrated that 17% have decay, and in many parts of the UK up to 50% of the child population has experience of decay by the time they are 5 years of age. Dental caries is associated with significant morbidity in children, and treatment of dental caries (and its sequelae) is currently the most common reason for a child's requiring general anaesthesia (GA) in the UK. Successfully managing decay in very young children presents the dentist with a number of significant challenges. This chapter will outline approaches to the management of the preschool child with dental caries. (See Key Points 7.1.)

Key Points 7.1

- Dental caries is one of the most prevalent diseases in the preschool child population of Western countries.
- By 5 years of age up to 50% of the child population have experienced dental decay.

7.2 Patterns of dental disease seen in preschool children

7.2.1 Early childhood caries

Early childhood caries (ECC) is a term used to describe dental caries presenting in the primary dentition of young children. Terms such as 'nursing bottle mouth', 'bottle mouth caries', or 'nursing caries' are used to describe a particular pattern of dental caries in which the upper primary incisors and upper first primary molars are usually most severely affected. The lower first primary molars are also often carious, but the lower incisors are usually spared—being either entirely caries free or only mildly affected (Fig. 7.1). Some children present with extensive caries that does not follow the 'nursing caries' pattern. Such children often have multiple carious teeth and may be slightly older (3 or 4 years of age) at initial presentation (Fig. 7.2). This presentation is sometimes called 'rampant caries'. However, there is no clear distinction between rampant caries and nursing caries, and the term 'early childhood caries' has been suggested as a suitable all-encompassing term.

In many cases, early childhood caries is related to the frequent consumption of a drink containing sugars from a bottle or 'dinky' type comforters (these have a small reservoir that can be filled with a drink) (Fig. 7.3). Fruit-based drinks are most commonly associated with nursing caries. Even many of those claiming to have 'low sugar' or 'no added

sugar' appear to be capable of causing caries. The sparing of the lower incisors seen in nursing caries is thought to result from shielding of the lower incisors by the tongue during suckling, whilst at the same time they are being bathed in saliva from the sublingual and submandibular ducts. The upper incisors, on the other hand, are bathed in fluid from the bottle/feeder.

Frequency of consumption is a key factor. Affected children often have a history of taking a bottle to bed as a comforter, or using a bottle as a constant comforter during the daytime. Research has shown that children who tend to fall asleep with the bottle in their mouths are most likely to get ECC, and this is probably a reflection of the dramatic reduction in salivary flow that occurs as a child falls asleep. However, the link between bottle habits and ECC is not absolute, and studies have suggested that other factors, such as linear enamel defects, malnutrition, and hypomaturation enamel defects on second primary molars, may play an important role in the aetiology of this condition in some children.

There is some circumstantial evidence that, in a few cases, ECC may be associated with prolonged on-demand breastfeeding. Breast milk contains 7% lactose and, again, frequent prolonged on-demand consumption appears to be an important aetiological factor. Most affected children sleep with their parents, suckle during the night, and are often

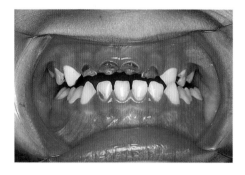

Figure 7.1 Early childhood caries presenting as nursing caries in a 2-year-old child.

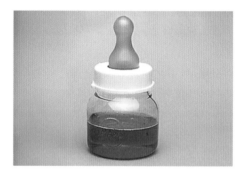

Figure 7.3 Dinky type comforter with a small reservoir that can be filled with something to drink.

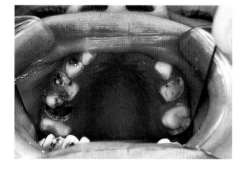

Figure 7.2 Extensive caries affecting primary molars in a 4-year-old child.

Key Points 7.2

- Early childhood caries (ECC) is an all-encompassing term that can be used to describe dental caries presenting in preschool children.
- The most commonly presenting pattern of ECC is often called 'nursing caries' or 'bottle mouth caries', where the upper anterior primary teeth are carious but the lower anterior teeth are usually spared.
- A prime aetiological factor is frequent consumption of a sweetened or fruit-based drink from a bottle or dinky feeder.
- Enamel defects and malnutrition may also play a role in the causation of ECC.

still being breastfed at 2 years of age or older. It is important to appreciate that this does not imply that normal breastfeeding up to around 1 year of age is bad for teeth, but that prolonging on-demand feeding beyond that age may carry a risk of causing dental caries. Experiments in animal models suggest that cows' milk (which contains 4% lactose) is not cariogenic, although some clinical studies have suggested that the night-time consumption of cows' milk from a bottle might be associated with early childhood caries in some children. Whether or not cows' milk has the potential to contribute to caries is currently uncertain. (See Key Points 7.2.)

7.3 Identifying preschool children in need of dental care

Identification of dental caries at an early stage is highly desirable if preventive measures and restorative care are to be successful. Many parents are under the misapprehension that they do not need to take their child for a dental check-up visit until age 4 or 5 years. Up to the end of the 1990s, the Community Dental Service in the UK (previously the School Dental Service) provided dental screening in schools. This often identified untreated caries in children who had not already had their first dental check-up. However, in recent years regular screening for dental disease in UK schools has been radically reduced or, in some areas, has ceased altogether, removing this 'safety net'. Therefore it is more important than ever that parents understand the need to seek oral health assessment for their children from an early age.

Parents should be encouraged to bring their child for a dental check (oral health assessment) as soon as he/she has teeth, usually around 6–12 months of age. This allows appropriate preventive advice regarding tooth-cleaning, fluoride toothpastes, and the avoidance of inappropriate bottle habits. It also allows the child to become familiar with the dental environment and enables the dentist to identify any carious deterioration of the teeth at an early stage. Other health professionals, such as health visitors, can also be valuable in delivering key preventive advice and helping to identify young children with possible decay. Hence making contact with local health visitors and delivering dental health messages via mother and toddler groups can be useful strategies. Recent guidelines published by the Department of Health, the Scottish Intercollegiate Guidelines Network (SIGN) and the Scottish Dental Clinical Effectiveness Programme (SDCEP) (see References) are valuable resources and provide information in a form suitable for sharing with other health professionals. (See Key Points 7.3.)

> **Key Points 7.3**
>
> - Parents should be encouraged to bring their children for a dental check-up as soon as the child has teeth (around 6 months of age).
> - Making contact with local health visitors, baby clinics, and mother-and-baby groups can be effective ways of getting dental information to the parents of preschool children.

7.4 Management of pain at first attendance

Unfortunately, the preschool child with caries has often already experienced pain when he/she first attends a dental surgery. Not only does this present the immediate problem of having to consider active treatment in a very young inexperienced patient, but also these problems are often compounded by the child's lack of sleep and the time constraints on the dentist.

Pulpitis can sometimes be effectively managed, in the short term, by gentle excavation of caries and dressing with a zinc oxide and eugenol based material, such as IRM (intermediate restorative material). Polyantibiotic and steroid pastes (e.g. Ledermix) may be useful beneath such dressings, and over/near exposure of the pulp.

The pulp chamber of abscessed teeth can sometimes be accessed by careful hand excavation, in which case placing a dressing of polyantibiotic paste on cotton wool within the pulp chamber will frequently lead to resolution of the swelling and symptoms. An acute and/or spreading infection or swelling may require the prescription of systemic antibiotics, although there is little rationale for the use of antibiotics in cases of toothache without associated soft tissue infection/inflammation.

Dental infection causing significant swelling of the face, especially where the child is febrile or unwell, constitutes a dental emergency and consideration should be given to referral to a specialized centre for immediate management. (See Key Points 7.4.)

> **Key Points 7.4**
>
> - Pain is a common presenting feature in preschool children.
> - Appropriate dressing of teeth will usually help to temporarily manage pain and localized infection.
> - Antibiotics should be prescribed where acute soft tissue swelling or signs of systemic involvement (e.g. pyrexia) are present.
> - Children with increasing facial swelling and/or significant systemic involvement should be referred to a specialized centre for urgent management.

7.5 Principles of diagnosis and treatment planning for preschool children

When planning dental treatment for preschool children, it is important to appreciate that dental caries of enamel is essentially a childhood disease and that progression of caries in the primary dentition can be rapid. Therefore early diagnosis and prompt instigation of appropriate treatment is important. Preschool children should be routinely examined for dental caries relatively frequently (at least two or three times per year). More frequent examination (e.g. every 3 months) may be justified for children in high-risk groups. Approximal caries is common in primary molars so, in children considered to be at increased risk of developing dental caries and where posterior contacts are closed, a first set of bitewing radiographs should be taken at 4 years of age, or as soon as practically possible after that (Fig. 7.4). In such children consideration should be given to repeating bitewings at least annually in the first instance. (See Key Points 7.5.)

> ### Key Points 7.5
>
> - Coronal enamel caries is essentially a childhood disease.
> - In children deemed to be at increased risk of developing caries, bitewing radiographs should be obtained at 4 years of age, or as soon as practically possible after that, and consideration should be given to repeating such radiographs at least annually.

7.6 Preventive care

Preventive measures are the cornerstone of the management of dental caries in children. There is often a failure to appreciate that those aspects of care we refer to as prevention are actually a fundamental part of the treatment of dental caries. Repairing the damage caused by dental caries is also important, but this will only be successful if the causes of that damage have been addressed. A good analogy is that of a burning house. Repairing the house (new windows, roof, furniture, etc.) is important, but all this will be of little benefit in the long term if the fire has not been put out! A structured approach to prevention should form a key part of the management of every preschool child. In the UK, a number of published guidelines focusing on the prevention of oral disease provide an invaluable resource (SIGN 2000, 2005; Department of Health 2009; SDCEP 2010). (See Key Point 7.6.)

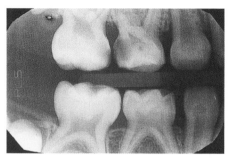

(a)

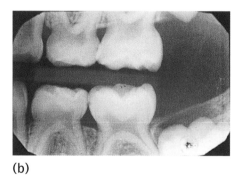

(b)

Figure 7.4 (a) Right and (b) left bitewing radiographs of a 4-year-old child. The caries in the upper right molars would be clinically obvious but the early approximal lesions in the lower left molars would not. Bitewing radiographs not only enable an accurate diagnosis, but also allow early lesions to be compared on successive radiographs to enable a judgement to be made about caries activity and progression.

> ### Key Point 7.6
>
> Preventive measures are the cornerstone to the successful treatment of dental caries in children.

7.6.1 Fluorides

Self-administered

Fluoride toothpaste

Parents should be advised to start brushing their child's teeth with a fluoride toothpaste as soon as the first tooth erupts, at around 6 months of age. A toothpaste containing 1000ppm fluoride should be advised for children considered to be at low risk of developing caries. Toothpastes with a lower fluoride concentration may be justified in areas receiving fluoridated water supplies, but the available evidence suggests that sub-1000ppm toothpaste has little or no caries-preventive effect if other sources of fluoride are not available. In the UK, the Department of Health now supports prescribing toothpastes containing higher concentrations of fluoride (i.e. 1350–1500ppm) to preschool children deemed to be at higher risk of developing caries, irrespective of their age. Where higher concentration toothpastes are prescribed for preschool children, parents should be counselled to ensure that brushing is supervised (see Section 7.6.4), small amounts of toothpaste are applied to the brush (up to 3 years a 'thin smear'; 3 years and above a 'small pea-size blob'), and that children spit out as well as possible (but avoid rinsing) after brushing. (See Key Point 7.7.)

Key Point 7.7

In areas without optimum levels of fluoride in the water supply, fluoride toothpaste is the most important method of delivering fluoride to preschool children.

Fluoride supplements

Supplementary fluoride, in the form of either drops or tablets, may be considered in those at high risk of caries and in children in whom dental disease would pose a serious risk to general health (e.g. children at increased risk of endocarditis). Such supplementation is only maximally effective if given long term and regularly. Unfortunately, studies have shown that long-term compliance with daily fluoride supplement protocols is poor, and consequently the most recent UK guidelines from the Department of Health and SDCEP no longer emphasize the routine prescription of fluoride supplements, focusing instead on the delivery of fluoride in toothpastes and professionally applied varnishes. Parental motivation and regular reinforcement are essential for such measures to be effective. If prescription is considered appropriate, dosage should follow the protocol advised by the British Society of Paediatric Dentistry (Table 7.1). No supplements should be prescribed if the water fluoride level is greater than 0.7ppm. The European Academy of Paediatric Dentistry still advocates dietary supplementation with fluoride, but with a lower maximum daily dose (0.5mg/day).

Fluoride mouth rinses

Fluoride mouth rinses are contraindicated in children less than 6 years of age because of the risk of excessive ingestion.

Table 7.1 Dosage schedule for fluoride supplements in areas where the water supply contains ≤0.3ppm as currently advised by the British Society of Paediatric Dentistry

Age	Fluoride dose per day (mg)
6 months to 3 years	0.25
3–6 years	0.50
≥6 years	1.00
In areas with water supplies containing more than 0.3ppm but less than 0.7ppm of fluoride dentists should consider a lower dosage, i.e. 6 months–3 years no supplementation, 3–6 years 0.25mg, and 6 years and over 0.5mg.	

Professionally applied fluorides

Fluoride can be applied professionally in the form of gels (acidulated phosphate fluoride (APF)), APF foams, and varnishes. APF gels and foams are not currently widely available in the UK and, in any case, are considered unsuitable for preschool children because of the risks of over-ingestion. Application of fluoride varnish can be effective at reducing caries experience and valuable in the management of early, smooth surface, and approximal carious lesions (Fig. 7.5). Regular professional application of fluoride varnish at least twice yearly for all children, increasing to three or four times yearly in children deemed to be at high caries risk, is advocated in the UK. The most popularly used varnishes contain 5% sodium fluoride (i.e. 22 600ppm fluoride). Hence, when using these products in young children, care should be taken to avoid overdosage (see below). Varnishes containing even higher concentrations of fluoride are available, but these are generally considered too concentrated for use in preschool children.

Fluoride overdosage

A dose of 1mg F/kg body weight can be enough to produce symptoms of toxicity and a dose of 5mg F/kg is considered to be potentially fatal. Symptoms of toxicity include nausea, vomiting, hypersalivation, abdominal pain (production of hydrogen fluoride (HF)), and diarrhoea. Subsequently, depression of plasma calcium levels results in convulsions, and cardiac and respiratory failure. The appropriate management of fluoride overdosage is detailed in Table 7.2.

Some of the terms used when describing fluoride toxicity are given in Table 7.3. In a 10kg, 18-month-old child, the ingestion of 0.5mL of a 2.26% fluoride varnish can produce toxicity, and slightly more than 2mL may be a potentially lethal dose (PLD). In this 10-kg child the safely tolerated dose (STD) would be 10mg F, the PLD 50g F, and the certainly lethal dose (CLD) 320–640mg F.

Toothpaste containing 1000ppm F will contain 1mg F per gram or per inch (25mm) of paste. Toothpaste tubes vary from 25g to 140g. Even if the larger tube was completely swallowed the amount of fluoride (140mg F) would still be less than the CLD for the 10-kg child, but would exceed the PLD. A container of 120 tablets (each 1mg) contains 120mg F. Again, this would be within the CLD but exceed the PLD. All containers with fluoride tablets should have childproof tops and be kept out of reach of young children.

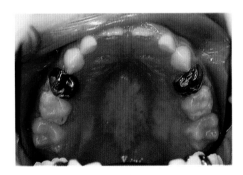

Figure 7.5 Site-specific application of fluoride varnish.

Table 7.2 Management of accidental fluoride overdosage

Amount swallowed (mg F/kg body weight)	Management
<5	Give milk to slow the absorption of fluoride.
5–15	The stomach contents need to be emptied unless other poisons were simultaneously swallowed. Ipecacuanha emetic mixture, paediatric BP (Ipecac syrup), at a dose of 10mL for a 6- to18-month-old child, 15mL for older children, and 30mL for adults should be given. In addition, milk, Epsom salts, or aluminium hydroxide antacid mixture will help to slow the absorption of any remaining fluoride.
>15	Urgent admission to a paediatric intensive care unit for neurological, cardiological, and respiratory support.

Table 7.3 Terms used in relation to fluoride toxicity

Safely tolerated dose (STD)	Dose below which symptoms of toxicity are unlikely to occur
	Usually considered to be 1mg/kg body weight
Potentially lethal dose (PLD)	Lowest dose associated with a fatality, i.e. 5mg/kg body weight
Certainly lethal dose (CLD)	Survival after consuming this amount of fluoride is unlikely
	Considered to be 32–64mg/kg body weight

7.6.2 Chlorhexidine gels

Clinical research in very young children is limited, but there is substantial agreement that daily professional applications of chlorhexidine followed by applications every few months can be significant in controlling caries. This probably results from chlorhexidine's ability to reduce the levels of *Streptococcus mutans* in both saliva and plaque.

7.6.3 Fissure sealants

Although not used routinely in the primary dentition, fissure sealants may be of value on primary molars (especially second primary molars) where one or more primary molars has already developed occlusal caries.

7.6.4 Toothbrushing

Plaque removal with a soft small-headed toothbrush in combination with a suitable fluoride toothpaste should start as soon as the child's first tooth erupts. Preschool children need help from their parents if effective oral hygiene is to be maintained, so parental involvement in

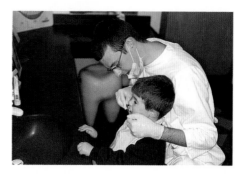

Figure 7.6 Standing or kneeling behind the child in front of the sink or mirror is often the easiest way to brush a young toddler's teeth effectively.

oral hygiene instruction is essential. Some toddlers can be resistant to parental (and professional!) attempts to brush their teeth. Parents should be encouraged to persevere through such difficulties, ensuring that their child's teeth are thoroughly cleaned at least once daily. Standing or kneeling behind the child in front of the sink or mirror is often the easiest way to brush a young toddler's teeth effectively (Fig. 7.6). Supervision of toothbrushing is also important to avoid over-ingestion of toothpaste. (See Key Points 7.8.)

Key Points 7.8

- Preschool children need help with toothbrushing.
- Parents should help with brushing to ensure effective cleaning and avoid over-ingestion of fluoride toothpaste.

7.6.5 Diet

Frequent consumption of drinks and food containing sugars is a key aetiological feature in many preschool children who present with caries. Hence reducing the frequency of sugar-containing food and drinks is a key dietary message to deliver to parents. For such advice to be effective, it must be delivered in an understanding way and should take into account some of the difficulties parents may face in making such changes to their child's diet. Young children have a high metabolic rate and their dietary calorific requirements are high. Some young children with early childhood caries are also 'poor eaters'; their parents report that the child does not eat well at meal times. Such children often make up the calories missed at meal times by consuming fruit-based drinks, which are high in calories, between meals. As well as helping to meet the child's nutritional requirements, this may suppress the appetite so that when the next mealtime approaches the child is not very hungry. Parents frequently misinterpret this and think that the child asks for drinks because of thirst. A history of poor sleeping is also common, with parents relating that the child 'will not sleep without the bottle'.

Once established, such cycles of behaviour can be difficult to break, and many parents have a sense of guilt that their child has dental decay, feeling that they must have done something wrong. For counselling to be effective it is essential to avoid making the parent feel excessively guilty, but to concentrate on the aetiology of the condition and practical strategies to deal with these problems. Stopping a night-time bottle habit can be achieved quickly by some parents, but can prove difficult for others. The idea of leaving the child to cry rather than giving him or her a bottle might seem a good idea whilst in the dental surgery, but it is a more challenging proposition at three o'clock in the morning! Weaning children from a night- or daytime bottle of juice can often be achieved by gradually making the juice in the bottle more dilute over a period of a few weeks until the contents become just water. At this point the child will either discard the bottle or continue to suckle on water alone, which is, of course, non-cariogenic. Thirsty children will always drink water. (See Key Points 7.9.)

> ### Key Points 7.9
>
> - Children have a high calorific requirement.
> - Children who are poor eaters at mealtimes and snack and drink frequently between meals are more likely to get decay.

7.7 Managing behaviour

7.7.1 Managing the preschool child's behaviour in the dental setting

The importance of establishing effective communication and adopting strategies which help to alleviate anxiety, in both child and parent, have already been fully discussed (Chapter 2). Where possible, restorative treatment should be carried out under local analgesia alone, but strategies such as sedation, by either the inhalation or oral route, or GA are sometimes indicated, especially in young children with extensive disease who are in acute pain, or where a non-pharmacological approach to behaviour management has failed (Chapter 4). Whichever strategy is chosen, it is essential to involve the parent in the decision and to obtain written consent.

The fundamental principles of effectively managing child behaviour in the surgery are fully covered in Chapter 2. However, there are some specific aspects that relate particularly to very young children.

7.7.2 Parental presence

This has been a topic of great controversy for many years. Dentistry for children is complicated by the fact that the dentist must establish a working relationship and communicate effectively with both child and parent. Virtually all studies designed to investigate the effect of parental presence in the surgery on the child's cooperation with dental treatment have failed to demonstrate any difference between behaviour with or without the parent present. Only one reasonably well-designed study, by Frankl *et al.* (1962) (from which came the useful Frankl scale), has ever suggested that parental presence might affect child behaviour. Their results indicated that children of around 4 years old and younger behaved more positively when parents were present. However, no difference was demonstrated in older children.

In most of the aforementioned studies, parents were carefully instructed to sit quietly in the surgery and not to interfere with dentist–child communication, so as to avoid the introduction of inconsistent variables. Frankl *et al.* commented on this in their concluding comments: 'the presence of a passively observing mother can be an aid to the child. This can be accomplished if the mother is motivated positively, is instructed explicitly and co-operates willingly in the role of a "silent helper"' (Frankl *et al.* 1962).

Certainly, having the parent present in the surgery when treating young children facilitates effective communication and helps to fulfil the requirements of informed consent. It also has the advantage that if any problems arise, or the child becomes upset during treatment, the parent is fully aware of the circumstances and of the dentist's approach to management. If a parent is sitting outside and hears their 3-year-old child start to cry in the surgery, events associated with the child's distress can easily be misinterpreted. Also, studies have shown that many parents wish to be present during dental treatment, especially at the child's first visit. Having said this, in the absence of any convincing evidence one way or the other, having the parent present during the treatment of preschool children remains a matter of individual choice.

7.7.3 Sedation

Sedation will not necessarily convert an uncooperative child into a cooperative one. However, it can help to alleviate anxiety, improve a child's tolerance of invasive procedures, and increase his/her ability to cope with prolonged treatment. Several routes of administration are available, but only inhalation sedation is considered to be generally suitable for delivery of dental care to preschool children in the primary dental care setting. Orally and/or nasally administered sedation is also practised in some centres, but its use is usually restricted to appropriately trained teams. Delivery of intravenous sedation for young children is considered to be highly specialized (usually only delivered by anaesthetists), and is currently considered to be of little value for the delivery of dental care. (See Key Points 7.10.)

> ### Key Points 7.10
>
> - Whether or not the parent is present does not seem to have a great effect on the child's behaviour in the surgery.
> - Very young children are probably more settled when the parent is present.
> - Parents should be encouraged to adopt the role of 'silent helper'.

Inhalation sedation with nitrous oxide and oxygen produces both sedation and analgesia. The reader is referred to Chapter 4 for a full review of this technique. The technique works most effectively on children who wish to cooperate but are too anxious to do so. Its use for preschool children is limited to those who are able to tolerate the nasal hood, but where this can be achieved, the technique is often effective.

Orally administered sedation has the advantage that, once administered, no further active cooperation from the child is required for the drug to take effect. However, unlike inhalation or intravenous sedation, it is impossible to titrate the dose of the drug to the patient's response, which results in some variation in effect from one patient to another.

Over the years, many agents have been advocated for use as oral sedative agents in dentistry, but none of these is ideal. In studies, most of the more popular agents produce a successful outcome in 60–70% of cases. For this reason, some workers, especially in the USA, advocate combinations of oral drugs, sometimes supplemented with inhaled nitrous oxide and oxygen, in order to achieve a more reliable result. However, administering multiple sedation drugs does not fall within the definition of 'simple dental sedation', where only a single sedative drug should be used. Many authorities consider such 'polypharmacy' to carry an increased risk and discourage the practice.

The most useful of the orally administered sedation agents available for preschool children are the chloral derivatives and some of the benzodiazepines.

Chloral derivatives

Chloral hydrate is a long-standing and effective sedative hypnotic. Its use in children's dentistry has been well researched; it has a good margin of safety, causes little or no respiratory depression at therapeutic levels, and has few serious side-effects. The optimum dosage is 30–50mg/kg, up to a maximum of 1.0g. However, its bitter taste makes it unpleasant to take and it is a potent gastric irritant, producing vomiting in many children. This not only has the potential to increase the child's distress, but also reduces the efficacy of the drug. Triclofos (discontinued in the UK), a derivative of chloral hydrate, causes less gastric irritation, but otherwise appears to produce similar results, although there has been little research to confirm this.

Benzodiazepines

Many benzodiazepines have been investigated as potential sedation agents for use in children's dentistry. They have a wide therapeutic index and can be reversed by flumazenil. Diazepam can be used for oral sedation, but produces prolonged sedation and has proved somewhat unpredictable in young children. Temazepam was popular some years ago, especially as its duration of action is shorter than that of diazepam. However, idiosyncratic reactions in some children have caused temazepam to fall from favour.

A number of studies using midazolam in young children, another short-acting benzodiazepine, have reported good results. Midazolam is easy to take orally and seems to offer safe and reliable sedation, with far fewer idiosyncratic reactions than temazepam. Onset of sedation is rapid (around 20 minutes) and recovery is also relatively quick. The optimum dose is 0.3–0.5mg/kg when given orally. The preparation designed for intravenous administration is used, often mixed into a small volume of a suitable fruit drink. Some studies also report successful delivery via the nasal mucosa, where doses of 0.2–0.3mg/kg have been advocated.

When using any sedative agent in children it is essential that suitable precautions are taken, that all staff involved are appropriately trained, and that appropriate emergency drugs and equipment are available. These important aspects are detailed fully in Chapter 4 and hence will not be further rehearsed here.

7.7.4 General anaesthesia

Dental extraction under GA has been used widely in the UK as a strategy for the treatment of dental caries in preschool children. Recently, the justification for such extensive use has been questioned. It is now widely agreed that GA should only take place in hospital and should only be employed where other behaviour management strategies have failed or are inappropriate. However, GA is indicated for some child patients. Comprehensive full-mouth care under intubated GA enables children with multiple carious teeth to be expediently rendered caries free in one procedure (Fig. 7.7). This approach has a place in the management of young, anxious, or disabled children with extensive caries, and in some medical conditions where multiple treatment episodes over a prolonged period increase the risks of systemic complications. Extractions under GA may be preferable to no treatment at all in the management of extensive caries in young children, especially when facilities for restorative care under GA are not available or parental motivation is poor and re-attendance for multiple visits is unlikely to occur. In addition, GA may be the only practical approach for children with acute infection.

Where GA is employed in the dental treatment of the preschool child, the emphasis must be on avoiding the need for repeated GA. Hence, each procedure needs careful planning with consideration being given to the management of all disease present in the child's mouth, while also considering the effect of premature extractions on the developing dentition. This may require the extraction plan to be quite radical, especially where facilities for restorative care under GA are not available. (See Key Points 7.11.)

Key Points 7.11

- Sedation can be a useful adjunct for anxious preschool children.
- GA should only be used where other management strategies have failed or are deemed inappropriate.

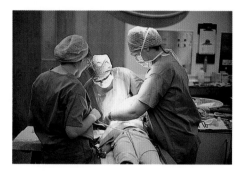

Figure 7.7 Comprehensive full-mouth care under intubated GA enables children with multiple carious teeth to be expediently rendered caries free in one procedure.

7.8 Treatment of dental caries

7.8.1 Temporization of open cavities

As an initial step in the management of caries, open cavities should be hand excavated and temporized with a suitable material such as a reinforced zinc oxide and eugenol cement, or, better still, a packable glass ionomer cement (Fig. 7.8). Carious exposures of vital or non-vital teeth can be dressed with a small amount of a polyantibiotic steroid paste (Ledermix) on cotton wool covered by a suitable dressing material.

Dressing open cavities has a number of advantages. It serves as a simple and straightforward way of introducing the child to dental procedures. By removing soft caries and temporarily occluding cavities, the oral loading of *Streptococcus mutans* is significantly reduced. It helps to reduce sensitivity, making toothbrushing and eating more comfortable, and also makes inadvertent toothache less likely. If a suitable material is used, it can produce a source of low-level fluoride release within the mouth. (See Key Points 7.12.)

> ### Key Points 7.12
>
> Temporization of teeth:
>
> - helps to reduce dental sensitivity and prevent toothache occurring before definitive care is complete;
> - reduces the oral load of *Streptococcus mutans*;
> - serves as an introduction to dental treatment;
> - provides a source for fluoride release if a glass-ionomer-based material is used.

7.8.2 Definitive restoration of teeth

The highly active nature of dental caries in the young primary dentition should be borne in mind when planning restorative care, but it is also important to plan to carry out such care in a way that the child can successfully accept. Approaches such as 'tell–show–do' (Chapter 2) and behaviour-shaping utilizing positive reinforcement to encourage appropriate behaviours are important. Communicating in terms the child can understand, and using vocabulary that avoids negative associations, is also important. For example, the term 'local anaesthetic' will mean nothing to most children, and words such as 'injection' and 'needle' may convey the suggestion of pain or discomfort. Suitable alternative terms might be 'sleepy juice' or 'jungle juice'. Such 'childrenese' can be developed for most routine dental equipment and procedures (Table 7.4).

The pace of treatment should take into account the preschool child's need to be familiarized with the dental environment and equipment. Starting treatment by temporizing any open cavities as described above serves as an easy introduction to operative care.

From that point on, planning to include both a preventive and a restorative component at each visit allows effective treatment to progress at a reasonable pace. Table 7.5 shows one way of constructing a treatment plan for a typical young child with caries. It is customary to start with treatment in the upper arch first as this is usually easier for both the child

and the dentist, although this approach may need to be modified if there are lower teeth in urgent need of attention. Appropriate use of local analgesia (Chapter 5) and rubber dam (Chapter 8) cannot be overemphasized, and any dentist treating young children needs to be proficient at both. Many preschool children are far more accepting of carefully delivered local analgesia than most dentists realize. Using techniques to

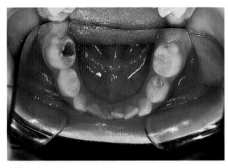

(a)

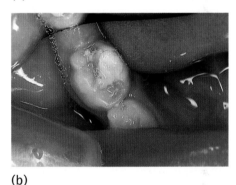

(b)

Figure 7.8 The large cavity in the lower-right second primary molar (a) has been hand excavated and temporized with a packable glass ionomer cement (b).

Table 7.4 Common terms used for introducing dental equipment to children

Item of equipment	Suitable term for children
Slow handpiece	Buzzy bee
	Buzzy brush
Airotor	Wizzy brush
	Tooth shower
Air/water syringe	Water spray
Local anaesthetic	Jungle juice
	Sleepy juice
Dental mirror	Spoon (with a mirror on the end)
Dental probe	Tickling stick
Rubber dam	Rubber raincoat
Inhalation sedation	Magic wind

Table 7.5 A typical visit-by-visit treatment plan for a young child with caries

	Preventive/other	Restorative
Visit 1	History and examination Bitewing radiographs Give diet sheet Baseline plaque score and OHI	Temporization of open cavities
Visit 2	Repeat plaque score plus reinforce OHI and advise 1350–1500ppm fluoride toothpaste Collect diet sheet Apply fluoride varnish	Restoration of 63b GIC (no LA/Rdam)
Visit 3	Dietary counselling	LA, Rdam intro Restn 64 pulpot and SSC Fissure seal 65
Visit 4	Fluoride varnish application	Restn 54 do Fissure seal 55
Visit 5	Repeat plaque score	Restn 74 do Restn 75 o
Visit 6	Review + reinforce diet/fluoride advice Apply fluoride varnish	Restn 84 o Fissure seal 85
Recall period Next bitewings	4 months 8 months	

LA, local anaesthetic; Rdam, rubber dam; OHI, oral hygiene instruction.

Table 7.6 Maximum dosage in children of commonly used local anaesthetic agents

Solution	Max. dose (mg/kg)	Max. dose by age of child (mL)		
		1 year (10kg)	3 years (15kg)	5 years (20kg)
2% lidocaine/L:80 000 adrenaline (20mg/mL lidocaine)	4.4	2.2	3.6	4.4
3% prilocaine/felypressin (30mg/mL prilocaine)	6.6	2.2	3.3	4.4
4% prilocaine (40mg/mL prilocaine)	5	1.2	1.8	2.5

The size of the cartridge of LA in the UK is commonly 2.2mL.

deliver local analgesia painlessly are crucial (Chapter 5, Section 5.6) and care should be taken to avoid overdosage with local analgesics (Table 7.6). For the most commonly prescribed local anaesthetic solutions (i.e. lidocaine 2% with 1:80 000 adrenaline and prilocaine 3% with felypressin), dosage should not exceed 1 cartridge (2.2mL) per 10kg body weight in the otherwise healthy child. It is also important to explain to the child the unusual feelings associated with soft tissue analgesia, and to warn both the child and parent of the need to avoid lip biting/sucking whilst these effects persist (Chapter 5, Section 5.7.3).

Placement of the rubber dam using a trough technique, where the clamp is placed on the tooth first and then the dam is stretched over (as described in Chapter 8), is, in the author's experience, the most straightforward approach in the young child. Careful attention to obtaining adequate analgesia of the gingival tissues, both buccally and lingually, ensures comfortable clamp placement. Intrapapillary injections are very useful for this (Chapter 5, Section 5.6.3). Encouraging the child to watch in a hand mirror helps to distract his/her attention from the intra-oral manipulations during actual placement of the dam (Fig. 7.9).

The techniques employed for definitive restoration in young children should take into account the often active nature of the disease in this age group. The use of plastic restorative materials should be limited to occlusal and small approximal lesions. Extensive caries, teeth with caries affecting more than two surfaces, and teeth requiring

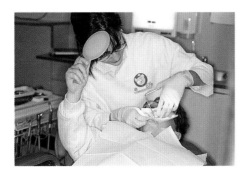

Figure 7.9 Encouraging the child to watch in a hand mirror helps to distract his/her attention from the intra-oral manipulations during rubber dam placement.

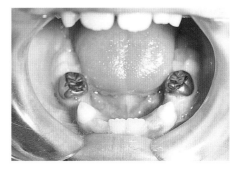

Figure 7.10 Extraction of the first primary molars with maintenance and restoration of the second primary molars.

pulpotomy or pulpectomy should be restored with stainless steel crowns. Amalgam is still widely used as a restorative material, but newer materials including glass ionomer cements, resin-modified glass ionomer cements, polyacid-modified resins (compomers), and composite resins may be preferred. However, all these materials are far more sensitive to moisture contamination and technique than amalgam, so adequate isolation, preferably with rubber dam, is essential. Cermet restorations perform poorly in primary teeth and are best avoided. A fuller discussion on material selection for the restoration of primary molars is given in Chapter 8. Composite strip crown restorations are the most effective way of repairing carious anterior teeth (Chapter 8). (See Key Points 7.13.)

analgesia—inhalation or oral sedation is a useful adjunct for anxious children. If more extractions are needed, these can sometimes be carried out at the same time as restoring adjacent teeth. However, GA is the only practical strategy for some children, in which case referral to an appropriate dental GA facility is mandatory.

When planning extractions, it is important to consider the need for balancing (Chapter 14). Factors such as the likelihood of the continued future attendance and cooperation of the child should also be borne in mind. In preschool children with extensive caries, extraction of first primary molars with maintenance and restoration of the second primary molars where possible is often a good plan (Fig. 7.10). Not only does this limit the risk of further decay by eliminating posterior primary contact areas, but also it minimizes the deleterious effect of early extraction on the developing dentition.

7.8.4 Replacing missing teeth

Where the child is motivated, dentures are surprisingly well tolerated. A simple removable acrylic denture with gum-fitted primary prosthetic teeth and clasps on the second molars can effectively restore aesthetics (Fig. 7.11). Even full dentures can be highly successful in cases where the child is keen to have teeth replaced. The methods of constructing dentures are essentially the same as those in adults. It is important that careful attention is given to cleaning such appliances to avoid them contributing to further disease. (See Key Points 7.14.)

Key Points 7.13

- Plan to carry out treatment at a pace that the child (and you) can cope with.
- Introduce young children to new equipment using a 'tell–show–do' approach.
- Make a comprehensive treatment plan at an early stage.
- Use local analgesia and rubber dam where possible.
- Select restorative material taking into account the high risk of further caries in the young child.
- Stainless steel crowns are the most effective restoration for primary molars with caries on more than two surfaces.

7.8.3 Extraction of teeth

Extraction is indicated for teeth that are unrestorable, and it may also be enforced by acute pain or infection. In preschool children the extraction of one or two teeth can often be accomplished under local

---

Key Points 7.14

- Balancing extractions should be considered when extracting in the primary dentition.
- Dentures to replace missing anterior teeth are well tolerated by motivated children.

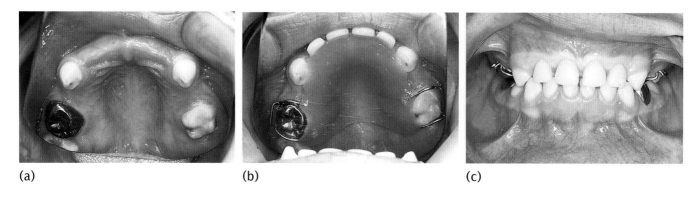

(a)   (b)   (c)

Figure 7.11 Extracted primary incisors (a) can be easily and effectively replaced by providing a removable acrylic denture (b) with gum-fitted primary prosthetic teeth (c) and clasps on the second molars.

7.9 Summary

1 Dental caries is a prevalent disease in the preschool population.

2 Nursing caries and rampant caries are common patterns of caries in preschool children.

3 Parents should be encouraged to bring their children for a dental check-up as soon as the child's first tooth has erupted.

4 Prevention is a cornerstone of the management of caries in the preschool child.

5 Planned treatment should be carried out at a pace the child can accept.

6 Preschool children need careful introduction to dental equipment and procedures.

7 Inhalation or oral sedation can be effective strategies for anxious preschool children.

8 GA should be reserved for those cases where other approaches to management either have failed or are deemed inappropriate.

9 Local analgesia is advisable for definitive restoration of all but small cavities, but care should be exercised to avoid overdosage in the small child.

10 Rubber dam makes good-quality treatment easier to achieve for both the child and dentist.

11 Choice of restorative materials should reflect the high risk of further caries in the young child.

12 Stainless steel crowns are the most effective restoration for primary molars with caries on more than two surfaces.

7.10 Further reading

British Society of Paediatric Dentistry (1997). A policy document on the dental needs of children. *International Journal of Paediatric Dentistry*, **7**, 203–7. (*BSPD consensus view document which reviews current standards of UK child dental care and suggests how these might be improved.*)

British Society of Paediatric Dentistry (2003). A policy document on oral healthcare in preschool children. *International Journal of Paediatric Dentistry*, **13**, 279–85. (*BSPD consensus document giving guidance for the delivery of oral healthcare to preschool children.*)

Duggal, M.S., Curzon, M.E.J., Fayle, S.A., Pollard, M.A., and Robertson, A.J. (2002). *Restorative techniques in paediatric dentistry* (2nd edn). Taylor & Francis, London. (*A practical guide to the restoration of carious primary teeth.*)

Seow, W.K. (1998). Biological mechanisms of early childhood caries. *Community Dentistry and Oral Epidemiology*, **26** (Suppl. 1), 8–27. (*An excellent review of the various aetiological factors involved in early childhood caries.*)

7.11 References

Department of Health (2009). *Delivering better oral health: an evidence-based toolkit for prevention* (2nd edn). Available online at:
**http://www.dh.gov.uk/en/Publicationsandstatistics/
Publications/PublicationsPolicyAndGuidance/DH_102331**

Frankl, S.N., Shiere, F.R., and Fogels, S.H.R. (1962). Should the parent remain with the child in the dental operatory? *Journal of Dentistry for Children*, **29**, 150–63.

SDCEP (2010). *Prevention and management of dental caries in children.* Available online at:
http://www.sdcep.org.uk/index.aspx?o=2332

SIGN (2000). *Preventing dental caries in children at high caries risk. Guideline no. 47.* Available online at:
http://www.sign.ac.uk/guidelines/fulltext/47/index.html

SIGN (2005). *Prevention and management of dental decay in the pre-school child. Guideline no. 83.* Available online at:
http://www.sign.ac.uk/guidelines/fulltext/83/index.html

8

Operative treatment of dental caries in the primary dentition

M.S. Duggal and P.F. Day

Chapter contents

8.1 Introduction

While there is no doubt that the best way to tackle the problem of dental caries is through an effective programme of prevention as outlined in the previous chapters, it is unfortunate that many children still suffer from the disease and its consequences. Hence there is a need to consider operative treatment to prevent the breakdown of the dentition. As discussed in earlier chapters, there are a number of different techniques and philosophies in treating dental caries. This chapter will concentrate mainly on the methods of complete caries removal. Research to support different philosophies, techniques, and materials frequently lacks evidence from randomized controlled trials, considered as the gold standard. Consequently, lower levels of evidence are used to support different techniques. More importantly dentists need to be skilled in different techniques and philosophies to ensure that appropriate care is provided to each and every child.

The removal of caries is not a new concept for the treatment of dental decay. Over the years the treatment of dental caries in children has been discussed and many attempts have been made to rationalize the management of the disease. Writing more than 150 years ago,

Harris (1839) was one of the first to address the problem of restoring the primary dentition. Even in those days he was emphasizing the importance of prevention by good toothbrushing. Caries could be arrested by 'plugging', but from his description he obviously found treatment for the young patient difficult and not as successful as in adults. However, he did emphasize the importance of looking after children's teeth: 'If parents and guardians would pay more attention to the teeth of their children, the services of the dentist would much less frequently be required', and, 'Many persons suppose that the teeth, in the early periods of childhood, require no attention, and thus are guilty of the most culpable neglect of the future well-being of those entrusted to their care'. Unfortunately, this statement still applies today.

Caries removal can be a stressful experience for the child, the parent, and the dentist. Therefore it is important that there is a positive health gain from any treatment that is provided. In this chapter we aim to outline the rationale for providing operative treatment, to give advice on the selection of appropriate ways of providing care, and to describe a few of the more useful treatment methods.

8.2 Philosophy of care

Any dental care provided for children should promote positive dental experiences, which in turn would promote positive dental attitudes in their later lives.

The importance of the history and examination cannot be underestimated. It is at this consultation that the dentist attempts to ascertain the motivation of the child and parent, the extent of decay, the age of the patient and the time that teeth are expected to survive until exfoliation, any symptoms associated with the decay, and the response of the underlying dental pulp. With this information the dentist can start to formulate a treatment plan and philosophy which is appropriate for each child.

When faced with a tooth that has caries, the first decision has to be whether it does in fact require treatment. It may be felt that the caries is so minor and prevention so effective that further progress of the lesion is unlikely. Less rationally, it may be felt that a carious tooth with a non-vital pulp is unlikely to cause great problems and may be left to

its own devices. There has been much discussion in the UK on whether most carious primary molars need to be restored at all! In the authors' view there is no doubt that untreated caries in the primary dentition causes abscesses, pain, and suffering in children. This can then need hospital admission and invasive treatment, sometimes under general anaesthesia, whereas a simple restoration, at the time when the caries was diagnosed, would have prevented this extremely distressing episode for the child. Therefore it is essential for all dentists involved in the care of young children to learn restorative techniques that give the best results in primary teeth, and this should always be alongside excellent preventive programmes. This chapter is devoted to the discussion of such techniques. Good-quality restorative care (Fig. 8.1), as and when caries is diagnosed, would also obviate the need for extractions of primary teeth under general anaesthesia for thousands of children, particularly in the UK. A treatment philosophy which the authors believe is effective in the management of caries in children is shown in Table 8.1.

8.3 Remove, restore, or leave

There are certain situations where the clinician might decide not to carry out invasive restorative procedures in primary teeth and instead use a rigorous preventive approach. Such an approach can be justified where it is likely that remineralization would occur or the tooth would be maintained in a state free from pain or infection until exfoliation. It

has been proposed (Pitts and Longbottom 1995) that it should be possible to divide lesions into those for which preventive care is advised (PCA) and those for which operative care is advised (OCA). More work is required on this concept, but the following sections discuss conflicting reasons to treat or not to treat particular carious lesions.

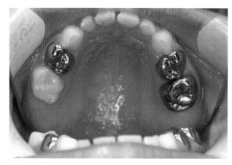

(a)

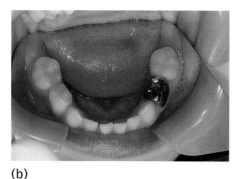

(b)

Figure 8.1 A well-restored primary dentition in a child: (a) upper arch; (b) lower arch. High-quality restorative care is supplemented with prevention in the form of sealants placed in other molars deemed to be susceptible to future carious attack.

8.3.1 Reasons not to treat

These can be divided into several distinct categories.

1. *The damage done by treatment to:*

   (a) *The affected tooth.* However conservative the technique, it is inevitable that some sound tooth tissue has to be removed when operative treatment is undertaken. This weakens the tooth and makes it more likely that problems such as cracking of the tooth or loss of vitality of the pulp may occur in the future. (See Key Point 8.1.)

Key Point 8.1

Every time that a restoration is replaced more sound tissue has to be removed, putting the tooth at further risk.

   (b) *The adjacent tooth.* It is almost inevitable when treating an approximal lesion that the adjacent tooth will be damaged. The outer surface has a far higher fluoride content than the rest of the enamel so that even a slight nick of the intact surface will remove this reservoir of fluoride. Additionally, it has been shown that early lesions that remineralize are less

Table 8.1 Five-point treatment philosophy for the provision of high-quality dental care for children

1.	Gain the cooperation and trust of the child and parent
2.	Make an accurate diagnosis and devise a treatment plan appropriate to the child's needs
3.	Comprehensive preventive care
4.	Deliver care in a manner that the child finds acceptable
5.	Use treatment methods and restorative techniques which produce a cost-effective long-lasting result

Key Points 8.2

- Early lesions that remineralize are less susceptible to caries.
- When preparing an interproximal cavity take great care not to damage the adjacent tooth.

susceptible to caries than intact surfaces, and these areas of the tooth are all too easily removed when preparing an adjacent tooth. The risk for an adjacent tooth has been demonstrated in the literature. (See Key Points 8.2.)

   (c) *The periodontal tissues.* Dental treatment can cause both acute and long-term damage to the periodontium. It is virtually impossible to avoid damaging the interdental papillae when treating approximal caries. The papillae can be protected by using rubber dam and/or wedges, and the tissues will heal fairly rapidly if well-fitting restorations are placed, but long-term damage can be more critical. Many adults can be seen to be suffering from overenthusiastic treatment of approximal caries in their youth, and while the relative importance of poor margins compared with bacterial plaque can be debated, the potential damage from approximal restorations is sufficient reason to avoid treatment unless a definite indication is present. Well-fitting stainless steel crowns in the primary dentition rarely cause gingivitis. However, when the same material is used for first permanent molars gingivitis is a common finding in late adolescence.

   (d) *The occlusion.* Poor restoration of the teeth can, over time, lead to considerable alteration of the occlusion. It is tempting when restoring occlusal surfaces to leave the material well clear of the opposing teeth to avoid difficulties, or to be unconcerned if the filling is slightly 'high'. However, this can allow the teeth to erupt into contact again or the interocclusal position to change and alter the occlusion. Often this is felt to be of little concern, but there are a large number of adults where the cumulative effect of many poorly restored teeth has severely disturbed the occlusion, thus making further treatment difficult, time-consuming, and expensive. The effect of occlusal rearrangement in the primary dentition appears to be less of an issue. The Hall technique of placing stainless steel crowns is one such example where the occlusion is left high. Currently, medium-term studies appear to show no detrimental effect with adjacent teeth over-erupting to accommodate the 'high' crown, although a significant amount of research is still required to show that this is indeed the case.

2. *The difficulty of diagnosis.* It is well known that it is difficult to diagnose dental caries accurately. Even when coarse criteria such as those developed for the UK Child Dental Health Surveys are used, there is variation between examiners. It is not just variations between examiners that need to be considered; there are also differences between the same examiner on different occasions. The implications need to be considered in relation to the decision to treat or not. The role of bitewing radiographs in the primary dentition leads to an approximate doubling in diagnostic yield for proximal caries.

3. *The slow rate of caries attack.* Caries usually progresses relatively slowly, although some individuals will show more rapid development than others. The majority of children and adolescents will have a low level of caries and progress of carious lesions will be slow. In general, the older the child at the time that the caries is first diagnosed, the slower the progression of the lesion. However, a substantial group of children will have caries that develops rapidly. This rate of caries attack will also determine how frequently bitewing radiographs in the primary and mixed dentition should be taken for children.

4. *The fact that remineralization can arrest and repair enamel caries.* It has long been known that early smooth-surface lesions are reversible. In addition, it is now accepted that the chief mechanism whereby fluoride reduces caries is by encouraging remineralization, and that the remineralized early lesion is more resistant to caries than is intact enamel. Although it is difficult to show reversal of lesions on radiographs, many studies have demonstrated that a substantial proportion of early enamel lesions do not progress over many years. (See Key Point 8.3.)

Key Point 8.3

When no plaque is present on a tooth, the caries process will stop. This emphasizes the importance of good brushing and flossing of proximal surfaces.

5. *The short life of dental restorations.* Surveys of dental treatment have often shown a rather disappointing level of success. In general, 50% of amalgam restorations in permanent teeth can be expected to fail during the 10 years following placement. Some studies have shown an even poorer success rate when looking at primary teeth, and this has been put forward as a reason for not treating these teeth. In one study, 61% of restorations placed in general practice had failed within a 23-month period.

8.3.2 Reasons to treat

1. *Adverse effects of neglect.* The fact that the treatment of approximal caries can cause damage to the affected tooth, the adjacent tooth, the periodontium, and the occlusion is a valid reason to think twice before putting bur to tooth. But a case can equally well be made that the neglect of treatment could cause as much or more damage. Lack of treatment can, and all too often does, lead to loss of contact with adjacent and opposing teeth, exposure of the pulp, resulting in the development of periapical infection, and/or loss of the tooth. At worst, the child may end up having a general anaesthetic for the removal of one or more teeth in combination with an associated facial swelling and several days in hospital on intravenous antibiotics, a process which has a significant morbidity. There is the occasional case of a child who develops lethal complications from their untreated decay.

2. *Unpredictability of the speed of attack.* While it is true that the rate of attack is usually slow, it is quite possible for the rate in any one individual to be sufficiently rapid that any delay in treatment would not then be in the best interests of the child.

3. *Difficulty in assessing whether a lesion is arrested.* Because of the normal slow rate of attack it is difficult to be sure if a lesion is arrested or merely developing very slowly. It is true that remineralization will arrest and repair early enamel lesions, but there is, in fact, little evidence that remineralization of the dentine or the late enamel lesion is common.

4. *Success when careful treatment is provided.* The majority of published studies show that class II amalgam or glass ionomer restorations in primary teeth have a poor life expectancy, but this is not the experience of the careful dentist. Some of these dentists have published their results, which show that the great majority of their restorations in primary teeth survive without further attention until they exfoliate. The treatment procedures used are not particularly difficult compared with others that dentists attempt on adults, and it is difficult to avoid the conclusion that the reasons for poor results in some studies are due to poor patient management and lack of attention to detail. It should be the aim of the profession to develop better and more effective ways of treating the disease, rather than throwing our hands up in surrender and expressing frustration just because so many restorations for primary teeth are placed without adherence to good principles of restorative dentistry.

5. *Early treatment is more successful than late treatment.* Small restorations are more successful than large restorations, and therefore if a carious lesion is going to need treatment it is better treated early rather than late. This was the rationale behind the early suggestions of a 'prophylactic filling' for pits and fissures, and for the modern versions in the form of fissure sealants and preventive resin restorations. The fact that small restorations are often more successful makes for difficult decisions when the management of caries involves preventive procedures which need both time to work and time to assess whether they have been effective.

8.3.3 Remove or restore

Once a decision has been made to treat a carious primary tooth a further decision has to be made as to whether to remove or restore it. This decision should take into account the following:

1. *The child.* Each child is an individual and treatment should be planned to provide the best that is possible for that individual. Too often treatment is given which is the most convenient for the parent or, more likely, the dentist. Is it really in the best interest of the child to remove a tooth which could be saved? A number of studies have identified tooth extraction under local anaesthetic as a significant cause of dental anxiety in children, which is not the case for restorative care. Furthermore, in the UK general anaesthesia is still widely used for removing the teeth of young children despite the risks of death, its unpleasantness, and the cost involved. (See Key Point 8.4.)

> **Key Point 8.4** !
>
> Treat the child—not the convenience of parents or dentist.

2. *The tooth.* It is not usually in a child's interest for a permanent tooth to be removed. However, if the pulp of a carious permanent tooth is exposed, a considerable amount of treatment may be required to retain it, and the prognosis for the tooth would still be poor. Therefore it may be in the child's long-term interest to lose it and to allow another tooth to take its place, either by natural drift or with orthodontic assistance. Primary teeth are often considered by parents and some dentists as being disposable items because there comes a time when they will be exfoliated naturally. However, it is an unusual child who thinks the same way! Loss of a tooth before its time has a considerable significance in a child's life. Losing a tooth early gives a message to the child that teeth are not valuable and not worth looking after. It can then be difficult to persuade a child to care for his/her teeth. Well-restored primary dentition can be a source of pride to young children and an encouragement for them to look after the succeeding teeth. It is usually more important, and fortunately rather easier, to save and restore a second primary molar than a first primary molar. While anterior teeth might be less important for the maintenance of space, their premature loss can cause low esteem in both child and parent.

3. *The stage of the disease.* It is easier for both child and dentist to restore teeth at an early stage of decay. Later, the pulp may become involved and subsequent restoration difficult, making loss of the tooth more likely.

4. *The extent of the disease.* Requirement of treatment for a large number of teeth may put a strain on a young child and, less importantly, on the parent and dentist.

The prevalence of caries in children is significantly less than it was 20 years ago, and it would be good to think that the dental profession would be able to provide effective restorative care for those who are still unfortunate enough to suffer from dental caries. Unfortunately, the care index (e.g. where teeth have been restored or extracted) is decreasing rather than increasing, suggesting that the opposite is true.

8.4 Diagnosis and treatment planning

This was discussed in Chapter 3 and will be only briefly outlined here. As stated above, the treatment of carious teeth should be based on the needs of the child. The long-term objective should be to help the child reach adulthood with an intact permanent dentition, no active caries, as few restored teeth as possible, and a positive attitude to their future dental health. If restorations are required, they should be carried out to the highest standard possible in order to maximize longevity of the restoration and avoid re-treatment prior to exfoliation.

8.4.1 Diagnosis

An accurate diagnosis of dental caries is important in the management of the primary dentition. The enamel of the primary tooth is thin compared with that of the permanent teeth and caries progresses quickly through it into the dentine, especially at the proximal area below the contact point, making an early diagnosis paramount. When caries is still confined to the enamel, preventive measures stand a chance of halting and reversing the lesion as discussed in Chapter 6.

Pulpal involvement

Once the caries is into the dentine, removal of the carious tissue and restoration of the tooth is required. Assessment of pulpal health both clinically and radiographically is essential. Caries can progress very rapidly through the primary dentine with early pulpal involvement. Because of the wide contact point in primary molars, clinical diagnosis is difficult when early dentinal caries is present. The collapse of the marginal ridge occurs once dentinal caries is well established. Research has shown that once the marginal ridge of a primary molar has broken away, the pulp of the tooth is significantly inflamed (Fig. 8.2).

Radiographs

The importance of radiographs for the diagnosis of caries in the primary dentition cannot be overemphasized (Fig. 8.3). As mentioned earlier, many early lesions may be halted or reversed by a rigorous preventive programme, but this depends on early diagnosis. While several techniques for caries diagnosis are available, bitewing (BW) radiography is by far the most acceptable and is widely available for use in general practice. Radiographs should form a routine part of any dental examination, and it is necessary to repeat radiographs for dental caries diagnosis at suitable intervals. The intervals that are appropriate to children vary according to caries risk. After an initial examination and BW radiographs, a second series should be taken within 12–24 months if the child is caries free but at 6–12 months if caries is active. Once it has been established that a child remains caries free, the interval

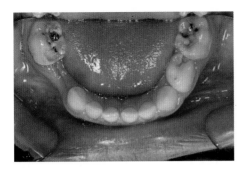

Figure 8.2 The marginal ridges of both the lower left first and lower right second primary molars have been involved in the carious process. The pulp in these teeth is likely to be inflamed.

between BWs can be increased to 24 months or even longer. However, if active caries remains a problem, 6-monthly intervals between BWs are necessary. (See Key Point 8.5.)

Key Point 8.5

Destruction of the marginal ridge of a primary molar by caries indicates probable pulpal involvement.

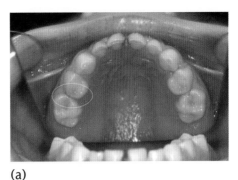

(a)

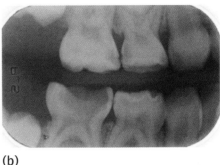

(b)

Figure 8.3 (a) A clinical examination in the upper arch gives a little clue to the presence of proximal carious lesions on both the upper right first and second primary molars. (b) However, extensive caries is evident when these are examined using BW radiographs.

8.4.2 Treatment planning

Treatment planning includes consideration of:

- the motivation of the child and parent, and their likely compliance with the preventive plan suggested;
- the extent of decay and the surfaces involved;
- the age of the patient and time that teeth are expected to survive until exfoliation;
- any symptoms associated with the decay;
- the health of the underlying dental pulp.

With this information the dentist can start to formulate a treatment plan and philosophy of care which is appropriate for the child. A logical treatment plan should be made which usually involves treating a quadrant of the mouth at a time. It used to be felt that multiple short visits placed least stress on a child, particularly if he/she was under 6 years of age. However, the most important aspect of child management is to gain the confidence of the child and make sure that there is as little discomfort as possible. Restorative care must be conducted with good pain control and management of a child's behaviour. Therefore local analgesia is mandatory, and is easily performed these days with topical analgesia, fine-gauge needles, and short-acting local analgesic agents.

Where an initial stabilization phase is planned to gain the confidence of the child and buy time for cooperation to develop, this should be clearly explained to the parents. No doubt, the least interventionist approach can be the correct one for some children, but it should be integrated within a treatment plan which is best in the long-term interest of the child and not an easy way out for the dentist. If this predisposes the child to repetitive treatment, and worse still pain, abscesses, and extractions under general anaesthesia, then it should be rejected in favour of comprehensive care using restorative techniques, such as those described in this chapter. A number of other clinical tips are useful when deciding the sequence and order of care.

Often a treatment plan should start with a relatively simple visit to introduce the child to the operative environment. This may include fissure sealant, preventive advice, or a simple buccal restoration of an anterior tooth which ideally does not require local anaesthetic.

Subsequent visits will invariably start with a simple visit using local anaesthetic (e.g. a small occlusal cavity). Where possible the order of quadrants will start with the upper arch, as this is easier to anaesthetize painlessly. If a lower quadrant is to be the starting point, consideration of using an articaine infiltration rather than a lidocaine inferior dental block may be an option as this will be a less painful injection. The presence of pain may change the order and priority of treatment visits, but wherever possible an extraction should be avoided as a first experience of operative dentistry.

Due consideration should be given to the use of a rubber dam that ensures a higher quality of restorations and can act as an aid in behaviour management. Once the tissues have been anaesthetized and the child is confident that there will be no pain, it is usually best to complete treatment on a whole quadrant. The number of visits can then be kept to a minimum and a reservoir of cooperation maintained. Where there is pulpal involvement of primary teeth, pulpotomies or pulpectomies are essential. Such teeth also need restoration with preformed metal crowns which should be placed on the same day, where clinical skill and patient cooperation allow. Finally, in each visit one or more items of preventive advice should be focused on.

8.5 Durability of restorations

Treatment decisions ought to be based on sound scientific evidence but, unfortunately, despite the great effort that has been made providing treatment over many years, little in the way of resources has been spent on clinical research into the success or otherwise of dental treatment methods. This is especially true with regard to the primary dentition. Slowly, more and more high-quality studies are being reported for different interventions, but many recommendations are based on retrospective case series and therefore need to be treated with caution.

The choice of restoration for primary teeth is based upon the criteria described in Section 8.4.2. For example, if the marginal ridge has broken away, simple proximal restoration will fail if the extent of pulpal inflammation is not considered when the choice of material is made.

8.5.1 Conventional restorative materials

Conventional restorative materials are mainly limited in use to occlusal lesions, small proximal lesions, and cavities on anterior teeth. Where caries is more extensive or involves more than two surfaces a stainless steel crown should be the default material for posterior primary molars. The benefits and disadvantages of different plastic materials are discussed in the following paragraphs. As with all materials, the operator's attention to detail and skill are paramount in ensuring optimal survival, no matter what restorative material is chosen.

Silver amalgam

Silver amalgam has been used for restoring teeth for over 150 years and, despite the fact that it is not tooth coloured and there have been repeated concerns about its safety (largely unfounded), it is still widely used. A recent randomized trial (New England Children's Amalgam Trial (NECAT)) could find no difference in neuropsychological or renal complications between the use of amalgam and compomer/composite when restoring posterior primary or permanent molars. However, amalgam has been discontinued in some Scandinavian countries because of environmental concerns.

Amalgam is relatively easy to use, is tolerant of operator error, and has yet to be bettered as a material for economically restoring posterior teeth. Modern non-gamma 2 alloy restorations have been shown to have extended lifetimes in permanent teeth when placed under good conditions, and have also been shown to be much less sensitive to poor handling than tooth-coloured materials.

In clinical trials and retrospective studies, no intracoronal material has so far performed more successfully than amalgam. This finding was confirmed in the NECAT study with amalgam outperforming compomer in primary molars and composite in permanent molars.

Stainless steel crowns

These were introduced in 1950 and have gained wide acceptance in North America. They have been less popular in Europe, being seen by most dentists as too difficult to use, although in reality they are often easier to place than some intracoronal restorations (Fig. 8.4). The recent development of the Hall technique, which simplifies placement, may increase their use, even though more research is required to assess the suitability of this technique. Because the entire crown of the tooth is covered, the stainless steel crown rarely needs to be replaced owing to recurrent caries or new caries at a site distant to the original filling.

All published studies have shown stainless steel crowns to have a higher success rate than all other restorative materials in primary teeth. They are certainly the preferred treatment option for primary molars with anything other than minimal caries.

Stainless steel crowns are also advocated for hypoplastic/hypomineralized or very carious first permanent molars, where they act as provisional restorations prior to either strategic removal at age 9–12 years or later restoration with a cast crown (Fig. 8.5). Etched retained castings can now be used for the definitive restoration of permanent teeth with developmental defects without involvement of the approximal surface or gingival margin; more conservative provisional restorations than stainless steel crowns should be considered if this is intended.

Composite resin

Composite resins came on the market in the early 1970s and have been modified since then in an attempt to improve their properties. The development of acid etching at the time that these materials were introduced has ensured that they have performed reasonably well in terms of marginal seal. They are sensitive to variations in technique and take longer to place than equivalent amalgam restorations. They must be placed in a dry field (Fig. 8.6).

The long-term success of composite resins is jeopardized by their instability in water. The best materials have maximum inorganic filler

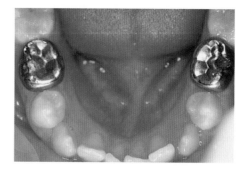

Figure 8.4 Restoration of lower second primary molars with stainless steel crowns 7 years after placement.

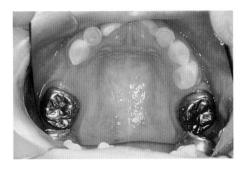

Figure 8.5 Temporary restoration of carious upper first permanent molars with stainless steel crowns in an 8-year-old child with a high caries rate.

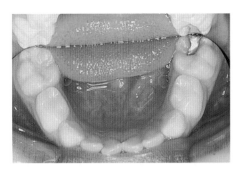

Figure 8.7 Distal–occlusal restorations on both lower second primary molars after 3 years. One is restored with conventional amalgam and the other with glass ionomer cement.

composite resins. As they are made from glasses with a high fluoride content, they not only provide a sustained fluoride release over an extended period but also act as a rechargeable fluoride reservoir, which may protect adjacent surfaces from caries progression.

Glass ionomers adhere to enamel and dentine without the need for acid etching, do not suffer from polymerization shrinkage, and, once set, are dimensionally stable in conditions of high humidity such as those existing in the mouth (Fig. 8.7). Similarly to composite resins, it is imperative that they are placed in a dry field. Glass ionomers should be seen as stabilization materials and have consistently shown poor results for proximal restorations over a time period of more than 12–24 months. (See Key Point 8.7.)

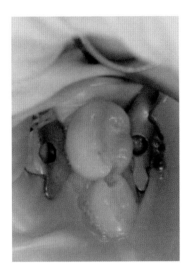

Figure 8.6 Rubber dam placement prior to restoration of approximal lesions with composite resin.

> ### Key Point 8.7
>
> Glass ionomer is not recommended for use in proximal cavities in the primary molars.

levels and low water absorption, but will deteriorate over time. The longevity of composite material appears to be similar to that of RMGIC or compomer for occlusal and small proximal restorations in primary teeth. The NECAT study showed inferior results compared with amalgam for the restoration of permanent molars in a population aged 6–10 years. (See Key Point 8.6.)

> ### Key Point 8.6
>
> All composite resin and glass ionomer restorations must be placed in a dry field and require excellent operator skill and attention to detail.

Glass ionomer

Glass ionomer cements came on to the market in the late 1970s and have been modified since then in order to enhance their properties. Current materials are much improved and have some advantages over

Resin-modified glass ionomer cements (RMGICs)

These consist of a glass ionomer cement to which has been added a resin system that will allow the material to set quickly using light or chemical catalysts (or both) while allowing the acid–base reaction of the glass ionomer to take place. Thus the materials will set, albeit rather slowly, without the need for the resin system and the essential qualities of a glass ionomer cement should be retained (Fig. 8.8).

Polyacid-modified composite resin (compomer)

These materials have a much higher resin content and the acid–base reaction of the glass ionomers does not take place. Therefore although they are easier to use (being premixed in capsules), there is some doubt as to the longer-term benefits compared with conventional composite resins (Fig. 8.9). Survival of compomer appears to be similar to RMGIC, composite, and amalgam in some studies (Marks *et al.* 1999; Welbury *et al.* 2000; Qvist *et al.* 2010), but its performance was poorer than that of amalgam in the NECAT study over a 5-year follow-up period. The NECAT study reported no clinical benefit over amalgam from the fluoride released by the compomer.

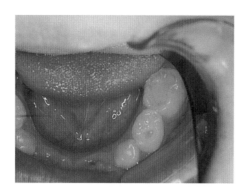

Figure 8.8 Resin-modified glass polymer restoration after 2 years in a lower second primary molar.

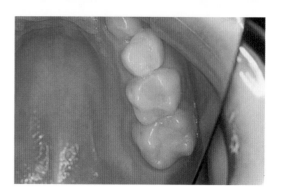

Figure 8.9 Mesial–occlusal restoration after 1 year in an upper second primary molar with polyacid-modified composite resin.

8.6 Rubber dam

Most texts that discuss operative treatment for children advocate the use of rubber dam, but it is used very little in practice despite many sound reasons for its adoption. In the UK fewer than 2% of dentists use it routinely. It is perceived as a difficult technique that is time-consuming and arduous for the patient. In fact, once mastered, the technique makes dental care for children easier and a higher standard of care can be achieved in less time than would otherwise be required. In addition, it isolates the child from the operative field, making treatment less invasive of their personal space. The benefits can be divided into three main categories as shown below.

8.6.1 Safety

Damage of soft tissues

The risks of operative treatment include damage to the soft tissues of the mouth from rotary and hand instruments and the medicaments used in the provision of endodontic and other care. Rubber dam will go a long way to preventing damage of this type.

Risk of swallowing or inhalation

There is also the risk that these items may be lost in the patient's mouth and swallowed or even inhaled, and there are reports in the literature to substantiate this risk.

Risk of cross-infection

There is considerable risk that the use of high-speed rotary instruments will distribute an aerosol of the patient's saliva around the operating room, putting the dentist and staff at risk of infection. This risk has been substantiated in the literature.

Nitrous oxide sedation

If this is used it is quite likely that mouth breathing by the child will increase the level of the gas in the environment, again putting dentist and staff at risk. The use of rubber dam in this situation will make sure that exhaled gas is routed via the scavenging system attached to the nose piece. Usually less nitrous oxide will be required for a sedative effect, increasing the safety and effectiveness of the procedure.

8.6.2 Benefits to the child

Isolation

One of the reasons that dental treatment causes anxiety in patients is that the operative area is very close to and involved with all the most vital functions of the body such as sight, hearing, breathing, and swallowing. When operative treatment is being performed, all these vital functions are put at risk and any sensible child would be concerned. It is useful to discuss these fears with child patients and explain how the risks can be reduced or eliminated.

Glasses should be used to protect the eyes and rubber dam to protect the airways and the oesophagus. By doing this, and provided that good local analgesia has been obtained, the child can feel themselves distanced from the operation. Sometimes it is even helpful to show the child their isolated teeth in a mirror. The view is so different from what they normally see in the mirror that they can divorce themselves from the reality of the situation.

Relaxation

The isolation of the operative area from the child will very often cause the child to become considerably relaxed—always provided that there is good pain control. It is common for both adult and child patients to fall asleep while undergoing treatment involving the use of rubber dam—a situation that rarely occurs without it (Fig. 8.10). This is a function of the safety perceived by the patient and the relaxed way in which the dental team can work with its assistance.

Latex free

Both rubber dam sheets and elasticated Wedjets are available in latex-free versions for children who are latex sensitive or allergic.

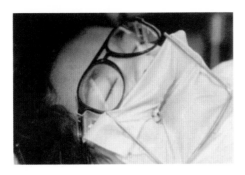

Figure 8.10 Rubber dam placed in a child. With the comfort it provides it is not unusual for children to fall asleep in the dental chair during treatment under rubber dam.

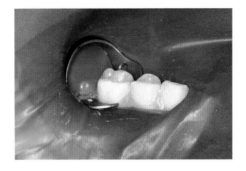

Figure 8.11 'Trough technique' of rubber dam placement.

8.6.3 Benefits to the dentist

Reduced stress

As noted above, once rubber dam has been placed the child will be at less risk from the procedures that will be used to restore their teeth. This reduces the effort required by the operator to protect the soft tissues of the mouth and airways. Treatment can be carried out in a more relaxed and controlled manner, therefore lessening the stress of the procedure on the dental team.

Retraction of tongue and cheeks

Correctly placed rubber dam will gently pull the cheeks and tongue away from the operative area, allowing the operator a better view of the area to be treated.

Retraction of gingival tissue

Rubber dam will gently pull the gingival tissues away from the cervical margin of the tooth, making it much easier to see the extent of any caries close to the margin and often bringing the cervical margin of a prepared cavity above the level of the gingival margin, thus making restoration considerably easier. Interdentally, this retraction should be assisted by placing a wedge firmly between the adjacent teeth as soon as the dam has been placed. This wedge is placed horizontally below the contact area and above the dam, thus compressing the interdental gingivae against the underlying bone. Approximal cavities can then be prepared, with any damage from rotary instruments being inflicted on the wedge rather than the child's gingival tissue.

It can often be difficult and time-consuming to take the rubber dam between the contacts because of dental caries or broken restorations. It is possible to make life easier by using a 'trough technique', which involves snipping the rubber dam between the punched holes. All the benefits of rubber dam are retained except for the retraction and protection of the gingival tissues (Fig. 8.11).

Moisture control

As mentioned previously, silver amalgam is probably the only restorative material that has any tolerance to being placed in a damp environment, and there is no doubt that it and all other materials will perform much more satisfactorily if placed in a dry field. Rubber dam is the only technique that readily ensures a dry field.

8.6.4 Technique

Most texts on operative dentistry demonstrate techniques for the use of rubber dam. It is not intended to duplicate this effort, but it would seem useful to point out features of the technique that have made life easier for the authors when using rubber dam with children.

Analgesia

Placement of rubber dam can be uncomfortable, especially if a clamp is needed to retain it. Even if a clamp is not required, the sharp cut edge of the dam can cause mild pain. Soft tissue analgesia can be obtained using infiltration in the buccal sulcus followed by an interpapillary injection. This will usually give sufficient analgesia to remove any discomfort from the dam. However, more profound analgesia may be required for the particular operative procedure that has to be performed.

Method of application

There are at least four different methods of placing the dam, but most authorities recommend a method whereby the clamp is first placed on the tooth and the dam is stretched over the clamp and then over the remaining teeth that are to be isolated. Because of the risk of the patient swallowing or inhaling a dropped or broken clamp before the dam is applied, it is imperative that the clamp is restrained with a piece of floss tied or wrapped around the bow. This adds considerable inconvenience to the technique, and the authors favour a simpler method whereby the clamp, dam, and frame are assembled together before application and taken to the tooth in one movement. Because the clamp is always on the outside of the dam relative to the patient there is no need to use floss to secure the clamp.

A 5-inch (about 12.5cm) square of medium dam is stretched over an Ivory frame and a single hole punched in the middle of the square. This hole is for the tooth on which the clamp is going to be placed and further holes should be punched for any other teeth that need to be isolated. A winged clamp is placed in the first hole and the whole assembly is carried to the tooth by the clamp forceps. The tooth that is going to be clamped can be seen through the hole and the clamp is applied to it. The dam is then teased off the wings using either the fingers or a hand instrument. It can then be carried forward over the other teeth with the interdental dam being 'knifed' through the contact areas. It may need to be stabilized at the front using floss, a small piece of rubber dam, a Wedjet (Figs 8.6 and 8.11), or a wooden wedge.

8.7 Operative treatment of primary teeth

8.7.1 Pit and fissure caries

Pit and fissure caries is less of a problem in primary teeth than in permanent ones. The fissures are usually much shallower and less susceptible to decay, so the presence of a cavity in the occlusal surface of a primary molar is a sign of high caries activity. Consequently, it is quite likely that the children who require treatment of these surfaces will be young. However, treatment is not difficult and can usually be accomplished without problems. Infiltration analgesia should be given together with supplemental intrapapillary injection. Caries is removed using a 330 bur in a high-speed handpiece. A number of materials can be used. Although, as discussed previously, silver amalgam has not been bettered in clinical trials so far, other materials have the benefit of sealing the remaining fissures of the tooth. As long as the sealant is inspected and 'topped up' if deficient, this will ensure that dental caries does not occur in other parts of the occlusal pattern (see Fig. 8.8).

8.7.2 Approximal caries

Silver amalgam

Failure of amalgam itself as well as faults in the cavity design have been the most commonly reported causes of failure of approximal restorations in primary teeth. Attempts to overcome these deficiencies and to improve durability have been made by altering cavity design and the choice of material used. A reduction in the size of the occlusal lock, rounded line angles, and minimum extension for prevention all result in less destruction of sound tooth tissue. In addition, the 'minimal' approximal cavity with no occlusal 'dovetail' has been described for both amalgam and adhesive restorations. It incorporates some mechanical retention in the form of small internal resistance grooves placed with a very small round bur just inside the enamel–dentine junction. Figure 8.12 demonstrates the clinical stages in the placement of two-surface amalgam restorations in the primary dentition.

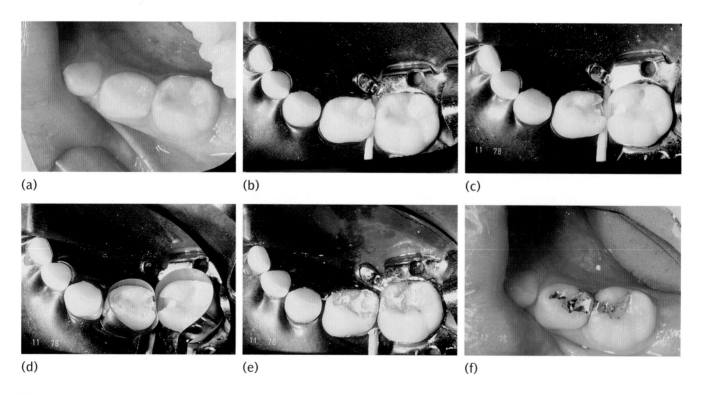

(a) (b) (c)

(d) (e) (f)

Figure 8.12 Technique sequence for the placement of two-surface amalgam restorations in lower primary molars. The first molar could have been restored with a stainless steel crown.

Because of the following anatomical features it is unlikely that the 'perfect cavity design' exists for an amalgam restoration in primary molars.

1. Widened contact areas make a narrow box difficult to achieve.

2. Thin enamel means that cracking and fracture of parts of the crown are more common.

3. Primary teeth may undergo considerable wear under occlusal stress themselves and this in turn will affect the restorations.

Therefore it is necessary to investigate other materials for use in restoring the primary dentition. The choice of alternative materials has been discussed earlier (Section 8.5.1) for small class II cavities. Where there is concern that further caries will develop at a distant site on the tooth, the cavity is larger than a small interproximal cavity, or care is provided under sedation or general anaesthetic, a stainless steel crown should be the default material. This will minimize the need for further restorative care for this tooth until exfoliation.

8.7.3 Stainless steel crowns

Stainless steel crowns should be considered whenever posterior primary teeth (especially first molars) require restoration. They were originally developed to provide a 'restoration of last resort' for those teeth that were not salvageable by any other means. At the time that they were introduced in the early 1950s, the only alternatives were silver or copper amalgam or a selection of cements, materials completely unsuited to the restoration of grossly carious teeth or those that had been weakened by pulp treatment. Over the years, it has become apparent that the life expectancy of these crowns is far better than any other restoration for primary posterior teeth and that they come close to the ideal of never having to be replaced prior to exfoliation. In addition, they are less demanding technically than intracoronal restorations in primary teeth. Therefore they should now be considered for any tooth where the dentist cannot be sure that an alternative would survive until the tooth is lost. It is unfair to put a child through further treatment visits than is necessary because a less successful material, which needs frequent replacement, was chosen.

The *indications* for stainless steel crowns are shown in Table 8.2.

The technique

The conventional preparation of a primary molar, which should currently be considered the most appropriate technique, is described in this section. An alternative, the 'Hall technique', has also been described. Wherever possible local anaesthesia should be given, although in certain situations (e.g. while preparing a non-vital tooth) this is not always necessary. Nevertheless, even in these teeth there will need to be some tooth preparation involving the gingival margin, which can cause some discomfort for which local anaesthesia is advisable. It is sometimes possible to use only a topical anaesthesia, such as a benzocaine ointment on the gingival cuff. In other instances, when the preparation for a crown is carried out at the same visit as a pulpotomy, local analgesia would already have been administered. Rubber dam is advisable as it is very easy for crowns to slip in the fingers and this protects the airway. Furthermore it facilitates restorative care, as

already described. Where the tooth to be prepared is also the tooth that is clamped, the rubber dam needs retracting for the distal slice.

Prior to preparation, all caries is removed and any pulp treatment that may be required is carried out. A recent preoperative radiograph must be available to make sure that the periapical and inter-radicular tissues are healthy and that the tooth is unlikely to be exfoliated in the near future.

The same bur can be used for the whole preparation, although it may be quicker to use a larger diamond wheel for the occlusal surface reduction of 1–2mm required between the prepared tooth and its opposite number. This ensures that the crown will fit with mimimal occlusal derangement. The use of wedges can help to protect the gingival tissues but is not essential. The mesial and distal surfaces of the tooth are removed using a fine tapered diamond bur (Fig. 8.13(b)). It is important to cut through the tooth, away from the contact area, to avoid damage to the adjacent tooth. It is essential that no shoulder is created at the gingival margin which will prevent a good seal or fit of the crown.

Many authorities advocate doing no more preparation than this, but it takes little further time to reduce the buccal and lingual surfaces sufficiently to remove any undercuts above the gingival margin. Any sharp line angles are rounded off to avoid interference that might prevent the crown from seating.

The mesial and distal preparation might seem rather radical compared with that required when a cast crown is constructed for a permanent tooth, but the principles of retention and resistance of the two types of crown are different. A cast crown is retained by friction between the walls of the prepared tooth and the internal surface of the crown. Therefore it is important to have near-parallel walls of adequate height. A stainless steel metal crown is retained by contact between the margins of the crown and the undercut portion of the tooth below the gingiva. The shape of the preparation above the gingiva is relatively unimportant, and difficulty in fitting these crowns most frequently occurs because of under-preparation. However, it is most important that a shoulder is not formed at the gingival margin as this would make the seating of a well-adapted crown impossible.

Table 8.2 Indications for stainless steel crowns

1.	Restoration of primary molars needing large multisurface restorations
2.	Restoration of primary molars in children with rampant caries
3.	Restorative care provided under sedation or general anaesthetic
4.	Restoration of teeth after pulp therapy
5.	Restoration of teeth with developmental defects, e.g. amelogenesis imperfecta
6.	Abutment for space maintainers
7.	Restoration of fractured primary molars
8.	Protection of molars in children with bruxism
9.	Restoration of hypomineralized young permanent molars

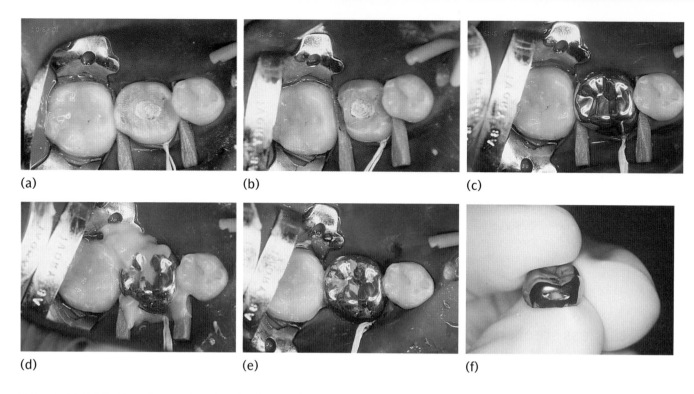

Figure 8.13 (a) Rubber dam and wedges in place; pulpotomy and coronal reduction completed. (b) Mesial and distal surfaces reduced. (c) Crown 'try-in'. (d) Cementation of crown. (e) Excess cement removed prior to rubber dam removal and occlusal analysis. (f) Some operators recommend perforating the approximal surface of the stainless steel crown to allow release of fluoride from GIC.

Try the crown on and check to feel that it is within the gingival crevice (Fig. 8.13(c)) by probing. If it rests on the gingival crevice, crimp in with some pliers. Again seat the crown. Wash and dry the tooth before cementation with a glass ionomer cement. Seat the crown from lingual to buccal, pressing down firmly (Fig. 8.13(d)). Remove excess cement when set with a probe and dental floss (Fig. 8.13(e)) before removing rubber dam and checking the occlusion.

Figure 8.14 shows how the restoration of heavily carious primary molars with stainless steel crowns has maintained arch space and prevented mesial drift of the posterior molars. This preservation of the mesial distal width helps to allow permanent premolars to erupt into ideal occlusion.

Success rates of stainless steel crown restoration

Over the last 20–30 years authors have consistently recorded and reported higher success rates for stainless steel crowns than for other restorations in primary molars. This is despite the stainless steel crowns being frequently used in more demanding clinical situations. Stainless steel crowns were by far the most durable restorations for primary molars, and the most remarkable fact is that, once placed, they seldom need replacing and they protect the entire surface of the tooth from further carious attack.

In a recent study, children expressed very positive opinions about the appearance of their stainless steel crowns and found the clinical procedure for their placement acceptable.

8.7.4 Anterior teeth

The treatment of decayed primary incisors depends on the stage of decay and the age and cooperation of the patient. In the preschool child, caries of the upper primary incisors is usually a result of 'nursing caries syndrome' due to frequent or prolonged consumption of fluids containing fermentable carbohydrate from a bottle or feeder cup (Chapter 6). The lower incisors are rarely affected as they are protected by the tongue during suckling and are directly bathed in secretions from the submandibular and sublingual glands. In 'nursing caries' the progression of decay is rapid, commencing on the labial surfaces and quickly encircling the teeth (Fig. 8.15). It is impossible to prepare satisfactory cavities for restoration, and after a comprehensive preventive programme the most suitable form of restoration is the 'strip crown technique'. This utilizes celluloid crown forms and a light-cured composite resin to restore crown morphology. High polishability hybrid composites make them aesthetically, as well as physically, suitable for this task.

Fractures of the incisal edges in primary teeth, as in permanent teeth, should be restored with composite resin.

The choice of how to repair anterior teeth depends on the child's cooperation, their symptoms, the extent of the destruction, pulpal assessment, and the parents' aspirations. In the authors' opinion, these crowns are excellent for building primary incisors where extensive tooth tissue has been lost due to either caries or trauma. The technique for their use is similar to that of such crowns used in permanent

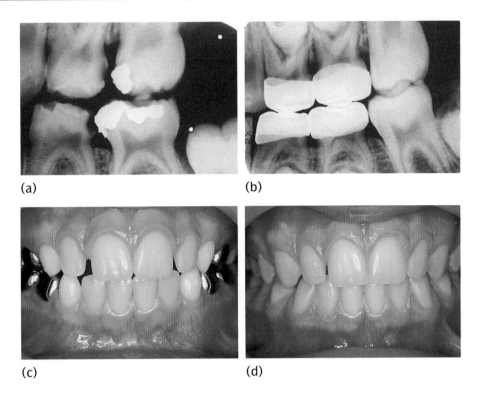

(a)

(b)

(c)

(d)

Figure 8.14 (a) Carious upper and lower primary molars. (b) After placement of stainless steel crowns. (c) Occlusion in the mixed dentition. (d) 'Ideal' final occlusion in the permanent dentition.

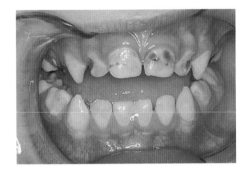

Figure 8.15 Labial and approximal caries in upper anterior primary teeth.

teeth; the crowns are easily trimmed with sharp scissors, filled with composite, and seated on a prepared and conditioned tooth. The celluloid crown form can be stripped off after the composite has been cured. Figure 8.16 shows that excellent results can be obtained using strip crowns. This technique needs significant cooperation from the child and, because of their young age, is frequently feasible only under a general anaesthetic with or without pulp treatment.

In older children (over 3 or 4 years of age) new lesions of primary incisors, although not usually associated with the use of pacifiers, indicate high caries activity (Fig. 8.15). Such lesions do not progress so rapidly and usually appear on the mesial and distal surfaces. In these situations a glass ionomer cement or composite resin can be used for

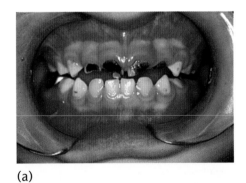

(a)

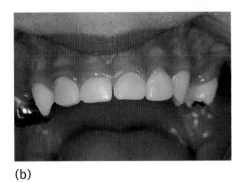

(b)

Figure 8.16 (a) Carious primary incisors that were (b) restored using strip crowns and composite resins to give an aesthetically pleasing result.

restoration. Glass ionomer lacks the translucency of composite resin but has the useful advantages of being adhesive and releasing fluoride. This care can be frequently provided without local anaesthetic depending on the extent of caries. The aesthetics is often not as optimal, with clinicians struggling with the retention of the material over the medium term and ensuring that there is no ledge at the gingival margin. Consequently, composite is the authors' preferred option, where possible, if good moisture control is present.

8.8 Pulp therapy in primary teeth

The principal goals of paediatric operative dentistry are to prevent the extension of dental disease and to restore damaged teeth to healthy function. To this end, a range of endodontic procedures provide an alternative to extraction for many pulpally compromised primary teeth. These are within the grasp of all practitioners and are central to the practice of paediatric dentistry. Failure to treat the carious process or refer to a provider who can is a missed opportunity. Once pain, sepsis, and infection have occurred, this cannot be ignored but must be treated. The endodontic treatment of non-vital primary teeth, which can be an alternative to extraction, is discussed in this section. Extraction has a number of consequences which are listed in Key Points 8.8. A thorough history and clinical and radiographic examination are essential to correct diagnosis and pulpal treatment planning (Box 8.1).

While many of the general principles and operative procedures in the primary dentition are shared with adult endodontics, a number of important differences exist which justify the special coverage given in this chapter. Failure to assess the underlying pulpal health may lead clinicians to frustration and lead to the opinion that treating primary teeth is futile.

8.8.1 Pulpal response to caries progression and the assessment of pulpal health

As caries progresses, the pulpal tissues mount a protective response. This includes the laying down of both hard tissue and tertiary dentine and inflammatory changes within the pulpal tissue. As the carious lesion progresses from the amelodentinal junction towards the pulp chamber so the inflammatory changes become more widespread within the pulp. Initally, only the odontoblasts adjacent to the carious lesion demonstrate signs of inflammation, but with progression of the lesion this extends to the pulp horn, the coronal pulp, and finally the radicular pulp tissue. The work by Helen Rodd has shown that the inflammatory process in the pulp tissue in the primary tooth is similar to that of the permanent tooth. This conclusion is based on occlusal caries; as discussed in the next section, proximal caries may show a more widespread inflammation at an earlier stage of the carious process.

The assessment of the pulp requires a careful history and a thorough clinical and radiographic examination. This information will help clinicians to identify the probable extent of any pulpal inflammation and how reversible it will be. Unfortunately, parents and children are not always the best historians of previous symptoms from a tooth, and frequently clinical and radiographic signs only appear once the pulp is infected and non-vital. Therefore it is essential to be aware of a number of histological studies which give an insight into the likely pulpal status as caries progresses. (See Key Point 8.9.)

Key Points 8.8

Disadvantages of unplanned extractions in the primary and mixed dentitions:

- loss of space, increasing the chances of developing a malocclusion;
- reduced masticatory function (especially posterior teeth);
- psychological disturbance (especially anterior teeth);
- extraction of teeth has been identified as a cause of future dental anxiety.

Box 8.1

Clinical history
- Reported history of pain and symptoms from the tooth

Clinical assessment
- The presence of an abscess, excessive mobility, swelling, or tenderness to percussion—this indicates that the tooth is infected and non-vital
- Is the tooth restorable?
- Extent of marginal ridge breakdown
- Site of caries—occlusal or proximal?

Radiograph assessment
- Root length
- Perifurcational radiolucency
- Internal resorption seen in root canal

Key Point 8.9

It is often difficult to asess the pulpal health as many clinical or radiographic signs may only appear once the tooth is infected.

Studies in the early 1970s showed that in over 50% of primary molars where loss of the marginal ridge had occurred, pulp inflammation was irreversible. More recent work (Duggal *et al.* 2002), in which the intercuspal distance (buccolingual) involved in the carious process was

Table 8.3 Relationship between the extent of marginal ridge breakdown and increasing involvement of the pulp with inflammation.

Pulp pathology	≤1/3 (N = 19)	≤2/3 (N = 19)	≥2/3 (N = 51)
Normal	1	1	0
Odontoblast layer	9	1	1
Pulp horn	9	17	34
Coronal pulp	0	0	9
Radicular pulp	0	0	7

measured, has shown that most teeth had pulp inflammation involving the pulp horn adjacent to the proximal carious lesion even when caries involved less than half the marginal ridge (Table 8.3). This suggests that inflammation of the pulp in primary molars develops at an early stage of proximal carious attack, and by the time most proximal caries is manifest clinically the pulp inflammation is significant and is often visible within the coronal pulp. What this study, and a subsequent investigation by Kassa *et al.* (2009), was unable to assess was whether the inflammation was reversible. (See Key Point 8.10.)

Key Point 8.10

With an increase in marginal ridge breakdown, pulpal inflammation is more widespread.

Kassa *et al.* (2009) compared the effect of proximal and occlusal caries on the amount of inflammation seen. This showed that when caries was greater than half the dentinal depth, pulpal inflammation was significantly more extensive for proximal caries than for similar sized occlusal lesions.

Monterio *et al.* (2009) examined the anatomical changes present within the coronal pulp with increasing physiological root resorption. They found no difference in primary teeth with respect to the apparatus to mount an inflammatory response with increasing physiological root resorption. This suggests that the tooth should respond in a similar way when under carious attack irrespective of the stage of root resorption. Clinical studies of carious primary molars in children of different ages, and therefore different stages of root resorption, report an opposite finding with less reported pain experienced with increasing root resorption. (See Key Points 8.11.)

The signs of this acute inflammation within the pulp are not obvious to the clinician apart from the development of pain. Only if the pulp is visualized, as occurs when the pulp tissue is exposed during a pulpotomy, can the clinician see other signs of inflammation. The most obvious of these is persistent bleeding. Consequently the exposure of the pulp chamber gives the clinician a better insight into the pulpal response to the carious process and whether the radicular pulp is inflamed. A recent study has shown that the use of direct pressure with saline

Key Points 8.11

- As a carious lesion progresses the pulpal inflammatory response involves a widespread area of tissue.
- The primary pulp mounts a similar response to occlusal caries progression as that of a permanent tooth.
- Deep proximal caries produces a more widespread inflammation than an occlusal lesion of similar size.
- The extent of breakdown of the marginal ridge gives an indication of how much of the pulp will be inflamed.
- It is unknown why with increasing root resorption the dental pulp is less likely to cause pain when there is no difference in pulpal architecture with respect to mounting an inflammatory response to caries.

cotton wool for 1 minute once the coronal pulp had been removed gave the highest success rates for four different pulpotomy techniques examined (Doyle *et al.* 2010). The authors felt that the use of ferric sulphate, which will be discussed in the pulpotomy section, may disguise inflammation extending into the radicular pulp and therefore lead to an inaccurate diagnosis of radicular pulpal health. (See Key Point 8.12.)

Key Point 8.12

A pulpotomy and use of sterile saline cotton wool applied for 1 minute over the pulp stumps may give a clinician a better insight into the health of the radicular pulp.

8.8.2 Treatment options for the inflamed pulp

There are a number of different treatment options for carious primary teeth with an inflamed pulp. For these to be successful, all clinical and radiographic findings must be collected and evaluated to ensure that the most appropriate treatment option is chosen. The indications for different pulp treatment techniques relating to clinical and radiographic signs and symptoms are shown in Table 8.4.

As the diagnosis of inflamed pulp is not an exact science there are certain patients for whom the consequences of a misdiagnosis and resulting infection are not worth the risk of retaining the tooth. Consequently, unless all caries has been removed and there is still a good depth of dentine left, the tooth is extracted. These patients include those at risk of endocarditis and those who are immunocompromised (e.g. during treatment for leukaemia).

8.8.3 Hall crown or no caries removal

As shown in Table 8.4 both the Hall technique with no caries removal and indirect pulp capping with partial caries removal rely on an

Table 8.4 Indications for different pulp treatment techniques relating to clinical and radiographic signs and symptoms

	No caries removal (e.g. Hall crown)	Indirect pulp cap	Direct pulp cap	Pulpotomy	Vital pulpectomy	Non-vital pulpectomy	Extraction
No history of pain or symptoms from tooth	Yes	Yes	No	Yes	Yes	NA	NA
History of reversible pulpitis	No	No	No	Yes	Yes	NA	NA
History of irreversible pulpitis	No	No	No	No	Yes	NA	NA
Marginal ridge breakdown <1/3rd	Yes	Yes	No	Yes	No	NA	No
Marginal ridge breakdown 1/3rd–2/3rd	Yes	?	No	Yes	Yes	NA	No
Marginal ridge breakdown >2/3rd	Yes	No	No	Yes	Yes	Yes	?
Occlusal caries	Yes	Yes	No	Yes	Yes	Yes	?
Proximal caries	Yes	?	No	Yes	Yes	Yes	If symptomatic or sepsis
Unrestorable	No	No	No	No	No	No	If symptomatic or sepsis
Sinus, swelling, tender to percussion, mobility	No	No	No	No	No	No	Yes
Root length >1/3rd	Yes	Yes	No	Yes	NA	NA	NA
Root length <1/3rd	No	No	No	No	No	No	If symptomatic or sepsis
Perifurcation radiolucency	No	No	No	No	No	No	Yes
Internal resorption of root	No	No	No	No	Yes	Yes	If symptomatic or sepsis
Caries extending to outer half of dentine	Yes	Yes	No	NA	NA	NA	NA
Caries extending to inner half of dentine	Yes	?	No	Yes	Yes	Yes	NA
Caries extending into pulp chamber	No	No	No	Yes	Yes	Yes	?

Extraction may not be an option in all clinical situations because of patient cooperation, medical history, or availability of treatments under sedation or general anaesthetic.

In some situations a Hall crown or indirect pulp cap may be undertaken even though the pulpal status may be suspect. This may be the only option the patient will tolerate and parents should be informed.

excellent coronal seal. Where this is achieved in the appropriate tooth, the inflammation present is reversible, and the pulp able to repair itself. These techniques both rely on an accurate assessment of pulpal health using the criteria described in Table 8.4 and the previous section. See Hall Technique electronic users manual in Further Reading section, Innes and Evans (2010).

8.8.4 Indirect pulp capping (IPC)

IPC is the equivalent of the stepwise excavation technique used in permanent teeth. In the majority of circumstances, carious lesions can and should be fully excavated before tooth restoration. A clinical dilemma is presented by a deep lesion in a vital symptom-free tooth where complete removal of softened dentine on the pulpal floor is likely to result

in frank exposure. The advancing front of a carious lesion contains very few cariogenic bacteria. Provided that the bulk of infected overlying dentine is removed, a small amount of softened dentine may often be left in the deepest part of the preparation without endangering the pulp. This is the basis of indirect pulp capping.

All caries is first cleared from the cavity margins with a steel round bur running at slow speed. Gentle excavation then follows on the pulpal floor, removing as much of the softened dentine as possible without exposing the pulp. Precisely how much dentine should be removed becomes a matter of experience and clinical judgement, although some have advocated the use of indicator dyes (e.g. 0.5% basic fuchsin) to show when all infected dentine has been eliminated. A thin layer of setting calcium hydroxide cement is then placed on the cavity floor to destroy any remaining micro-organisms and to promote the deposition of reparative secondary dentine. In its classical application, the indirect pulp cap was covered with zinc oxide–eugenol cement or glass ionomer and, after observation for several weeks, the cavity was re-entered to remove all remaining softened dentine. A more modern adaptation of this technique commonly used is to permanently restore the tooth at the same visit. The material that is placed over remaining caries has also been debated, with advocates for resin bonding systems, glass ionomer, and non-setting calcium hydroxide. As has been demonstrated by an number of studies, the coronal seal is the most important reason for success and therefore a stainless steel crown is the optimal option. Periodic clinical and radiographic review is then undertaken to monitor the pulp response.

In light of the study by Kassa *et al.* (2009), where it was shown that deep proximal caries cause more widespread inflammation of the pulp compared with occlusal caries of the same depth, IPC should be carefully applied for very deep proximal cavities in primary molars, if at all. It is the authors' view that although many primary teeth with deep occlusal caries will be suitable for IPC, most primary teeth with deep proximal caries will be better restored with a pulpotomy, where the inflamed pulp has been removed.

8.8.5 Direct pulp capping (DPC)

As discussed in the previous sections, the pulp is deemed to be inflamed, prior to clinical exposure. Consequently direct pulp capping following pulpal exposure has a poor success rate as applying a medicament is less likely to stimulate a reparative response in an area of inflamed pulpal tissue. Thus the success rates for DPC are poorer than other pulpal treatments and are therefore not recommended. (See Key Points 8.13.)

Key Points 8.13

- Direct pulp capping is not recommended in the primary dentition because of poor success rates.
- IPC and the Hall technique rely on an accurate diagnosis of pulpal health.

8.8.6 The vital pulpotomy

A pulpotomy involves the removal of the inflamed coronal pulp tissue. This usually leaves an intact radicular pulp tissue to which a medicament is applied before placing a coronal restoration.

The pulpotomy technique

The various steps involved in carrying out a pulpotomy in a primary molar are shown in Fig. 8.17.

As already described, the health of the radicular pulp can be assessed once the coronal pulp has been removed. Bleeding can be stopped with either a medicament or direct pressure with a cotton-wool ball soaked in sterile saline. If bleeding is persistent, this suggests that the radicular pulp is inflamed and a vital pulpectomy, or more frequently an extraction, is required. If a pulpotomy is carried out on an inflamed

radicular pulp internal resorption will appear over the medium term. This is often, but not necessarily, symptomless. If on opening up the pulp chamber there is no pulpal tissue, either a pulpectomy or an extraction is indicated. (See Key Points 8.14.)

Key Points 8.14

- If, on accessing the pulp chamber, no pulpal tissue or bleeding is encountered, a pulpotomy is not the appropriate pulpal treatment. A non-vital pulpectomy or an extraction is indicated.
- If a pulpotomy is carried out on an inflamed radicular pulp, internal resorption will be seen in the medium term.

Pulpotomy medicament

Ferric sulphate is the current gold standard for application onto the radicular pulp. Ferric sulphate has been widely used to control gingival bleeding prior to impression taking and also in endodontics. It is an excellent haemostatic agent, forming a ferric ion–protein complex on contact with blood, which then stops further bleeding by sealing the vessels (Fig. 8.21). It has also been shown to be as effective as formocresol in a number of medium-term studies with strict inclusion criteria and in a randomized controlled trial. Ferric sulphate is available commercially as Astringident, at a concentration of 15.5%. Guidelines advise that it is either burnished onto the pulp stumps or applied on a sterile cotton wool ball for 15 seconds. If bleeding continues, ferric sulphate is reapplied for another 15 seconds. If this still proves unsuccessful, a vital pulpectomy or an extraction are the two options available.

There are some concerns that ferric sulphate is too effective at stopping bleeding and may hide an inflamed radicular pulp. Historically, formocresol (both full strength and one-fifth dilution) was used. This and a number of other medicaments are no longer used because of worries over their carcinogenic potential. Interestingly, when ferric sulphate was first proposed as an alternative to formocresol there were concerns that it would not be as efficacious as it was unable to fix the remaining radicular pulpal tissue. Consequently, a more accurate pulpal diagnosis was needed. Formocresol fixed the radicular pulp irrespective of whether it was inflamed or not.

Material used to fill up the pulp chamber and coronal seal

The classical material used to fill the coronal pulp space is zinc oxide–eugenol. This has a long history of use. Concerns have been voiced that placing eugenol directly onto the radicular pulp may itself cause inflammation. This has been investigated by Doyle *et al.* (2010). A non-eugenol-containing cement had the worst performance out of four techniques tested, including the current gold standard of placing zinc oxide–eugenol after the application of ferric sulphate. The technique with the best outcome at a median follow-up of 2 years was the use of mineral trioxide aggregate (MTA) following direct pressure with cotton wool soaked in sterile saline. Many recent studies have also shown that the use of MTA after removal of the coronal pulp gives a better outcome in the medium term. However, MTA is expensive and its routine use for pulp therapy cannot always be justified from a cost-effectiveness viewpoint.

Administer local analgesia and apply rubber dam wherever possible.

Remove caries and identify the site of pulp exposure (Fig. 8.18). If there is no pulp exposure, then access to the pulp chamber is made from the base of the cavity.

Remove roof of the pulp chamber. When the bur passes through the roof of the chamber a 'dip' is felt. Once this is felt the bur is not taken any deeper but moved sideways to remove the roof of the pulp chamber.

Remove coronal pulp with a large round bur or large excavators (Fig. 8.19(a)). Excavators are safer to avoid perforation in the furcation region (Fig. 8.20).

Apply medicament to the radicular pulp on a cotton pledget (Fig. 8.19(b)).

Remove the cotton pledget and check that there is no haemorrhage from the remaining pupal tissue (Fig. 8.19(c)).

Fill chamber with zinc oxide–eugenol cement, pressing on the zinc oxide with a damp pledget to make sure that it is well condensed in the pulp chamber (Fig. 8.19(d)).

Place coronal restoration, preferably a stainless-steel crown.

Figure 8.17 The pulpotomy technique.

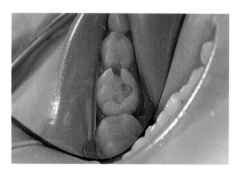

Figure 8.18 On removal of caries an exposure of the pulp below the mesiolingual cusp is clearly evident.

Following the sealing of the coronal pulp chamber, the tooth should be restored with a stainless steel crown. One study has demonstrated the benefit of a stainless crown over amalgam to optimize the coronal seal. A further two studies have identified the importance of completing all the treatment in one visit rather than temporizing the pulpotomy and restoring the tooth with a stainless steel crown at a later time. (See Key Points 8.15.)

Key Points 8.15

- Ferric sulphate is a suitable medicament for pulpotomy in primary molars when the inflammation is diagnosed to be restricted only to the coronal pulp.

- Ferric sulphate should be applied for 15 seconds at the site of amputation of the coronal pulp. If bleeding continues, one further application should be made.

- Ferric sulphate followed by the placement of zinc oxide–eugenol may soon be replaced by the use of direct pressure with sterile saline cotton wool pellet for 1 minute followed by placement of MTA onto the radicular pulp.

- If the radicular pulp continues to bleed, the tissue is still inflamed and alternative treatment with either a vital pulpectomy or an extraction is indicated.

- A stainless steel crown should be used to restore the tooth, and this should be applied on the same day.

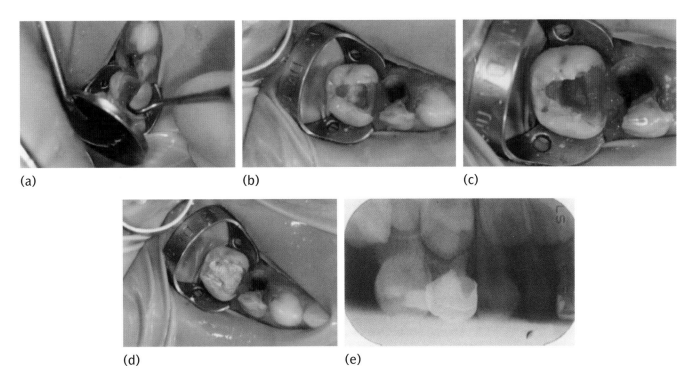

(a)   (b)   (c)

(d)   (e)

Figure 8.19 (a) A lower right second primary molar where, after removing the roof of the pulp chamber, the coronal pulp is being completely removed using excavators. (b) A cotton pledget with the medicament placed over the radicular pulp tissue to control the bleeding. (c) On removal of the cotton pledget, bleeding from the amputation sites has stopped. (d) Kalzinol (or any other zinc oxide–eugenol preparation) placed in the pulp chamber prior to placing the coronal restoration. (e) Periapical radiograph of right upper first primary molar showing a completed pulpotomy. Note the excellent condensation of cement in the pulp chamber and coronal restoration with stainless steel crown.

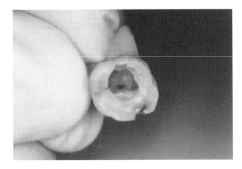

Figure 8.20 Perforation in the floor of the pulp chamber in a second primary molar. If this happens extraction is indicated.

Follow-up

Teeth that have undergone pulpotomy should be reviewed clinically and radiographically. Clinically, the following criteria indicate success:

- absence of symptoms;
- absence of any abscess or draining sinus;
- no excessive mobility or tenderness;
- retention of tooth until it would exfoliate naturally.

Radiographically, the following should be observed.

1. No evidence of bone loss in the furcation region is seen. Figure 8.19(e) demonstrates good bone condition in the bifurcation region 6 months after the pulpotomy was performed.

2. No evidence of internal resorption. Internal resorption indicates chronic inflammation and the activity of giant cells causing resorption of the dentine. It creates few symptoms and is usually detected as an incidental finding on radiographic examination. It should be considered as a form of irreversible pulpitis (Fig. 8.22). Treatment (e.g. extraction of the tooth) is only indicated if the resorption extends to the external surface of the root canal or signs or symptoms of infection develop.

8.8.7 Vital pulpectomy

Where inflammation extends into the radicular pulp, two options are open to the clinician—root canal treatment or extraction. This section will concentrate on vital root canal therapy. The success rates are excellent, with Casas *et al.* (2003, 2004) reporting similar or higher success

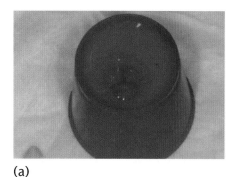

(a)

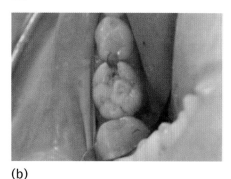

(b)

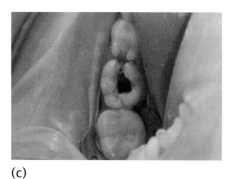

(c)

Figure 8.21 (a) Ferric sulphate in a concentration of 15.5% solution is available commercially as Astringident (Ultradent in the USA). (b) Ferric sulphate being applied to the root canal tissue after the amputation of coronal pulp in the upper right second primary molar. (c) Bleeding stops almost immediately on application of ferric sulphate.

rates than ferric sulphate pulpotomies in 2- and 3-year outcome studies. The technique is very similar to that described in the next section for non-vital pulpectomies except for the following:

- the remaining inflamed radicular pulp is first extirpated with a Hedstrom file;
- the duration of the disinfection phase can be shortened as no infection is present in the root canals.

The disadvantage of the technique is that extra time is needed and therefore excellent behaviour management techniques are required. Consequently, this technique may be reserved for strategic teeth such as retaining the second primary molars or where there is a missing

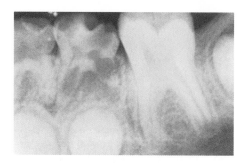

Figure 8.22 Internal inflammatory resorption identified as an incidental finding on routine radiographic examination.

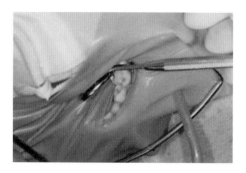

Figure 8.23 A non-vital left lower primary molar.

second premolar and the decision has been made with orthodontic colleagues to retain the second primary molar.

In some situations, because of either loss of patient cooperation or hyperaemic pulp tissue which cannot be successfully anaesthetized, a Ledermix dressing can be left *in situ* for a couple of weeks. Following this time period the tooth will need either an extraction or a vital (perhaps now non-vital) pulpectomy to be completed.

8.8.8 Management of non-vital and abscessed primary molars—the pulpectomy technique

Primary molars with abscesses are usually indicated for extractions. Persistent and chronic infection in primary molars can cause damage to the developing permanent tooth-germs and such foci of infection should be removed.

In some cases the non-vital primary molars (Fig. 8.23) or primary molars with a chronic discharging sinus might need to be retained for the following reasons:

- orthodontic;
- medical, where extraction is not appropriate such as in severe haemophiliacs;
- parents' refusal to accept extraction.

In such cases these teeth can be retained by carrying out a non-vital pulpectomy procedure. In the UK there is reluctance among many

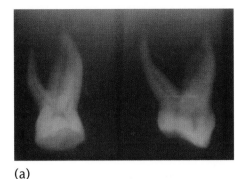

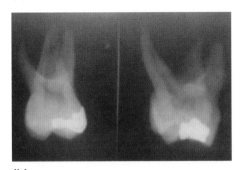

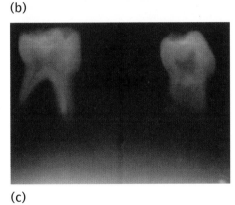

Figure 8.24 Root canal morphology of primary molars: (a) maxillary first primary molar; (b) maxillary second primary molar; (c) mandibular primary molars. (Reproduced with the kind permission of Professor H.S. Chawla, PGIMER, India.)

dentists to carry out a pulpectomy as it is perceived to be difficult in a young child, with extraction being preferred. The authors feel that this is a misconception. This technique should be learnt by all paediatric dentists, as it can often save the child from the trauma of a general anaesthetic for extraction of primary teeth. Pulpectomy involves accessing the root canal system of primary molars, disinfecting the root canals as well as possible, and then using an appropriate material, usually pure zinc oxide–eugenol, to obturate the root canals. Pure zinc oxide–eugenol is preferred as it is entirely resorbable and is easily removed as the roots of the primary teeth undergo resorption. Also, if it is extruded through the apices, it is completely resorbed by the apical tissues. Other materials, such as iodoform paste (KRI), calcium hydroxide, or a combination paste of iodoform and calcium hydroxide (Vitapex, Endoflax), are available.

In the lower primary molars there are always two mesial root canals—mesiobuccal and mesiolingual—with one or sometimes two distal root canals. In upper primary molars there are three root canals—mesiobuccal, distobuccal, and palatal (Fig. 8.24). The root canals are often flared or flame-shaped and consequently are difficult to clean thoroughly using mechanical instrumentation. The clinician should stay within the root canal by 2mm, thereby avoiding potential damage to the developing tooth bud. The most important part of the procedure is disinfection of the root canal space using either hypochlorite or chlorhexidene; again, the irrigant should be limited to within the root canal system. After drying the root canal a paste, as described earlier, is applied throughout the root canal system.

Indications for a non-vital pulpectomy

- Non-vital/infected primary molars or incisors that need to be maintained in the arch.
- Abscessed primary molars.
- Primary molars with radiographic evidence of furcation pathology.
- The tooth is restorable with at least two-thirds of root length remaining.

The steps for performing a pulpectomy are shown in Fig. 8.25. Figure 8.26 shows a diagrammatic representation of the technique.

In some cases where there is acute infection or persistent discharge from the root canals, it may be necessary to disinfect the root canal over two visits. Similar to adult endodontics, an inter-visit paste such as non-setting calcium hydroxide can be used to help with disinfection of the root canal. At the second visit, the root canal is instrumented, disinfected further, and then obturated.

Follow-up and review

Although the pulpectomy technique has a good prognosis, the outcome is not as good as a vital pulpotomy or pulpectomy. Clinical follow-up augmented by one periapical radiograph on a yearly basis is required (Fig. 8.27). The following clinical and radiographic parameters can be taken as indications of success:

- Clinical:
  - alleviation of acute symptoms
  - tooth free from pain and mobility.
- Radiographic:
  - improvement or no further resorption of bone in the furcation area.

Pulp treatment of primary incisors

The pulpotomy, vital pulpectomy, and non-vital pulpectomy techniques described can be used to treat inflamed or non-vital and abscessed primary incisors. Increasingly, parents are reluctant to have their child's upper anterior teeth extracted. In a modern society, where a child's self-esteem is important, it is the duty of the dentist to maintain aesthetics wherever possible. Many primary incisors with abscesses that are extracted can be retained with the help of a pulpectomy technique, and the root canal morphology is such that this can easily be performed (Fig. 8.28); the only limiting factor is the child's cooperation.

Access pulp chamber as described for the pulpotomy procedure.

Identify root canals.

Debride root canals gently with Hedstrom files and copious irrigation with chlorhexidine or 0.5% solution of sodium hypochlorite. With the help of a good preoperative radiograph, care should be taken to keep files 2–3mm short of apex to avoid damage to developing tooth germ.

Prepare the canals to no more than file size 30.

Dry root canals with paper points.

Select a spiral root canal filler that is two-sizes smaller than the last file used in the root canal (to avoid it being caught in the root canal), thereby minimizing the risk of it fracturing in the root canal.

Mix zinc oxide–eugenol as a slurry and with the help of spiral paste fillers spin this into the root canals. Alternatively, the paste can be carried into the root canals with gutta percha points.

Fill the pulp chamber with cement.

Restore the crown, with a stainless steel crown.

Figure 8.25 The pulpectomy technique.

Indications for a pulpectomy in primary incisors include carious or traumatized primary incisors with pulp exposures or acute or chronic abscesses. Figure 8.29 shows an example of primary central incisors treated with a pulpectomy.

8.9 Treatment of a child with high caries rate

It is absolutely true that restoration of children's teeth without adequate prevention is like replacing windows in a burning house. When presented with a child with a high caries rate, establishing a good preventive regime should be the first and foremost item in the treatment plan. However, it would be folly to think that prevention alone will maintain the child in a pain-free state. Restorative treatment or extraction of decayed teeth that are not suitable for restoration should be planned alongside securing good prevention. Therefore, when dealing with a high-caries-risk child, a comprehensive visit-by-visit treatment plan that deals with the preventive and restorative care of the child should be established. One of the findings from the NECAT study was that in this high-caries-risk population only 11% (48 children, aged 6–10

years) did not develop further caries over the duration of the 5-year study. Therefore without a comprehensive preventive regime to go hand in hand with the restorative treatment, clinicians, children, and parents will not achieve an optimal result. The study found that older children with more caries at the start of the trial and less frequent reported toothbrushing were at most risk of developing further caries.

The type of treatment instituted for patients with rampant caries depends on patients' and parents' motivation towards dental treatment, the extent of decay, and the age and cooperation of the child. Initial treatment, including temporary restorations, diet assessment, oral hygiene instruction, and home and professional fluoride treatments, should be performed before any comprehensive restorative programme commences.

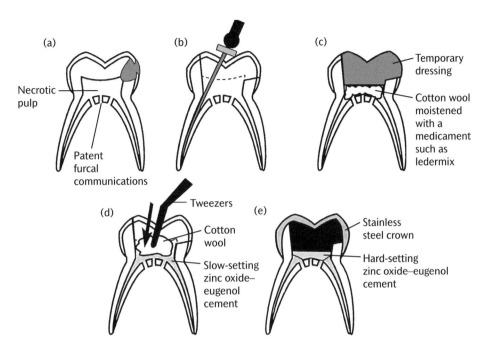

Figure 8.26 Non-vital pulp therapy—primary tooth. (a) A carious, but restorable, non-vital primary molar. (b) Caries is eliminated and access made to the pulp. Gentle canal debridement is undertaken with small files and irrigation. (c) Disinfection of the canal system: a pledget of cotton wool is sealed into the pulp chamber for 7–10 days. (d) The tooth is reopened at a second visit and, after irrigation and drying, a soft mixture of slow-setting zinc oxide–eugenol cement is gently packed into the canals with a cotton wool pledget. (e) The pulp chamber is packed with accelerated zinc oxide–eugenol cement before definitive restoration of the tooth.

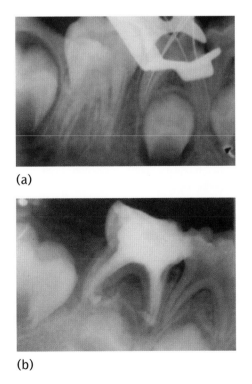

(a)

(b)

Figure 8.27 (a) Periapical radiograph showing files placed in the root canals of left lower second primary molar. (b) Root canals have been filled with pure zinc oxide–eugenol. (Reproduced with the kind permission of Professor H.S. Chawla, PGIMER, India.)

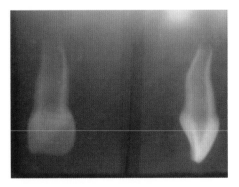

Figure 8.28 Radiograph showing the typical morphology of the root canal in upper primary incisors.

The use of serial plaque scores is a good way to monitor parent and/or child compliance with the preventive plan devised. However, immediate treatment is indicated in patients presenting with acute and severe signs and symptoms of gross caries, pain, abscess, sinus, or facial swelling. This may involve extractions and even a general anaesthetic in a young child. At this point, it is wiser to extract all the teeth with a dubious prognosis under one general anaesthetic rather than have an acclimatization pro-gramme interrupted by a painful episode in the future.

Once rampant caries is under control, comprehensive restorative treatment can be undertaken. This should aim to retain the primary dentition with the methods described in this chapter and in Chapter 7, and to deliver the child pain free and motivated to access oral care into adolescence and adulthood.

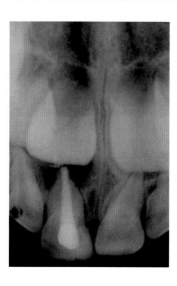

Figure 8.29 Root canal filling in an upper primary central incisor. (See Key Points 8.16.)

Key Points 8.16

- A vital or non-vital pulpectomy should be considered wherever it is essential to preserve a primary tooth that cannot be treated by other means, such as a pulpotomy.
- Both primary molars and incisors can be treated with a pulpectomy technique.

8.10 Summary

1 A full preventive programme must be instituted before any definitive restorations are performed in a child with a high caries rate.

2 Repetitive treatment should be avoided. With careful treatment planning and the use of appropriate restorative materials and techniques, the restoration will last for the lifetime of the tooth.

3 Sepsis and/or pain must be treated, no matter which restorative philosophy is being followed.

4 Stainless steel metal crowns are the most durable restoration in the primary dentition for large cavities and endodontically treated teeth.

5 Resin-modified glass ionomers, compomers, and polyacid-modified composite resins have similar results to amalgam for occlusal and small proximal restorations over the medium term (3–4 years). Cavities beyond this size should be restored with stainless steel crowns.

6 Glass ionomer cements are not appropriate for restoration of proximal lesions in primary teeth.

7 If at all possible, rubber dam should be placed prior to the restoration of all teeth.

8 Careful evaluation of the pulpal inflammation is essential before undertaking any restorative treatment.

9 There are multiple options for treatment of the inflamed pulp depending on the reported symptoms and the clinical and radiographic examination.

10 Ferric sulphate is currently the medicament of choice for pulpotomies. It is likely that there will be a move away from this material and zinc oxide–eugenol for pulp treatment in the primary dentition to direct pressure with a wet sterile cotton ball and the use of MTA as it is felt that this gives a better indication of the extent of inflammation in the radicular pulp.

11 The Hall Technique offers a viable treatment alternative in the absence of symptoms and of clinical or radiographic infection when patient tolerance is poor.

8.11 Acknowledgement

Some parts of this text have been reproduced from *Dental Update* with the kind permission of George Warman Publications.

8.12 Further reading

Curzon, M.E.J. and Roberts, J.S. (1996). *Kennedy's paediatric operative dentistry* (4th edn). Wright, London. (*A comprehensive text on the technical aspects of operative dentistry for children.*)

Dental Practice Board (1997). *Setting standards in dental care for children*. Dental Practice Board, Eastbourne. (*An attempt to give guidance to dentists in general dental practice.*)

Duggal, M.S., Curzon, M.E.J., Fayle, S.A., Toumba, K.J., and Robertson, A.J. (2002). *Restorative techniques in paediatric dentistry* (2nd edn). Taylor & Francis, London. (*A superb colour atlas and pictorial guide.*)

Duggal, M.S., Gautum, S.K., and Nicol, R. (2003). Paediatric dentistry in the new millennium. 4: Cost effective restorative techniques for primary molars. *Dental Update*, **30**, 410–15.

Faculty of Dental Surgery Clinical Effectiveness Committee (1999). *UK national clinical guidelines in paediatric dentistry. 1. Stainless steel pre-formed crowns for primary molar.* Dental Practice Board for England and Wales, Eastbourne. (*Invaluable clinical guideline and aide-memoire.*)

Faculty of Dental Surgery Clinical Effectiveness Committee (1999). *UK national clinical guidelines in paediatric dentistry. 2. Management of the stained fissure in the first permanent molar.* Dental Practice Board for England and Wales, Eastbourne. (*Invaluable clinical guideline and aide-memoire.*)

Faculty of General Dental Practice (UK) (1998). *Selection criteria for dental radiography.* FGDP (UK), London. (*An excellent guide to when to take radiographs for the diagnosis of caries in children.*)

Innes, N.P. and Evans, D.J. (2010). The Hall technique, a minimal intervention, child centred approach to managing the carious primary molar. A user's manual. Available online at: **http://wcm-live.dundee.ac.uk/media/dundeewebsite/dentalschool/documents/Hall%20manual3rdEd111110.pdf**

Kidd, E.A.M., Smith, B.G.N., and Watson, T. (2003). *Pickard's manual of operative dentistry* (8th edn). Oxford University Press, Oxford. (*An ideal reference manual for the restoration of permanent teeth.*)

Paterson, R.C., Watts, A., Saunders, W.P., and Pitts, N.B. (1991). *Modern concepts in the diagnosis and treatment of fissure caries.* Quintessence, London. (*A very practical and clear approach to the problem.*)

Reid, J.S., Challis, P.D., and Patterson, C.J.W. (1991). *Rubber dam in clinical practice.* Quintessence, London. (*This guide will prove to you that you can easily use rubber dam.*)

8.13 References

Casas, M.J., Layug, M.A., Kenny, D.J., Johnston, D.H., and Judd, P.L. (2003). Two-year outcomes of primary molar ferric sulfate pulpotomy and root canal therapy. *Pediatric Dentistry*, **25**, 97–102.

Casas, M.J., Kenny, D.J., Johnston, D.H., and Judd, P.L. (2004). Long-term outcomes of primary molar ferric sulfate pulpotomy and root canal therapy. *Pediatric Dentistry*, **26**, 44–8.

Doyle, T., Casas, M., Kenny, D., and Judd, P (2010). Mineral trioxide aggregate produces superior outcomes in vital primary molar pulpotomy. *Pediatric Dentistry*, **32**, 41–7.

Duggal, M.S., Nooh, A., and High, A. (2002). Response of the primary pulp to inflammation: a review of the Leeds studies and challenges for the future. *European Journal of Paediatric Dentistry*, **3**, 111–14.

Harris, C.A. (1839). *The dental art.* Armstrong and Berry, Baltimore, MD.

Huth, K.C., Paschos, E., Hajek-Al Khatar, N., *et al.* (2005). Effectiveness of 4 pulpotomy techniques—randomized controlled trial. *Journal of Dental Research*, **12**:1144–8.

Innes, N.P.T., Evans D.J.P., and Stirrups D.R. (2010). Sealing caries in primary molars: Hall Technique RCT 5-year results. Available online at: **http://iadr.confex.com/iadr/2010barce/webprogramcd/Paper138838.html**

Kassa, D., Day, P., High, A., and Duggal, M. (2009). Histological comparison of pulpal inflammation in primary teeth with occlusal or proximal caries. *International Journal of Paediatric Dentistry*, **19**, 26–33.

Marks, L.A.M., Weerheijm, K.L., and van Amerongen, W.E. (1999). Dyract versus Tylin class II restorations in primary molars: 36 months evaluation. *Caries Research*, **33**, 387–92.

Monterio, J., Day, P., Duggal, M., Morgan, C., and Rodd, H. (2009). Pulpal status of human primary teeth with physiological root resorption. *International Journal of Paediatric Dentistry*, **19**, 16–25.

Pitts, N.B. and Longbottom, C. (1995). Preventative care advised (PCA)/operative care advised (OCA)—categorising caries by the management option. *Community Dentistry and Oral Epidemiology*, **23**, 55–9.

Qvist, V., Poulsen, A., Teglers, P.T., and Mjör, I.A. (2010). The longevity of different restorations in primary teeth. *International Journal of Paediatric Dentistry*, **20**, 1–7.

Welbury, R.R., Shaw, A.J., Murray, J.J., Gordon, P.H., and McCabe, J.F. (2000). Clinical evaluation of paired compomer and glass ionomer restorations in primary molars: final results after 42 months. *British Dental Journal*, **189**, 93–7.

9

Operative treatment of dental caries in the young permanent dentition

J.A. Smallridge

Chapter contents

9.1 Introduction

Caries is a chronic disease. If it starts to affect the permanent teeth the child patient is drawn into a cycle requiring **ongoing** care for the rest of his/her life. Therefore when treating the young permanent dentition we have to adopt an approach that considers and addresses the whole disease process and not just treat the outcome of the disease.

Caries is still a considerable problem in children and adolescents. The 2002–2003 British Association for the Study of Community

Dentistry (BASCD) surveys which looked at dental disease levels in 77 693 14-year-old children in England and Wales (Pitts *et al.* 2004) found that, on average, half of the children examined had dentinal decay, with a mean of three permanent teeth decayed into dentine. Other studies have shown a low care index in UK children. The average care index for 11-year-old children is 41%, i.e. 59% of caries is left untreated, and in some parts of the country 80% is untreated. These children are at high risk of pain and discomfort relating to their teeth. Interviews with 8-year-old children showed that 47.5% had experienced toothache, 7.6% of whom had had pain in the previous 4 weeks!

Caries prevalence declined in the later decades of the twentieth century. As it dropped, a concentration of the disease occurred, with a small percentage of the population experiencing most of the disease. Caries prevalence is greatest in the occlusal surfaces of the first permanent molars and buccal grooves of the lower first molars, and the prevalence in these sites has dropped by the smallest proportion. The least susceptible sites are the approximal surfaces of the incisors, so if caries is seen in these permanent teeth you are dealing with rampant caries (Sheiham and Sabbah 2010).

The first permanent teeth erupt into the mouth at approximately 6 years of age, but may appear as early as the age of 4 years. The eruption of the anterior teeth usually causes great excitement, as it is associated with 'the fluttering of tooth fairy wings'. However, the eruption of the first permanent molars goes largely unnoticed until there is a problem. The mean eruption time for first permanent molars has been determined as 6.1 years in girls and 6.3 years in boys, but there is a tremendous variation in both the time of eruption and the time it takes for the tooth to emerge into the mouth. It takes 12–18 months for a first or second molar to erupt fully.

The first permanent molars are teeth that commonly exhibit disrupted enamel; the reported incidences of defects range from 3.6% to 25%. The occlusal surfaces of these molar teeth account for about 90% of caries in children. The most rapid rise in DMFT rates occurs during late childhood and adolescence, a time when the enamel is still immature but when responsibility for oral hygiene and dietary choices is changing from parent to child. The rate of increase slows as young adulthood is reached.

Restoration of the young permanent dentition is part of a continuum and cannot be regarded in isolation. Restoration is only one small part of the child's treatment. Essentially it is 'surgery' to remove the carious infected area of the tooth and insertion of a suitable substitute to restore the missing structure. It does nothing to cure the disease and must form part of a much wider treatment modality, which includes identification of the risk factors contributing to the disease followed by introduction of specific prevention counter-measures.

Effort must be applied in all of these areas to attempt to provide the optimum conditions for future tooth survival. The risk factors and preventive measures are addressed in detail in other chapters; this chapter will confine itself to appraisal of methods of treatment of caries in the young permanent dentition. It cannot hope to completely cover every aspect of operative treatment and there are other texts that the dentist should read to give a fuller account of the available techniques. However, the authors intend to give an outline of some of the options available.

9.2 Assessment of caries risk

Caries risk assessment is essential for producing a holistic dental management plan specific for the individual child. There are many questions to consider when planning treatment of caries:

- Is there caries?
- Is it into dentine?
- When to monitor?
- When to treat?
- What is the family attitude to teeth?
- What cooperation can you expect?
- Are they at low risk of further caries?
- Are they at high risk of more caries developing?

The idea of a caries risk assessment for each child patient is to ensure that the chosen diagnostic tests, preventive treatment, and any restorations are geared specifically to the needs for that individual patient. Factors requiring consideration are:

1. present caries activity
2. past caries activity
3. parent/sibling caries activity
4. sugar consumption (food and drink)
5. oral hygiene
6. fluoride exposure
7. tooth morphology
8. *Streptococcus mutans* levels
9. saliva characteristics, flow rate, and consistency.

Factors (1)–(7) will become clear when a full history and examination are carried out (Fig. 9.1). Factors (8) and (9) will only come into play if there is rampant caries that cannot be explained by the history.

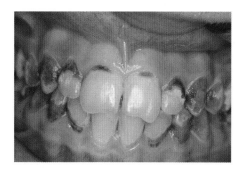

Figure 9.1 An example of caries in a 12-year-old girl, who sucked Polo mints non-stop—'six packets per day'.

9.3 Treatment decisions

The clinician must **always** give consideration to whether it is better to treat a carious lesion or to remineralize it.

9.3.1 Important points in relation to treatment

1. Gaining access to the caries inevitably means destruction of sound tooth tissue. The operator must keep this to a minimum consistent with complete caries eradication.

2. Once the operator places an initial restoration, he/she cannot 'undo' it and that tooth will inevitably require further restoration in its lifetime.

3. **Every** time an operator places a restoration, he/she destroys more of the original tooth structure, thereby weakening the tooth.

4. Even though the occlusion in a young person changes as growth occurs and teeth erupt, it is important to realize that when the operator places restorations, he/she must replicate the original occlusal contacts in the tooth. Although it may be tempting to keep the restoration totally out of the occlusion, teeth will move back into the occlusion, which will thereafter be slightly different and the cumulative effect of a lot of little changes can severely disrupt the occlusion in the long term.

5. When treating an approximal lesion on one tooth with an adjacent neighbour, the operator will almost certainly damage the latter. The important surface layer of the neighbouring tooth, which contains the highest level of fluoride, is the most resistant, so damage inflicted increases the chances of the adjacent surface of the neighbouring tooth becoming carious. It also creates an area of roughness on that surface, which in turn will accumulate more plaque, thereby increasing the risk of further decalcification.

6. When placing a class 2 restoration it is inevitable that there is some damage to the periodontal tissues. There is the transient damage caused by placement of the matrix band and wedge, and there is also an enduring effect, caused by the presence of the restoration margin. The very presence of the new restoration margin results in a contour change of the interstitial space. However smooth the operator attempts to make it, the altered state will increase plaque accumulation.

7. Repair and refurbishment of restorations instead of replacement saves tooth structure.

(See Key Points 9.1.)

9.3.2 Important points in relation to remineralization

1. Early smooth surface lesions are **reversible** in the right conditions.

2. There is little evidence to suggest that remineralization occurs in lesions already into dentine.

Key Points 9.1

- The surface layer of enamel contains most fluoride and is most resistant to caries.
- Every time an operator places a restoration, he/she destroys more of the original tooth structure, thereby weakening the tooth.
- Repair and refurbishment of restorations instead of replacement saves tooth structure.

3. It is very difficult to **predict** the rate of progression of a caries lesion. The rate of caries progression is usually slow, but can be rapid in some individuals, particularly younger children. In general, the older the child is when a carious lesion is diagnosed, the slower the progress of the lesion, assuming constancy of other risk factors.

4. The remineralized tissue of early caries is **less** susceptible to further caries.

5. **Small** restorations are generally more successful than large restorations, so a balance has to be struck between allowing preventive procedures adequate time to function and the risk of lesion enlargement.

The progression rate of approximal caries can vary from tooth to tooth within the same mouth (Figs 9.2 and 9.3). It is thought that if the circumstances for remineralization are favourable, clinicians should use this modality as opposed to a restoration that has a finite but limited lifespan.

The operator can achieve remineralization with the aid of:

- fluoride rinse
- fluoride varnish
- chlorhexidine varnish
- CPP-ACP

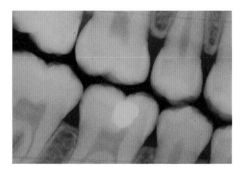

Figure 9.2 A bitewing radiograph of a 13-year-old boy showing early caries in the upper right first permanent premolar and molar and in both lower molars.

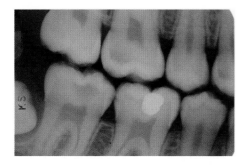

Figure 9.3 Radiograph of the same boy 18 months later showing rapid progress of caries in the upper first premolar, molar, and lower second molar, with little or no change in the lower second premolar and molar.

- oral hygiene measures
- adjacent glass ionomer restorations.

Determination of the most effective method of retarding the progression of approximal caries requires identification of not only the most effective remineralizing agent but also the frequency with which to employ it.

Current studies indicate that fluoride varnishes, solutions, and toothpastes all have a significant effect on the progression of approximal caries in permanent molars when assessed radiographically. Chlorhexidine varnish does not appear to add any additional benefit to this. CPP-ACP shows some early promise as a remineralization tool, but further random controlled trials are needed. (See Key Point 9.2.)

Key Point 9.2

At present, 4-monthly application of fluoride varnish seems to provide the best chance of remineralization.

Some questions still remain:

- Would the lesions have developed to the restorative stage if remineralizing techniques had not been employed?
- For how long should remineralization techniques be used?
- What is an acceptable frequency of monitoring the lesions radiographically if this is the only acceptable way of determining progress?
- Is the cost of remineralization therapy less than that of restorative treatment, particularly if it entails multiple attendances by the patient?

The progress of caries through the enamel seems to be fairly slow, but once the dentine is reached it accelerates. Therefore, as a rule of thumb, restore approximal surfaces once the lesion reaches the enamel–dentine interface.

9.4 Diagnosis

Whilst most dentists would agree that approximal caries is best diagnosed from bitewing radiographs, detection of occlusal caries is much more difficult. Where there is no overt or open cavity, diagnosing the status of a discoloured or stained fissure can be extremely difficult, if not impossible on occasions. Many methods have been proposed, both alone and in combination. These include:

- visual methods (dry tooth)
- probe/explorer (used only to remove debris)
- bitewing radiographs (see Box 9.1)
- electronic
- fibreoptic trans-illumination
- laser diagnosis.

When two or three methods are used in combination, there is greater accuracy and higher rates of detection of caries. The most widely used combination is visual inspection to examine a dry tooth (for stains, opacities, etc.) with a good light, along with a good-quality bitewing radiograph. Drying the tooth to be examined is **essential**, as early lesions, where the demineralization is minimal, will only become visible when there is a dry surface. (See Key Point 9.3.)

Key Point 9.3

Teeth should be dried prior to examination for caries.

Additionally, flossing to clear any interstitial plaque and temporary separation of the teeth with either wedges or orthodontic separators may aid diagnosis by providing some direct vision to approximal areas (Figs 9.4 and 9.5). Different recommendations are made for the timing of bitewing radiographs in published guidelines, as discussed in Chapter 6. Conformity to these guidelines may not be good; a recent study

Box 9.1 Benefits of bitewing radiographs for caries diagnosis

- Detect caries that cannot otherwise be detected
- Help estimate the extent of lesions
- Provide a baseline for monitoring lesions

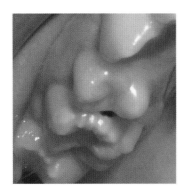

Figure 9.4 Decalcification on the mesial surface of the upper first molar. Radiographs show lesion confined to enamel.

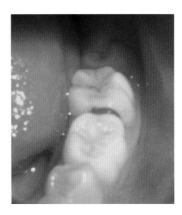

Figure 9.5 Insertion of a separator may allow examination of the suspicious surface.

found that only 72% of a group of Scottish dentists used radiography as a caries diagnostic tool in children. When planning which radiographs to take, the orthodontic implications that treatment of the caries may raise must also be taken into consideration. Young *et al.* (2009) reported that only 46.2% of children referred for removal of permanent teeth

under general anaesthetic had undergone a previous radiographic assessment!

Bitewing radiographs (see Box 9.1) will show dentinal caries in teeth that are designated as clinically sound. The prevalence of 'hidden caries', i.e. radiographically visible dentine caries under a seemingly sound surface on visual inspection, in teenagers is reported to be between 10% and 15%. There will also be teeth visually designated as carious in which there are no radiological signs of caries, hence the need for more than one method of diagnosis.

In making a diagnosis of caries, the operator has to decide not only that there is a lesion present but also:

- whether demineralization is present
- the depth of the lesion
- the rate of progression of the lesion
- whether it is an arrested or active lesion.

It would be useful to have a method of quantifying these factors. Measurements of electrical conductance and laser fluorescence have the potential to chart lesion progression/retardation as they provide a quantitative record which, if repeated over several appointments, will demonstrate whether the lesion is active or arresting. They can be repeated safely more frequently than radiographs. However, it should be remembered that the electrical conductance and laser fluorescence methods will incorrectly interpret hypomineralization as caries and that the laser-based instrument will routinely interpret staining as caries. (See Key Points 9.4.)

Key Points 9.4

- Early diagnosis of caries is important to be able to plan the whole treatment modality.
- Bitewing radiographs are recommended as an essential adjunct to a patient's first clinical examination.

9.5 Recurrent caries

Visual examination and radiographs are the most common ways of **detecting** recurrent caries.

Recurrent caries is most commonly found at the gingival margins of class II restorations, but often restorations will look a little 'tatty' at recall so careful examination in good light is essential.

Visually it is important to differentiate recurrent lesions from stained margins on resin-based composite restorations. Alternatives such as polishing or exploratory preparations adjacent to the lesion and repair

may be appropriate rather than replacing the whole restoration. (See Key Point 9.5.)

Key Point 9.5

Repair and refurbishing of lesions saves tooth structure.

9.6 Fissure sealants

A fissure sealant is a material that is placed in the pits and fissures of teeth in order to **prevent** the development of dental caries.

Fissure sealants cannot be discussed in isolation from caries diagnosis or treatment of pit and fissure caries. Fissure sealants can be used both preventively and therapeutically.

Toothbrush bristles cannot access the pit and fissure system because the dimensions of the fissures are too small. As a result micro-organisms remain within the fissure system undisturbed. The tooth is most susceptible to plaque stagnation during eruption, i.e. a period of 12–18 months. During this time, children need extra parental help in maintaining their oral hygiene. (See Key Point 9.6.)

Key Point 9.6

Sealing with a resin-based sealant is a recommended procedure for preventing caries of the occlusal surface of permanent molars.

Lesion formation takes place in the plaque stagnation area at the entrance to the fissure and commences with subsurface demineralization. Demineralized enamel is **more** porous than sound enamel. The more demineralized and porous the affected enamel, the more it shows up both clinically and on radiographs. (See Key Point 9.7.)

Key Point 9.7

To detect the earliest white spots the tooth must be dried to render them more obvious.

Once the initial lesion has developed, caries may spread laterally so that a small surface lesion may hide a much greater area of destruction below the surface (Figs 9.6 and 9.7).

Remineralization of occlusal lesions is much more difficult to achieve. Fissure sealing, application of 2.26% fluoride varnish every 6 months with oral hygiene instruction, and a weekly 0.2% sodium fluoride rinse have all been found to help stabilize the disease and retard the progress of occlusal caries, but fissure sealing the teeth is most effective. Many studies have shown that as caries rates decline, the proportion of pit and fissure caries of molar teeth has generally increased, and that the caries appears to be concentrated in a smaller cohort of children, with most of the decay occurring in 25% of the child population. This predilection has meant that correct application of fissure sealants should have a maximal effect.

There is no dispute that when **correctly applied** and **monitored** fissure sealants are highly effective at preventing dental caries in pit and fissures, but interpretation of the correct application and monitoring require scrutiny. (See Key Points 9.8.)

Key Points 9.8

- Fissure sealants reduce caries incidence but must be carefully monitored and maintained.
- The relative caries risk reduction pooled estimate for resin-based sealants on permanent first molars has been reported as 33%. The effect depends on the retention of the sealant.
- 4.5 years after sealing permanent molar teeth in children aged 5–10 years there was a reduction in decay in over 50% of biting surfaces compared with teeth without sealants.

9.6.1 Who will benefit?

Not every fissure will become carious if it is not sealed. Therefore each tooth for each child must be assessed on its own merits. The clinician must assess the risk factors for that tooth developing pit or fissure

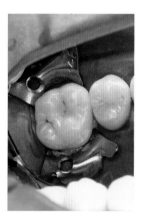

Figure 9.6 Hidden caries. Although the occlusal surface looks mostly intact it hides extensive caries.

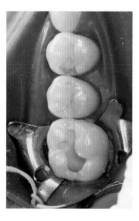

Figure 9.7 Caries has been removed. The size of the cavity emphasizes the extent of the lesion.

Table 9.1 Factors to consider for sealant recommendation

Patient factors	Tooth factors
Caries in primary teeth	Depth of fissures
Caries in other permanent molar	Hypomineralization
Patients with underlying medical, physical, or emotional problems	Hypoplasia
	Inaccessible for cleaning
Risk factors (e.g. diet)	

caries (Table 9.1). As a general guide to who will benefit, review the British Society of Paediatric Dentistry (BSPD) guidelines (Smallridge 2010). (See Key Point 9.9.)

> **Key Point 9.9**
>
> In areas of high caries prevalence it has been shown that treatment costs can be reduced by sealing susceptible surfaces, and even where sealant retention is incomplete there is sufficient caries inhibition to endorse the use of sealants.

The main beneficiaries are the following:

1. Children and young people with impairments such that their general health would be jeopardized by either the development of oral disease or the need for dental treatment. In such children all susceptible sites in both the primary and permanent dentitions should receive consideration.

2. The operator should seal all susceptible sites on permanent teeth in children and young people with caries in their primary teeth (decayed, filled, and missing tooth surfaces (DMFS) ≥2).

3. Where occlusal caries affects one permanent molar, the operator should seal the occlusal surfaces of the other molars.

4. If the anatomy of the tooth is such that surfaces are deeply fissured, the operator should seal that surface.

5. Where potential risk factors such as dietary factors or oral hygiene factors indicate a high risk of caries, seal all at-risk sites.

6. Where there is doubt about the caries status of a fissure or it is known to have caries confined to the enamel, fissure sealants may be used therapeutically but it is essential to monitor the surface both clinically and radiologically after application.

(See Key Point 9.10.)

> **Key Point 9.10**
>
> Even in a fluoridated community sealants may be cost effective.

Sealant use must be based on personal, tooth, and surface risk, and the clinician must **assess** these risks at intervals since they might

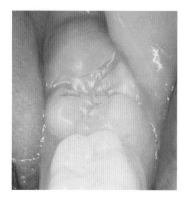

Figure 9.8 It is too early to seal this tooth with resin. Therefore it should be painted with fluoride varnish, or if the caries risk is very high it should be sealed with glass ionomer until further eruption has taken place.

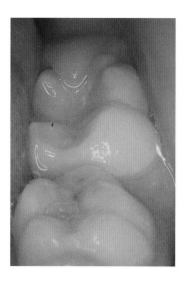

Figure 9.9 This molar is just at the correct stage to apply fissure sealant. The very small operculum of gingival tissue can gently be held away from the tooth with a flat plastic spatula.

change at any time in the life of the patient. Therefore, whereas it was traditionally stated that dentists should complete sealant application up to a year or two after eruption, he/she should assess the potential risk factors regularly, and place sealant when indicated (Figs 9.8 and 9.9).

Failure rates are higher when sealants are placed on newly erupted teeth and in mouths with high previous caries experience. Monitoring the integrity of the sealant is vital in these circumstances, and any deficiencies should be corrected. It is important that parents are made aware of this, and the fact that a sealant does not protect all surfaces of a tooth, so that their expectations are realistic and they bring their child for regular checks.

9.6.2 Clinical technique

Pre-treatment prior to sealant application

Tooth preparation with pumice and a rotary brush results in good clinical retention rates. Dry brushing achieves similar results. Air polishing using a Prophy-Jet, an early air abrasion system that uses sodium bicarbonate particles as the abrasive medium, provides good bond strength and sealant penetration, but has not received general acceptance probably because most dental surgeries do not possess this item of equipment.

Some researchers have advocated the use of 'enameloplasty', a more aggressive intervention into the tooth, i.e. mechanical enlargement of the fissures with a bur or with air abrasion, to improve sealant penetration and reduce micro-leakage. Although some studies have confirmed these claims, the authors feel that this submits the child to an unnecessary extra procedure and do not recommend it.

Etching

Etching for just 20 seconds with a range of concentrations of acid, but usually 35–37.5% phosphoric acid, is the tried and tested method. Its one drawback is the susceptibility of the etched surface to saliva/moisture contamination, which reduces the bond strength. Salivary contamination results in significantly reduced bond strengths unless the salia is removed by thorough washing. Re-etching of the surface is usually necessary.

Bonding agents

Use of a bonding agent under a resin fissure sealant **aids** bond strength. A bonding agent used as an additional layer under a resin sealant yields bond strengths significantly greater than the bond strength obtained when using sealant without a bonding agent. The initial results of clinical trials also show increased retention of the sealant when an intermediate bond is used. New bonding techniques are proving to be less technique sensitive with respect to moisture control than previous procedures.

The use of a bonding agent under sealant on wet contaminated surfaces yields bond strengths equivalent to the bond strength obtained when sealant is bonded directly to clean etched enamel without contamination. Most of the data on the use of a bonding agent as part of the sealant procedure support its use.

Use of a bonding agent tends to increase the time and cost of the sealant application, but in cases where maintaining a dry surface is difficult or where there are areas of hypomineralization on the surface it has many advantages.

Logically, combination of these technologies to achieve better penetration with fewer steps in the application sequence would be beneficial. The big bonus of the self-etching primer–adhesive system is the speed with which the operator can apply it. The operator brushes the self-etching adhesive onto the surface, where air thins it, and follows this by immediate placement of the sealant and polymerization. In the study, the average time operators took for the procedure was 1.8 minutes compared with 3.1 minutes with the conventional technique. Such time-saving is very useful in young fidgety children. However, there are conflicting results with these systems at present, and conventional separate etch and bond systems still appear to give superior retention of the sealant.

A Cochrane review (Ahovuo-Saloranto et al. 2004) **recommends** sealing with a resin-based sealant to prevent caries of the occlusal surface of permanent molars. Resin-based sealants have a good track record. Many clinical trials have demonstrated their effectiveness, and several long-term studies have show their benefits. A 28% complete retention and 35% partial retention of sealants on first permanent molars after a single application have been shown. Where researchers re-applied sealant to deficient surfaces, as determined by annual examinations, 65% complete retention was obtained and only 13% of the surfaces had caries or restorations after 20 years.

Re-treatment

Sealants placed in the first permanent molars of 6-, 7-, and 8-year-old children and in second permanent molars in 11- and 12-year-old children required more re-application than those placed in the teeth of older children. If the clinician places fissure sealant in newly erupted teeth, it is more likely to fail, but it should still be placed as **early** as possible because the teeth are so vulnerable to caries at this time. Parents must be aware of the possible loss and the importance of regular monitoring.

Modifying the resin to incorporate fluoride is a logical rationale. However, fluoride release occurs for only a very short time and at a very low level. Many studies over 2- to 3-year periods have reported good retention but similar caries incidence to conventional sealant. Since the addition of fluoride to sealant resin does not have any detrimental effect it could certainly be used, but until the chemistry can be adapted to unlock the fluoride readily, the anti-cariogenicity cannot be attributed to the fluoride.

A greater release of fluoride can be achieved by using a glass ionomer (poly-alkenoate). Such cements have high levels of fluoride available for release but they suffer from the drawback of poor retention. Even with their very poor retention rates, sealing with glass ionomer does seem to impart some caries-protective effect. This may be due to both the fluoride released by the glass ionomer and residual material retained in the bottom of the fissure, which is invisible to the naked eye. Hence glass ionomers used as sealants can be classified as fissure sealants but more realistically as fluoride depot materials. Resin and glass ionomer sealants are compared in Table 9.2

Glass ionomer sealants can also be used in partially erupted teeth and where cooperation is too limited for a resin sealant. They can be usefully employed to seal partially erupted molars in high-risk children since eruption of the molars takes 12–18 months and during this time they are often very difficult to clean. Once the teeth are sufficiently

Table 9.2 Resin sealants versus glass ionomer sealants

Resin sealant	Glass ionomer sealant
Better retention	Poorer retention
Technique-sensitive application	Easier application
Longer time to apply	Short application time
Act as barrier only; no residual effect if lost	Release of fluoride; some effect even if lost

erupted the operator can place a resin sealant. They are also useful in children in whom there are difficulties with the level of cooperation as the technique does not depend on absolute moisture control.

Both RMGIs and compomers have been used as sealants. As yet, studies of these materials used as fissure sealants show no improvement over resin-based sealants and so there is nothing to recommend them in preference to resins.

Filled or unfilled resins?

Retention is better for unfilled resins probably because it penetrates into the fissures more completely. In addition, it does not need occlusal adjustment as it abrades very rapidly. If a filled resin is not adjusted there is a perceptible occlusal change, possible discomfort, and wear of the opposing antagonist tooth.

Coloured or clear material?

Opaque sealants have the advantage of high visibility at recall (Fig. 9.10). It has been found that the identification error for opaque resin was only 1% whilst for clear resin the corresponding figure was 23%, with the most common error being false identification of the presence of clear resin on an untreated tooth. The disadvantage of opaque sealant is that the dentist cannot visually examine the fissure at future recalls (Fig. 9.11). Both camps have a case, so it really comes down to personal choice.

Safety issues

There has only been one report of an allergy to the resin used for pit and fissure sealing.

Concern has been raised about the oestrogenicity of resin-based composites. The proposed culprit, bis-phenol A (BPA), is not a direct ingredient of dental sealants but is a chemical that appears in the final product if the raw materials fail to react fully. The amount released orally is undetectable in the systemic circulation and concerns about potential oestrogenicity are probably unfounded.

Sealant bulk in relation to application

With respect to the method of application, it is important to remember that the sealant must be kept to a minimum consistent with coverage of the complete fissure system including buccal and lingual pits. Over-filling can lead to reduction in retention and increased micro-leakage.

Sealant monitoring

Once the sealant has been placed the operator must monitor it at recall appointments and repair or replenish as necessary. Teeth lose 5–10% of sealant bulk each year. Partial loss of resin sealant allows ingress of bacteria into the fissure system, which leaves that surface equally at risk from caries as one that has not been sealed at all (Figs 9.12 and 9.13).

Cost-effectiveness

Cost-effectiveness will depend on the caries rate of the children in the population. Where there is a high caries rate, generalized sealing will protect more surfaces that would become carious in the future. However, if the caries rate is very high, the risk of developing interproximal lesions is also high and may lead to restoration even when the fissure-sealed surfaces remain caries free. In low-caries populations, the cost-effectiveness of sealant application *en masse* is questionable, and obviously the dentist should assess each child's individual risk factors when they attend the surgery.

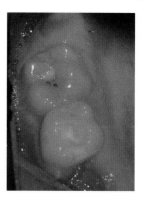

Figure 9.12 Partial loss of sealant with caries in the occlusal fissure.

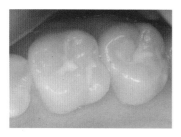

Figure 9.10 White fissure sealants can easily be seen to check at recall. They are also visible to show the patient and parent to help them understand the procedure.

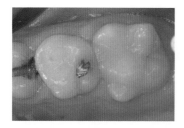

Figure 9.11 Clear fissure sealant is less easy to see but its presence can be checked by etching if an area is giving cause for concern.

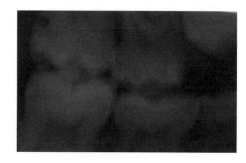

Figure 9.13 Radiograph of the tooth showing that the caries has extended into the dentine so a preventive resin restoration (PRR) is indicated.

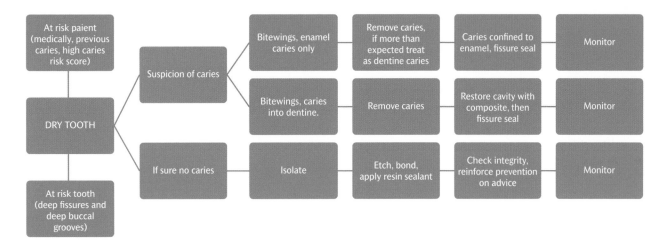

Figure 9.14 Algorithm for treating caries.

In contrast with this general concept, one study has shown that it costs 1.6 times as much to restore carious lesions in the first permanent molars in an unsealed group of 5- to 10-year-old children living in a fluoridated area than to prevent the lesions with a single application of pit and fissure sealant. The study also revealed a greater number of lesions if sealants were not utilized.

Sealing over caries

As stated earlier, diagnosis of caries in pits and fissures can be difficult. Once caries has been diagnosed, it is important to determine its extent. If there is clear unequivocal evidence that the lesion does not extend beyond the enamel, the surface can be sealed and monitored both clinically and radiologically. If the lesion extends into the dentine, the dentist must place either a PRR or, if in an area of occlusal load, a conventional restoration.

Several studies have shown that carious lesions do not progress under sealants as long as the sealant stays intact. However, if the sealant were to fail immediately or shortly after application, the lesion would have 4–6 months to progress before the next review, so the authors do not advocate sealing over caries except in very exceptional circumstances. (See Key Points 9.11.)

An algorithm for treating caries is shown in Fig. 9.14.

> **Key Points 9.11**
>
> - If the caries is confined to enamel, the surface should have a resin-based sealant placed to reduce the chance of progress of the lesion.
> - As long as cooperation permits, all suspected caries lesions should be investigated and the caries removed and restored prior to sealing.

9.7 Rubber dam

Although rubber dam is often perceived as difficult to apply on children, its use creates a better working environment for both the dentist and the child (Fig. 9.15). Once the technique is mastered, it can be applied both quickly and with minimal discomfort.

1. It protects the soft tissues (tongue, cheeks, and gingivae) from damage by instruments or medicaments.
2. It reduces the risk of swallowing and/or inhalation of instruments, particles, and debris.
3. It makes the salivary aerosol produced by high-speed rotary instruments easier to control, thereby reducing the risk of infection to dental staff.
4. If used with inhalation sedation it will reduce the amount of mouth breathing, so that less nitrous oxide is needed and the gas level in the general environment of the dental surgery is reduced.

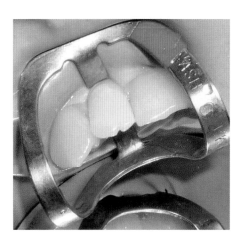

Figure 9.15 Rubber dam in place protecting gingivae and eliminating moisture.

5. It often makes the child feel isolated from the treatment. This can make the child feel more relaxed and able to cope.

6. It provides the best possible dry field. Its use is imperative for materials where moisture control is essential.

Other texts give fuller details of rubber dam application techniques and these should be consulted so the operator can apply rubber dam quickly and efficiently. It must be remembered that good analgesia is very important as placement of rubber dam is painful, particularly when a clamp is used. An infiltration backed up by intra-papillary injections is usually needed.

9.8 Anterior caries

Caries of anterior teeth is not very common in childhood and adolescence. It usually occurs either where there is defect in the formation of the teeth, leading to plaque accumulation, or in children with rampant caries where the sugar intake is so high that the dentition is overwhelmed.

The best material for restoring anterior teeth is composite resin. The use of this material in the treatment of patients affected by trauma or as a solution for cosmetic problems is described in Chapters 10 and 12.

In patients suffering from 'normal' caries, with class III cavities, composite restoration is the material of choice. In patients with rampant caries it may be preferable to use glass ionomer to restore the lesions as an interim measure whilst the risk factors are addressed.

9.9 Occlusal caries

Where the dentist has established a diagnosis that a stained fissure is a carious lesion into dentine, restorative treatment is indicated. If the lesion is limited to areas of the tooth not bearing occlusal loads, a preventive resin restoration is appropriate. If the lesion is more extensive, the clinician should consider a composite or amalgam class I restoration.

9.9.1 Preventive resin restoration

Clinical technique

1. Administer local analgesia, after application of topical anaesthetic paste at the injection site.

2. Place rubber dam.

3. Explore the suspect area of the fissure system with a high-speed small bur, removing only enough enamel to gain access to the caries. The access must by wide enough to ensure that the operator can remove caries from the peripheral tissue. If the radiographs show dentinal caries, even if the enamel seems intact, access must progress into dentine. Undermined enamel can be left *in situ* as the bis-GMA resin restoration virtually restores the original strength of the tooth.

4. Line the cavity with calcium hydroxide if the pulp is close. There is some debate as to whether it is necessary to line these cavities. Some studies report no pulpal problems in teeth where the operator has directly etched and bonded the dentine.

5. Etch. Precise details dependent on the chosen 'restorative' system for steps 5–8.

6. Wash.

7. Dry.

8. Bond.

9. Place the chosen composite in the cavity as a sandwich. Glass ionomer cement (GIC) is an alternative in smaller cavities.

10. Seal all the remaining fissure system with fissure sealant.

11. Check the occlusion and adjust if necessary.

12. Review the integrity of the sealant at the routine recall appointments. If the visual appearance is inconclusive, re-etch the surface to identify sealant retention.

The technique is illustrated in Figs 9.16–9.26.

Where the diagnostic methods are inconclusive, the clinician should explore the fissure to validate caries-free status or eradicate occult caries. Depending on the extent of any lesion, restoration by fissure sealing or composite completes the procedure.

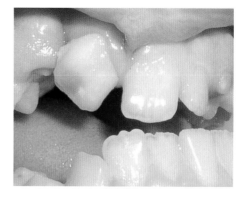

Figure 9.16 Anterior caries in a child with a cleft lip and palate. Teeth that are malformed or malpositioned are more susceptible to caries.

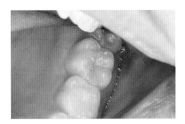

Figure 9.17 Unrestored carious first molar. Caries identified in mesial fossa on radiograph.

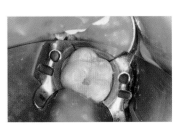

Figure 9.18 Cavity preparation commenced after local analgesia and application of rubber dam. Access and outline form should only be of a size to enable removal of caries.

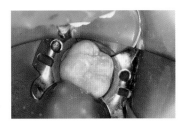

Figure 9.19 Tooth restored with glass ionomer.

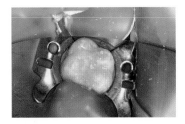

Figure 9.20 Restoration covered with fissure sealant.

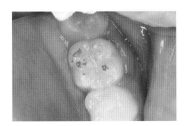

Figure 9.21 Rubber dam removed and occlusion checked.

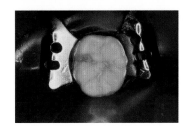

Figure 9.22 The same principles can apply with a slightly larger lesion.

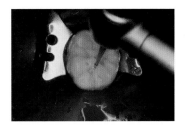

Figure 9.23 Undermined enamel can be left as long as the operator can reach all the caries.

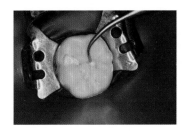

Figure 9.24 Place a calcium hydroxide lining in the deep parts of the cavity.

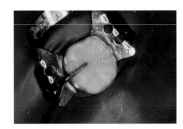

Figure 9.25 After etching and bonding, place composite resin incrementally.

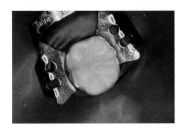

Figure 9.26 Finish the restoration with fissure sealing.

Materials: what to use?

Properties of the materials used are summarized in Table 9.3.

9.9.2 Class I restorations in young permanent teeth

If caries affects most of the occlusal fissure system, the clinician should place a class I restoration. The choice of material for this restoration depends on the choice of the operator and appropriately informed parents. The plethora of available tooth-coloured materials together with the continuing development and introduction of new materials makes choice both extensive and difficult.

Silver amalgam

Silver amalgam is the standard material against which the success of alternative materials is often judged. Amalgam has a known track record. Dentists have used it for restoring teeth for more than 150 years. When consulting the literature it must be remembered that amalgam technology has evolved over a very long period and that the amalgam alloys available today are probably very different in composition from those used even as recently as 20 years ago. (See Key Point 9.12.)

Key Point 9.12

Amalgam is an effective filling material that is easy to handle and less technique-sensitive than tooth-coloured materials.

Amalgam has many useful properties.

1. It is easy to handle.
2. It has good durability.
3. It has a relatively low cost.
4. It exhibits reducing micro-leakage with time. It should be remembered that it can take up to 2 years for a marginal seal to be produced with high-copper amalgams, and double the time for low-copper amalgams, but high-copper amalgams are not as susceptible to corrosion phenomena and resulting porosity and therefore retain their strength.
5. It is less technique-sensitive than other restorative materials.

It is still important to control moisture as excess moisture causes delayed expansion, particularly in zinc-containing alloys, and for this reason rubber dam should always be used if possible.

Despite these good properties, amalgam has two main disadvantages:

- it is not aesthetic
- it contains mercury, a known poison.

Little can be done to combat the poor aesthetics. Remember to polish amalgams as this does improve characteristics, including appearance, and leads to a significant reduction in their replacement.

Table 9.3 Key research into choosing materials

Soncini et al. 2007	5-year follow-up occlusal lesions 6- to 10-year-olds Replacement rate: composite, 14.9% amalgam, 10.8%
Hickel and Manhart 2001	Annual failure rates: composite, up to 14.4% amalgam, up to 9%
Mjor et al. 2000	Median age of failed restorations in <18-year-olds: GIC, 2 years RMGIC, 2 years composite, 3 years amalgam, 5 years
Forss and Widstrom 2003	Mean age of failure: 3.5 years (58.7% composite, 0.6% amalgam, 40% RMGIC)

GIC, glass ionomer cement; RMGIC, resin-modified glass ionomer cement.

Clinicians concerned about the toxicity of silver amalgam seek reassurance on the continuing use of the alloy. There are four main areas of concern:

- inhalation of mercury vapour or amalgam dust
- ingestion of amalgam
- allergy to mercury
- environmental considerations.

Inhalation of amalgam dust is most likely to occur during removal of a previous restoration. This effect is transient and the effects are minimized if the operator uses rubber dam and high-speed aspiration. It is not disputed that mercury is released from amalgam restorations at placement, polishing, during chewing, and during removal, but the amounts are very small and come nowhere near the amounts ingested daily from other sources (e.g. air, water, and diet). True allergy to amalgam is rare; only 50 cases have been reported in 100 years. Many countries are trying to reduce all industrial uses of mercury for environmental reasons and better mercury hygiene in dental practice is one of the areas targeted.

In small class I restorations the only difference needed in tooth preparation between composite and amalgam is that when an amalgam is to be placed, undermined enamel must be removed. In both cases a resin sealant material should be placed over the margins of the restoration and the remaining fissure system (Fig. 9.27). Researchers report very high success rates when amalgam is used in this way.

Composite resins

Many dentists advocate the use of composite resins as a restorative in the treatment of children. Since their introduction in the 1970s there have been many modifications. The abrasive wear of many composite

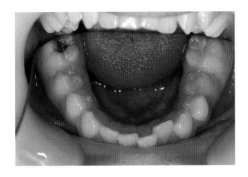

Figure 9.27 After restoration with amalgam, place fissure sealant to cover the amalgam and seal the fissure system.

systems is comparable to that of silver amalgam (in the region of 10–20μm/year), and colour stability is now excellent compared with earlier materials.

After placement and occlusal adjustment of the restorative material, the operator should place a layer of sealant on the finished surface to fill any micro-cracks within the surface of the resin, followed by curing of the latter to ensure maximal polymerization. (See Key Point 9.13.)

Key Point 9.13

Composite resin restorations are extremely technique sensitive. Clinicians should only place them when they can guarantee isolation.

Before making decisions concerning the most appropriate restorative material in the treatment of children, the clinician should consider the following:

1. Moisture exclusion. Is it realistic for this patient?
2. Patient compliance. Will the patient sit still during the restoration?
3. The size of the cavity. Lesion extent determines operative duration.
4. Patient compliance after the procedure. Will he/she return for monitoring and review?

As long as the responses to questions 1, 2, and 4 are in the affirmative and the restoration is relatively small, composite can be used with confidence that it will survive well.

Dentine bonding systems have enabled clinicians to achieve bonding of materials to dentine as well as to enamel, thereby improving the strength of the restoration. Dentine bonding is very technique sensitive. Adherence to the manufacturer's instructions is axiomatic at all times. Initially the technique consisted of etching and rinsing followed by application of primer containing a solvent resin monomer to wet and penetrate the collagen meshwork. Finally, the operator applied a bonding agent which penetrated into the primed dentine.

One-bottle systems in which the primer and bonding agent are combined within one solution are most commonly used. They require a moist dentine surface (moist but no visible shine) to facilitate bonding, so it is important not to over-dry after etching. The bond strength produced also depends on evaporation of the solvent and residual monomers prior to polymerization, so a steady air stream that aids evaporation but is not so strong that it removes the bond leaving denuded dentine is needed. Systems where the etch, prime, and bond solutions are combined in a single solution are available. The potential time-saving advantage of these solutions would, of course, be very welcome, but at present these materials appear to have a lower initial bond strength and exhibit more degradation than other systems. Research continues and it is important that dentists keep their knowledge up to date on the composition, characteristics, and mechanisms of adhesion of available bonding systems in order to make informed choices in their usage to provide the best long-term bond strengths. (See Key Points 9.14.)

Key Points 9.14

- When bonding, it is very important to follow the manufacturer's instructions carefully for best results.
- New techniques and materials will always come to market, but it is essential for the busy practitioner to be sceptical until researchers report clinical trials of adequate form and duration. Extrovert exponents of a particular technique or material frequently sway us into purchasing a material prematurely, to our later cost.

Glass ionomer cements

These materials tend to be more brittle than composites but have the advantage of adherence to tooth substance, both enamel and dentine, without etching. The coefficient of expansion of glass ionomer is very close to that of dentine, and once set these materials remain dimensionally stable even in the mouth where the moisture and temperature levels are constantly changing. Their greatest advantage over composites is that they are able to release fluoride over an extended period of time. Their lack of strength limits their use in the permanent dentition, but they can be used in PRRs where there is no occlusal load and as an interim restoration whilst caries is brought under control (Figs 9.28 and 9.29). They are also the authors' choice of material for cementing stainless steel crowns.

Resin-modified glass ionomer

Reinforcement of glass ionomer with resin has been used to produce a fast-setting cement, but these materials require etching prior to placement. Fracture toughness/resistance and abrasion resistance all improve in these modified materials, but they still retain biocompatibility, fluoride ion hydrodynamics, and favourable thermal expansion and contraction characteristics. Most importantly, they still retain physicochemical bonding to tooth structure.

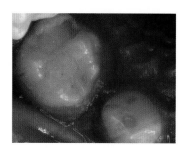

Figure 9.28 A deficient glass ionomer restoration seen after a year.

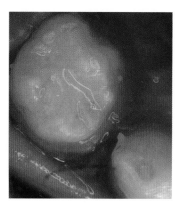

Figure 9.29 The operator simply adds more glass ionomer to the deficient restoration.

Compomer (polyacid-modified resin-based composite)

These materials are a combination of composite and ionomer. They have better aesthetics than glass ionomer as a single material and have the advantage of some fluoride release, but there is still a need to etch during the restorative procedure. However, they appear to suffer from the disadvantages of loss of retention and gap formation between the material and tooth substance.

Restoration failure

The principal reasons for failure of restorations are:

- secondary caries
- fracture
- marginal deficiencies
- wear
- postoperative sensitivity.

It is always important to look carefully at an unsatisfactory restoration and consider if it is possible to repair it rather than replace it completely. This can only be done if all recurrent caries is removed and the tooth is not left vulnerable to the same sort of failure in the future. It was found in a Cochrane review (Sharif *et al*. 2010) that there are no randomized controlled trials that have established whether it is better to replace or repair defective composite restorations, so sound clinical judgement must be used.

9.10 Approximal caries

It is well known that caries in children occurs more often occlusally than approximally, and that the relative level of approximal caries increases as they progress to adulthood. Occlusal caries should be managed immediately by sealing or PRR or restoration; approximal caries should be managed with remineralization techniques as an early intervention approach unless the lesion has reached the dentine. (See Key Point 9.15.)

Key Point 9.15

Approximal lesions in enamel only should have fluoride varnish applied and be closely monitored.

More recently sealing of non-cavitated approximal posterior carious lesions has been proposed and initial results, which at present only follow the teeth for up to 2 years, show some promise of reducing the rate of progress of the lesions compared with fluoride varnish or flossing as controls. Whichever way the clinician chooses to restore approximal caries, it will always entail loss of some sound tooth tissue. It also has

the potential to damage the adjacent interproximal surface in almost 70% of cases, leaving this surface more liable to develop caries. (See Key Point 9.16.)

Key Point 9.16

Damage to surrounding tissues occurs when a cavity is cut.

In class II restorations, tooth preparation need only be sufficient to gain access to the carious dentine. Shape the outline form to include just the carious dentine and to remove demineralized enamel. Finish the cavo-surface margins to remove unsupported enamel (slot preparation). The technique is illustrated in Figs 9.30–9.34.

Amalgam works well in this situation, but clinicians are increasingly using composite resins in class II restorations of young permanent teeth. Although some studies have reported good success rates, the overall consensus seems to be that tooth-coloured restorations are prone to earlier failure than amalgam restorations and operators should

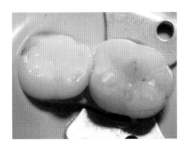

Figure 9.30 Mesial caries in a lower first molar. The lesion is not readily apparent.

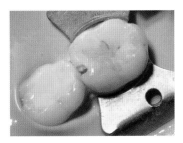

Figure 9.31 The lesion is opened. This view shows the extent of the caries more clearly. The operator does not need to extend for prevention.

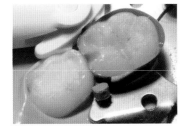

Figure 9.32 The caries has been removed, a band placed with wedge, and the cavity lined.

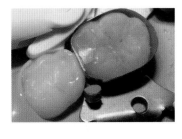

Figure 9.33 The operator has packed amalgam into the mesial slot.

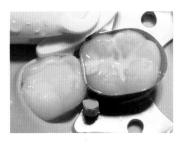

Figure 9.34 The operator has sealed the remainder of the fissure system.

inform parents of this proviso when discussing the choice of restorative material. (See Key Points 9.17.)

A flowchart illustrating treatment decision-making when approximal caries is detected is shown in Fig. 9.35.

Key Points 9.17

- Remember: the progression rate of lesions in the inner half of the enamel of the mesial surface of the first permanent molar is relatively fast between 6 and 12 years of age. About 20% progress into dentine within a year.
- The progression rate of caries is considerably faster in dentine than in enamel.

9.11 Extensive/deep caries

9.11.1 Extensive/deep caries in young teeth

Unfortunately, the situation sometimes arises where the caries is already extensive prior to the initial consultation, and the clinician needs to consider preservation versus extraction issues.

Rampant caries occurs in the permanent dentition as well as the primary dentition and once again treatment planning has to consider the whole person, not only with children, but sometimes the whole family, rather than just the teeth involved of one particular individual. This involves making decisions on:

- the advisability of restoration versus planned extraction;
- how to restore if that is the favoured modality;
- how to prevent onset of further lesions, i.e. reduce the risk factors by examining diet, oral hygiene, fissure sealing, fluoride treatment, and a rigid recall regime.

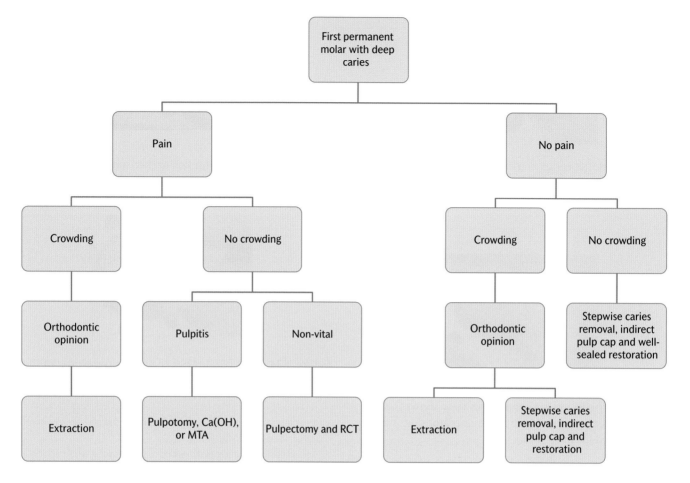

Figure 9.35 Treatment decision-making when approximal caries is detected.

9.11.2 Extraction considerations

(see Key Point 9.18)

Key Point 9.18

When a child presents with extensive caries in a molar you have to decide whether it is best to preserve the tooth or to extract it as part of a strategy to relieve crowding.

If there is extensive caries affecting the first permanent molars it may be expedient to consider extraction rather than restoration. However, it is important to check for the presence and development of the second premolars before prescribing extraction of the first permanent molars since lack of premolars means that all possible measures must be made to attempt to retain the first permanent molars. The decision on extraction depends on the age of the child, the stage of development of the dentition, and the occlusion. This is discussed fully in Chapter 14.

Whereas there are two options in treatment planning relating to first permanent molars, the clinician should invariably attempt to retain incisors and/or canines with extensive caries whenever possible.

9.11.3 Conservative treatment options

(see Key Point 9.19)

Key Point 9.19

Both the caries process and the trauma of caries removal can cause detrimental inflammatory changes within the pulp.

Various techniques are used to conserve teeth with deep caries:

- indirect pulp capping
- direct pulp capping
- pulpotomy
- pulpectomy.

(See Key Point 9.20.)

Key Point 9.20

Pulp preservation is important to ensure that the tooth is able to form full-length mature roots.

When the tooth erupts its roots are incompletely formed and are 20–40% shorter than the mature root. It takes up to 5 years after eruption for the root to complete its formation and develop an apical constriction. (See Key Point 9.21.)

Key Point 9.21

Whenever it is thought that caries removal might result in a pulpal exposure, clinicians should consider the most efficacious way to preserve pulp vitality in order to enable root maturation to occur, i.e. a state with continued physiological dentine deposition and complete root development.

Indirect pulp capping

If caries is deep and exposure is likely to occur, it is expedient to leave caries in the deepest part of the lesion when it is felt that further removal would lead to pulp exposure. Place a radio-opaque biocompatible base over the remaining carious dentine to stimulate healing and repair. It is important to remove caries completely from all the lateral walls of the cavity before restoration, since failure to do so will result in secondary spread and the need for future intervention. The technique is illustrated in Figs 9.36–9.40.

A Cochrane review (Ricketts *et al.* 2006) reported only four papers fitting their criteria, but found no difference in the progression of decay, longevity of restorations, or incidence of damage to the tooth pulp between ultra-conservative and complete decay removal.

Traditionally, operators use calcium hydroxide for indirect pulp capping which has a good success rate. Alternatives suggested include adhesive resins and glass ionomer cements, but as yet there are no studies looking at these techniques in permanent teeth. Whichever material is utilized, the crucial factor is to isolate the pulp well from the oral environment with a restoration of sufficient integrity to keep any remaining bacteria isolated from their source of nutrition such that they either remain dormant or die. Re-investigation of such affected teeth after about 6 months when the pulp has had an opportunity to

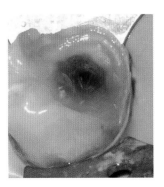

Figure 9.37 Remove caries from the amelodentinal junction.

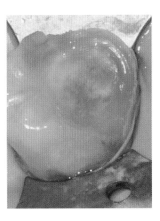

Figure 9.38 Remove further caries from all areas except where the operator considers that such removal will expose the pulp.

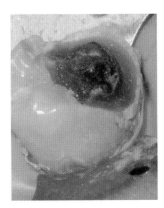

Figure 9.36 A very large carious lesion with a definite risk of pulp exposure.

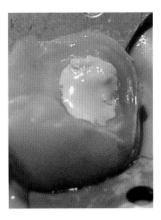

Figure 9.39 Place a calcium hydroxide dressing.

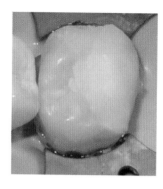

Figure 9.40 Cover the dressing with glass ionomer prior to preparation for a stainless steel crown.

lay down reparative dentine used to be the standard approach. Studies have found that the remaining carious dentine mostly remineralizes and hardens and caries progression does not occur in the absence of micro-leakage. Returning to the operative site to complete caries removal increases the risk of pulp exposure. Therefore indirect pulp capping and definitive restoration should be performed in one appointment. (See Key Point 9.22.)

> ### Key Point 9.22
>
> Stepwise removal of caries and indirect pulp capping is the treatment of choice for symptomless immature molars with extensive caries.

Direct pulp capping

When a small exposure is encountered during cavity preparation the operator can place a direct pulp cap. Again, the aim is to preserve the vitality of the pulp. Calcium hydroxide has traditionally been used as the remedial agent. Total etching and sealing with a dentine bonding agent has been tried, but this resulted in increased non-vitality and so it is contraindicated. Successful results have been reported with MTA as a pulp capping agent. However, disappointing results have been obtained with pulp capping in traumatic exposures; 5-year success rates were only 37% compared with 91–93% for partial pulpotomy so this technique should only be used if a partial pulpotomy cannot be performed.

For all techniques in which the pulp is preserved it is important to assess the situation correctly before embarking on the treatment. It is important that:

- there is no history of spontaneous pain;
- there is no swelling, mobility, or discomfort to percussion;
- there is a normal periodontal appearance radiographically;
- pulp tissue appears normal and vital;
- cessation of bleeding from the pulp exposure site with isotonic irrigation occurs within 2 minutes.

Partial pulpotomy

Pulpotomies are successful in young teeth because of their increased pulpal circulation and ability to repair. The procedure consists of applying rubber dam after local analgesia and then clearing all lateral margins around the exposure and the pulpal floor of any caries. The superficial layer of the exposed pulp and the surrounding dentine are excised to a depth of 2mm using a high-speed diamond bur. The technique is the same as the Cvek pulpotomy described in Chapter 12 for pulp exposure in traumatised teeth.

Only tissue judged to be inflamed should be removed. Whether sufficient tissue has been removed is ascertained by gently irrigating the remaining pulp surface with isotonic saline until bleeding stops. If bleeding does not cease easily, it is probable that the tissue is still inflamed and a further millimetre of pulp tissue is removed. After haemostasis has been obtained, a soluble paste of calcium hydroxide is applied to the wound surface. It is important that there is no blood clot between the wound surface and the dressing as this will prevent repair and reduce the chances of success. MTA has been proposed for pulp capping and pulpotomy dressings, and the results are very promising but long-term studies are not yet available. In order to aid repair, the clinician should carefully apply dry sterile cotton wool pellets with modest pressure to adapt the medicament to the prepared cavity and remove excess water from the paste. The technique is illustrated in Figs 9.41–9.45.

As in pulp capping, it is essential that the operator fills the cavity with a material that provides a good hermetic seal. The latter can be the final

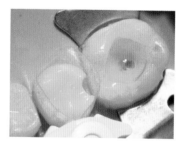

Figure 9.41 Where a pulp exposure occurs in an immature permanent molar, cut out the superficial pulp tissue (about 2mm) with a high-speed diamond bur. Bleeding should cease easily.

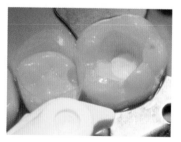

Figure 9.42 Pressure with saline-soaked cotton wool pledget consolidates the position. It is important to stress that the haemorrhage must cease before placing the lining.

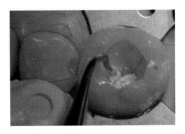

Figure 9.43 Place a calcium hydroxide lining.

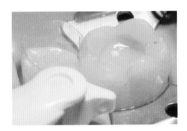

Figure 9.44 Place a glass ionomer base over the calcium hydroxide.

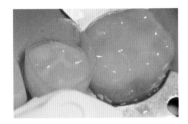

Figure 9.45 Restore with etched bonded composite resin to provide a hermetic seal. There is no need to re-investigate the site, so consider the restoration as definitive.

restoration as there is no need to re-enter the wound site. Although the presence of a dentinal bridge radiographically represents a success, its absence does not indicate failure. After a year, success is confirmed by a tooth where there are no signs of clinical or radiographic pathology and where the root has developed apically and thickened laterally.

The pulpotomy technique has much to recommend it, namely a good success rate and continued root development. Therefore it is considered the treatment of choice when there has been a pulp exposure in an immature permanent tooth. (See Key Point 9.23.)

> **Key Point 9.23**
>
> MTA or calcium hydroxide pulpotomy is the treatment of choice for an immature molar with pulpal exposure.

Pulpectomy

Root canal therapy following pulpectomy has a poor success rate in young permanent molars. In a recent study only 36% of young root-filled molar teeth were considered a success. Hence pulpectomy should be reserved for cases exhibiting symptoms of irreversible pulp damage where extraction is not indicated as part of a long-term orthodontic plan.

As with all endodontic work, the outcome is improved if:

- there are no voids in the root filling;
- the root filling extends to within 2mm of the radiographic apex;
- there is no preoperative periapical radiolucency;
- there is a satisfactory coronal restoration providing a good marginal seal.

A flowchart illustrating treatment decision-making for a first permanent molar with extensive caries is shown in Fig. 9.46.

9.12 Treatment for hypomineralized, hypomature, or hypoplastic first permanent molars

As caries has declined generally, it has become more apparent that there is another problem that commonly affects first permanent molars—molar incisor hypomineralization (MIH). This term covers a range of developmental anomalies from a small white, yellow, or brown patch to extensive loss of tissue from almost the whole enamel surface. (See Key Points 9.24.)

> **Key Points 9.24**
>
> - MIH affects up to 25% of the population.
> - Hypomineralized molars can be extremely sensitive.

MIH is characterized by very rapid breakdown of the enamel, which can be extremely sensitive; often the breakdown occurs in just a few months even while the tooth is still erupting. The difficulties of cleaning a partially erupted tooth are then compounded by the sensitivity. This produces an area where plaque builds up which leads to rapid carious attack. As is always the case with first adult molars, exfoliation of primary molars does not precede their eruption, so children and parents are often unaware of their presence and thus they do not seek treatment until the teeth start to cause problems or until the next recall. (See Key Points 9.25.)

MIH has been defined as 'hypomineralization of systemic origin of one to four permanent molars frequently associated with affected incisors'. The expression of the phenomenon can vary in severity between

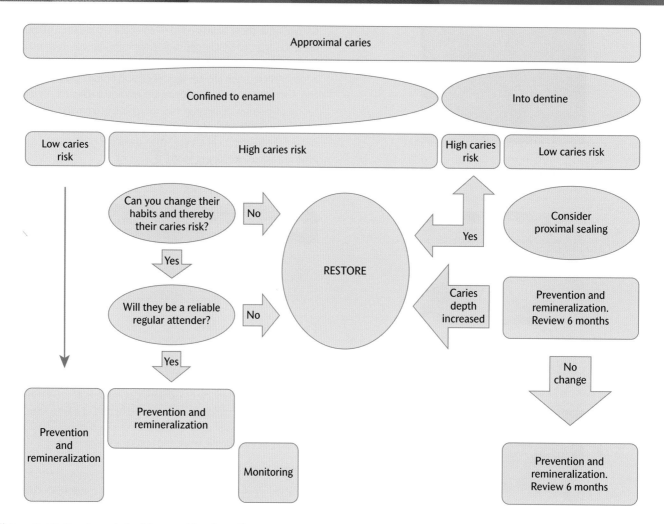

Figure 9.46 Treatment decision-making for a first permanent molar with extensive caries in a young person.

Key Points 9.25

- Teeth affected by MIH frequently show acute sensitivity to hot/cold/sweet stimuli even in the absence of apparent surface breakdown.
- Cleaning is often poor because of the sensitivity.
- Treatment is difficult. Often local anaesthesia has a limited effect.

The precise **aetiology of MIH** is unknown, but the following have been reported as possible factors:

- asthma
- pneumonia
- upper respiratory tract infections
- otitis media
- tonsillitis
- antibiotics
- dioxins in mother's milk
- problems in pregnancy
- chickenpox at age <3 years.

Formation defects may occur from the **calcification start dates** until the crown is formed approximately 3 years later. Calcification start dates for permanent teeth are:

- upper central incisors, 3–4 months
- lower central incisors, 3–4 months
- lower lateral incisors, 4–5 months

patients but also within a mouth, so that in one quadrant there may only be a small hypomineralized area and in others almost total destruction of the occlusal surface (Figs 9.47, 9.48, and 9.49).

Usually the incisors do not suffer the same breakdown of the surface and sensitivity as the molars. Of course, they often have cosmetic defects. This can be treated as the child becomes conscious of it as a problem by either coverage with composite or partial removal of the defect and coverage with composite. Details of these treatment techniques are given in Chapter 10.

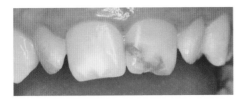

Figure 9.47 Effects of MIH on the incisors: a mild white patch on one tooth can occur in the same mouth as more severe brown discolouration with some surface breakdown.

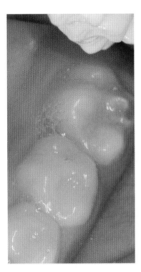

Figure 9.48 MIH affecting the first permanent molars; some breakdown of the hypomineralized enamel is already occurring.

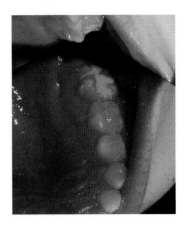

Figure 9.50 Glass ionomer placed on a hypoplastic molar as a temporary measure to reduce sensitivity.

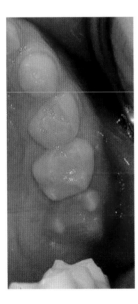

Figure 9.49 Severely affected first molar. A gross defect is apparent even with the tooth partially erupted.

The first problem to remedy in molars is the sensitivity. The following desensitizing agents help theoretically and anecdotally, but no clinical trials specifically related to MIH have been reported:

- repeated application of 5% sodium fluoride varnish (Duraphat®);
- commercially available 'sensitive tooth toothpastes';
- daily use of 0.4% stannous fluoride gels;
- CPP-ACP.

Fissure sealants can be useful where the affected areas are small and the enamel is intact. The use of bonding agents as described for resin sealants in Section 9.6.2 should help with bonding if the margin of the sealant is left on an area of hypomineralized enamel. As a digression, the application of the bonding agents, once polymerized, appears to reduce the sensitivity in the affected teeth themselves. It is important to remember to monitor the fissure sealant very carefully as there is a high chance of breakdown of the margin.

If there is surface breakdown the tooth will require some form of restoration. The first decision to make is whether the clinician needs to maintain the tooth throughout life or if it is more pragmatic to consider extraction. In the case of MIH there is evidence that planned extraction may avoid long-term restorative problems. Mejare *et al.* (2005) found that when patients with MIH were examined at 18 years, 48% had at least one unacceptable restoration, whereas space closure was acceptable in 87% of individuals where the molars had been extracted.

If the decision is that the first molars will be extracted in the future as part of a longer-view orthodontic plan, it is probable that they will still need temporization to render them comfortable because of the high level of sensitivity. It must also be remembered that these teeth are very difficult to anaesthetize, often staying sensitive when the operator has given normal levels of analgesic agent. If a child complains during treatment of a hypomineralized molar tooth, credibility should be given to their grievance. If a child experiences pain or discomfort during treatment, they will become increasingly anxious in successive treatments. This has been shown to be true for 9-year-old children,

- upper lateral incisors, 12 months
- first permanent molars, birth.

Problems associated with MIH are listed in Table 9.4 and the staging of MIH is summarized in Table 9.5.

Table 9.4 Problems associated with MIH

Effects of MIH	Associated problems
Enamel more porous	Ingress of bacteria leading to inflammation of the pulp and **sensitivity**
Hypomineralization	Weaker enamel prone to breakdown under occlusal forces, common failure of restorations
Sensitivity	Difficulties in obtaining good anaesthesia and consequent fear of dental procedures
Discolouration	Cosmetic defect

Table 9.5 Stages for MIH molars

Stage 1	Identify affected teeth early
Stage 2	Desensitization and remineralization
Stage 3	Prevention of caries and post-eruptive breakdown
Stage 4	Decide whether to opt for long-term restoration or extraction
Stage 5	Maintenance

where dental fear, anxiety, and behaviour problems were far more common in children with severely hypomineralized first permanent molars than in unaffected controls.

Therefore a balance has to be made between using simpler methods such as dressing with a glass ionomer (Fig. 9.50) which may well often need replenishment on several occasions before the optimum time for extraction, or deciding early within the programme to provide a full-coverage restoration, such as a stainless steel crown which should last without requiring replacement prior to extraction time. All adjuncts to help analgesia, such as inhalation sedation, should be used if indicated. It is also helpful to use rubber dam for all the usual reasons plus the protection afforded by exclusion of spray from the other three non-anaesthetized molars, contact with which would undoubtedly exacerbate the sensitivity.

If the intention is long-term maintenance of the molar, the choice of restorative techniques expands. If the area of breakdown of hypomineralized enamel is relatively confined, the operator should use conventional restorative techniques. However, it is difficult to determine where the margins of a preparation should be left as seemingly normal enamel (to visual examination) sometimes breaks down (Fig. 9.51).

Amalgam is of limited use because further breakdown often occurs at the margins, and as it is non-adhesive it does not restore the strength of the tooth. Composite resins should have a good success rate when used with an appropriate bonding agent in well-demarcated lesions. Again, it is the problem of deciding where to leave the margin that presents difficulty. Fayle (2003) described an approach of investigating abnormal-looking enamel at the margins of the defect with a slowly rotating steel bur and extending into these areas until good resistance is detected. Currently, this approach is not supported by clinical studies but the technique has been adopted by many

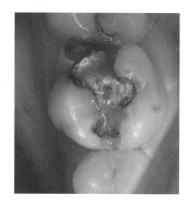

Figure 9.51 Caries and further breakdown around an amalgam in a hypomineralized molar.

dentists and could help avoid unnecessary sacrifice of sound tissue. (See Key Point 9.26.)

Key Point 9.26

When restoring teeth with MIH, investigate the enamel at the margins of the defect with a slowly rotating steel bur, extending into these areas until good resistance is felt, to reduce the chance of further enamel breakdown.

Most hypomineralized molars with surface breakdown involving one cusp or more will need a restoration with greater coverage. Stainless steel crowns or cast adhesive copings provide the most satisfactory options.

9.12.1 Preformed metal crowns (stainless steel crowns)

The advantages of stainless steel crowns are as follows:

- They require one visit for placement.
- The procedure is relatively quick and simple to perform.
- They usually reduce sensitivity totally, because they cover the whole tooth.
- They are inexpensive compared with cast restorations.
- They have a good retention rate.

However, they have the following disadvantages:

- More preparation of the tooth is required than with cast restorations.
- Once a tooth has been prepared for a stainless steel crown, it will eventually need a full-coverage restoration. Placing orthodontic separators 1–2 weeks prior to preparation reduces the amount of tissue that needs to be removed. However, some reduction is usually necessary.
- The gingival margins are sub-gingival.

Operative technique

A week before the procedure, insert orthodontic separators mesial to the affected permanent molar if possible to decrease the need to reduce this surface with burs.

1. Obtain adequate anaesthesia.
2. Isolate the tooth to be crowned.
3. Select the crown size.
4. Remove any carious dentine and enamel.
5. Replace tooth bulk with glass ionomer.
6. Reduce the occlusion minimally.
7. Reduce the mesial and distal surfaces, slicing with a fine tapered bur.
8. Try the selected crown. Adjust the shape cervically, such that the margins extend approximately 1mm below the gingival crest evenly around the whole of the perimeter of the crown. Sharp BB scissors usually achieve this most easily, followed by crimping pliers to contour the edge to give spring and grip. Permanent molar preformed metal crowns need this because they are not shaped accurately cervically. This is because there is such a variation in the crown length of the first permanent molars.
9. After contouring, smooth and polish to ensure that the crown does not attract excessive amounts of plaque.
10. After test fitting the crown remove the rubber dam to check the occlusion and then reapply for cementation.
11. Cement the crown (usually with a glass-ionomer-based cement).
12. Remove excess cement carefully with an explorer and floss. Finally, recheck the occlusion.

The technique is illustrated in Figs 9.52–9.56.

9.12.2 Cast adhesive copings

Restorations of this type offer two main advantages over preformed metal crowns:

- they avoid unnecessary approximal restoration;
- they enable the margins to remain supra-gingival.

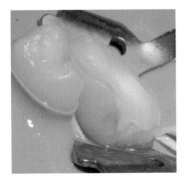

Figure 9.52 Stainless steel crown preparation: the occlusal surface is reduced minimally just enough to allow room to place the crown without disrupting the occlusion.

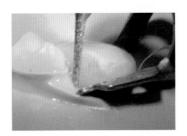

Figure 9.53 Obtain mesial and distal reduction with a fine tapered diamond bur with minimal buccal and palatal reduction just sufficient to allow the operator to place the crown. It is tempting not to effect any distal reduction if there is no erupted second permanent molar, but remember that it is important not to change the proportions of the tooth or create an overhang that will impede second molar eruption.

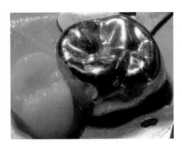

Figure 9.54 The stainless steel crown is tried in and the fit is determined. This crown will now need to be contoured and smoothed around the margins so that they fit evenly 1mm below gingival level around the whole periphery. It is important that the crown has a good contact point mesially. Contour the tooth with the correct pliers.

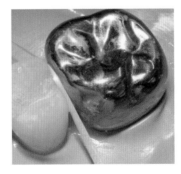

Figure 9.55 Glass ionomer cement is placed in the crown and overfilled to prevent voids forming under the crown. Excess cement is removed with cotton wool rolls and hand instruments, and the interstitial area is cleared with dental floss.

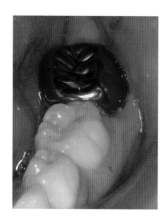

Figure 9.56 A stainless steel crown that was placed a year previously.

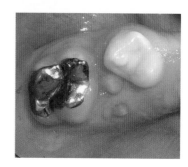

Figure 9.57 An etched coping covering the occlusal surface of a hypoplastic molar.

However, they have the following disadvantages:

- they still need local analgesia;
- they take two visits to complete;
- the technique is more expensive.

The technique
(Harley and Ibbetson 1993)

Visit 1

1. Local analgesia.
2. Rubber dam.
3. Preparation to remove any carious or softened enamel.
4. Gingival retraction with cords (to prevent crevicular fluid and other moisture contaminating the preparation site and impressions).
5. Take impression with rubber base material.
6. Temporization if much tooth tissue has been removed.

The casting is constructed in the laboratory and the fit surface is sandblasted.

Visit 2

7. Local analgesia.
8. Rubber dam.
9. Tooth is brushed with pumice, washed, and dried.

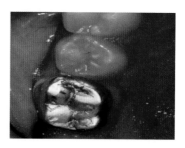

Figure 9.58 A gold coping with good extension over a hypomineralized tooth.

10. Casting is tried to check marginal adaptation and fit.
11. Casting is re-sandblasted to obtain optimum conditions for bonding.
12. Tooth is etched, washed, and dried.
13. Cement is applied to the fit surface of casting ensuring that there are no bubbles.
14. The casting is held in position under pressure for 3 minutes.
15. Excess cement is removed.
16. Oxygen-inhibiting material (Oxyguard™) is applied over the margins of the casting and maintained in position for a further 3 minutes.
17. The Oxyguard™ is removed by washing; the margins are rechecked and the occlusion is checked.

The technique is illustrated in Figs 9.57 and 9.58.

9.13 Alternatives to conventional cavity preparation

Alternative methods of cavity preparation are summarized in Table 9.6.

9.13.1 Air abrasion

Several different commercial air abrasion units are available. With air abrasion machines, aluminium oxide particles (27 or 50μm) are blasted against the teeth under a range of pressures (30–160psi) with variable particle flow rates.

One very obvious concern is the safety aspect of the presence of quantities of free aluminium oxide in the surgery environment. In theory, aluminium oxide is considered harmless. It is found in a wide variety of products from toothpastes to polishing wheels. The

Table 9.6 A summary of alternatives to conventional cavity preparation

Method	Advantages	Disadvantages
Air abrasion	Less need for LA Less vibration, noise, and pressure Less fracture and crazing of enamel or porcelain	**Dust** (particles in the air) Will not remove very soft caries Not efficient at removing large amalgam restorations Risk of soft tissue laceration, air dissection, and emboli
Ozone	Painless	'There is no reliable evidence that application of ozone gas to the surface of decayed teeth stops or reverses the decay process' (Rickard *et al.* 2004)
Chemomechanical	Less painful and less need for local anaesthetic More conservative of dental tissue as only carious dentine is softened for removal	Need to use burs to gain access for the gel Time taken using gel application and excavation is more than twice that needed for conventional methods
Lasers (Er:YAG)	Smear-layer-free cavity walls Selective and localized removal of tooth structure Reduced need for LA Higher resistance of cavity walls to secondary decay	Still require acid etching for bonding Risk of rise in pulpal temperature if not used correctly

LA, local anaesthetic.

size of the particles is considered to be too large to enter the distal airways or alveoli of the lungs. What dust does enter the lungs should easily be removed by ciliary action. However, anyone who has used one of these units will know that control of dust is an ongoing challenge. Rubber dam and very good suction help, but it still seems to spread.

Air abrasion produces a cavity preparation with both rounded cavo-surface margins and internal line angles. The surface it creates is irregular with many fine voids and defects. Initially it was considered that this surface might provide enough retention without etching but studies have show that this is erroneous.

Some of the clear advantages proposed for air abrasion are:

- elimination of vibration, less noise, and decreased pressure;
- reduction in pain during cavity preparation (85% of patients do not require local analgesia);
- less damaging pulpal effects than with conventional handpiece when used at higher pressures (160psi) and smaller particle size (27μm);
- less fracture and crazing of enamel and dentine during cavity preparation;
- root canal access through porcelain crowns without fracturing porcelain.

Therefore air abrasion has been proposed for:

- cleaning and removing stains and incipient caries from pits and fissures prior to sealant and PRRs;
- small class I, III, IV, and V cavity preparations and selected class II preparations;
- repair and removal of composites, glass ionomers, and porcelain restorations;
- cleaning and preparation of castings, orthodontic bands, and brackets prior to cementation.

What air abrasion cannot do is remove leathery dentinal caries or prepare extensive cavities requiring classical retentive form.

To use air abrasion successfully the clinician must learn a new technique, as the tip does not touch the tooth and therefore there is no tactile feedback. The tip width and the tip-to-tooth distance seem to have the most influence on the cavity width and depth. Increasing the distance produces larger shallower cuts. Increasing the tip diameter produces larger deeper cuts. Therefore the most precise removal of tooth tissue is achieved with a tip with a small inner diameter (0.38mm) held 2mm from the tooth surface. If cutting a class II cavity, it is essential to protect the adjacent tooth. Care must also be taken around the soft tissues to prevent surgical emphysema. As mentioned previously, dust is a problem, so glass/mirror surfaces may be damaged.

The technique gives as good a result as conventional methods in the preparation of PRRs. It was thought that cavities would be smaller with air abrasion but this has not been found to be correct.

In conclusion, air abrasion may be useful in the preparation of small cavities, with reduced patient discomfort, when combined with acid etching to obtain a good bond with adhesive materials, and when correctly and carefully used. However, the dust is a practical problem. (See Key Point 9.27.)

Key Point 9.27

Dust created during air abrasion is a major problem.

9.13.2 Ozone

A Cochrane review (Rickard *et al.* 2004) found no reliable evidence that the application of ozone gas to the surface of decayed teeth stops or reverses the decay process. No new data have emerged since to support its use.

9.1.3.3 Chemomechanical caries removal

Solutions that are able to soften carious dentine, making it easy to remove with hand instruments, have been available for a long time. Although they purport to be painless they did not catch on because they took a very long time to work, and frequently burs were still needed to gain full access to the caries. In some parts of the world there has been a resurgence of chemomechanical caries removal with the advent of a gel containing papain, chloramines, and toluene blue to make it visible. Papain is an endoprotein with bactericidal and anti-inflammatory action that interacts with the exposed collagen in the demineralized dentine, further softening it so that it can be scooped out with excavators.

The advantage of chemomechanical caries removal is that it is far less painful than conventional burs and so reduces the need for local anaesthetic. Because it only removes carious dentine, it is very conservative of dental tissue and produces cavities with rounded internal angles. Because it only uses hand instrumentation, there is no chance of pulpal heat damage. However, the time taken to remove the carious dentine is more than twice the time needed using burs, and burs are still needed to gain sufficient access to the dentine, so potentially this technique can still be problematic unless cooperation is good.

9.13.4 Lasers in dentistry

Lasers produce light energy within a narrow frequency range. They are named after the active element within them, which determines the wavelength of the light emitted. The wavelengths of some of the more common lasers are as follows:

- neodymium:yttrium aluminium garnet (Nd:YAG), 1.064μm
- carbon dioxide (CO_2), 10.6μm
- erbium:yttrium aluminium garnet (Er:YAG), 2.94μm
- argon, 457–502nm
- gallium arsenide (GaAs) (diode), 904nm
- holmium:yttrium aluminium garnet (Ho:YAG), 2.1μm

The wavelength of the emitted light is the primary determinant of the degree to which the target material absorbs light. The deeper the laser energy penetrates, the more it scatters and distributes throughout the tissue; for example, a CO_2 laser penetrates 0.01–0.03mm into the tissue whilst an Nd:YAG laser penetrates 2–5mm. The light from dental lasers is absorbed and converted to heat; the thermal effects caused depend on the tissue composition and the time that the beam is focused on the target tissue. The temperature increases may cause the tissue to change in structure and composition (e.g. denaturation, vaporization, carbonization, and melting followed by recrystallization).

The argon laser has a major advantage over the other lasers in that the wavelength at which it operates is absorbed by haemoglobin and therefore provides excellent haemostasis.

The public perception of lasers in dentistry is that they can do remarkable things painlessly, so obviously this appeals to a large number of people. However, the number of dentists offering lasers as an option in their practices is still small. The cost of the equipment is obviously a significant factor, and as with all new technologies, it is important that each dentist considers the proven clinical outcomes, i.e. what the recorded literature states regarding safety, efficacy, and effectiveness. This is further complicated by the fact that there are many different types of laser, with different uses, and new types and applications being produced constantly. (See Key Point 9.28.)

> **Key Point 9.28**
>
> Lasers don't do anything conventional techniques can't do!

Laser types and uses

- Carbon dioxide lasers:
  - soft tissue incision/ablation
  - gingival troughing
  - aesthetic contouring of gingivae
  - treatment of oral ulcers
  - fraenectomy and gingivectomy
  - de-epithelization of gingival tissue during periodontal regenerative procedures.
- Nd:YAG:
  - similar to the above plus removal of incipient caries, but because of the depth of penetration there is a greater risk of collateral damage than with carbon dioxide lasers.
- Er:YAG:
  - caries removal
  - cavity preparation in both enamel and dentine
  - preparation of root canals.
- Argon laser:
  - resin curing
  - tooth bleaching
  - treatment of ulcers
  - aesthetic gingival contouring
  - fraenectomy and gingivectomy.

Using an Er:YAG laser for cavity preparation and caries removal

Advantages

- Clean sharp margins in enamel and dentine.
- The pulp is protected and safe as the depth of energy penetration is negligible. (There is a study that shows deeper damage to nerve terminals and fibres which is visible under electron microscope examination but its clinical significance is unknown.)

- Patients report little or no pain during cavity preparation.
- The time taken for cavity preparation is short.

Disadvantages

- Cost.
- The need to learn a new technique in which there is no proprioceptive feedback since the laser tip does not impinge on dental tissue.

In order for a procedure to be deemed safe, collateral damage must be within acceptable limits, i.e. the risk–benefit ratio must be small with the benefit to the patient being significant. For example, laser-induced tissue trauma to the surgical site can add several more days to the healing process and cause dramatically abnormal appearances for up to 10–14 days postoperatively. Balanced against this, postoperative pain is usually minimal.

Laser caries detection/laser fluorescence

This is a low-power laser application which does not raise safety concerns. The system is commercially available and known as Diagnodent. Many workers have studied it and reported that the laser fluorescence system over-scores lesions whilst the conventional visual method under-scores them. The problem with the laser fluorescence instrument is that it cannot differentiate between caries and hypomineralization. Furthermore, staining is interpreted as caries and the presence of plaque deleteriously affects performance. Therefore it should only be used as an adjunct to clinical examination and diagnosis.

Argon laser irradiation as a preventive treatment

At certain settings Nd:YAG laser irradiation of sound enamel has been reported to increase surface micro-hardness. Some researchers have reported that argon laser irradiation produces a surface with enhanced caries resistance.

Several authors have looked at these effects by creating plaque-retentive areas on teeth destined to be removed for orthodontic reasons and recorded the effect of different pre-treatments prior to 6 weeks of plaque accumulation. Pre-treatment with an argon laser led to less lesion formation, with further improvement if combined with topical fluoride application. The results seem very impressive but need replication in the long term in the form of controlled clinical trials to determine the significance in a population as a whole instead of in specific artificially created caries-prone areas. If the results are validated, they may yield a simple non-invasive and pain-free technique for reducing the susceptibility of enamel to caries.

Resin curing

Argon lasers are able to polymerize composite resins in a shorter time than conventional light sources. The use of this type of laser has the additional advantage of increasing the ability of tooth structure to resist cariogenic challenges and may well increase the resistance of the enamel surrounding the polymerized resin. In addition, laser polymerization reduced the proportion of non-polymerized monomer and slightly improved the physical properties of the resin compared with curing using visible light methods. It is important to remember that resins cured with lasers do not necessarily have superior physical properties, and it is particularly important to check that the initiators within the resin activate at the specific wavelength of the laser. Again, there are few clinical studies to support these concepts.

Laser bleaching

Both CO_2 and argon lasers have been suggested as a method of tooth whitening. There have been no controlled clinical studies and there are concerns in relation to pulpal safety in connection with CO_2 lasers so the use of this type of laser for tooth bleaching is not recommended.

In one study an argon ion laser produced a lower temperature rise than conventional quartz tungsten lights when used to increase the activity of a bleaching gel and therefore may be acceptable.

Enamel etching

It has been suggested that laser irradiation may eliminate the need for etching, but as yet there is not enough scientific evidence to support this claim.

Lasers in paediatric dentistry

Possible uses of lasers in paediatric dentistry are as follows:

- caries prevention
- tooth preparation
- caries detection
- margin finishing
- pit and fissure sealing
- root canal decontamination
- curing
- dentine sealing
- pulp decontamination and coagulation
- pulpotomy
- haemostasis
- minor oral surgery (e.g. frenectomy)
- gingivectomy
- bleaching.

Some of the preliminary reports on the use of lasers give much room for optimism. They suggest that it might be possible not only to use lasers to help to prevent decay but also to perform certain types of surgery and to prepare cavities with little pain for the patient. However, much fuller clinical trial validation of these claims is needed before lasers can be considered so superior to conventional methods that failure to utilize the former will be considered to be rendering our patients a disservice. As yet, the cost of the equipment and the need to use different types of laser for different types of treatment prohibit their use by most UK dentists.

9.14 Rampant caries

It is important to consider the many factors that determine the treatment of a child with a high caries rate (Fig. 9.59). If the child presents with an acute problem of pain or swelling, immediate treatment is indicated to take the child out of pain. After that, it is important that the clinician considers the attitude of the child and parents, together with motivation towards dental treatment, the cooperation of the child, the age of the child, and the extent of decay.

It may be possible to place temporary restorations whilst preventive strategies are commenced as follows:

- dietary analysis and appropriate advice to the child and parent;
- plaque control, oral hygiene instruction to the child (depending on age) and the parent, and demonstration of the techniques of tooth brushing and disclosure;
- fluoride:
  - toothpaste
  - mouth rinse
  - varnish application every 6 months;
- fissure sealants;
- regular recall.

Once the caries is under control, definitive restorative treatment can commence.

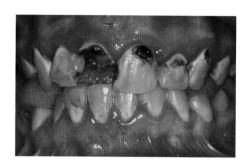

Figure 9.59 Rampant caries in a 13-year-old girl. She only attended because the incisor had fractured. Her whole attitude to dentistry needs to change in order to treat her successfully.

9.15 Summary

1 A full preventive programme to attempt to treat the cause of the caries must accompany any restorative treatment.

2 Utilize rubber dam if at all possible prior to the restoration of all teeth.

3 Early treatment of occlusal surface caries saves tooth tissue, but with early approximal lesions use remineralization wherever the lesion has not reached the dentine.

4 Consideration should be given to pulp preservation in deep lesions in immature permanent teeth.

5 Hypomineralized first molars deteriorate rapidly, can be extremely sensitive, and require early treatment.

6 New materials and technologies constantly present for evaluation. Treat with caution until the results of long-term clinical trials verify the claims of the initial researchers.

9.16 Acknowledgement

The editors thank Dr Brian Williams for his contributions to this chapter in previous editions.

9.17 References

Ahovuo-Saloranta, A., Hiiri, A., Norblad, A., Makela, M., and Worthington, H.V. (2004). Pit and fissure sealants for preventing dental decay in the permanent teeth of children and adolescents. *Cochrane Database of Systematic Reviews*, **4**, CD001830.

Fayle, S.A. (2003). Molar incisor hypomineralisation: restorative management. *European Journal of Paediatric Dentistry*, **4**, 121–6. (*A good practical approach to treatment of MIH*).

Forss, H. and Widstrom, E. (2003). The post amalgam era: a selection of materials and their longevity in the primary and young permanent dentitions. *International Journal of Paediatric Dentistry*, **13**, 158–64.

Harley, K.E. and Ibbetson, R.J. (1993). Dental anomalies: are adhesive castings the solution? *British Dental Journal*, **174**, 15–22. (*Outlines the steps needed well.*)

Hickel, R. and Manhart, J. (2001). Longevity of restorations in posterior teeth and reasons for failure. *Journal of Adhesive Dentistry*, **3**: 45–64.

Mejare, I., Bergman, E., and Grindefjord, M. (2005) Hypomineralised molars and incisors of unknown origin: treatment outcome at age 18 years. *International Journal of Paediatric Dentistry*, **15**, 20–8. (*A long-term look at outcomes of different treatment choices for hypomineralised molars.*)

Mjor, I.A., Moorhead, J.E., and Dahl, J.E. (2000). Reasons for replacement of restorations in permanent teeth in general dental practice. *International Dental Journal*, **50**, 361–6.

Pitts, N.B., Boyles, J., Nugent, Z.J., Thomas, N., and Pine, C.M. (2004). The dental caries experience of 14-year-old children in England and Wales. Surveys co-ordinated by the British Association for the Study of Community Dentistry in 2002/2003. *Community Dental Health*, **21**, 45–57. (*Good figures of the levels of dental disease affecting UK children.*)

Rickard, G.D., Richardson, R., Johnson, T., McColl, D., and Hooper, L. (2004). Ozone therapy for the treatment of dental caries. *Cochrane Database of Systematic Reviews*, **3**, CD004153.

Ricketts, D.N., Kidd, E.A., Innes, N., and Clarkson, J. (2006). Complete or ultraconservative removal of decayed tissue in unfilled teeth. *Cochrane Database of Systematic Reviews*, **3**, CD003808.

Sharif, M.O., Catleugh, M., Merry, A., *et al.* (2010). Replacement versus repair of defective restorations in adults: resin composite; amalgam. *Cochrane Database of Systematic Reviews*, **2**, CD005970, CD005971.

Sheiham, A. and Sabbah, W. (2010). Using universal patterns of caries for planning and evaluating dental care. *Caries Research*, **44**, 141–50. (*Interesting look at the patterns of dental disease within the mouth.*)

Smallridge, J.; British Society of Paediatric Dentistry (2010). Guideline for the use of fissure sealants including management of the stained fissure in the first permanent molars. *International Journal of Paediatric Dentistry*, **20** (Suppl 1), 3. (*Consensus guideline for fissure sealing.*)

Soncini, J.A., Maserejian, N.N., Trachtenberg, F., Tavares, M., and Hayes, C. (2007). The longevity of amalgam versus compomer/composite restorations in posterior primary and permanent teeth: findings from the New England Children's Amalgam Trial. *Journal of the American Dental Association*, **138**, 763–72. (*Interesting large study of restorations in children.*)

Young, N.L., Rodd, H.D., and Craig, S.A. (2009). Previous radiographic experience of children referred for dental extractions under general anaesthesia in the UK. *Community Dental Health*, **26**, 29–31. (*Shows how guidelines are often ignored to the detriment of the patient.*)

10 Advanced restorative dentistry

N.M. Kilpatrick and L.A.L. Burbridge

Chapter contents

10.1 Introduction

The aim of this chapter is to cover the management of more complicated clinical problems associated with children and adolescents: tooth discolouration, inherited enamel and dentine defects, hypodontia, and tooth surface loss. As there is considerable overlap in the application of the various restorative techniques, the chapter is divided into two parts. The first outlines the clinical steps involved in the various procedures, while the second covers the more general principles of management of particular dental problems.

10.2 Advanced restorative techniques

It is not the remit of this chapter to cover advanced restorative dentistry in detail, but many of the techniques used in children are the same as those for adults (Boxes 10.1 and 10.2).

With the aid of some clinical examples, seven of the restorative procedures will be described in simple stages. Omitted from this list are the stages involved in the provision of full crown restorations and

> **Box 10.1 Advanced restorative techniques**
>
> Hydrochloric acid–pumice micro-abrasion technique
> Non-vital bleaching
> Vital bleaching—chairside and nightguard
> Localized composite resin restorations
> Composite veneers—direct and indirect
> Porcelain veneers
> Adhesive metal castings
> Full crowns
> Bridgework—adhesive and fixed

> **Box 10.2 Ideal features of restorative treatments**
>
> - Resolve sensitivity
> - Restore function
> - Aesthetic
> - Have proven durability
> - Cause insignificant loss of tooth structure, i.e. are minimally invasive
> - Preserve dental hard tissues
> - Enhance periodontal health
> - Simple, quick, and tolerable to the patient

bridgework, which are the specific remit of a restorative dentistry textbook. However, the provision of porcelain veneers, more commonly associated with adult patients, will be mentioned briefly.

10.2.1 The hydrochloric acid–pumice micro-abrasion technique

This is a controlled method of removing surface enamel in order to improve discolourations that are limited to the outer enamel layer. It is achieved by a combination of abrasion and erosion—the term 'abrosion' is sometimes used. In the clinical technique that will be described no more than approximately 100mm of enamel is removed. Once completed, the procedure should not be repeated again in the future. Too much enamel removal is potentially damaging to the pulp and cosmetically the underlying dentine colour will become more evident. This approach is described in further detail in the BSPD guideline on treatment of intrinsic discolouration in permanent anterior teeth in children and adolescents (Wray and Welbury 2004).

Indications

- Fluorosis
- Idiopathic speckling
- Post-orthodontic treatment demineralization
- Prior to localized composite restorations or veneer placement for well-demarcated stains
- White/brown surface staining, e.g. secondary to primary predecessor infection or trauma (Turner teeth)

Armamentarium

- Bicarbonate of soda/water
- Soft white paraffin
- Fluoridated toothpaste
- Pumice
- Rubber dam
- Rubber prophylaxis cup
- Soflex discs (3M)
- 18% hydrochloric acid

Technique

1. Perform preoperative vitality tests; take radiographs and photographs (Fig. 10.1(a)).
2. Clean the teeth with pumice and water, wash, and dry.
3. Isolate the teeth to be treated with rubber dam, including placement of soft white paraffin under the dam.
4. Place a mixture of sodium bicarbonate and water on the dam behind the teeth as protection in case of spillage (Fig. 10.1(b)).
5. Mix 18% hydrochloric acid with pumice into a slurry and apply a small amount to the labial surface for 5 seconds using either a rubber cup rotating slowly or a wooden stick (Fig. 10.1(c)), before washing for 5 seconds directly into an aspirator tip. Repeat until the stain has reduced up to a maximum of ten 5-second applications per tooth. Any improvement that is going to occur will have done so by this time.
6. Remove the rubber dam.
7. Polish the teeth with the finest Soflex discs.
8. Polish the teeth with fluoridated toothpaste in a rubber cup for 1 minute.
9. Review in a month to assess the outcome and to undertake vitality tests and clinical photographs (Fig. 10.1(d)).
10. Review biannually, checking pulpal status.

Critical analysis of the effectiveness of the technique should not be made immediately, but delayed for at least a month as the appearance of the teeth will continue to improve over this time. Experience has shown that brown mottling is removed more easily than white, but even where white mottling is incompletely removed it often becomes less perceptible. This phenomenon has been attributed to the relatively prismless layer of compacted surface enamel produced by the 'abrosion' technique, which alters the optical properties of the tooth surface.

Long-term studies of the technique have found no association with pulpal damage, increased caries susceptibility, or significant prolonged thermal sensitivity. Patient compliance and satisfaction is good, and any dissatisfaction is usually due to inadequate preoperative explanation. The technique is easy to perform for the operator and patient and is

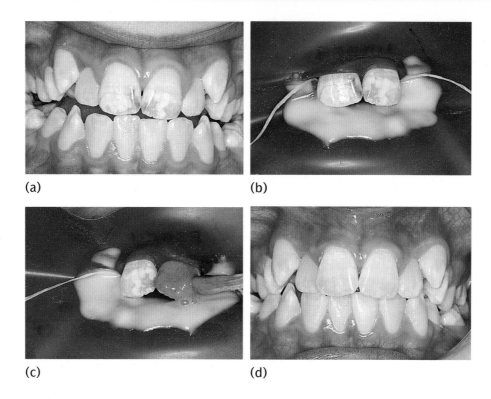

Figure 10.1 (a) Characteristic appearance of fluorotic discolouration. (b) Rubber dam isolation with bicarbonate of soda in position. (c) Application of hydrochloric acid–pumice slurry with a wooden stick. (d) Appearance 2 years after treatment.

not time-consuming. Removal of any mottled area is permanent and is achieved with an insignificant loss of surface enamel. Failure to improve the appearance by the hydrochloric acid–pumice micro-abrasion technique has no harmful effects and may make it easier to mask some lesions with veneers or composite restorations.

10.2.2 Non-vital bleaching

This technique describes the bleaching of teeth that have become discoloured by the diffusion into the dentinal tubules of haemoglobin breakdown products from necrotic pulp tissue.

Indications

- Discoloured non-vital teeth.
- Well-condensed gutta percha root filling.
- No clinical or radiological signs of periapical disease.

Contraindications

- Heavily restored teeth.
- Staining due to amalgam.

Armamentarium

- Rubber dam
- Glass ionomer or IRM cement

- 37% phosphoric acid
- Bleaching agent, e.g. sodium perborate, hydrogen peroxide, or carbamide peroxide
- Cotton wool
- White gutta percha
- Composite resin
- Non-setting calcium hydroxide

Technique

1. Take preoperative periapical radiographs. These are essential to check for an adequate root filling (Fig. 10.2(a)).

2. Clean the teeth with pumice and make a note of the shade of the discoloured tooth.

3. Place rubber dam, isolating the single tooth. Ensure adequate eye and clothing protection for the patient, operator, and dental nurse.

4. Remove palatal restoration and pulp chamber restoration.

5. Remove root filling to 1mm below the level of the dentogingival junction. You may need to use adult burs in a miniature head (Figs 10.2(b) and 10.2(c)).

6. Place 1mm of cement over the gutta percha.

7. Gently freshen dentine with a round bur. Do not remove excessively.

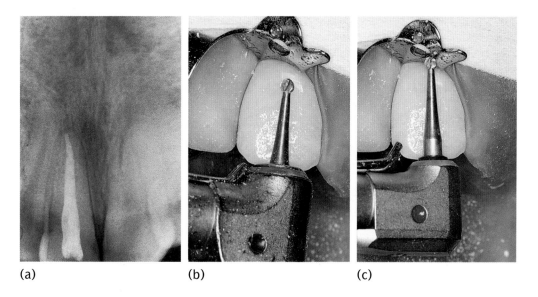

(a)   (b)   (c)

Figure 10.2 (a) Radiograph of upper right central incisor with a well-condensed root filling. (b) A standard bur in a contra-angled head may not reach the dentogingival junction. (c) Correct depth is achieved using a standard bur in a miniature head.

8. Etch the pulp chamber with 37% phosphoric acid for 30–60 seconds, wash, and dry. This will facilitate the ingress of the hydrogen peroxide.

9. Place the bleaching agent, either alone or on a cotton wool pledget, into the pulp chamber.

10. Place a dry piece of cotton wool over the mixture.

11. Seal the cavity with glass ionomer cement.

12. Repeat the process at weekly intervals until the tooth is slightly over-bleached.

13. Place non-setting calcium hydroxide into the pulp chamber for 2 weeks. Seal with glass ionomer cement.

14. Finally, restore the tooth with white gutta percha (to facilitate reopening the pulp chamber again, if necessary, at a later date) and composite resin.

Figures 10.3(a) and (b) show an example of a highly successful result. If the colour of a tooth has not significantly improved after three changes of bleach, it is unlikely to do so and further bleaching should be abandoned. The maximum number of bleach applications is usually accepted as ten. Failure of a tooth to bleach could be due to either inadequate removal of filling materials from the pulp chamber or 'time expired' bleaching agent. Both these factors should be checked before abandoning a procedure.

Slight over-bleaching is desirable, but the patient should be instructed to attend the surgery before the next appointment if marked over-bleaching has occurred.

Non-vital bleaching has a reputation of causing brittleness of the tooth. This is probably the result of the endodontic treatment along with previous injudicious removal of dentine (which only needs to be 'freshened' with a round bur) rather than a direct effect of the bleaching procedure itself.

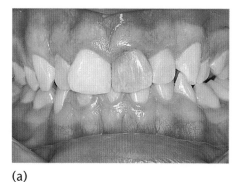

(a)

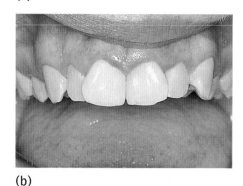

(b)

Figure 10.3 Intensely darkened non-vital upper left central incisor (a) treated by four changes of bleach (b).

This method of bleaching has been associated with the later occurrence of external cervical resorption. The exact mechanism of this association is unclear, but it is thought that the hydrogen peroxide diffuses through the dentinal tubules to set up an inflammatory reaction in the periodontal ligament around the cervical region of the tooth. For this reason the use of hydrogen peroxide mixed with sodium perborate crystals in this technique is now recommended to be used with caution. In a small number of teeth there is a gap between the end of the enamel and the beginning of the cementum, and in these cases the above explanation is tenable. The purpose of the 1mm layer of cement is to cover the openings of the dentinal tubules at the level where there may be a communication to the periodontal ligament. In the same way, non-setting calcium hydroxide is placed in the pulp chamber for 2 weeks prior to final restoration in order to eradicate any inflammation that may have been initiated in the periodontal ligament.

Clinical studies have demonstrated that regression can be expected with this technique. The longest study gave a 21% failure rate after 8 years.

The advantages of the technique are many: easy for operator and patient; conservation of tooth tissue and maintenance of the original crown morphology; no irritation to gingival tissues; no problems with changing gingival level in young patients compared with veneers or crowns; no technical assistance required.

10.2.3 Vital bleaching—chairside

This technique involves the external application of hydrogen peroxide to the surface of the tooth followed by its activation with a heat source. The technique has become increasingly popular in recent years, but it is a lengthy and time-consuming procedure that requires a high degree of patient compliance and motivation.

Indications

- Very mild tetracycline staining without obvious banding
- Mild fluorosis
- Yellowing due to ageing
- Single teeth with sclerosed pulp chambers and canals

Armamentarium

- Rubber dam with clamps and floss ligatures
- Orabase® paste
- Topical anaesthetic
- Gauze
- 37% phosphoric acid
- Heating light with rheostat
- 30–35% hydrogen peroxide
- Polishing stones

Technique

1. Take preoperative periapical radiographs and perform vitality tests. Replace any leaking restorations.
2. Clean the teeth with pumice and water to remove extrinsic staining. Take preoperative photographs with a tooth from a Vita shade guide, registering the shade adjacent to the patient's teeth.
3. Apply topical anaesthetic to gingival margins.

4. Coat the buccal and palatal gingivae with Orabase® paste as extra protection from the bleaching solution.
5. Isolate each tooth to be bleached using individual ligatures. The end teeth should be clamped (usually from second premolar to second premolar).
6. Cover the metal rubber dam clamps with damp strips of gauze to prevent them from getting hot under the influence of the heat source.
7. Etch the labial and a third of the palatal surfaces of the teeth with phosphoric acid for 60 seconds, wash, and dry. Thoroughly soak a strip of gauze in the hydrogen peroxide and cover the teeth to be bleached.
8. Position the heat lamp 13–15 inches (33–38cm) from the patient's teeth. Set the rheostat to a mid-temperature range and increase it until the patient can just feel the warmth in their teeth; then reduce it slightly until no sensation is felt.
9. Keep the gauze damp by reapplying the hydrogen peroxide every 3–5 minutes using a cotton bud. Make sure that the bottle is closed between applications as the hydrogen peroxide deactivates on exposure to air.
10. After 30 minutes remove the rubber dam, clean off the Orabase® paste, and polish the teeth using the Shofu stones. Apply the fluoride drops for 2–3 minutes.
11. Note that postoperative sensitivity may occur and should be relieved with paracetamol.
12. Assess the change—it may be necessary to repeat the process three to ten times per arch. Treat one arch at a time. Keep the patient under review as rebleaching may be required after a year or more.
13. Take postoperative photographs with the original Vita shade tooth included.

This technique is very time-consuming and re-treatment may be necessary, so the patient must be highly motivated. The technique can be used in the treatment of discolouration caused by pulp chamber sclerosis (Fig. 10.4). These cases require isolation of the single tooth.

10.2.4 Vital bleaching—nightguard

This technique involves the daily placement of carbamide peroxide gel into a custom-fitted tray on either the upper or the lower arch. As the name suggests, it is carried out by the patient at home and is initially done on a daily basis.

Indications

- Mild fluorosis
- Moderate fluorosis as an adjunct to hydrochloric acid–pumice micro-abrasion
- Yellowing of ageing
- Single teeth with sclerosed pulp chambers and canals
- Selective bleaching for aesthetic purposes

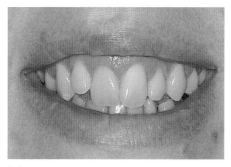

(a)

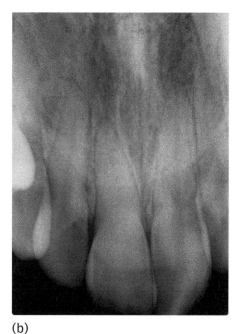

(b)

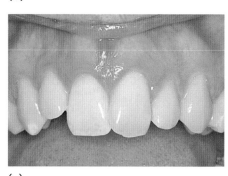

(c)

Figure 10.4 (a) A discoloured upper right central incisor with (b) a radiograph confirming sclerosis of the pulp chamber and root canal. (c) Appearance of upper right central incisor after four chairside bleaching treatments.

Armamentarium

- Upper impression and working model
- Soft mouthguard—avoiding the gingivae
- 10% carbamide peroxide gel.

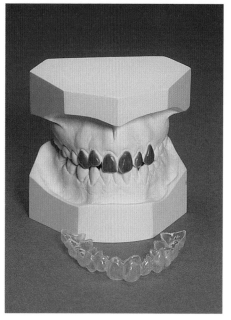

(a)

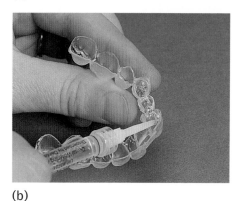

(b)

Figure 10.5 (a) Model of upper arch with wax relief for construction of a nightguard. (b) Mouthguard being loaded with carbamide peroxide gel.

Technique

1. Take an alginate impression of the arch to be treated and cast a working model in stone.
2. Relieve the labial surfaces of the teeth by about 0.5mm and make an acrylic pull-down vacuum-formed splint as a mouthguard with or without reservoirs for bleaching agent on the teeth requiring lightening (Fig. 10.5(a)). The splint should be no more than 2mm thick and should not cover the gingivae. It is only a vehicle for the bleaching gel and is not intended to protect the gingivae.
3. Instruct the patient on how to floss their teeth thoroughly. Perform a full-mouth prophylaxis and instruct them how to apply the gel into the mouthguard (Fig. 10.5(b)).
4. Note that the length of time the guard should be worn depends on the product used.

5. Review about 2 weeks later to check that the patient is not experiencing any sensitivity, and then at 6 weeks by which time 80% of any colour change should have occurred.

Carbamide peroxide gel (10%) breaks down to 3% hydrogen peroxide and 7% urea in the mouth. Both urea and hydrogen peroxide have low molecular weights, allowing them to diffuse rapidly through enamel and dentine. This explains the transient pulpal sensitivity occasionally experienced with home bleaching systems.

Pulpal histology with regard to these materials has not been assessed, but no clinical significance has been attributed to the changes seen with 35% hydrogen peroxide over 75 years of usage, except where teeth have been overheated or traumatized. By extrapolation, 3% hydrogen peroxide in the home systems should be safe.

Although most carbamide peroxide materials contain trace amounts of phosphoric and citric acids as stabilizers and preservatives, no indication of etching or a significant change in the surface morphology of enamel has been demonstrated by scanning electron microscopy analysis. There was early concern that bleaching solutions with a low pH would cause demineralization of enamel when the pH fell below the 'critical' value of 5.2–5.8. However, no evidence of this process has been noted to date in any clinical trials or laboratory tests, possibly because the urea (and subsequently the ammonia) and carbon dioxide released on degradation of the carbamide peroxide elevate the pH.

There is an initial decrease in bond strengths of enamel to composite resins immediately after home bleaching, but this returns to normal within 7 days. This effect has been attributed to the residual oxygen in the bleached tooth surface which inhibits polymerization of the composite resin. The home-bleaching systems do not affect the colour of restorative materials. Any perceived effect is probably due to superficial cleansing.

Minor ulceration or irritation may occur during the initial treatment. It is important to check that the mouthguard does not extend onto the gingivae and that the edges of the guard are smooth. If ulceration persists, a decreased exposure time may be necessary. If there is still a problem, allergy is a possibility.

There are no biological concerns regarding the short-term use of carbamide peroxide. It has a similar cytotoxicity on mouse fibroblasts to zinc phosphate cement and Crest toothpaste, and has been used for a number of years in the USA to reduce plaque and promote wound healing. However, there are no long-term studies of its safety. Laboratory studies have shown that carbamide peroxide has a mutagenic potential on vascular endothelium and there may be harmful effects on the periodontium, together with delayed wound healing.

Published clinical studies of 1–2 years' duration have shown that the yellowing of ageing responds best to this treatment. Although this would appear to take home bleaching out of the remit of paediatric dentistry, it may still have a part to play in cases of mild fluorosis. Irrespective of the clinical application, evidence suggests that annual re-treatment may be necessary to maintain any effective lightening. This further highlights the importance of more research into the long-term effects of this treatment on the teeth, mucosa, and periodontium.

The exact mechanism of bleaching in any of the methods described is unknown. Theories of oxidation, photo-oxidation, and ion exchange have been suggested. Conversely, the cause of re-discolouration is also unknown. This may be a combination of chemical reduction of the oxidation products previously formed, marginal leakage of restorations, allowing ingress of bacterial and chemical by-products, and salivary or tissue fluid contamination via permeable tooth structure.

There is currently, and has been for some years, continued confusion relating to the legal position of dentists using tooth-whitening techniques which involve the use of bleach. The situation at the time of publication is that it is illegal in the UK to supply a product for the purpose of tooth-whitening if that product contains or releases more than 0.1% hydrogen peroxide. When considering such products for clinical use it is advisable to seek medico-legal advice.

10.2.5 The inside–outside bleaching technique

An alternative approach to the management of the discoloured endodontically treated tooth has been described. Known as the inside–outside bleaching technique, it is essentially a combination of the walking and vital bleaching techniques. Tooth preparation is the same as described for the walking bleach technique (Section 10.2.2) with particular attention being paid to removal of the gutta percha below the cemento-enamel junction followed by the placement of a barrier (usually a glass ionomer cement or IRM cement) to seal the root canal from the oral cavity. A custom-made tray (see Fig. 10.5(b)) is constructed as a vehicle for the bleaching gel. However, rather than creating space labially as in the vital bleaching technique, a small reservoir is created palatal to the affected tooth only. The gel (10% carbamide peroxide) is placed by the patient into both the access cavity of the non-vital tooth and the tray. The tray is then worn full time for up to 4 days, with the gel being replaced every 2–4 hours. Once an aesthetically acceptable result is achieved, the access cavity is refilled appropriately. Long-term results for this approach are not yet available, but relapse is as likely as for any of the other bleaching techniques.

10.2.6 Localized composite resin restorations

This restorative technique uses recent advances in dental materials science to replace defective enamel with a restoration that bonds to and blends with enamel.

Indications

- Well-demarcated white, yellow, or brown hypomineralized enamel such as those seen in MIH (see Section 10.6 and Fig. 10.25(c))

Armamentarium

- Rubber dam/contoured matrix strips
- Round and fissure diamond burs
- Enamel–dentine bonding kit
- New-generation highly polishable hybrid composite resin
- Soflex discs (3M) and interproximal polishing strips.

Technique

1. Take preoperative photographs and select the shade (Fig. 10.6(a)).

2. Apply rubber dam and contoured matrix strips if required.

3. Remove full extent of demarcated lesion with a round diamond bur down to the amelodentinal junction (ADJ).

4. Chamfer the enamel margins with a diamond fissure bur to increase the surface area available for retention if required.

5. Etch the resultant cavity margins. Wash and dry.

6. Apply the prime and bonding agent as per the manufacturer's instructions.

7. Apply the chosen shade of composite, use a brush lubricated with the bonding agent to smooth and shape, and light-cure for the recommended time.

8. Remove the matrix strip/rubber dam.

9. Polish with graded Soflex discs (3M), finishing burs, and interproximal strips if required. Add characterization to the surface of the composite.

10. Take postoperative photographs (Fig. 10.6(b)).

The localized restoration is quick and easy to complete. Despite the removal of defective enamel down to the ADJ, there is often no significant sensitivity and therefore no need for local anaesthesia. If the hypoplastic enamel has become carious and this extends into dentine, administration of local anaesthesia will be necessary. Advances in bonding and resin technology make these restorations simple and obviate the need for a full labial veneer. Disadvantages are marginal staining, accurate colour match, and suboptimal aesthetics if the full extent of the demarcated lesion is not removed to the ADJ.

10.2.7 Composite resin veneers

Although the porcelain jacket crown (PJC) may be the most satisfactory long-term restoration for a severely hypoplastic or discoloured tooth, it is not an appropriate solution for children for two reasons: the large size of the young pulp horns and chamber, and the immature gingival contour.

Composite veneers may be direct (placed at the initial appointment) or indirect (placed at a subsequent appointment having been fabricated in the laboratory). Conservative veneering methods may offer not just a temporary solution, but a satisfactory long-term alternative to the PJC. Most composite veneers placed in children and adolescents are of the 'direct' type, as these can be placed in a single visit and outcomes for both techniques are equivocal.

Before proceeding with any veneering technique, the decision must be made as to whether to reduce the thickness of labial enamel before placing the veneer. Certain factors should be considered.

1. Increased labiopalatal bulk makes it harder to maintain good oral hygiene. This may be courting disaster in the adolescent with a dubious oral hygiene technique.

2. Composite resin has a better bond strength to enamel when a surface layer of 200–300mm is removed.

3. If a tooth is very discoloured, some sort of reduction and/or use of an opaqueing agent may be desirable as a thicker layer of composite will otherwise be required to mask the intense stain.

4. If a tooth is already instanding or rotated, its appearance can be enhanced by a thicker labial veneer. However, this may not be appropriate in cases where orthodontic treatment is planned as the natural anatomy of the tooth will be changed.

New-generation highly polishable hybrid composite resins can replace relatively large amounts of missing tooth tissue as well as being used in thin sections as a veneer. Combinations of shades can be used to simulate natural colour gradations and hues.

Indications

- Discolouration
- Enamel defects
- Diastemata
- Malpositioned teeth
- Large restorations

Relative contraindications

- Insufficient tooth tissue available for bonding
- Oral habits, e.g. woodwind musicians
- Occlusal factors

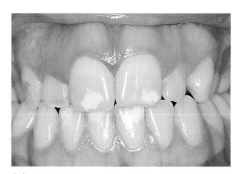

(a)

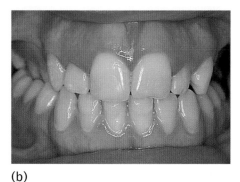

(b)

Figure 10.6 Well-demarcated white opacities on the upper central incisors (a) treated by localized composite restorations (b).

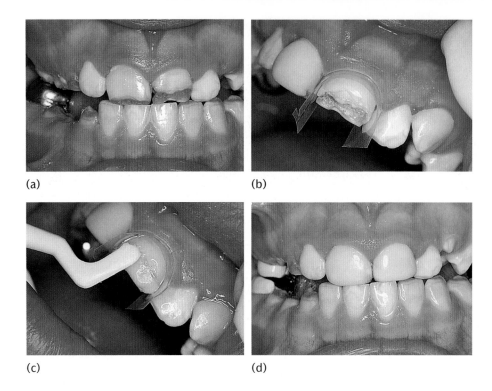

Figure 10.7 (a) A young patient with amelogenesis imperfecta. (b) Contoured matrix strip in position. (c) Incremental placement of dentine shade composite. (d) Postoperative view showing final composite veneers.

Armamentarium

- Rubber dam/contoured matrix strips
- Preparation and finishing burs
- New-generation highly polishable hybrid composite resin
- Soflex discs (3M) and interproximal polishing strips

Technique

1. Use a tapered diamond bur to reduce labial enamel by 0.3–0.5mm if appropriate. Identify the finish line at the gingival margin and also mesially and distally just labial to the contact points.

2. Clean the tooth with a slurry of pumice in water. Wash and dry, and select the shade (Fig. 10.7(a)).

3. Isolate the tooth with rubber dam and a contoured matrix strip. Hold this in place by applying unfilled resin to its gingival side against the gingiva and curing for 10 seconds (Fig. 10.7(b)).

4. Etch the enamel as per the manufacturer's instructions.

5. Apply a thin layer of priming and bonding resin to the labial surface with a brush as per manufacturer's instructions. It may be necessary to use an opaquer at this stage if the discolouration is intense.

6. Apply composite resin of the desired shade to the labial surface and roughly shape it into all areas with a plastic instrument; then use a brush lubricated with unfilled resin to 'paddle' and smooth it into the desired shape. Cure for 40 seconds gingivally, 40 seconds mesio-incisally, 40 seconds disto-incisally, and 40 seconds from the palatal aspect if incisal coverage has been used. Different shades of composite can be combined to achieve good matches with adjacent teeth and a transition from a relatively dark gingival area to a lighter more translucent incisal region (Fig. 10.7(c)).

7. Flick away the unfilled resin holding the contour strip and remove the strip.

8. Finish the margins with diamond finishing burs and interproximal strips, and the labial surface with graded sandpaper discs. Characterization should be added to improve light reflection properties (Fig. 10.7(d)).

The exact design of the composite veneer will depend on each clinical case but will usually be one of four types: intra-enamel or window preparation, incisal bevel, overlapped incisal edge, or feathered incisal edge (Fig. 10.8). Tooth preparation will not normally expose dentine, but this will be unavoidable in some cases of localized hypoplasia or with caries.

Figure 10.9 shows an example of successful composite veneers that have been in place for 5 years. Studies have shown that composite veneers are durable enough to last through adolescence until a more aesthetic porcelain veneer can be placed. This is normally only considered at about the age of 18–20 years when the gingival margin has matured to an adult level and the standard of oral hygiene and dental motivation are acceptable.

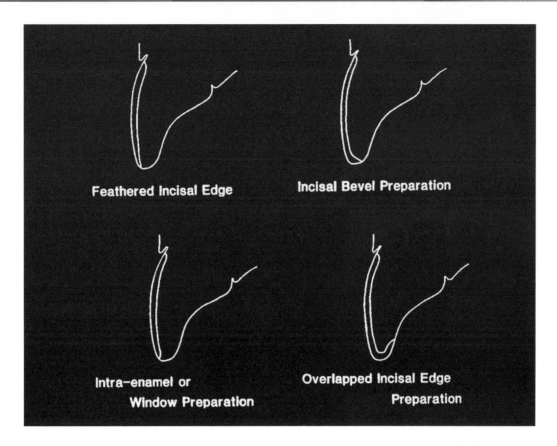

Figure 10.8 Types of veneer preparation.

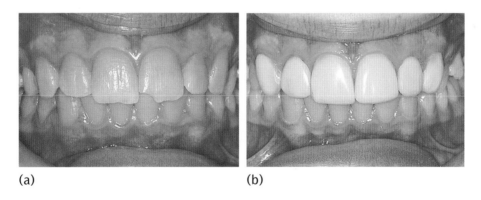

(a)   (b)

Figure 10.9 (a) Teenage girl with dark tetracycline discolouration and an enamel fracture. (b) Five years after placement of composite veneers.

10.2.8 Porcelain veneers

Porcelain has several advantages over composite as a veneering material: its appearance is superior, it has a better resistance to abrasion, and it is well tolerated by the gingival tissues. However, it is vital that the porcelain fits exactly and that the film thickness of the luting cement is kept to a minimum. Luting cements are only moderately filled composite resins, and they absorb water, hydrolyse, and stain. This, coupled with the apical migration of the gingival margin in young patients, can result in an unacceptable aesthetic appearance in a relatively short time.

Instruction in standard porcelain veneer preparation is covered in restorative dentistry textbooks. If there are occasions when they are used at an earlier age, the same principles apply. However, a non-standard application that is being used more frequently at a younger age is the restoration of the peg lateral incisor if placement of a direct composite resin restoration is considered unsuitable (Fig. 10.10(a)). This utilizes a no-preparation technique, and the

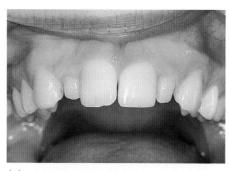

(a)

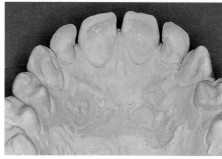

(b)

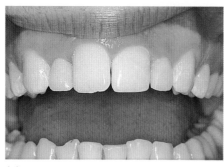

(c)

Figure 10.10 (a) Peg-shaped lateral incisors in a 15-year-old patient. (b) Laboratory model showing three-quarter wrap-around porcelain veneers on the upper laterals. (c) Final restorations on the upper laterals 2 years after cementation.

technician is asked to produce a three-quarter wrap-around veneer finished to a knife edge at the gingival margin (Fig. 10.10(b)). An elastomeric impression is taken after gingival retraction to obtain the maximum length of crown, and cementation should be under rubber dam (Fig. 10.10(c)).

10.2.9 Adhesive metal castings

The development of acid-etched retained cast restorations has allowed the fabrication of cast occlusal onlays for posterior teeth and palatal veneers for incisors and canines. These restorations are manufactured with minimal or no tooth preparation and are ideal for cases where there is a risk of tooth tissue loss.

Indications

- Amelogenesis imperfecta
- Dentinogenesis imperfecta
- Dental erosion, attrition, or abrasion
- Enamel hypoplasia

Armamentarium

- Gingival retraction cord
- Elastomeric impression material
- Facebow system
- Semi-adjustable articulator
- Rubber dam
- Panavia-Ex (Kuraray)

Technique

1. Obtain study models (these are essential) and photographs if possible.
2. Perform a full-mouth prophylaxis.
3. Ensure good moisture isolation.
4. Place a retraction cord into the gingival crevices of the teeth to be treated and remove immediately prior to taking the impression.
5. Take an impression using an elastomeric impression material (a putty–wash system is best) and check that the margins are easily distinguishable.
6. Take a facebow transfer and interocclusal record in the retruded axis position.
7. Mount the casts on a semi-adjustable articulator.
8. Construct cast onlays a maximum of 1.5mm thick occlusally in either nickel–chrome or gold.
9. Grit-blast the fitting surfaces of the occlusal onlays.
10. Return to the mouth and check the fit of the onlays and sandblast before fitting.
11. Polish the teeth with pumice and isolate under rubber dam where possible.
12. Cement onlays using Panavia-Ex.
13. Check occlusion and record extent of discrepancies.
14. Review in a week to check occlusion and other problems, and regularly thereafter.

Figure 10.11 shows gold onlays cemented onto the lower first permanent molars of a 16-year-old boy with erosive tooth surface loss. Such cast restorations can be provided for both posterior and anterior teeth with very little or no tooth preparation. Nevertheless, some children may find this treatment challenging as it demands high levels of patient cooperation. Local anaesthesia may be needed as the hypoplastic teeth are often sensitive to the etching and washing procedure, and the placement of gingival retraction cord can be uncomfortable. Furthermore, moisture control can be difficult and, while preferable, rubber dam is not

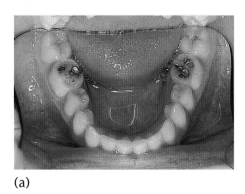

(a)

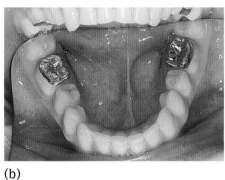

(b)

Figure 10.11 (a) Marked occlusal enamel loss of lower first permanent molars. (b) Cast occlusal onlays *in situ* after replacement of amalgam restorations with composite resin.

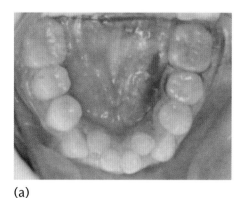

(a)

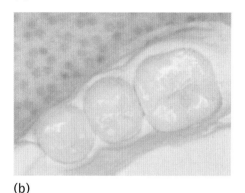

(b)

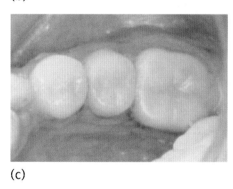

(c)

Figure 10.12 Direct composite onlays made for lower posterior quadrants. (a) Lower occlusal view, (b) lower right quadrant on model, (c) *in situ*.

always feasible. Disruption of the occluso-vertical dimension should be anticipated. However, this is usually well tolerated by young patients.

When used to protect the palatal aspect of the upper anterior teeth there may be an aesthetic problem as the metal may 'shine through' the translucent incisal tip of young teeth if an opaque luting cement is not used. The durability of this form of restoration has now been confirmed by 10-year evaluation studies.

10.2.10 Indirect composite resin onlays

Indirect composite onlays and porcelain onlays are an alternative to cast metal onlays. In addition to the obvious aesthetic advantages, composite restorations can be modified relatively easily. This is particularly useful for conditions such as erosion where the disease process may well be ongoing and therefore the tooth and/or restoration may require repair or additions. Studies suggest that these restorations are durable in the anterior region. However, in response to patient demand, tooth-coloured restorations are increasingly being used in the posterior region

(Fig. 10.12) where their durability is currently unclear. The disadvantage of these restorations is that they need to be thicker than their cast counterparts, are bulkier, and can cause greater increases in vertical dimension. However, provided that the occlusion remains balanced and there is no periodontal pathology, increases in vertical dimension appear to be well tolerated in young patients.

10.3 Tooth discolouration

The colour of a child's teeth can be of great importance. Peer-group pressure can be very strong, and teasing about the size, position, and colour of the teeth can be very harmful to a child or adolescent.

The causes of discoloured teeth may be classified in a number of ways: congenital/acquired; enamel/dentine; extrinsic/intrinsic; systemic/local. The most useful method of classification for the clinical

Table 10.1 The aetiology of tooth discolouration

Extrinsic discolouration	
Beverages/food	
Smoking	
Poor oral hygiene (chromogenic bacteria): green/orange stain	
Drugs	
Iron supplements: black stain	
Minocycline: black stain	
Chlorhexidine: brown/black stain	
Intrinsic discolouration	
Enamel	
Local causes	Caries
	Idiopathic
	Injury/infection of primary predecessor
	Internal resorption
Systemic causes	Amelogenesis imperfecta
	Drugs (e.g. tetracyclines)
	Fluorosis
	Idiopathic
	Systemic illness during tooth formation
Dentine	
Local causes	Caries
	Internal resorption
	Metallic restorative materials
	Necrotic pulp tissue
	Root-canal-filling materials
Systemic causes	Bilirubin (haemolytic disease of newborn)
	Congenital porphyria
	Dentinogenesis imperfecta
	Drugs (e.g. tetracyclines)

management of discolouration is one that identifies the main site of discolouration (Table 10.1). Once the aetiology of the discolouration had been identified, the most appropriate method of treatment can be chosen. Ideal and permanent results may not be realistic in the young patient, but significant improvements are achievable which do not compromise the teeth in the long term.

The approach to treatment for all forms of discolouration should be cautious, with the emphasis on minimal tooth preparation. For example, in a case of fluorosis the micro-abrasion technique may produce some improvement but the patient/parent may still be dissatisfied. Composite veneers can then be placed, although if the child requires subsequent fixed appliance treatment these may be damaged and require replacement before placing porcelain veneers as the definitive restoration in the late teenage years.

Discolouration originating in the dentine is often difficult to treat. The single non-vital dark incisor presents particular problems. In the young patient, the apex may be immature, root canal therapy incomplete, and therefore non-vital bleaching precluded. A composite veneer can improve the aesthetics but may fail to adequately disguise the discolouration even with the use of opaqueing agents. Ultimately, a jacket crown may be the best option in the older patient. Similarly, moderate to severe tetracycline discolouration, which fortunately is much less common today, is very difficult to treat in the young patient. Long-term full crowns or porcelain veneers often provide definitive treatment, but composite veneers can be acceptable in the adolescent without completely masking the underlying discolouration (Fig. 10.13). Indirect composite veneers, placed with minimal tooth preparation, may be useful in the management of this problem but this technique has yet to be evaluated. (See Key Points 10.1.)

Key Points 10.1

- Micro-abrasion should be the first line of treatment in all cases of enamel opacities.
- Composite should be used in preference to porcelain in children.

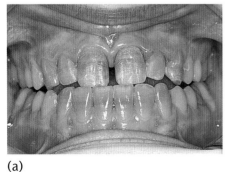
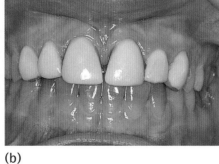
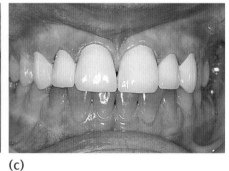

(a)   (b)   (c)

Figure 10.13 (a) Severe tetracycline discolouration in a 14-year-old. (b) Composite veneers placed over opaqueing agents to mask the discolouration. (c) Porcelain jacket crowns were provided at 20 years of age.

Finally, it is very important to bear in mind the expectations of the patient and, often more importantly, the parent. An unrealistically high expectation of brilliant white 'film star' teeth will result in postoperative disappointment. For instance, in fluorosis cases it is the excessively white mottled areas which will be removed by the micro-abrasion technique, resulting in a uniform colour that is the same as the original background colour, and some patients will feel that their treated teeth are 'too yellow'. Adequate preoperative explanation, preferably with photographic examples, may help to minimize this problem. Nevertheless, a group of dissatisfied patients will remain and for medico-legal reasons careful documentation (preferably photographic) of all cases of cosmetic treatment should be kept.

10.4 Tooth surface loss

Dentists have been aware of the problem of tooth surface loss (TSL) or non-carious loss of tooth tissue for a long time. However, it is only more recently that it has been increasingly associated with the younger population. Three processes make up the main contribution to the phenomenon of TSL:

- *attrition*—wear of the tooth as a result of tooth-to-tooth contact;
- *erosion*—irreversible loss of tooth substance brought about by a chemical process that does not involve bacterial action;
- *abrasion*—physical wear of tooth substance produced by something other than tooth-to-tooth contact.

Abrasion is relatively uncommon in children. The most frequent cause of abrasion is overzealous toothbrushing, which tends to develop with increasing age. Attrition during mastication is common, particularly in the primary dentition where almost all upper incisors show some signs of attrition by the time they exfoliate (Fig. 10.14). However, over the past decade the contribution of erosion to the overall process of tooth wear in the younger population has been highlighted. While erosion may be the predominant process, attrition and abrasion may be compounding factors. For example, toothbrush abrasion may be increased if brushing is carried out immediately after the consumption of erosive foodstuffs or drinks. It is often difficult to identify a single causative agent in a case of tooth wear, so the general term 'tooth surface loss' may be more appropriate.

10.4.1 Prevalence

The problem with trying to assess the prevalence of tooth wear is that a degree of tooth tissue loss is a part of the normal physiological process of ageing; however, when it is likely to prejudice the survival of the teeth, it can be said to be pathological. Smith and Knight (1984) described a tooth wear index (TWI), which included certain features that they felt were diagnostic of pathological tooth wear. These features are shown in Box 10.3.

There is very little published evidence on the prevalence or severity of TSL in children. In the 2003 National Children' Dental Health Survey (Office for National Statistics 2003), 53% of 5-year-old children had evidence of TSL involving the palatal surfaces of their primary incisors, with 22% showing progression into the dentine if not also into the pulp (Fig. 10.15). The prevalence of erosion in adolescents is more worrying, with a third (33%) of 15-year-olds having some evidence of TSL on the

---

Box 10.3 Clinical signs of tooth wear

- Pulp exposure
- Loss of vitality attributable to tooth wear
- Exposure of secondary dentine
- Exposure of dentine on buccal or lingual surfaces
- Cupped occlusal or incisal surfaces
- Wear in one arch more than the other
- Restorations projecting above the surface of the tooth
- Wear producing sensitivity
- Reduction in length of incisal teeth so that the length is out of proportion to the width

Smith and Knight (1984)

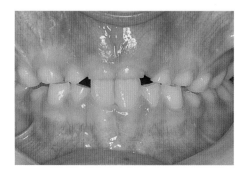

Figure 10.14 Primary incisors showing physiological wear.

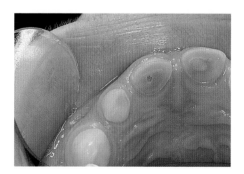

Figure 10.15 Primary incisors showing pathological wear and pulp exposure

palatal surfaces of their incisors, with 5% progressing in to the dentine and pulp. These figures represent a 6% increase over the past decade.

10.4.2 Aetiology

In young patients there are three main causes of TSL:

- dietary
- gastric regurgitation
- parafunctional activity.

In addition to these three factors, certain environmental factors have been linked to tooth wear. However, with the exception of frequent use of chlorinated swimming pools, most environmental and occupational hazards do not apply to children.

Dietary causes of TSL

The most common cause of erosive TSL is an excessive intake of acidic food or drink. Box 10.4 shows the types of foodstuffs implicated in erosive TSL in young patients.

Acidic drinks, in particular, are available to children of all age groups. Pure 'baby' fruit juices are marketed for consumption by infants and these have been shown to have pH values below the critical value for the dissolution of enamel (pH 5–5.5). Many of these drinks are given to infants in a feeding bottle, and the combination of the highly acidic nature of the drink and the prolonged exposure of the teeth to the acidic substrate may result in excessive TSL as well as dental caries. Although a wide range of foods and drinks are implicated in the aetiology of TSL, soft drinks make up the bulk of the problem. Soft drink consumption has increased dramatically over the past 40 years to a staggering annual value of 229 litres per head of the population in the UK in 2009. Pure fruit juices do contribute to this figure, but carbonated drinks make up 43% of these purchases, particularly through the younger population's intake. Such drinks are widely available in vending machines located in schools, sports centres, and other public areas. Both normal and so-called diet carbonated drinks have very low pH values and are associated with TSL, although unflavoured carbonated mineral water has negligible erosive potential. While there is no direct relationship between the pH of a substrate and the degree of TSL, pH

does give a useful indication of the potential to cause damage. Other factors such as titratable acidity, the influence on plaque pH, and the buffering capacity of saliva will all influence the erosive potential of a given substrate. In addition, it has been shown that erosive TSL tends to be more severe if the volume of drink consumed is high or the intake occurs at bedtime. (See Key Points 10.2.)

Key Points 10.2

The degree of erosive tooth-surface loss may be related to:

- the frequency of intake
- the timing of intake
- toothbrushing habits.

The pattern of dietary erosive TSL depends on the manner in which the substrate is consumed. Carbonated drinks are not uncommonly held in the mouth for some time as the child 'enjoys' the sensation of the bubbles around the mouth. This habit may result in a generalized loss of surface enamel (Fig. 10.16). Note the chipping of the incisal edges of the upper anterior teeth in Fig. 10.16—this is an example of attrition contributing to the overall pattern of TSL. A generalized loss of the surface enamel of posterior teeth is often evident, particularly on the first permanent molars, and characteristic saucer-shaped lesions

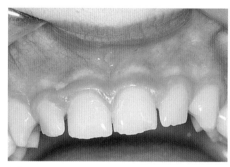

(a)

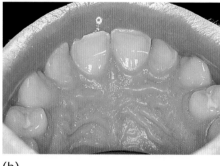

(b)

Figure 10.16 Teeth of a teenager who consumed considerable amounts of carbonated drinks. (a) Note chipping of the incisal edges and (b) characteristic palatal TSL.

Box 10.4 Examples of foods and drinks with erosive potential

Citrus fruits (e.g. lemons, oranges, grapefruit)
Tart apples
Vinegar and pickles
Yoghurt
Sauces (e.g. ketchup, brown sauce)
Fruit juices and herbal teas
Carbonated drinks, including low-calorie varieties and 'sports drinks'
Certain alcoholic drinks (e.g. Alcopops, cider, white wine)
Vitamin C tablets

develop on the cusps of the molars. This phenomenon is known as perimolysis. More peculiar habits are not uncommon; Fig. 10.17 shows the dentition of a young cyclist who very frequently consumed a lemon drink via a straw in his bicycle's drink bottle. Figure 10.18 is an example of a young adult who, for many years, consumed 2 pounds (almost 1kg) of raw Bramley cooking apples daily. The extent of TSL has left his amalgam restorations standing 'proud'.

Gastric regurgitation and TSL

The acidity of the stomach contents is below pH 1.0 and therefore any regurgitation or vomiting is potentially damaging to the teeth. As many as 50% of adults with signs of TSL have a history of gastric reflux. The aetiology of gastric regurgitation can be divided into two categories: those with upper gastrointestinal disorders, and those with eating disorders.

Long-term regurgitation in young patients is associated with a variety of underlying problems (Box 10.5). In addition, there are a group of patients who suffer from gastro-oesophageal reflux disease (GORD). This may be either symptomatic, in which case the individual knows what provokes the reflux, or, more insidiously, asymptomatic, where the patient is unaware of the problem and continues to ingest reflux-provoking foods.

Unexplained erosive TSL is one of the principal signs of an eating disorder. There are three such disorders to be aware of: anorexia nervosa, bulimia nervosa, and, more rarely, rumination (this is a condition of unknown aetiology in which food is voluntarily regurgitated into the oral cavity and either expelled or swallowed again).

Anorexia nervosa is a sociocultural disease affecting predominantly white middle-class intelligent females between 12 and 30 years of age.

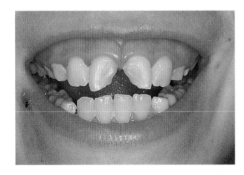

Figure 10.17 A 12-year-old with an unusual pattern of TSL.

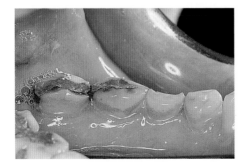

Figure 10.18 Marked TSL may eventually leave an amalgam restoration standing 'proud'.

Box 10.5 Conditions in children associated with chronic regurgitation

Gastro-oesophageal reflux
Oesophageal strictures
Chronic respiratory disease
Disease of the liver/pancreas/biliary tree
Overfeeding
Feeding problems/failure to thrive conditions
Neuromuscular disability (e.g. cerebral palsy)
Reye's syndrome
Rumination

Like bulimia nervosa, it is a secretive disease with sufferers denying illness and refusing therapy. People with anorexia exhibit considerable weight loss (up to 25% of their body weight in severe cases), and have a fear of growing fat and a distorted view of their body shape. Those with bulimia suffer characteristic binges on 'junk foodstuffs' and follow this with self-induced vomiting, overzealous exercise, and the use of laxatives to prevent weight gain. They may subsequently develop GORD, which causes typical signs of heartburn and oesophagitis.

The pattern of erosive TSL seen in all patients who suffer from chronic gastric regurgitation is similar, with marked erosion of the palatal surface of upper incisors and premolars. There is a surprising lack of tooth sensitivity. Over time, the buccal and occlusal surfaces of the lower molars and premolars also become affected (Fig. 10.19).

As a result of the asymptomatic nature of some of the gastrointestinal disorders and the secretive nature of the eating disorders, dentists may well be the first professionals to see the signs of gastric regurgitation. The presence of erosive TSL may be the only sign of an underlying disorder, and such a finding should be taken seriously and handled carefully in communication with medical colleagues.

Parafunctional activity

Localized TSL frequently occurs in patients who exhibit abnormal parafunctional habits. The excessive grinding that is a feature of this problem is not always apparent to the patient. However, apart from the marked tooth tissue loss, other signs of bruxism may be evident including hypertrophy of the muscles of mastication, cheek biting, and tongue faceting. An example of erosion and parafunction having a disastrous effect on the dentition may be seen (and heard) in children who have cerebral palsy. These children often have chronic gastric regurgitation and also severe bruxism, resulting in excessive TSL.

10.4.3 Management

Immediate

The most important aspect of the management of TSL is early diagnosis. While it is important to treat any dental sensitivity resulting from TSL, it is essential to establish the aetiology and, where possible, eliminate the cause. This may not always be possible—the existence of an underlying eating disorder cannot be resolved quickly or simply. Indeed, as with all forms of behaviour modification, the elimination of dietary causes of

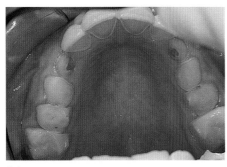

(a)

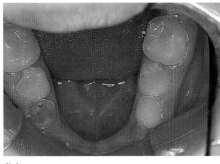

(b)

Figure 10.19 (a) Upper and (b) lower arches of a 10-year-old boy with chronic GORD.

erosion will often be difficult, particularly in young adolescents who are no longer under parental control and who often find it hard to adjust to alternative lifestyles and dietary habits. Ideally, the cause of TSL should be eliminated before restorative treatment is started. In order to achieve this, all patients and parents should be given dietary counselling which should be personal, practical, and positive. It is important not to simply advise against all carbonated drinks, but to offer positive alternatives, and to suggest that such drinks may be taken as a treat occasionally and that intake should be limited to meal times. Box 10.6 gives some practical suggestions which may be made to patients depending on the aetiology of the problem.

Dental sensitivity may be a problem in young patients. Erosive TSL may be rapid and, with the large pulp chambers, pulpal inflammation is common and secondary dentine does not have time to form. Promoting mineralization of affected teeth through the uptake of calcium and phosphate may reduce both sensitivity and susceptibility to further tissue loss. The development of casein phosphopeptide-amorphous calcium phosphate (CPP-ACP) technology provides a way of delivering calcium and phosphate to the tooth surface in a supersaturated medium stabilized by the CPP. One product that incorporates this technology is Tooth Mousse (GC Corporation, 76-1 Hasunuma-cho, Itabashi-ku, Tokyo 174-8586, Japan). Whilst clinical data on this product are currently limited, the application of Tooth Mousse digitally directly onto affected teeth by the patient is anecdotally associated with a reduction in sensitivity.

The use of glass ionomer cements or resin-based composites as temporary coverage may also resolve the sensitivity. There is some controversy in the literature about the value of glass ionomer cements in these

cases as they themselves dissolve in an acidic environment. However, the affected teeth are often so hypersensitive, at least initially, that placing a resin-based material with its associated drying requirements is simply not clinically possible as it is too painful for the child. Placement of a glass ionomer may provide temporary relief and facilitate ongoing review.

Definitive treatment

If TSL is diagnosed early, preventive counselling may be sufficient in many cases. It is a good idea to make study casts of all patients with signs of TSL and to give these to the patient to keep. The rate of progression of wear can then be monitored. However, in more advanced cases, where there are sensitivity or cosmetic problems, active intervention is required. Table 10.2 shows the relative merits of the options available. (See Key Points 10.3.)

Key Points 10.3

Main treatment objectives for tooth surface loss:

- resolve sensitivity
- restore missing tooth surface
- prevent further tooth tissue loss
- maintain a balanced occlusion.

In some cases there will be only localized tooth wear and an incomplete overbite, leaving enough space to place the restorations. Figure 10.20 shows the same patient as shown earlier in Fig. 10.16 who consumed considerable quantities of carbonated drinks in association with sporting activities. This habit caused considerable palatal wear of his upper incisors, with characteristic chipping of the incisal edges. Cast adhesive veneers were placed on the palatal aspect of the upper incisors to protect from further wear, and direct resin-based composite labial veneers were used to restore the aesthetics. Note in this case the slight grey 'shine-through' effect on the incisal tips due to the placement of cast restorations without the use of an opaque luting cement.

Table 10.2 Treatment techniques for tooth surface loss

Technique	Advantages	Disadvantages
Cast metal (nickel–chrome or gold)	Fabricated in thin section—requires only 0.5mm space Very accurate fit possible Very durable Suitable for posterior restorations in parafunction Does not abrade opposing dentition	May be cosmetically unacceptable because of 'shine-through' of metallic grey Cannot be simply repaired or added to intra-orally
Composite Direct	Adequately durable for labial veneers only Least expensive Can be used as a diagnostic tool	Technically difficult for palatal veneers Limited control over occlusal and interproximal contour Inadequate as a posterior restoration
Indirect	Can be added to and repaired relatively simply intra-orally Aesthetically superior to cast metal Control over occlusal contour and vertical dimension	Requires more space—minimum of 1.0mm Unproven durability
Porcelain	Best aesthetics Good abrasion resistance Well tolerated by gingival tissues	Potentially abrasive to opposing dentition Inferior marginal fit Very brittle—has to be used in bulk section Hard to repair

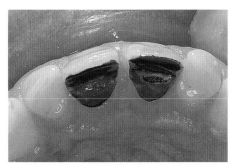

(a)

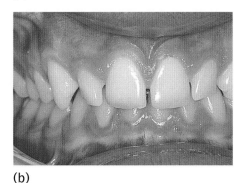

(b)

Figure 10.20 (a) Cast palatal veneers on upper central incisors. (b) Note the 'shine-through' despite placement of labial composite veneers.

In many other cases compensatory growth, which will help to maintain the occlusal vertical dimension, or the presence of a significant malocclusion may result in inadequate space for the necessary restorations. Figure 10.21(a) shows a case of a 12-year-old boy who has a class II, division II malocclusion and who consumed three cans of carbonated drinks every day. The combination of the erosive drink and the attrition brought about by the close tooth-to-tooth contact has resulted in a loss of palatal tooth tissue from the upper central incisors. There is insufficient space palatally to place any form of restoration, but a simple removable appliance with a flat anterior bite plane can be used to reduce the overbite by virtue of the Dahl principle (Fig. 10.21(b)). In children this occurs relatively quickly (within 6 weeks), principally by compensatory over-eruption of the posterior segments. Once sufficient space has been created, cast metal palatal veneers can be placed. Alternatively, palatal veneers can be placed without the initial use of an appliance to directly produce the Dahl effect on the occlusion.

Alternatively, if there has been marked wear of the posterior teeth, as shown in Fig. 10.22(a), it will be necessary to restore the occlusal surfaces and protect them from further wear prior to placing anterior restorations. Cast adhesive occlusal onlays are recommended in such cases (Fig. 10.22(b)). Young patients will accommodate the increase in vertical dimension easily, provided that a balanced occlusal contact is achieved. The use of a facebow record facilitates this. The main advantage of using cast metal onlays is the minimal thickness of material needed and its resistance to abrasive wear. Indirect

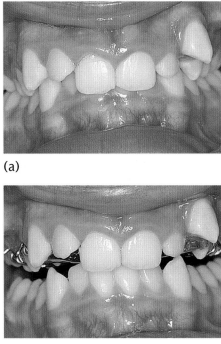

(a)

(b)

Figure 10.21 (a) Skeletal pattern II with deep overbite compounding palatal erosion in a 12-year-old boy. (b) An upper removable appliance in position to reduce the overbite.

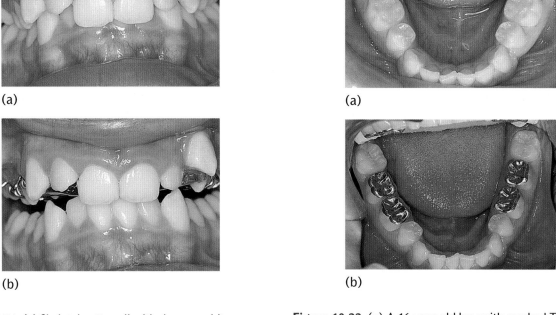

(a)

(b)

Figure 10.22 (a) A 16-year-old boy with marked TSL of lower permanent molars. Note the perimolysis of the first molars. (b) Post-cementation of gold onlays on the permanent molars.

composite veneers are a recent addition to our armamentarium and they offer considerable advantages, particularly in cases where the aetiology is unclear or the patient cannot stop the habit/problem. These restorations facilitate future additions and repairs (using direct composite) if the erosion continues or restarts. Median survival times in excess of 4 years have been reported for such indirect restorations in the anterior dentition. However, if there is an element of attrition or signs of parafunction, composite onlays may not be adequately durable in the posterior segments, so cast restorations are still the preferred option.

Long-term review

All patients with TSL should be reviewed regularly for three reasons:

- to monitor future TSL

- to maintain the existing restorations
- to provide support for the patient.

Patients with eating disorders in particular are prone to periods of relapse and the dentist is in an ideal position to diagnose these periods. The dentist can develop a special and trusting relationship with the young patient over the longer term, which is based on seeing the patient not simply when they are 'ill', and therefore admonishing them, but also when they are well, to support and encourage them. Likewise, in patients with dietary erosion, continual reinforcement of good dietary habits is needed throughout the child's life and into adulthood. People change their diet as they get older—one example is the young adolescent who manages to stop drinking Coca Cola but starts drinking lager to excess instead, and the erosion continues!

10.5 Inherited anomalies of enamel and dentine

Chapter 13 covers the whole range of dental anomalies. However, the treatment of amelogenesis imperfecta and dentinogenesis imperfecta poses specific challenges to the dentist. In view of the wide variety of presentations and the degree to which each case is affected, it is difficult to make generalizations. Early diagnosis of these conditions is important to their long-term prognosis; parents need to be educated as to the

implications of the condition, monitoring of the amount of tooth wear can start early, and, where necessary, teeth can be protected. Four main clinical problems are associated with inherited enamel and dentine defects:

- poor aesthetics
- chipping and attrition of the enamel

- exposure and attrition of the dentine, causing sensitivity
- poor oral hygiene, gingivitis, and caries.

Although it is impossible to draw up a definitive treatment plan for all cases, it is possible to define the principles of treatment planning for this group of patients. It is important to realize that not all children with amelogenesis imperfecta or dentinogenesis imperfecta are affected equally. Many will not have marked tooth wear or symptoms and will not require advanced intervention. Table 10.3 summarizes the principles of treatment with respect to the age of the child/adolescent and the three aspects of care—prevention, restoration, and aesthetics. (See Key Points 10.4.)

Key Points 10.4

Main treatment objectives for dental anomalies
- to alleviate symptoms
- to maintain/restore occlusal height
- to improve aesthetics.

Prevention

Prevention is an essential part of the management of children with enamel and dentine anomalies. Oral hygiene in these children is often poor due in part to the rough enamel surface which promotes plaque retention and in some cases to the sensitivity of the tooth to brushing. As a result there may be marked gingival inflammation and bleeding. The combination of gingival swelling and enamel hypoplasia can result in areas of food stagnation and a generally low level of oral health. Oral hygiene instruction must be given sympathetically, with plenty of encouragement, and should be continually reinforced. In some cases it may be necessary to carry out some restorative/cosmetic treatment before good oral hygiene measures can be practised. For example, the placement of anterior composite veneers may reduce dentine sensitivity and improve the enamel surface so that the patient can brush their

teeth more effectively. Conventional caries prevention with diet advice, fluoride therapy, and placement of fissure sealants is mandatory. In this group of children it is particularly important to preserve tooth tissue and not allow caries to compromise the dental hard tissues further.

Restoration

Restorative treatment varies considerably depending on the age of the child and the extent of the problem. The basic principle of treatment is that of minimal intervention. If there is sensitivity or signs of enamel chipping, techniques to cover and protect the teeth should be considered. In the very young child it is often impossible to carry out extensive operative treatment, but the placement of glass ionomer cement over areas of enamel hypoplasia is simple and effective. In older/more cooperative children stainless steel (or nickel–chrome) preformed crowns should be placed on the second primary molars to minimize further wear due to tooth-on-tooth contact (Chapter 8). It is advisable (and usually possible) to place such restorations with minimal or no tooth preparation because of the pre-existing tooth tissue loss.

Young children with dentinogenesis imperfecta often pose the greatest problems. The teeth undergo such excessive wear that they become worn down to gingival level and are unrestorable. Teeth affected by dentinogenesis imperfecta are also prone to spontaneous abscesses because of the progressive obliteration of the pulp chambers. In these cases pulp therapy is unsuccessful and extraction of the affected teeth is necessary.

As the permanent dentition develops, close monitoring of the rate of tooth wear will guide the decision about what intervention is needed. Cast occlusal onlays on the first permanent molars not only protect the underlying tooth structure but also maintain function and control symptoms. The resulting increase in the vertical dimension is associated with a decrease in the vertical overlap of the incisors. Full occlusion is usually re-established within a few weeks, and the whole procedure is well tolerated by young patients. As the premolars erupt, similar castings may be placed if wear is marked (Fig. 10.23). Alternatively, localized composite or glass ionomer cement restorations can be placed over areas of hypoplasia.

The emphasis should remain on minimal tooth preparation until the child attains adulthood. At this point, if clinically indicated, full-mouth

Table 10.3 Principles of treatment for amelogenesis and dentinogenesis imperfecta

	Prevention	Restoration	Aesthetics
Primary dentition (0–5 years)	Diet advice	GIC	Minimal intervention
	Fluoride supplements	SSCs (particularly on Es)	GICs
	Oral hygiene instruction		
Mixed dentition (6–16 years)	Diet advice	SSCs on primary molars	Direct composite veneers
	Fluoride therapy	Adhesive castings on first permanent molars	Indirect composite or porcelain veneers
	Oral hygiene instruction ± chlorhexidine	Localized composite/GIC	Dentures
Permanent dentition (16+ years)	Oral hygiene instruction	Adhesive castings on premolars	Porcelain veneers
	Fluoride therapy	Full mouth rehabilitation	Full crowns
			Overdentures
			Complete dentures

GIC, glass ionomer cement; SSC, stainless steel crown.

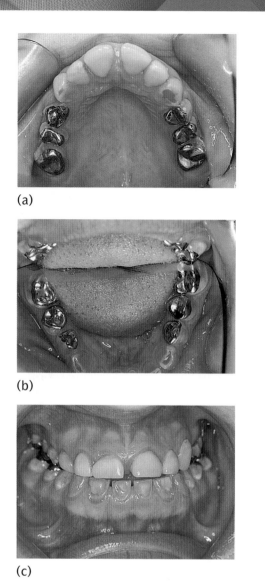

(a)

(b)

(c)

Figure 10.23 (a) Upper and (b) lower arches of a 14-year-old girl with dentinogenesis imperfecta showing cast onlays on the second permanent molars and premolars, and (c) labial and (a) palatal composite veneers on the upper incisors.

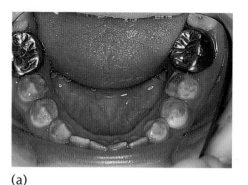

(a)

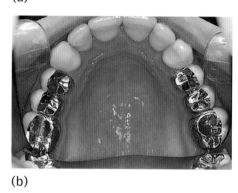

(b)

Figure 10.24 (a) A 14-year-old boy with severe amelogenesis imperfecta. Stainless steel crowns were placed on the first permanent molars at 9 years of age (lower arch). (b) At 20 years of age a full-mouth rehabilitation was completed (upper arch).

Aesthetics

Aesthetics is not usually a problem in the primary dentition. Where the child is sufficiently cooperative, the use of glass ionomer cements to restore and improve the appearance of primary incisors can be useful in gaining respect and support from the patient and the parent. In a few exceptional cases the loss of primary teeth may cause upset, but can be compensated for by constructing dentures. In cases of dentinogenesis imperfecta where the teeth are very worn but remain asymptomatic, overdentures can be constructed to which young children adapt remarkably well. These will need to be remade regularly as the child grows.

As the permanent incisors erupt they must be protected from chipping of the enamel. The placement of composite veneers not only improves the appearance but also promotes better gingival health and protects the teeth from further wear. In a few cases the quality of the enamel is so poor that the bond between composite and tooth will be unsuccessful. It should be noted that in these cases porcelain veneers are also likely to be unsuccessful and full coronal restorations are the only option.

Early consultation with an orthodontist and restorative dentist is advisable in order to keep long-term treatment requirements realistic. Orthodontic treatment for these patients is possible and in many cases proceeds without problems. The use of removable appliances, where appropriate, and orthodontic bands rather than brackets will minimize the risk of damage to the abnormal enamel. The problem is twofold: there may

rehabilitation may be considered and should have a good prognosis in view of the conservative approach that has been adopted throughout the early years (Fig. 10.24). Patients with dentinogenesis imperfecta should be treated with caution. The characteristic form of the teeth in this condition is unfavourable for crowning, as they are supported by short thin roots. The permanent dentition, like the primary dentition, is prone to spontaneous abscesses and the prognosis for endodontic treatment is very poor. The long-term plan for these patients is often some form of removable prosthesis, either an overdenture placed over the worn permanent teeth or a more conventional complete denture. The role of implants in these patients is often to provide retention for complete prostheses.

be frequent bond failure during active treatment, or the enamel may be further damaged during debonding. Some orthodontists prefer to use bands even for anterior teeth, while others will use glass ionomer cement as the bonding agent in preference to more conventional resin-based agents. In other instances cosmetic restorative techniques (veneers and crowns) may be more appropriate than orthodontic treatment.

10.6 Molar incisor hypomineralizaton

Molar incisor hypomineralization (MIH) is a term used to refer to hypomineralization of one or more of the first permanent molars and often, but not necessarily also, involving incisor teeth. Clinically, MIH may present as discrete opaque lesions that are often asymmetrically distributed with marked variation in severity between and within affected individuals (Fig. 10.25). The enamel is soft and, on eruption, chips away easily, leading to exposed dentine. These teeth are not only porous and more susceptible to plaque accumulation but also often very sensitive, making effective oral hygiene difficult. Therefore affected individuals are at increased risk of caries. The specific prevalence of MIH is unclear because of differences in diagnostic criteria across studies. However, figures between 5% and 31% have been reported.

10.6.1 Management of MIH

The key to successful management of this condition is early identification. Careful review is needed around the time of eruption of the first permanent molars to identify affected teeth. When incisors erupt prior to the molars, the presence of an opacity on the surface of a newly erupted incisor is a strong indicator of MIH. Once a child is diagnosed as having MIH, they should be considered at 'high caries risk' and an associated proactive preventive plan developed. Promoting mineralization of affected enamel through the uptake of calcium and phosphate will potentially enhance its mechanical properties and reduce susceptibility to further breakdown. The development of CPP-ACP technology provides a way of delivering calcium and phosphate to the tooth surface in a supersaturated medium stabilized by the casein phosphopeptide. In addition to promoting mineralization, CPP-ACP will further inhibit carious demineralization. Products incorporating this technology include Tooth Mousse or MI Paste Plus (GC Corporation, 76-1 Hasunuma-cho, Itabashi-ku, Tokyo 174-8586, Japan). Whilst clinical data on these products are currently scarce, the application of these pastes at least twice daily is associated with a rapid reduction in sensitivity in affected children which in turn optimizes oral hygiene.

In arriving at a definitive treatment plan, consideration needs to be given to the long-term prognosis of the affected molar teeth, the malocclusion, and the aesthetic impact of any lesions involving the anterior teeth. The restoration of MIH-affected molars poses significant challenges as the success of conventional restorative techniques is compromised because of the poor mechanical and physical properties of the affected enamel. Furthermore, not only are these teeth often extremely sensitive, requiring robust local analgesia, but also they are difficult to access physically in young patients. As a result careful consideration should be given to whether attempting to restore these teeth is in the best interests of the child. The indications for, and outcomes associated with, removing first permanent molars are covered elsewhere (Chapter 14). However, the presence of significant post-eruptive breakdown and/or caries in a hypomineralized tooth should at least raise the question of extraction.

However, in many cases it may be desirable to try to retain the first permanent molars, at least in the short to medium term if not in the long term. However, there are challenges associated with most restorative options. Amalgam, being non-adhesive, requires the removal of excessive

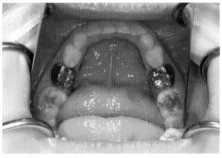

(a)

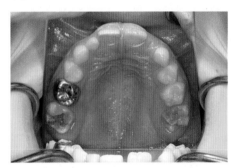

(b)

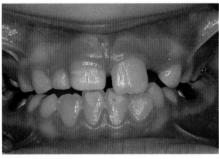

(c)

Figure 10.25 The characteristic presentation of a young child with MIH in the early mixed dentition. Note the caries superimposed upon the hypomineralized first permanent molars. (a) Lower arch, (b) upper arch, and (c) labial view. (Images by kind permission of Dr J. Winters.)

tooth tissue for mechanical retention, leaving the residual tooth vulnerable to fracture. The quality and integrity of the interface between resin-based restorative materials, such as composites, and hypomineralized enamel is inadequate, leading to microleakage, marginal breakdown, sensitivity, re-infection, and further deterioration. Temporization and maintenance of existing tooth structure can be achieved through the use of glass ionomer cements such as the low-viscosity high-fluoride chemically curing materials (Fig. 10.26). Although such materials are promoted for fissure protection, they can facilitate preservation of these compromised teeth asymptomatically for many years if regularly maintained.

If longer-term retention of the affected molar is needed, a preformed metal crown (PMC) is the preferred option. However, placement of a PMC requires excellent analgesia and patient cooperation, which may not be forthcoming. In addition, consideration needs to be given to the long-term management of teeth restored in this fashion. If the tooth is maintained into adulthood, it can present significant challenges to the adult prosthodontist and may still require extraction and replacement with other forms of prostheses such as an implant.

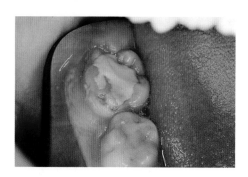

Figure 10.26 An example of a hypomineralized first permanent molar temporized using a glass ionomer cement material. Image by kind permission of Dr J. Winters.

If a child is disturbed by the appearance of their incisors, aesthetic improvements can often be achieved using more conservative approaches such as micro-abrasion ± bleaching. However, some of the more severe brown or white opacities may require localized composite veneers.

10.7 Hypodontia

Individuals with missing teeth may present at any age requesting replacement of their missing teeth for both aesthetic and functional reasons. A detailed discussion of the management of hypodontia is beyond the remit of this text, but a few principles can be considered here. During infancy and early school years there is rarely a need for any active intervention. An exception may be adolescents with ectodermal dysplasia who can have multiple missing teeth (Fig. 10.27). In such cases, the provision of removable partial or even complete dentures can be very successful at a young age. However, as children move through the mixed and permanent dentition phases, aesthetics become increasingly important. Replacing one or two teeth may be relatively straightforward using either removable partial dentures or adhesively retained bridges. However, those individuals with multiple missing teeth often have associated skeletal and dento-alveolar discrepancies which demand a multi-disciplinary approach (Fig. 10.28). The multidisciplinary team (MDT) should include at least a paediatric dentist, orthodontist, and prostho-dontist, but access to a periodontist and a maxillofacial surgeon is also useful.

Early referral to such an MDT is essential for discussion and prelimi-nary planning. Consideration needs to be given to the number and posi-tion of the missing dental units, the age of the child, their level of and attitude towards oral health, and importantly the wishes and expecta-tions of the individual and their family. The aim of orthodontic treat-ment is to consolidate the spacing and place the existing teeth in the optimum position to support the definitive restorations. However, con-sideration also needs to be given to any underlying skeletal discrepancy or dento-alveolar deficiency that may require a more surgical approach.

Interim restorative solutions, such as removable dentures, composite veneer, or partial veneer restorations, can be placed during the mixed dentition phase but will require maintenance throughout adolescence. Proactive preventive strategies need to be supported in order to achieve optimum dental and periodontal health. This is essential for the long-term success of definitive prosthodontic solutions which may include removable dentures, porcelain veneers or crowns, fixed conventional or adhesively retained bridges, and osseo-integrated implants. Finally, access to a geneticist with expertise in orofacial anomalies can be ben-eficial as adolescents begin to contemplate the implications of their dental anomaly on family planning. (See Key Points 10.5.)

Key Points 10.5

- Children with multiple missing teeth should be:
  - referred early to an MDT
  - exposed to proactive prevention to optimize their perio-dontal health.
- Treatment options may include:
  - interim measures—partial dentures or composite veneers in childhood and adolescence
  - definitive restorations—crowns, bridges, veneers, and den-tal implants post growth
  - surgical interventions—orthognathic surgery and bone grafting.

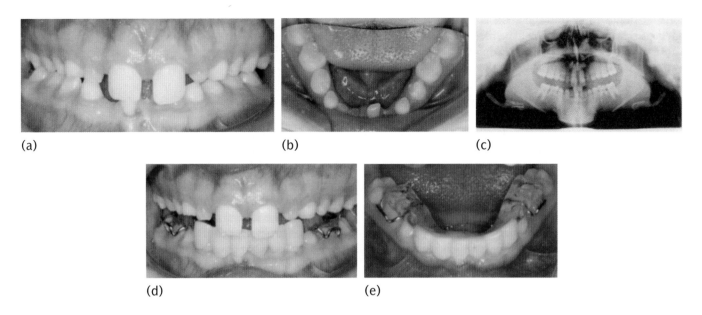

Figure 10.27 (a) Anterior view of an adolescent with hypodontia. (b) Lower arch of the same adolescent with hypodontia. (c) OPG radiograph confirming multiple missing teeth. (d), (e) Lower partial interim denture *in situ* increasing the vertical dimension and providing a more balanced occlusion.

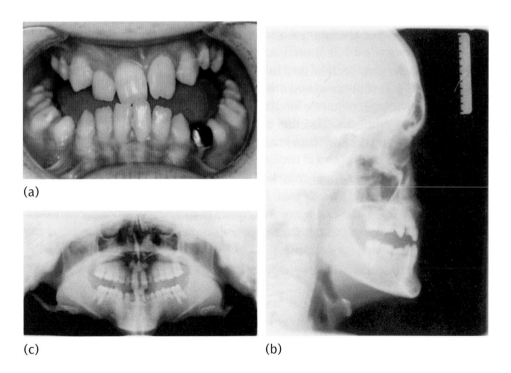

Figure 10.28 (a) Anterior clinical view of a 15-year-old male with a significant skeletal discrepancy, posterior open bites, and multiple missing teeth. (b), (c) Radiographs of the same 15-year-old male.

10.8 Summary

1 The management of children with advanced restorative problems should be viewed as a long-term commitment.

2 Advanced restorative problems in children should be treated as conservatively as possible.

3 Identification of the aetiology of tooth discolouration is essential for selecting the most appropriate treatment technique.

4 Micro-abrasion should be the first treatment option in all cases of enamel surface discolouration.

5 Porcelain veneers should be delayed until a mature gingival contour is attained.

6 A third of all 15-year-olds have experience of erosive TSL.

7 The cause of TSL should be determined and eliminated before active treatment is started.

8 Maintenance of occlusal face height is essential in patients with amelogenesis or dentinogenesis imperfecta.

10.9 Further reading

Bishop, K., Briggs, P., and Kelleher, M. (1994). The aetiology and management of localized anterior tooth wear in the young adult. *Dental Update*, **21**, 153–60. (*A good review with a lot of references and clinical examples.*)

Dahl, J.E. and Pallesen, U. (2003). Tooth bleaching: a critical review of the biological aspects. *Critical Reviews in Oral Biology and Medicine*, **14**, 292–304. (*A well-referenced review on the efficacy of tooth bleaching.*)

Harley, K.E. and Ibbetson, R.J. (1993). Dental anomalies—are adhesive castings the solution? *British Dental Journal*, **174**, 15–22. (*A well-written study covering the clinical technique and the follow-up of 12 children with amelogenesis or dentinogenesis imperfecta.*)

Kilpatrick, N.M. and Welbury, R.R. (1993). Hydrochloric acid–pumice microabrasion technique for the removal of enamel pigmentation. *Dental Update*, **20**, 105–7. (*A clinical study assessing the effectiveness of the micro-abrasion technique.*)

King, P.A. (1999). Tooth surface loss: adhesive techniques. *British Dental Journal*, **186**, 321–6. (*A good description of current techniques.*)

Lygidakis, N.A., Wong, F.S., Jalevik, B., *et al.* (2010). Best clinical practice guidance for clinicians dealing with children presenting with molar-incisor-hypomineralisation. *European Archives of Paediatric Dentistry*, **11**, 75–81.

Nunn, J.H., Carter, N.E., Gillgrass, T.J., *et al.* (2003). The interdisciplinary management of hypodontia: Parts 1–5. *British Dental Journal*, **194**, 245–51, 299–304, 361–6, 423–7, 479–82. (*A comprehensive series of papers addressing the complexities of management of hypodontia.*)

O'Sullivan, E. and Milosovic, A. (2008). UK National Clinical Guidelines in Paediatric Dentistry: diagnosis, prevention and management of dental erosion. *International Journal of Paediatric Dentistry* **18** (Suppl 1), 29–38. (*Contemporary guidelines for dental erosion.*)

Poyser, N.J., Kelleher, M.G., and Briggs, P.F. (2004). Managing discoloured non-vital teeth: the inside/outside bleaching technique. *Dental Update*, **31**, 204–10. (*A simple report of the technique.*)

10.10 References

Office for National Statistics (2003). *National Children's Dental Health Survey*. Available online at:
www.statistics.gov.uk

Smith, B.G. and Knight, J.K. (1984). An index for measuring the wear of teeth. *British Dental Journal*, **156**, 435–8.

Wray, A.P.M. and Welbury, R.R. (2001, revised 2004). Treatment of intrinsic discolouration in permanent anterior teeth in children and adolescents. Available online at:
www.rcseng.ac.uk

11

Periodontal diseases in children

P.A. Heasman and P.J. Waterhouse

Chapter contents

11.1 Introduction

Periodontal diseases comprise a group of infections that affect the supporting structures of the teeth: marginal and attached gingiva, periodontal ligament, cementum, and alveolar bone.

Acute gingival diseases—primarily herpetic gingivostomatitis and necrotizing gingivitis—are ulcerative conditions which result from specific viral and bacterial infection. Chronic gingivitis, however, is a nonspecific inflammatory lesion of the marginal gingiva which reflects the bacterial challenge to the host when dental plaque accumulates in the gingival crevice. The development of chronic gingivitis is enhanced when routine oral hygiene practices are impaired. Chronic gingivitis is reversible if effective plaque control measures are introduced. If left untreated, the condition invariably converts to chronic periodontitis which is characterized by resorption of the supporting connective tissue attachment and apical migration of the junctional epithelia. Slowly progressing chronic periodontitis affects most of the adult population to a greater or lesser extent, although the early stages of the disease are detected in adolescents.

Children are also susceptible to aggressive periodontal diseases that involve both the primary and permanent dentitions and present in localized or generalized forms. These conditions, which are distinct clinical entities affecting otherwise healthy children, must be differentiated from the extensive periodontal destruction that is associated with certain systemic diseases, degenerative disorders, and congenital syndromes.

Periodontal tissues are also susceptible to changes that are not, primarily, of an infectious nature. Factitious stomatitis is characterized by self-inflicted trauma to oral soft tissues, and the gingiva are invariably involved. Drug-induced gingival enlargement is becoming increasingly more prevalent with the widespread use of organ transplant procedures and the use of long-term immunosuppressant therapy. Localized enlargement may occur as a gingival complication of orthodontic treatment.

Table 11.1 A classification of periodontal diseases in children

Gingival conditions without loss of connective tissue attachment	Periodontal conditions with loss of connective tissue attachment
Acute gingivitis	Chronic periodontitis
Herpetic gingivostomatitis	Plaque-induced
Necrotizing ulcerative gingivitis	Complication of orthodontic treatment
Chronic gingivitis	Aggressive periodontitis
Plaque-induced	
Puberty gingivitis	
Gingival enlargement	Periodontitis as a manifestation of systemic disease
Drug-induced (generalized)	
Traumatic gingivitis	Papillon–Lefèvre syndrome
Mucogingival problems	Ehlers–Danlos syndrome
	Hypophosphatasia
	Chediak–Higashi syndrome
	Leucocyte adhesion deficiency syndrome
	Neutropenias
	Langerhans' cell histiocytosis

A classification of periodontal diseases in children is given in Table 11.1.

11.2 Anatomy of the periodontium in children

Marginal gingival tissues around the primary dentition are more highly vascular and contain fewer connective tissue fibres than tissues around the permanent teeth. The epithelia are thinner with a lesser degree of keratinization, giving an appearance of increased redness that may be interpreted as mild inflammation. Furthermore, the localized hyperaemia that accompanies eruption of the primary dentition can persist, leading to swollen and rounded interproximal papillae and a depth of gingival sulcus exceeding 3mm.

During eruption of the permanent teeth the junctional epithelium migrates apically from the incisal or occlusal surface towards the cemento-enamel junction (CEJ). While the epithelial attachment is above the line of maximum crown convexity, the gingival sulcus depth often exceeds 6 or 7mm, which favours the accumulation of plaque. When the teeth are fully erupted, there continues to be an apical shift of junctional epithelium and the free gingival margins. Stability of the gingiva is achieved at about 12 years for mandibular incisors, canines, second premolars, and first molars. The tissues around the remaining teeth continue to recede slowly until about 16 years. Thus the gingival margins are frequently at different levels on adjacent teeth that are at different stages of eruption. This sometimes gives the erroneous appearance that gingival recession has occurred around those teeth that have been in the mouth longest.

A variation in sulcus depths around posterior teeth in the mixed dentition is common. For example, sulcus depths on the mesial aspects of Es and 6s are greater than those on the distal of Ds and Es, respectively. This is accountable to the discrepancy in the horizontal position of adjacent CEJs because of the difference in the occluso-apical widths of adjacent molar crowns.

The attached gingiva extends from the free gingival margin to the mucogingival line minus the sulcus depth in the absence of inflammation. Attached gingiva is necessary to maintain sulcus depth, to resist functional stresses during mastication, and to resist tensional stress by acting as a buffer between the mobile gingival margin and the loosely structured alveolar mucosa. The width of attached gingiva is less variable in the primary than in the permanent dentition. This may partly account for the scarcity of mucogingival problems in the primary dentition.

The periodontal ligament space is wider in children, partly as a consequence of thinner cementum and alveolar cortical plates. The ligament is less fibrous and more vascular. Alveolar bone has larger marrow spaces, greater vascularity, and fewer trabeculae than adult tissues, features that may enhance the rate of progression of periodontal disease when it affects the primary dentition.

The radiographic distance between the CEJ and the healthy alveolar bone crest for primary canine and molar teeth ranges from 0 to 2mm. Individual surfaces display distances of up to 4mm when adjacent permanent or primary teeth are erupting or exfoliating, respectively, and eruptive and maturation changes must be considered when radiographs are used to diagnose periodontal disease in children. When

> **Key Points 11.1**
>
> Anatomy:
> - junctional epithelium
> - marginal gingiva
> - attached gingiva
> - alveolar bone
> - differences between the primary and permanent dentitions

such changes are excluded, a CEJ–alveolar crest distance of more than 2mm should arouse suspicion of pathological bone loss in the primary dentition. (See Key Points 11.1.)

11.3 Acute gingival conditions

The principal acute gingival conditions that affect children are primary herpetic gingivostomatitis and necrotizing ulcerative gingivitis. The latter is most frequently seen in young adults, but it also affects teenagers.

11.3.1 Primary herpetic gingivostomatitis

Herpetic gingivostomatitis is an acute infectious disease caused by *Herpesvirus hominis*. The primary infection is most frequently seen in children between 2 and 5 years of age, although older age groups can be affected. A degree of immunity is transferred to the newborn from circulating maternal antibodies, so an infection in the first 12 months of life is rare. Almost 100% of urban adult populations are carriers of, and have neutralizing antibodies to, the virus. This acquired immunity suggests that the majority of childhood infections are subclinical.

Transmission of the virus is by droplet infection and the incubation period is about a week. The child develops a febrile illness with a raised temperature of 37.8–38.9° C (100–102° F). Headaches, malaise, oral pain, mild dysphagia, and cervical lymphadenopathy are the common symptoms that accompany the fever and precede the onset of a severe oedematous marginal gingivitis. Characteristic fluid-filled vesicles appear on the gingiva and other areas such as the tongue, lips, and buccal and palatal mucosa. The vesicles, which have a grey membranous covering, rupture spontaneously after a few hours to leave extremely painful yellowish ulcers with red inflamed margins (Fig. 11.1). The clinical episode runs a course of about 14 days and the oral lesions heal without scarring. Rare but severe complications of the infection are aseptic meningitis and encephalitis.

The clinical features, history, and age group of the affected children are so characteristic that diagnosis is rarely problematic. However, if in doubt smears from recently ruptured vesicles reveal degenerating epithelial cells with intranuclear inclusions. The virus protein also tends to displace the nuclear chromatin to produce enlarged and irregular nuclei.

Herpetic gingivostomatitis does not respond well to active treatment. Bed rest and a soft diet are recommended during the febrile stage and the child should be kept well hydrated. Pyrexia is reduced using a paracetamol suspension and secondary infection of ulcers may be prevented using chlorhexidine. A chlorhexidine mouth rinse (0.2%, two to three times daily) can be used in older children who are able to expectorate, but in younger children (under 6 years of age) a chlorhexidine

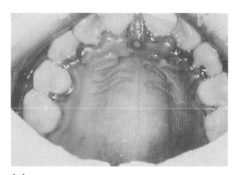

(a)

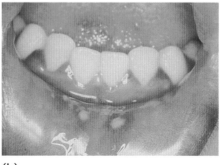

(b)

Figure 11.1 Ulcerative stage of primary herpetic gingivostomatitis: (a) palatal gingiva; (b) lower lip mucosa.

spray can be used (twice daily) or the solution applied using a sponge swab. In severe cases of herpes simplex infection, systemic aciclovir can be prescribed as a suspension (200mg) swallowed five times daily for 5 days. In children under 2 years the dose is halved. Aciclovir is active against the herpesvirus but is unable to eradicate it completely. The drug is most effective when given at the onset of the infection. (See Key Points 11.2 and 11.3.)

Key Points 11.2

Herpetic gingivostomatitis—clinical:

- primary/recurrent
- viral
- vesicular lesions
- complications rare.

Key Points 11.3

Herpetic gingivostomatitis—treatment:

- symptomatic
- rest and soft diet
- fluids
- paracetamol suspension
- aciclovir.

After the primary infection the herpesvirus remains dormant in the host's epithelial cells. Reactivation of the latent virus or re-infection in subjects with acquired immunity occurs in children and adults. Recurrent disease presents as an attenuated intra-oral form of the primary infection or as herpes labialis, i.e. the common 'cold sore' on the mucocutaneous border of the lips (Fig. 11.2). Cold sores are treated by applying aciclovir cream (5%) five times daily for about 5 days. To prevent auto-inoculation and spread of the lesions onto hands and the face, children should be discouraged from touching the vesicles.

11.3.2 Necrotizing ulcerative gingivitis

Necrotizing ulcerative gingivitis (NUG) is one of the most common acute diseases of the gingiva. In the USA and Europe, NUG affects young adults in the 16–30 age range with a reported incidence of 0.7–7%. In developing countries, NUG is prevalent in children as young as 1 or 2 years of age, when the infection can be very aggressive leading to extensive destruction of soft and hard tissues (Fig. 11.3). Epidemic-like occurrences of NUG have been reported in groups such as army recruits and first-year college students. These outbreaks are more likely to be a consequence of the prevalence of common predisposing factors rather than communicability of infection between subjects.

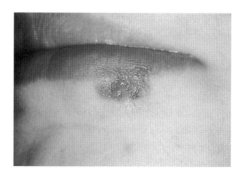

Figure 11.2 Herpetic 'cold sore' at the vermilion border of the lower lip.

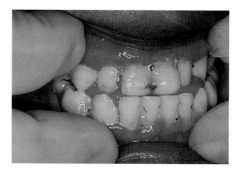

Figure 11.3 A 5-year-old Ethiopian boy with necrotizing ulcerative gingivitis.

Clinical features

NUG is characterized by necrosis and ulceration, which first affect the interdental papillae and then spread to the labial and lingual marginal gingiva. The ulcers are 'punched out', covered by a yellowish-grey pseudomembranous slough, and extremely painful to the touch (Fig. 11.3). The acute exacerbation is often superimposed upon a pre-existing gingivitis, and the tissues bleed profusely on gentle probing. The standard of oral hygiene is usually very poor. A distinctive halitosis is common in established cases of NUG, although fever and lymphadenopathy are less common than in herpetic gingivostomatitis.

The clinical course of NUG is such that the acute stage enters a chronic phase of remission after 5–7 days. However, recurrence of the acute condition is inevitable, and if this acute–chronic cycle is allowed to continue the marginal tissues lose their contour and appear rounded. Eventually, the inflammation and necrosis involve the alveolar crest and the subsequent necrotizing periodontitis leads to rapid bone resorption and gingival recession. Progressive changes are also a consequence of inadequate or incomplete treatment.

Aetiology

A smear taken from an area of necrosis or the surface of an ulcer will reveal numerous dead cells, polymorphonuclear leucocytes, and a sample of the micro-organisms that are frequently associated with NUG. Fusiform bacteria and spirochaetes are both numerous and easy to detect. A fusospirochaetal complex has been strongly implicated as the causative organisms in NUG. Other Gram-negative anaerobic organisms, including *Porphyromonas gingivalis*, *Veillonella* species, and *Selenomonas* species, have been detected, which suggests that NUG could be a broad anaerobic infection.

A viral aetiology has also been suggested, primarily because of the similarity between NUG and known viral diseases. For example, the restriction of the disease to children and young adults may imply that older subjects have undergone seroconversion (and thus are immune) as a consequence of clinical or subclinical viral infection in earlier life. The recurring episodes of the disease may also be explained by a viral hypothesis. The ability to undergo latent infection that is subject to reactivation is a characteristic of the herpesvirus. Therefore the argument for the implication of a virus in NUG is valid and novel, although a specific virus has yet to be isolated from oral lesions.

Predisposing factors

Poor oral hygiene and pre-existing gingivitis invariably reflect the patient's attitude to oral care. Many young adults with NUG are heavy smokers. The effect of smoking on the gingiva may be mediated through a local irritation or by the vasoconstrictive action of nicotine, thus reducing tissue resistance and making the host more susceptible to anaerobic infection. Smoking is obviously not a predisposing factor in young children. However, children in underdeveloped countries are often undernourished and debilitated, which may predispose to infection. Outbreaks of NUG in groups of subjects who are under stress has implicated emotional status as an important predisposing factor. Elevated plasma levels of corticosteroids as a response to an emotional upset are thought to be a possible mechanism.

It is conceivable that all the predisposing factors have a common action to initiate or potentiate a specific change in the host such as lowering the cell-mediated response. Indeed, patients with NUG have depressed phagocytic activity and chemotactic response of their polymorphonuclear leucocytes. (See Key Points 11.4.)

Treatment

It is important that the patient is informed at the outset of the nature of NUG and the likelihood of recurrence of the condition if the treatment is not completed. Smokers should be advised to reduce the number of cigarettes smoked. A soft multi-tufted brush is recommended when a medium-textured brush is too painful.

Key Points 11.4

Necrotizing ulcerative gingivitis—clinical:

- yellow-grey ulcers
- fusospirochaetal infection
- possible viral aetiology
- well-established predisposing factors.

Mouth rinses may be recommended but only for short-term use (7–10 days). Rinsing with chlorhexidine (0.2%) for about a minute reduces plaque formation, and the use of a hydrogen peroxide or sodium hydroxyperborate mouth rinse oxygenates and cleanses the necrotic tissues.

Mechanical debridement should be undertaken at the initial visit. An ultrasonic scaler with its accompanying water spray can be effective with minimal discomfort for the patient. Further, if NUG is localized to one part of the mouth, local anaesthesia of the soft tissues can allow some sub-gingival scaling to be undertaken.

In severe cases of NUG, a 3-day course of metronidazole (for children over 10 years of age: 200mg three times daily) alleviates the symptoms, but the patients must be informed that they are required to reattend for further treatment.

Occasionally, it is necessary to surgically recontour the gingival margin (gingivoplasty) to improve tissue architecture and facilitate sub-gingival cleaning. (See Key Points 11.5.)

Key Points 11.5

Necrotizing ulcerative gingivitis—treatment:

- intense oral hygiene
- remove predisposing factors
- mechanical debridement
- metronidazole.

11.4 Chronic gingivitis

National Surveys (1973, 1983, 1993, and 2003) of children's dental health in the UK show that the prevalence of chronic gingivitis increases steadily between the ages of 5 and 12 years and is closely associated with the amount of plaque, debris, and calculus present (Fig. 11.4). For example, in 2003, 32% of 5-year-olds had some signs of gingivitis, and the proportion increased to 65% at the age of 12. The prevalence of gingivitis peaks at about 12 years (65%) and then decreases slightly with age to 15 years (52%). In terms of gingivitis, there has been no improvement over the decades between surveys.

Indeed, in 2003, 13–19% more children of all ages between 5 and 12 years had signs of gingivitis when compared with 1983. However, these differences were not maintained with increasing age, as 52% of 15-year-olds had gingivitis in both 1993 and 2003. These data suggest that the gingival condition of children in the UK has deteriorated over the 20 years between 1983 and 2003. Certainly, changes in gingival health do not mirror the dramatic improvement in the prevalence of caries over the same period. Children's mouths tended to be cleaner in 1983 than in 1973. This trend was reversed by 1993 when

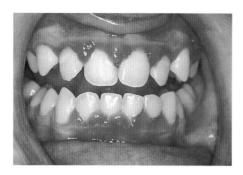

Figure 11.4 Chronic marginal gingivitis in a 10-year-old girl.

Key Points 11.6

Chronic gingivitis:

- plaque-associated
- lymphocyte-dominated
- linked to the onset of puberty
- potentially a key role in predicting future attachment and tooth loss.

10–20% more children of all ages had plaque deposits, and in 2003 this had deteriorated even further (by 5–6%) across all age groups. Levels of calculus in 8-, 12-, and 15-year-olds increased between 1993 and 2003.

The onset of puberty and the increase in circulating levels of sex hormones is one explanation for the increase in gingivitis seen in 11-year-olds. Oestrogen increases the cellularity of tissues and progesterone increases the permeability of the gingival vasculature. Oestradiol also provides suitable growth conditions for species of black pigmenting organisms which are associated with established gingivitis.

Histopathology

The inflammatory infiltrate associated with marginal gingivitis in children is analogous to that seen in adults during the early stages of gingival inflammation. The dominant cell is the lymphocyte, although small numbers of plasma cells, macrophages, and neutrophils are in evidence. There is a relative absence of plasma cells, which are found in abundance in more established and advanced lesions in adults.

Microbiology

The first organisms to colonize clean tooth surfaces are the periodontally harmless Gram-positive cocci. A more complex flora of filamentous and fusiform organisms indicates a conversion to a Gram-negative infection which, when established, comprises significant numbers of *Capnocytophaga*, *Selenomonas*, *Leptotrichia*, *Porphyromonas*, and *Spirochaete* species. These species are also cultivable from established and advanced periodontal lesions in cases of adult periodontitis.

The role of gingival inflammation

It is well established that gingivitis is a precursor of chronic periodontitis, although the role that gingival inflammation may have in predicting the development of chronic periodontitis may have been understated. There is little evidence in the literature to implicate specific bacteria in predicting when gingivitis will progress to a state of chronic attachment loss and a cause-and-effect relationship is certainly not clear. Indeed, the inflammatory lesion itself may be crucial in changing the composition of the sub-gingival microflora, a concept that is consistent with evidence from long-term epidemiological studies which shows that the severity of gingivitis rather than the presence of specific pathogens is the more reliable predictor of long-term tooth loss. (See Key Points 11.6.)

Home-based oral healthcare

The treatment and prevention of chronic plaque-induced gingivitis are dependent on achieving and maintaining a standard of plaque control which, on an individual basis, is compatible with health. Toothbrushing is the principal method of removing dental plaque.

Toothbrushing should start as soon as the first primary tooth erupts, and it is recommended that teeth are brushed twice daily with a smear or small pea-sized amount of fluoride toothpaste. Children who are younger than 3 years should have their teeth brushed by an adult using toothpaste containing no less than 1000ppm fluoride. If older than 3 years, toothpaste containing 1350–1500ppm fluoride is recommended.

Data from the Child Dental Health Survey 2003 showed that an adult carer either brushed or helped with brushing the teeth for approximately 50% of 5-year-olds and 15% of 8-year-olds. Within the group of 5-year-olds who brushed their own teeth without adult help, a significantly greater proportion had plaque compared with those children receiving adult help. It is generally recommended that toothbrushing should be supervised until the child is at least 7 years old or until their manual dexterity is sufficiently developed.

The Child Dental Health Survey 2003 also revealed that the use of powered toothbrushes was widespread (50–75% of all children reported using them). Powered toothbrushes now provide a widely available alternative to the more conventional manual toothbrushes for cleaning teeth. There is considerable evidence in the literature to suggest that powered toothbrushes are beneficial for specific groups: patients with fixed orthodontic appliances, for whom there is also evidence that powered toothbrushes are effective in reducing decalcification; children and adolescents; and children with special needs. It remains questionable whether children who are already highly motivated with respect to tooth-cleaning will benefit from using a powered toothbrush. It is possible that, particularly in children, any improved plaque control as a consequence of using a powered toothbrush may result from the 'novelty effect' of using a new toothbrush rather than because the powered toothbrush is a more effective cleaning device.

A systematic review evaluating manual and powered toothbrushes with respect to oral health has made some important conclusions. Compared with manual toothbrushes, rotating/oscillating designs of powered toothbrushes reduced plaque and gingivitis by 7–17%, although the clinical significance of this could not be determined. Therefore powered brushes are at least as effective and equally as safe as their manual counterparts with no evidence of increased incidence of soft tissue abrasions or trauma. No clinical trials have looked at the durability, reliability, and relative cost-effectiveness of powered and manual brushes, so it is not possible to make any recommendation regarding overall toothbrush superiority.

The use of dental floss by children is not widespread, although floss-holders specifically designed for children's use are available. It is recommended that flossing in young children is supervised by an adult carer, and it has been shown to be of some benefit for children with a high caries risk status. Flossing should only be introduced into a child's own

oral hygiene regime when manual dexterity is sufficiently developed. (See Key Point 11.7.)

Key Point 11.7

Effective toothbrushing alongside professional prophylaxis and scaling (if required) are the key factors aiding the maintenance of good gingival and periodontal health in children.

11.5 Drug-induced gingival enlargement

Enlargement of the gingiva is a well-recognized unwanted effect of a number of drugs. The most frequently implicated are phenytoin, ciclosporin, and nifedipine.

11.5.1 Phenytoin

Phenytoin is an anticonvulsant used in the management of epilepsy. Gingival enlargement (Fig. 11.5) occurs in about 50% of dentate subjects who are taking the drug, and is most severe in teenagers and those who are cared for in institutions. The exact mechanism by which phenytoin induces enlargement is unclear. The gingival enlargement reflects an overproduction of collagen (rather than a decrease in degradation), and this may be brought about by the action of the drug on phenotypically distinct groups of fibroblasts that have the potential to synthesize large amounts of protein. Phenytoin-induced enlargement has been associated with a deficiency of folic acid, which may lead to impaired maturation of oral epithelia.

11.5.2 Ciclosporin

Ciclosporin is an immunosuppressant drug that is used widely in organ transplant patients to prevent graft rejection. Approximately 30% of patients taking the drug demonstrate gingival enlargement, with children being more susceptible than adults. The exact mechanism of the drug in causing enlargement is unknown. There is evidence to suggest a stimulatory effect

on fibroblast proliferation and collagen production as well as an inhibitory effect on collagen breakdown by the enzyme collagenase.

11.5.3 Nifedipine

Nifedipine is a calcium-channel blocker that is used in adults for the control of cardiovascular problems. It is also given to post-transplant patients to reduce the nephrotoxic effects of ciclosporin. The incidence of gingival enlargement in dentate subjects taking nifedipine is 10–15%. The drug blocks the calcium channels in cell membranes—intracellular calcium ions are a prerequisite for the production of collagenases by fibroblasts. The lack of these enzymes could be responsible for the accumulation of collagen in the gingiva.

11.5.4 Clinical features of gingival enlargement

The clinical changes seen in drug-induced enlargement are very similar irrespective of the drug involved. The first signs of change are seen after 3–4 months of drug administration. The interdental papillae become nodular before enlarging more diffusely to encroach upon the labial tissues. The anterior part of the mouth is most severely and frequently involved, so that the patient's appearance is compromised. The tissues can become so abundant that oral functions, particularly eating and speaking, are impaired.

Enlarged gingiva is pink, firm, and stippled in subjects with a good standard of oral hygiene. When there is a pre-existing gingivitis, the enlarged tissues compromise an already poor standard of plaque control. The gingiva then exhibit the classical signs of gingivitis (Fig. 11.5).

11.5.5 Management of gingival enlargement

A strict programme of oral hygiene instruction, scaling, and polishing must be implemented. Severe cases of gingival enlargement inevitably need to be surgically excised (gingivectomy) and then recontoured (gingivoplasty) to produce an architecture that allows adequate access for cleaning.

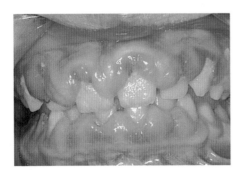

Figure 11.5 Drug-induced (phenytoin) gingival enlargement in a 12-year-old boy.

A follow-up programme is essential to ensure a high standard of plaque control and to detect any recurrence of the enlargement. As the causative drugs need to be taken on a long-term basis, recurrence is common. When a phenytoin-induced enlargement is refractory to long-term treatment, the patient's physician may be requested to modify or change the anticonvulsant therapy to drugs such as sodium valproate or carbamazepine, which do not cause gingival problems. (See Key Points 11.8.)

Key Points 11.8

Gingival enlargement:

- drug-induced
- collagen accumulation
- surgical treatment
- superimposed gingivitis.

11.6 Traumatic gingivitis (gingivitis artefacta and factitious gingivitis)

Gingivitis artefacta has minor and major variants. The minor form results from rubbing or picking the gingiva using the fingernail, or perhaps from abrasive foods such as crisps, and the habit is usually provoked by a locus of irritation such as an area of persistent food packing or an already inflamed papilla (Fig. 11.6). The lesions resolve when the habit is corrected and the source of irritation is removed.

The injuries in gingivitis artefacta major are more severe and widespread and can involve the deeper periodontal tissues (Fig. 11.7(a)). Other areas of the mouth, such as the lips and tongue may be involved, and extra-oral injuries may be found on the scalp, limbs, or face (factitious dermatitis) (Fig. 11.7(b)). The lesions are usually viewed with complete indifference by the patient who is unable to recall details of their time of onset or possible cause.

The treatment of these patients, other than the dressing and protection of oral wounds, does not lie with the dentist. Psychological reasons for inflicting the lesions may be complex and obscure. A psychological or psychiatric consultation, rarely welcomed either by older children or by their parents, is necessary if the patient is to be prevented from ultimately inflicting serious damage upon themselves. (See Key Points 11.9.)

Key Points 11.9

Gingivitis artefacta:

- minor/major
- self-inflicted
- habitual
- psychological.

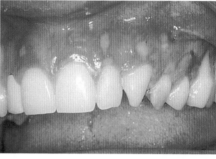

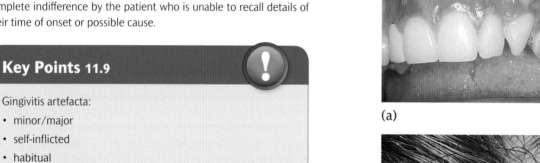

(a)

(b)

Figure 11.7 (a) Generalized self-inflicted ulceration of the attached gingiva and extensive loss of attachment around 26. (b) Ulcerative lesion at the hairline on the scalp. The lesions were produced by rubbing with a fingernail. (Reproduced from Heasman, P.A., Factitious gingival ulceration: a manifestation of Munchausen's syndrome, *Journal of Periodontology*, 1994. With permission of the American Academy of Periodontology.)

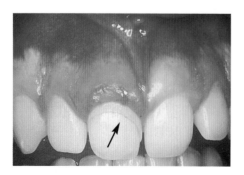

Figure 11.6 Traumatic gingival injury inflicted by the fingernail (arrowed) that has been teased from the gingival crevice of 11. (Reproduced by permission from MacMillan Publishers Ltd: *British Journal of Dentistry* © 1994.)

11.7 Mucogingival problems in children

In adults much attention has focused on whether recession is more likely to occur locally where there is a reduced width of keratinized gingiva (KG). Conversely, of course, gingival recession inevitably leads to a narrowing of the zone of KG. Therefore it is often difficult to determine unequivocally whether a narrow zone of KG is the cause or the effect of recession. A narrow or finite width of KG is compatible with gingival health, provided that the tissues are maintained free from inflammation and chronic traumatic insult. A wider zone of KG is considered more desirable to withstand gingival inflammation, trauma from mastication, toothbrushing, and forces from muscle pull.

Anterior teeth with narrow zones of KG are frequently encountered in children, as the width of KG varies greatly during the mixed dentition. For example, when permanent teeth erupt labially to their predecessors they frequently appear to erupt through alveolar mucosa with a complete absence of KG (Fig. 11.8). When the tooth has fully erupted an obvious width of KG is present.

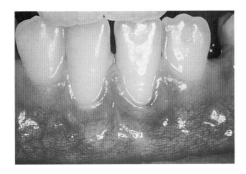

Figure 11.8 Lower central incisors that have erupted somewhat labially to the partially erupted 32 and 42. There is only a minimal width of KG buccal to 31 and 41.

The width of KG alone should not be the sole indicator of potential sites of gingival recession in children. The position of a tooth in the arch is a better guide, as studies have shown that about 80% of those permanent incisors with recession are displaced labially. Aggravating factors such as gingivitis or mechanical irritation from excessive and incorrect toothbrushing further increase the likelihood of recession.

Gingival recession is also a common periodontal complication of orthodontic therapy when labial tipping of incisors is undertaken. When roots move labially through the supporting envelope of alveolar bone the potential for recession increases.

When gingival recession occurs in children, a conservative approach to treatment should be adopted. The maximum distance from the gingival margin to the CEJ should be recorded. Over-enthusiastic toothbrushing practices should be modified and a scale and polish given if necessary. The recession must then be monitored carefully until the permanent dentition is complete. Longitudinal studies of individual cases have shown that, as the supporting tissues mature, the gingival attachment tends to creep spontaneously in a coronal direction to cover at least part of the previously denuded root surface. This cautious approach is preferred to corrective surgical intervention to increase the width of KG. (See Key Points 11.10.)

> ## Key Points 11.10
>
> Gingival recession:
> - narrow keratinized gingiva
> - local trauma
> - post orthodontics
> - conservative treatment approach.

11.8 Chronic periodontitis

A number of epidemiological studies (Table 11.2) have investigated the prevalence of chronic periodontitis in children. The variation in prevalence between studies is considerable and is attributable to different methods of diagnosing attachment loss and the use of different cut-off levels to determine disease presence. Some researchers use intra-oral radiographs to measure from the CEJ to the alveolar crest (AC), while others use a periodontal probe to determine clinically the distance from the CEJ to the base of the periodontal crevice or pocket. Radiographic studies of children with a primary or a mixed dentition indicate that loss of attachment is uncommon under the age of 9 years. However, a microscopic examination of the root surfaces of 200 extracted molars demonstrated a mean attachment loss of 0.26mm on two-thirds of the surfaces on 94% of teeth. Clinically, such small changes are insignificant and difficult to detect.

Cut-off levels at which disease is diagnosed in adolescents have been set at 1, 2, or 3mm. Larger cut-off values provide more stringent criteria for the detection of attachment loss and consequently the disease appears less prevalent. An exception to this trend was seen in a study of 602 14- to 15-year-olds in the UK: 51.5% of the subjects were diagnosed as having periodontal disease determined by a CEJ–AC distance of 3mm. Additional radiographic features were also used, namely an irregular contour of the AC and a widened coronal periodontal ligament space. Such observations may result from minor tooth movements following eruption of the second molars and consolidation of the occlusion, or from remodelling of bone after orthodontic treatment. Therefore it is likely that 51.5% is a considerable overestimate of disease prevalence in this age group. If a cut-off value of 2mm is deemed acceptable, the majority of studies put the prevalence of disease in adolescents at 1–11%. This suggests that chronic adult periodontitis begins and progresses during the early teenage years.

Table 11.2 Key studies to determine the prevalence of periodontal disease (ALOSS) in children

Study (country)	Subjects	Method of diagnosis of ALOSS	Periodontal disease prevalence	Observations
Lennon and Davis 1974 (UK)	590 15-year-olds	Probing from CEJ: ≥1mm ≥2mm	 46% 11%	Evidence of social class gradient: lower class, higher disease prevalence
Hull *et al.* 1975 (UK)	602 14-year-olds	Radiographs: CEJ–AC >3mm	51.5%	Disease also diagnosed by irregular AC and widened ligament space
Hansen *et al.* 1984 (Norway)	2409 15-year-olds	Radiographs: CEJ–AC >2mm	11%	Maxillary first molars primarily affected
Keszthelyi and Szabó 1987 (Hungary)	200 extracted primary molars	Microscopic examination of root surface	Mean ALOSS: 0.26mm on two-thirds of surfaces of 94% of teeth	More ALOSS on maxillary (than mandibular) molars and adjacent to carious tooth surfaces
Aass *et al.* 1988 (Norway)	2767 14-year-olds	Radiographs: CEJ–AC >2mm	4.5%	Previous orthodontic treatment may increase prevalence of ALOSS
Clerehugh *et al.* 1990 (UK)	167 14-year-olds	Probing from CEJ: ≥1mm ≥2mm	 3% 0%	Subgingival calculus closely correlates with future ALOSS
Bimstein *et al.* 1994 (New Zealand)	317 5-year-olds	Radiographs: CEJ–AC >2mm	2.1% Definite bone loss	Bone loss more likely with higher DMFT
Sjodin and Matsson 1994 (Sweden)	8666 7- to 9-year-olds	Radiographs: CEJ–AC >2mm	2–5%	Children with bone loss had more calculus and higher DMFS

CEJ, cemento-enamel junction; ALOSS, attachment loss; AC, alveolar crest; DMFT/S, decayed, missing, filled teeth/surfaces.

Observations made with respect to periodontal disease in children include the following:

- When loss of attachment occurs at interproximal sites, it is a consequence of pathological change and correlates closely with the presence of sub-gingival calculus.
- The prevalence of periodontal destruction correlates positively with DMF teeth or surfaces. This suggests either that carious or broken down surfaces predispose to plaque accumulation or, perhaps more likely, that periodontal disease and caries progress independently in the absence of oral healthcare.
- When the loss of attachment occurs on buccal or palatal surfaces, it is more often associated with trauma from an incorrect brushing technique than with an inflammatory response.

(See Key Points 11.11.)

Key Points 11.11

Loss of attachment:

- plaque-induced
- trauma-induced
- detected radiographically
- decayed, missing, and filled (teeth) link.

11.9 Screening for periodontal diseases in children

In the 1980s, the British Society of Periodontology introduced a policy statement for the introduction of a screening system for periodontal diseases to be used in general dental practice: the Basic Periodontal Examination (BPE). The system involves recording the single most severe code for each sextant of the dentition after probing the gingival and periodontal pockets with a 0.5mm ball-ended WHO 621 probe which has a black band between 3.5 and 5.5mm from the tip of the ball end. The codes are in the range 0–4 defined as follows:

0 Healthy gingiva with no pockets or bleeding after probing.

1 Bleeding after probing but no calculus present and the entire black band remains visible.

2 Calculus and other plaque-retentive factors such as overhanging or deficient restoration margins; bleeding after probing may also be present and the black band remains completely visible.

3 Shallow pocket with the band only partly visible above the gingival margin.

4 Deep pocket where the band disappears entirely sub-gingivally.

An asterisk was also introduced into the system to denote a sextant that has a tooth with furcation involvement or where the pocket depth and the degree of gingival recession is ≥7mm.

The codes help to inform the clinician of the treatment need in each quadrant, with plaque control measures being indicated for lower scores and sextants with higher scores requiring scaling, root surface instrumentation, and possibly referral to a specialist periodontist.

The British Society of Periodontology and British Society of Paediatric Dentistry have made some adaptations to this screening examination so that it can be used in those under 18 years of age by taking into consideration the presence of false pockets that are associated with the developing dentition and periodontium. This simplified BPE involves the following (Fig. 11.9):

- Using six index teeth—16, 11, 26, 36, 31, and 46.
- Using codes 0, 1, and 2 for children between 7 and 11 years of age as false pockets are particularly prevalent and likely to overestimate the treatment need.

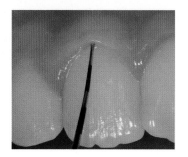

Figure 11.9 Basic Periodontal Examination of index tooth 11. The ball-tip of the screening probe is just in the gingival sulcus as the probe is being swept around the tooth. There is no sub-gingival calculus and probing causes no bleeding from the sulcus. The entire width of the 3.5–5.5mm black band is visible. This equates to code 0, indicating no need for treatment.

- Using the full range of codes for children and adolescents between 12 and 18 years. If codes 3 or 4 are found, an intra-oral radiograph may be indicated to check for bone loss.
- Using the system for patients who are under 18 years and about to undergo orthodontic treatment.

11.10 Risk factors for periodontal conditions and diseases

A risk factor can be defined as a state or occurrence that increases the probability that an individual will develop a disease. Risk factors for periodontal disease can be classified as local or general. Local factors (e.g. an instanding lateral incisor) may serve to compromise local plaque control by hindering effective cleaning and resulting in accumulation of dental plaque. On the other hand, general risk factors, such as an inherited disorder, may predispose an individual to periodontal disease despite a good level of plaque control.

It is important to understand that if a child possesses a risk factor for periodontal disease, it does not necessarily follow that he/she will develop the condition. Conversely, a patient may appear to have no risk factors, but the disease may develop subsequently. Bearing this in mind, risk factors (both local and general) should be considered when assessing, diagnosing, treating, and maintaining child patients with periodontal disease.

11.10.1 Local risk factors

These can be grouped simply into four areas. There may be overlap between these areas.

- malocclusions
- traumatic dental injuries
- plaque retentive factors

Malocclusions

An instanding or rotated tooth may be difficult to clean and can cause increased plaque retention. A traumatic occlusion may result in direct damage to the periodontal support. Angle's class II, division ii, malocclusions with increased and complete overbites may predispose to damage of the gingiva palatal to the upper incisor teeth. Similarly, severely retroclined upper incisor teeth may damage the labial gingiva of the lower teeth.

Traumatic dental injury

Luxation, intrusion, and avulsion injuries all result in varying degrees of damage to the periodontal ligament and, if severe, the alveolar bone. This results in increased tooth mobility which is managed by providing the affected teeth with a splint. If a traumatized tooth is left in a severely mobile state or in traumatic occlusion, the periodontal ligament fibres will not heal and further damage may ensue.

Plaque retentive factors

There are a multitude of plaque retentive factors which may serve to compromise the health of the periodontium. They may be naturally occurring (in the case of a dental anomaly) or iatrogenic.

Examples of dental anomalies include:

- erupted supernumerary teeth (localized malocclusion);
- invaginated odontomes;
- talon cusps;
- pitted and grooved amelogenesis imperfecta (with sensitivity);
- enamel pearls or root grooves.

Examples of iatrogenic factors include:

- orthodontic appliances;
- partial dentures;
- ledges and overhangs on poorly fitting preformed metal crowns;
- ledges and overhangs on intracoronal restorations.

11.10.2 General risk factors

General risk factors for periodontal disease may have a genetic basis, with certain inherited conditions possessing periodontal manifestations (e.g. Papillon–Lefèvre syndrome). These genetic conditions are dealt with later in this chapter. There are also metabolic, haematological, and environmental risk factors within the general category. A full discussion of each is outwith the scope of this chapter, so only the two most prevalent examples of general risk factors, diabetes mellitus and smoking, will be discussed.

Diabetes mellitus

Children with type 1 diabetes, especially when poorly controlled, are at risk of developing periodontal disease. Diabetes, like chronic periodontitis, is an inflammatory condition, and it is likely that the pathogenesis of both conditions may be linked through the following:

- Defective or altered polymorphonuclear leucocyte function (chemotaxis, phagocytosis, and adherence).
- Disruption of the host's immune and inflammatory networks, for example those regulating the cytokine interleukin 6.
- Deposition of insoluble glycosalated protein molecules of the connective tissue matrix (so-called advanced glycation end-products) which then interact with receptors on macrophages to enhance and upregulate inflammatory cytokines which cause local damage in the tissues.

The overall severity of periodontal disease may increase with duration of diabetes and there is emerging evidence from longitudinal trials to suggest that treatment of the periodontal condition may lead to improved control of the diabetes.

Tobacco smoking

Smoking is now thought to be a significant environmental risk factor for periodontal disease. Smokers have three to six times the level of periodontal disease as non-smokers, and young people are thought to be more vulnerable. The signs of disease are often masked because nicotine and other tobacco products cause vasoconstriction, reducing the blood supply to the gingivae and lowering the tendency to bleed.

There are a number of smoking-related mechanisms pertaining to smoking as a risk factor for periodontal disease. These include:

- increased prevalence of some periodontal pathogens;
- reduction in the levels of salivary IgA;
- reduction in effective phagocytosis;
- alterations in the numbers of certain T-cell populations.

If an individual stops smoking, this will allow an improved response to the management of periodontal disease, but the time taken for this 'recovery' to occur is unclear.

The underlying defect associated with general risk factors is compromised phagocytosis and/or chemotaxis. The importance of polymorphonuclear leucocyte (neutrophil) function to the host response is also demonstrated in less common conditions such as the neutropenias (see p. 215).

11.11 Periodontal complications of orthodontic treatment

Orthodontic treatment in adolescents, particularly with fixed appliances, can predispose to a deterioration in periodontal health and a number of well-recognized complications.

11.11.1 Gingivitis

Access for interproximal toothbrushing is reduced considerably during fixed appliance therapy, and the accumulation of plaque induces gingivitis (Fig. 11.10). The problem is compounded when teeth are banded rather than bonded as periodontal health is more easily maintained when the gingival sulcus is not encroached upon by metal bands.

When supra-gingival plaque deposits are present on teeth that are being repositioned orthodontically, the type of movement used may play an important part in the development of periodontal problems. Supra-gingival plaque deposits are shifted into a sub-gingival location by tipping movements. Conversely, bodily movements are less likely to induce a relocation of supra-gingival plaque.

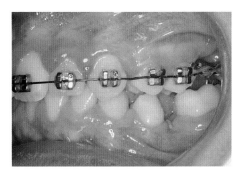

Figure 11.10 Chronic marginal gingivitis associated with fixed appliance therapy.

11.11.2 Gingival enlargement

The anterior palatal gingiva and mucosa have a propensity for enlargement when tissues are 'rolled up' between incisors that are being retracted and the fixed anterior margin of the acrylic plate of a removable appliance (Fig. 11.11). These changes may resolve when appliances are removed, but surgical elimination of the enlarged tissues may be indicated.

11.11.3 Attachment and bone loss

The mean annual rate of coronal attachment loss during appliance therapy ranges from 0.05 to 0.30mm, which compares favourably with the mean annual attachment loss in untreated populations. A well-recognized complication of orthodontic tooth movement is apical root resorption, particularly when excessive forces are used (Fig. 11.12). Such changes must also be regarded as loss of attachment, albeit at an apical rather than a coronal site.

11.11.4 Gingival recession

The response of the facial periodontal tissues to labial tooth movement in anterior segments is unpredictable. Labial movement of incisors is sometimes associated with gingival recession. The risk of recession is greater when the alveolar bone plate is thin or where there are dehiscences or fenestrations in the bone.

11.11.5 Trauma

Direct local irritation of the soft tissues by components of a fixed appliance can be minimized if due care and attention is exercised during bonding, banding, and placement of wires and elastics. If chronic irritation of the gingiva does occur, a localized acute inflammatory reaction will quickly follow. This may develop further into a region of gingival enlargement or a fibrous epulis that is superimposed upon a burrowing infra-bony lesion. (See Key Points 11.12.)

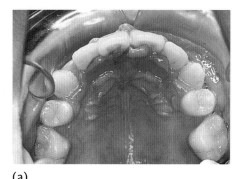

(a)

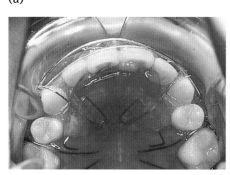

(b)

Figure 11.11 (a) Gingival enlargement on the palatal aspect of retracted maxillary incisors. (b) Appliance *in situ*. (Reproduced by kind permission of Mr N.E. Carter.)

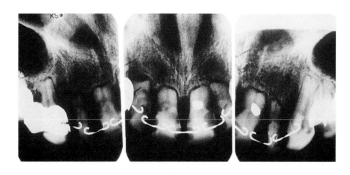

Figure 11.12 Apical root resorption of 13–23 following orthodontic treatment. (Reproduced by kind permission of Professor I.L. Chapple, Birmingham, UK.)

> **Key Points 11.12**
>
> Orthodontic problems:
> - gingivitis
> - enlargement
> - root resorption
> - gingival trauma.

11.12 Aggressive periodontal diseases

Aggressive periodontal diseases comprise a group of rare, but rapidly progressing, infections that affect the primary and permanent dentitions. The disorders are associated with a more specific microbial challenge and an inherent defect in the host's immunological response. The nature of these diseases can lead to premature tooth loss at an early age. Prompt diagnosis is essential if treatment is to be successful, and the periodontal status must be monitored regularly to ensure that the treated disease remains quiescent.

Aggressive periodontal diseases were previously known as early-onset diseases, namely prepubertal and juvenile periodontitis. A classification system for periodontal diseases and conditions published in 1999 effectively combined these two diseases into one—aggressive periodontitis (see Further reading). This classification, which is used in this chapter, removed the arbitrary age limitations that were previously implied by terms such as prepubertal, juvenile, and even adult periodontitis. It is now recognized that aggressive periodontitis can affect the primary and permanent dentitions in both localized and generalized forms.

11.12.1 Primary dentition

The disease may present immediately after the teeth have erupted. In the generalized form the gingiva appear fiery red, swollen, and haemorrhagic. The tissues become hyperplastic with granular or nodular proliferations that precede gingival clefting and extensive areas of recession. Gross deposits of plaque are inevitable as the soft tissue changes make it difficult to maintain oral hygiene. The disease progresses extremely rapidly, with primary tooth loss occurring as early as 3–4 years of age. However, the entire dentition may not be affected as the bone loss may be restricted to one arch. Children with generalized disease are susceptible to recurrent general infections, principally otitis media and upper respiratory tract infections.

Localized disease progresses more slowly than the generalized form, and bone loss characteristically affects only incisor and molar teeth. Plaque levels are usually low; consequently soft tissue changes are minimal with gingivitis and proliferation involving only the marginal tissues.

The predominant micro-organisms that have been identified are aggressive periodontopathogens: *Aggregatibacter* (previously *Actinobacillus*) *actinomycetemcomitans*, *Porphyromonas gingivalis*, *Fusobacterium nucleatum*, and *Eikenella corrodens*. This suggests that there is an infective component to the disease, although defects in the host's response have also been identified. Profound abnormalities in chemotaxis and phagocytosis of polymorphonuclear neutrophils and monocytes are frequently reported in these patients. These immunological defects are heritable risk factors that help to define the disease entity phenotypically. Conversely, they may also be associated with more serious and life-threatening conditions, and thus a full medical screen is indicated.

Oral hygiene instruction, scaling, and root surface instrumentation should be undertaken. Bacterial culturing of the pocket flora identifies specific periodontopathogens. If pathogens persist after oral debridement, an antibiotic such as metronidazole or amoxicillin should be given systemically (after sensitivity testing) as a short course over 1–2 weeks. Generalized disease responds poorly to treatment. Extraction of involved teeth has produced some improvement in neutrophil chemotaxis, which suggests that the defect may be induced by certain organisms in the periodontal flora. Furthermore, in severe cases of generalized periodontitis, extraction of all primary teeth (and the provision of a removable prosthesis) can limit the disease to the primary dentition. Presumably, anaerobic pathogens are unable to thrive in the absence of teeth. When the permanent teeth erupt, bacterial culturing of the sub-gingival flora ensures that re-infection is detected early. (See Key Points 11.13.)

> ### Key Points 11.13
>
> Primary dentition:
> - localized/generalized
> - aggressive pathogens
> - intense treatment.

11.12.2 Permanent dentition

In the permanent dentition, aggressive periodontitis involves severe periodontal destruction with an onset around puberty. The localized form occurs in otherwise healthy individuals, with destruction classically localized around the first permanent molars and incisors, and not involving more than two other teeth. Generalized periodontitis also occurs in otherwise healthy individuals but involves more than 14 teeth, i.e. generalized to an arch or the entire dentition. Some reports have monitored children suffering from aggressive periodontitis of the primary dentition and found that, at around puberty, the disease became generalized to involve the entire dentition.

Epidemiology

Studies show a prevalence of about 0.1% in developed countries and about 5% in underdeveloped nations, although some variation may be due to different methods of screening and different criteria used to define the disease. The disease is clearly more prevalent in certain ethnic groups. In the UK, an epidemiological study of 7266 schoolchildren in Coventry and Birmingham showed an overall prevalence of 0.02% in Caucasians, 0.2% in Asians, and 0.8% in the African Caribbean population. There was no difference in prevalence between males and females, which does not concur with the data from many earlier epidemiological studies of the disease which reported a female to male ratio of 3:1.

Clinical and radiographic features

The age of onset is between 11 and 15 years. The clinical features are pocket formation and loss of attachment associated with the permanent incisors and first molar teeth. The radiographic pattern of bone loss

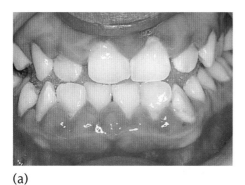

(a)

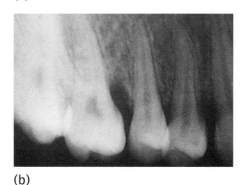

(b)

Figure 11.13 (a) Clinical appearance of a 13-year-old girl with localized aggressive periodontitis. (b) Radiographic appearance of vertical bone loss on the mesial aspect of 16. (Reproduced by kind permission of Mr D.G. Smith, Consultant in Restorative Dentistry, Newcastle upon Tyne.)

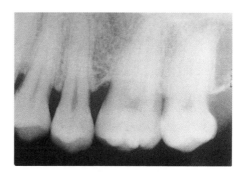

Figure 11.14 Radiographic view of 27 that has erupted and tipped mesially into the 16 extraction site. The contour of the bone crest on the mesial of 27 gives the impression of a vertical bony defect.

to the mouth during a sporting activity, causes unexpected loosening of teeth.

Bacteriology and pathogenesis

The sub-gingival microflora comprises loosely adherent Gram-negative anaerobes including *Eikenella corrodens*, *Capnocytophaga* species, and *Prevotella intermedia*. The most frequently implicated organism is *A. actinomycetemcomitans*, which has been found in over 90% of patients. Sufferers also have raised IgG titres to *A. actinomycetemcomitans*, but levels of bacteria fall significantly following successful treatment of the condition. (See Key Points 11.14.)

Key Points 11.14

Permanent dentition:

- onset around puberty
- localized/generalized
- *Aggregatibacter actinomycetemcomitans*
- neutrophil chemotaxis defect.

is quite distinctive. Bilateral angular bone defects are identified on the mesial and/or distal surfaces of molars (Fig. 11.13). Angular defects are sometimes seen around the incisors, although the very thin interproximal bone is resorbed more evenly to give a horizontal pattern of resorption. The bone loss around the molars can be detected on bitewing radiographs. However, the films must be interpreted with a sound knowledge of the patient's dental history, as localized angular defects are found adjacent to teeth with overhanging or deficient interproximal restorations and teeth that have tilted slightly (Fig. 11.14). The gingiva can appear healthy when the levels of plaque are low, but a marginal gingivitis will be present if a good standard of plaque control is not evident.

The generalized form may also present at puberty. Severe generalized bone loss is the characteristic feature (Fig. 11.15). The pattern may be a combination of angular and horizontal resorption, producing an irregular alveolar crest. When patients have good plaque control, the degree of bone resorption is not commensurate with the level of oral hygiene. The more generalized nature of the disease predisposes to multiple and recurrent abscess formation, which is a common presenting feature.

Invariably, one of the presenting signs is tooth migration or drifting of incisors. Tooth movement is not necessarily a consequence of advanced disease as drifting may occur when only a fraction of a tooth's periodontal support is lost. Conversely, extensive bone loss can occur with no spontaneous movement of teeth, and the subject may only be alerted to the problem when a minor traumatic episode, such as a blow

The extreme pathogenicity of *A. actinomycetemcomitans* is due to its ability to invade connective tissues and the wide range of virulence factors that it produces. These include a potent lipopolysaccharide that induces bone resorption, collagenase, an epitheliotoxin, a fibroblast-inhibiting factor, and a leucotoxin that kills neutrophils and so dampens the host's first line of defence against bacterial challenge.

About 70% of patients have defects in neutrophil chemotaxis and phagocytosis. The chemotactic defect is linked to reduced amounts of cell-surface glycoproteins and is transmitted as a dominant trait. About 50% of siblings of patients who have both aggressive periodontitis and chemotactic defects also demonstrate impaired neutrophil function.

Treatment

A combined regimen of regular scaling and root surface instrumentation with a 2-week course of systemic tetracycline therapy (250mg, four

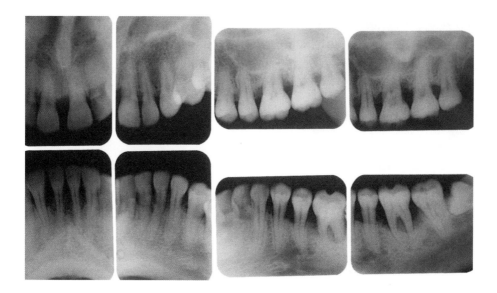

Figure 11.15 Aggressive periodontitis with generalized bone loss in a 16-year-old male.

times daily) has been used extensively in the management of this condition. *A. actinomycetemcomitans* is sensitive to tetracycline, which also has the ability to be concentrated up to 10 times in gingival crevicular fluid when compared with serum. A combination of metronidazole (250mg) and amoxicillin (375mg) three times daily for a week, in association with sub-gingival scaling, has also been found to be effective.

A more radical approach is to undertake flap surgery so that better access is achieved for root surface instrumentation and the superficial infected connective tissues are excised. An antimicrobial regimen can also be implemented in conjunction with a surgical approach. (See Key Points 11.15.)

> ### Key Points 11.15
>
> Permanent dentition (juvenile periodontitis)—treatment:
> - plaque control
> - mechanical debridement
> - systemic antimicrobials
> - periodontal surgery.

11.12.3 Genetic factors and aggressive diseases

The increased prevalence of aggressive periodontitis in certain ethnic groups and within families strongly suggests that susceptibility to these diseases may be influenced by a number of genetic determinants. Furthermore, genetic factors are implicated in the pathogenesis of the diseases as many affected patients have functionally defective neutrophils.

The mode of transmission has not been determined unequivocally. The apparent increased incidence in females suggests an X-linked dominant mode of inheritance with reduced penetrance. However, the association with females may reflect epidemiological bias as females are more likely to seek dental attention. Large family studies of subjects with aggressive periodontitis suggest an autosomal-recessive pattern of inheritance.

The role of hereditary components in periodontal diseases has been supported by the link with specific tissue markers. The major histocompatibility complex (MHC) determines the susceptibility of subjects to certain diseases. Class I and II genes in the MHC encode for specific human leucocyte antigens (HLA I and HLA II), which account for individual variation in immunoresponsiveness. There are clear associations between HLA serotypes and diabetes mellitus and rheumatoid arthritis. A strong link between an HLA serotype and aggressive diseases has still to be determined, although a mild association between the HLA-A9 antigen and aggressive periodontitis has been found. (See Key Points 11.16.)

> ### Key Points 11.16
>
> Genetic components of periodontitis:
> - family associations
> - ethnic associations
> - major histocompatibility complex link
> - link with syndromes.

11.13 Periodontitis as a manifestation of systemic disease

The genetic basis for aggressive periodontitis in particular is substantiated by the definite association between the condition and a number of rare inherited medical conditions and syndromes (see Table 11.1). The pattern of inheritance reflects a single-gene disorder, commonly involving inherited defects of neutrophils, enzyme reactions, or collagen synthesis.

11.13.1 Papillon–Lefèvre syndrome (PLS)

This syndrome is characterized by palmar–plantar hyperkeratosis, premature loss of primary and permanent dentitions, and ectopic calcifications of the falx cerebri. Some patients show an increased susceptibility to infection. The syndrome is an autosomal recessive trait with a prevalence of about 1–4 per million of the population. Consanguinity of parents is evident in about one-third of cases.

Rapid and progressive periodontal destruction affects the primary dentition with an onset at about 2 years (Fig. 11.16). Exfoliation of all primary teeth is usual before the permanent successors erupt, and patients may be edentulous by the mid to late teens. Cases of a late-onset variant of PLS have also been described in which the palmar–plantar and periodontal lesions are relatively mild and only become evident in the permanent dentition. An extensive family dental history supported by clinical, laboratory, and radiographic examinations confirms the diagnosis.

11.13.2 Neutropenias

The neutropenias comprise a heterogeneous group of blood disorders which are characterized by a periodic or persistent reduction in the number of circulating polymorphonuclear neutrophils. Neutropenias can be drug-induced or be secondary to severe bacterial or viral infections or autoimmune diseases such as lupus erythematosus. Cyclic neutropenia, benign familial neutropenias, and severe familial neutropenias are all heritable conditions transmitted as autosomal dominant traits, and diagnoses are often made during early childhood. The chronic benign neutropenia of childhood is diagnosed between 6 and 24 months of age and is characterized by frequent and multiple pyogenic infections of the skin and mucous membranes.

The periodontal problems associated with the neutropenias are very similar, and in many cases the patient presents with a localized or generalized aggressive periodontitis. Occasionally, the primary dentition may not be involved, and clinical signs do not appear until the permanent dentition has erupted. The gingiva are inflamed and oedematous; gingival recession, ulceration, and desquamation can also occur.

The treatment of a neutropenic-induced periodontitis involves local removal of plaque and calculus. Strict plaque control measures are difficult to achieve in younger children, so use of an antibacterial mouth rinse may prove useful.

11.13.3 Chediak–Higashi syndrome

This is a rare and very often fatal disease inherited as an autosomal recessive trait. Clinical features include partial albinism, photophobia, and nystagmus. The patients suffer from recurrent pyogenic infections and malignant lymphoma, which is accompanied by neutropenia, anaemia, and a thrombocytopenia. The neutrophils show defects in migration, chemotaxis, and phagocytosis, producing a diminished bactericidal capacity.

Periodontal changes associated with the syndrome include severe gingival inflammation and rapid and extensive alveolar bone resorption that can lead to premature exfoliation. The nature of the changes has not been fully established, but they may be plaque induced, secondary to infection, or related to the underlying defect in neutrophil function.

11.13.4 Leucocyte adhesion deficiency syndrome (LAD)

This autosomal recessive trait is characterized clinically by a delayed separation of the umbilical cord, severe recurrent bacterial infections, impaired wound healing, formation of pus, and an aggressive gingivitis, which may be the presenting sign of the disorder. Consanguinity

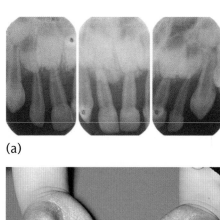

(a)

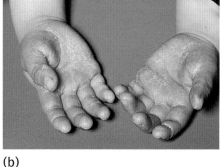

(b)

Figure 11.16 Papillon–Lefèvre syndrome in a 3-year-old boy: (a) radiographic appearance showing almost total bone loss around maxillary anterior teeth; (b) hyperkeratosis of the palms of the hand.

between the parents of affected children confirms the mode of the inheritance as autosomal recessive.

The syndrome demonstrates the important role of leucocytes (and other white blood cells) in protecting the host against periodontal disease. However, moderate phenotypes may appear relatively disease free, but then develop symptoms and progress 'downhill' extremely rapidly. The majority of patients do not survive beyond 30 years. The progressive periodontal condition is very difficult to control and is often of secondary importance to other life-threatening infections.

11.13.5 Ehlers–Danlos syndrome

The syndrome is an autosomal dominant trait with nine variants that display defects in the synthesis, secretion, or polymerization of collagen. The variants of the syndrome exhibit extensive clinical heterogeneity and collectively represent the most common of the heritable disorders of connective tissues. The clinical findings are principally excessive joint mobility, skin hyperextensibility, and susceptibility to scarring and bruising of the skin and oral mucous membranes (Fig. 11.17). Defective type IV collagen supporting the walls of small blood vessels predisposes to persistent post-extraction haemorrhage.

Gingival tissues are fragile and have a tendency to bleed on toothbrushing. The type VIII syndrome is associated with advanced periodontal disease. Periodontitis has also been linked with the type IV variant, although other variants do not appear to be affected. Ultrastructural changes also occur in the teeth, with abnormalities of the amelodentinal junction, vascular inclusions in dentine, fibrous degeneration of the pulp, and disorganization of cementum.

Type VIII patients require a thorough preventive periodontal programme as root debridement can cause extensive trauma to the fragile soft tissues. Periodontal surgery should be avoided because of the risk of haemorrhage and the potential problems encountered with suturing soft tissue flaps.

11.13.6 Langerhans' cell histiocytosis (LCH)

Langerhans' cell histiocytosis (LCH) is a non-malignant granulomatous childhood disorder that is characterized pathologically by uncontrolled proliferation and accumulation of Langerhans' cells mixed with varying proportions of eosinophils and multinucleated giant cells. LCH replaced the term 'histiocytosis X' and the closely related syndromes eosinophilic granuloma, Hand–Schuller–Christian disease, and Letterer–Siwe disease. The clinical hallmark of LCH is the presence of lytic bone lesions that may be single or multiple. When lesions are widespread, they can affect the pituitary gland and retro-orbital region, thus causing diabetes insipidus and exophthalmos, respectively. The disseminated form of LCH is extremely aggressive and has a poor prognosis. It is often diagnosed in the first 6 months of life before becoming widespread by about 3 years of age.

The periodontal manifestations of LCH, which include a marginal gingivitis, bleeding gingiva, abscess formation, pain, and drifting and mobility of the teeth, may be the presenting signs. Radiographs show localized or generalized bone loss, characteristic osteolytic lesions, and 'floating teeth' with no alveolar bone support (Fig. 11.18).

A biopsy will confirm the diagnosis and full radiographic screening determines the severity of the syndrome. Local lesions that are confined to bone respond well to curettage and excision. The mortality rate increases in the more widely disseminated forms of the syndrome and when overlying soft tissues are involved. Treatment is by radiotherapy and chemotherapy.

11.13.7 Hypophosphatasia

Hypophosphatasia is a rare inborn error of metabolism characterized by defective bone mineralization, a deficiency of alkaline phosphatase (ALP) activity, and an increased excretion of phosphoethanolamine in the urine. ALP plays a major part in the mineralization of hard tissues, and so the absence of the enzyme predisposes to a range of bone and cartilage defects. The condition is an autosomal recessive trait, although

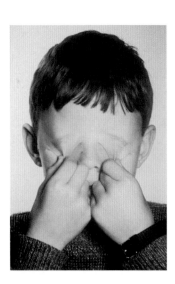

Figure 11.17 Cutaneous hyperextensibility of the upper eyelids in a 9-year-old child with Ehlers–Danlos syndrome.

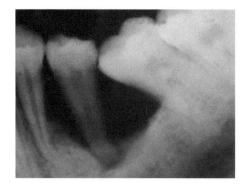

Figure 11.18 Extensive bone loss around the mandibular left premolars in a 15-year-old child with Langerhans' cell histiocytosis. (Reproduced by kind permission of Professor I.L. Chapple, Birmingham, UK.)

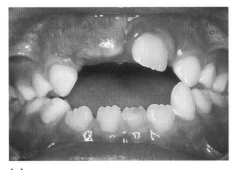

(a)

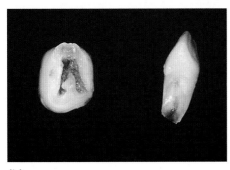

(b)

Figure 11.19 (a) Premature loss of upper primary incisors in a 3-year-old child with hypophosphatasia. The 21 and the lower permanent incisors have already erupted. (b) Extensive root resorption led to exfoliation of primary teeth at 4 years of age. (Reproduced by kind permission of Professor I.L. Chapple, Birmingham, UK.)

the inheritance pattern of some milder forms of hypophosphatasia may be autosomal dominant.

The lesions of juvenile or childhood hypophosphatasia become apparent before 2 years of age. Bone defects are usually quite mild, with bowing of the legs, proptosis, and wide-open fontanelles being prominent signs. Dental features are resorption of alveolar bone (in the absence of marked gingivitis), premature exfoliation of anterior primary teeth, hypoplasia or complete absence of cementum, and the presence of 'small teeth' that have enlarged pulp chambers as a consequence of defective mineralization (Fig. 11.19). The aplastic or hypoplastic cementum and weakened periodontal attachment is thought to render the patients susceptible to infection with periodontopathogens.

The diagnosis of hypophosphatasia is confirmed biochemically by low activity of serum ALP and a raised level of phosphoethanolamine in a 24-hour urine sample. (See Key Points 11.17.)

Key Points 11.17

Systemic diseases:

- very rare
- autosomal mode of inheritance
- aggressive periodontal destruction.

11.13.8 Down syndrome

Children with Down syndrome (trisomy 21) do not suffer aggressive periodontal disease. However, a significant number of local and general risk factors may exist as a result of the syndrome. Local factors that may serve to increase dental plaque retention are:

- Angle's class III malocclusions with crowding;
- lack of an anterior lip seal;
- anterior open bites.

General risk factors for periodontal disease are mainly centred on leucocyte defects and may include:

- defects of polymorphonuclear leucocyte function (chemotaxis, killing, and phagocytosis);
- reduced T-cell activity.

11.14 Summary

1. Anatomical variation, which occurs during tooth eruption, and the maturation of the periodontal tissues can mimic signs of gingivitis, recession, and bone loss.

2. Herpetic gingivostomatitis is most frequently seen in children under 5 years of age, whereas necrotizing ulcerative gingivitis is more prevalent in young adults.

3. Although the prevalence of dental caries has declined in the UK and other European countries, the prevalence of plaque-induced gingivitis in children has not reduced over the last 20 years.

4. Chronic gingivitis in children is highly prevalent and is an established precursor of chronic periodontitis.

5. Gingival changes can also occur in children who are prescribed drugs to control epilepsy or following transplant surgery, during orthodontic therapy, and at sites of self-inflicted trauma.

6. Early signs of chronic periodontitis are sometimes seen during adolescence, and targeting this age group with a primary prevention strategy may help to reduce tooth loss in later life.

7. Extreme vigilance is necessary to diagnose aggressive periodontal diseases and those periodontal conditions that may be associated with systemic disease. Bleeding after gentle probing in the presence of apparently healthy gingiva indicates the need for further investigation.

11.15 Further reading

Armitage, G.C. (1999). Development of a classification system for periodontal diseases and conditions. *Annals of Periodontology*, **4**, 1–6.

Clerehugh, V. (2008). Periodontal diseases in children and adolescents. *British Dental Journal*, **204**, 469–71.

Oh, T.-J., Eber, R., and Wang, H.-L. (2002). Periodontal diseases in the child and adolescent. *Journal of Clinical Periodontology*, **29**, 400–10.

Preshaw, P.M. (2008). Diabetes and periodontal disease. *International Dental Journal*, **58**, 237–43.

Robinson, P.G., Deacon, S.A., Deery, C., *et al.* (2005). Manual versus powered tooth brushing for oral health. *Cochrane Database of Systematic Reviews (Issue 2)*. Wiley, Chichester.

Sabiston, C.B., Jr (1986). A review and proposal for the etiology of acute necrotising gingivitis. *Journal of Clinical Periodontology*, **13**, 727–34. (*An overview of the epidemiology of NUG with an emphasis on a viral rather than a bacterial aetiology.*)

Van Dyke, T. (2011) Proresolving lipid mediators: potential for prevention and treatment of periodontitis. *Journal of Clinical Periodontology*, **38**, 119–25.

White, D. and Lader, D. (2004). *Periodontal condition, hygiene behaviour and attitudes to oral health. Children's Dental Health in the United Kingdom, 2003.* Office of National Statistics, London. (*Data relating to oral hygiene and gingival health from the Children's Dental Health Survey 2003.*)

11.16 References

Aass, A.M., Alabandar, J., Aasenden, R., Tollefsen, T., and Gjermo, P. (1988). Variation in prevalence of radiographic alveolar bone loss in subgroups of 14-year-old schoolchildren in Oslo. *Journal of Clinical Periodontology*, **15**, 130–3.

Bimstein, E., Treasure, E.T., Williams, S.M., and Dever, J.G. (1994). Alveolar bone loss in 5-year-old New Zealand children: its prevalence and relationship to caries prevalence, socio-economic status and ethnic origin. *Journal of Clinical Periodontology*, **21**, 447–50.

Clerehugh, V., Lennon, M.A., and Worthington, H.V. (1990). 5-year results of a longitudinal study of early periodontitis in 14- to 19-year-old adolescents. *Journal of Clinical Periodontology*, **17**, 702–8.

Hansen, B.F., Gjermo, P., and Bergwitz-Larsen, K.R. (1984). Periodontal bone loss in 15-year-old Norwegians. *Journal of Clinical Periodontology*, **11**, 125–31.

Heasman, P.A. (1994). Factitious gingival ulceration: a manifestation of Munchausen's syndrome. *Journal of Periodontology*, **65**, 442–7

Hull, P.S., Hillam, D.G., and Beal, J.F. (1975). A radiographic study of the prevalence of chronic periodontitis in 14-year-old English schoolchildren. *Journal of Clinical Periodontology*, **2**, 203–10.

Keszthelyi, G. and Szabó, I. (1987). Attachment loss in primary molars. *Journal of Clinical Periodontology*, **14**, 48–51.

Lennon, M.A. and Davies, R.M. (1974). Prevalence and distribution of alveolar bone loss in a population of 15-year-old schoolchildren. *Journal of Clinical Periodontology*, **1**, 175–82.

Sjodin, B. and Matsson, L. (1994). Marginal bone loss in the primary dentition. A survey of 7–9-year-old children in Sweden. *Journal of Clinical Periodontology*, **21**, 313–19.

12
Traumatic injuries to the teeth

R. Welbury, J.M. Whitworth, and M.S. Duggal

Chapter contents

12.1 Epidemiology

Dental trauma in childhood and adolescence is common (Fig. 12.1). At 5 years of age 31–40% of boys and 16–30% of girls, and at 12 years of age 12–33% of boys and 4–19% of girls, will have suffered some dental trauma. Boys are affected almost twice as often as girls in both the primary and the permanent dentitions.

The majority of dental injuries in the primary and permanent dentitions involve the anterior teeth, especially the maxillary central incisors. Concussion, subluxation, and luxation are the most common injuries in the primary dentition (Fig. 12.2), while uncomplicated crown fractures are most common in the permanent dentition (Fig. 12.3).

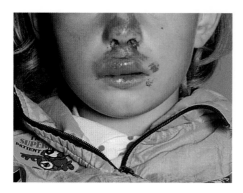

Figure 12.1 A 7-year-old girl who fell off her bicycle and sustained orofacial injuries.

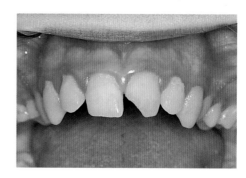

Figure 12.3 A fracture of the upper left central incisor involving enamel and dentine.

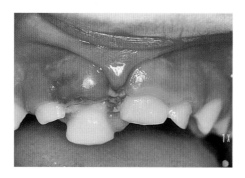

Figure 12.2 A 3-year-old child with a combination of injuries to her upper anterior teeth.

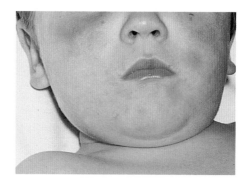

Figure 12.4 A 3-year-old boy with bruises and abrasions resulting from non-accidental injury.

Prognosis of traumatic injuries has improved significantly in the last 20 years. This has been largely due to a greater understanding and knowledge of pulpal procedures.

12.2 Aetiology

Children are most accident prone between 2 and 4 years for the primary dentition and between 7 and 10 years for the permanent dentition. Coordination and judgement are incompletely developed in children with primary dentition, and the majority of injuries are due to falls in and around the home as the child becomes more adventurous and explores his/her surroundings. In the permanent dentition most injuries are caused by falls and collisions while playing and running, although bicycles are a common accessory. The place of injury varies in different countries according to local customs, but accidents in the school playground remain common. Sports injuries usually occur in the teenage years and are commonly associated with contact sports. Injuries due to road traffic accidents and assaults are most commonly associated with the late teenage years and adulthood, and are often closely related to alcohol abuse.

One form of injury in childhood that must never be forgotten is child physical abuse or non-accidental injury (NAI). More than 50% of these children will have orofacial injuries (Fig. 12.4). See also Chapter 18.

Accidental injuries can be the result of either direct or indirect trauma. Direct trauma occurs when the tooth itself is struck. Indirect trauma is seen when the lower dental arch is forcefully closed against the upper, for example by a blow to the chin. Direct trauma implies injuries to the anterior region, while indirect trauma favours crown or crown–root fractures in the premolar and molar regions as well as the possibility of jaw fractures in the condylar regions and symphysis. The factors that influence the outcome or type of injury are a combination of energy impact, the resilience of the impacting object, the shape of the impacting object, and the angle of direction of the impacting force.

Increased overjet with protrusion of upper incisors and insufficient lip closure are significant predisposing factors to traumatic dental injuries. Injuries are almost twice as frequent among children with protruding incisors, and the number of teeth affected in a particular incident for an individual patient also increase.

12.3 Classification

The classification of dento-alveolar injuries based on the World Health Organization (WHO) system is summarized in Table 12.1.

Table 12.1 Classification of the nature of dento-alveolar injuries based upon World Health Organization (WHO) System.

Type of injury	Description of injury
Injuries to hard dental tissues and pulp	
Enamel infraction	Incomplete fracture (crack) of enamel without loss of tooth substance
Enamel fracture	Loss of tooth substance confined to enamel
Enamel–dentine fracture	Loss of tooth substance confined to enamel and dentine not involving the pulp
Complicated crown fracture	Fracture of enamel and dentine exposing the pulp
Uncomplicated crown–root fracture	Fracture of enamel, dentine, and cementum but not involving the pulp
Complicated crown–root fracture	Fracture of enamel, dentine, and cementum exposing the pulp
Root fracture	Fracture involving dentine, cementum, and pulp
	Can be subclassified into apical, middle, and coronal (gingival) thirds
Injuries to the periodontal tissues	
Concussion	No abnormal loosening or displacement but marked reaction to percussion
Subluxation (loosening)	Abnormal loosening but no displacement
Extrusive luxation (partial avulsion)	Partial displacement of tooth from socket
Lateral luxation	Displacement other than axially with comminution or fracture of alveolar socket
Intrusive luxation	Displacement into alveolar bone with comminution or fracture of alveolar socket
Avulsion	Complete displacement of tooth from socket
Injuries to supporting bone	
Comminution of mandibular or maxillary alveolar socket wall	Crushing and compression of alveolar socket
	Found in intrusive and lateral luxation injuries
Fracture of mandibular or maxillary alveolar socket wall	Fracture confined to facial or lingual/palatal socket wall
Fracture of mandibular or maxillary alveolar process	Fracture of the alveolar process which may or may not involve the tooth sockets
Fracture of mandible or maxilla	May or may not involve the alveolar socket
Injuries to gingiva or oral mucosa	
Laceration of gingiva or oral mucosa	Wound in the mucosa resulting from a tear
Contusion of gingiva or oral mucosa	Bruise not accompanied by a break in the mucosa
	Usually causes submucosal haemorrhage
Abrasion of gingiva or oral mucosa	Superficial wound produced by rubbing or scraping the mucosal surface

12.4 History and examination

A history of the injury followed by a thorough examination should be completed in any situation.

12.4.1 Dental history

1. When did injury occur? The time interval between injury and treatment significantly influences the prognosis of avulsions, luxations, crown fractures with or without pulpal exposures, and dento-alveolar fractures.

2. Where did injury occur? This may indicate the need for tetanus prophylaxis.

3. How did injury occur? The nature of the accident can yield information on the type of injury expected. Discrepancy between history and clinical findings raises suspicion of physical abuse.

4. Lost teeth/fragments? If a tooth or fractured piece cannot be accounted for when there has been a history of loss of consciousness, a chest radiograph should be obtained to exclude inhalation.

5. Concussion, headache, vomiting, or amnesia? Brain damage must be excluded and referral to a hospital for further investigation organized.

6. Previous dental history? Previous trauma can affect pulpal sensibility tests and the recuperative capacity of the pulp and/or periodontium. Alternatively, are there suspicions of physical abuse? Previous treatment experience, age, and parental/child attitude will affect the choice of treatment.

12.4.2 Medical history

1. Congenital heart disease, a history of rheumatic fever, or severe immunosuppression? These may be contraindications to any procedure that is likely to require prolonged endodontic treatment with a persistent necrotic/infected focus. Not all congenital heart defects carry the same risks of bacterial endocarditis, and the child's paediatrician/cardiologist should be consulted before a decision regarding endodontic treatment is made.

2. Bleeding disorders? Very important if soft tissues are lacerated or teeth are to be extracted.

3. Allergies? Penicillin allergy requires alternative antibiotics.

4. Tetanus immunization status? Referral for tetanus toxoid injection is necessary if there is soil contamination of the wound and the child has not had a 'booster' injection within the last 5 years.

12.4.3 Extra-oral examination

When there are associated severe injuries a general examination is made with respect to signs of shock (pallor, cold skin, irregular pulse, hypotension), symptoms of head injury suggesting brain concussion, or maxillofacial fractures.

Facial swelling, bruises, or lacerations may indicate underlying bony and tooth injury. Lacerations will require careful debridement to remove all foreign material and suturing. Antibiotics and/or tetanus toxoid may be required if wounds are contaminated. Limitation of mandibular movement or mandibular deviation on opening or closing the mouth indicate either jaw fracture or dislocation.

Crown fracture with associated swollen lip and evidence of a penetrating wound suggests retention of tooth fragments within the lip. Clinical and radiographic examinations should be undertaken (Fig. 12.5).

12.4.4 Intra-oral examination

This must be systematic and the following should be recorded:

1. Laceration, haemorrhage, and swelling of the oral mucosa and gingiva (Fig. 12.6). Any lacerations should be examined for tooth fragments or other foreign material. Lacerations of lips or tongue require suturing, but those of the oral mucosa heal very quickly and may not need suturing.

2. Abnormalities of occlusion, tooth displacement, fractured crowns, or cracks in the enamel.

The following signs and reactions to tests are particularly helpful:

1. *Mobility*. Degree of mobility is estimated in a horizontal and a vertical direction. When several teeth move together *en bloc*, a fracture of the alveolar process is suspected. Excessive mobility may also suggest root fracture or tooth displacement.

2. *Reaction to percussion* in a horizontal and vertical direction compared with a contralateral uninjured tooth. A duller note may indicate root fracture.

3. *Colour of tooth*. Early colour change associated with pulp breakdown is visible on the palatal surface of the gingival third of the crown.

4. *Reaction to sensitivity tests*. Thermal tests with warm gutta percha (GP) or ethyl chloride (EC) are widely used. However, an electric pulp tester (EPT) in the hands of an experienced operator is more reliable. Nevertheless, sensitivity testing is notoriously unreliable, especially in children, and should never be assessed in isolation from the other clinical and radiographic information. Neither negative nor positive responses immediately after trauma should be trusted. A positive response does not rule out later pulpal necrosis, and a negative response, while indicating pulpal damage, does not necessarily indicate a necrotic pulp. The negative reaction is often due to a 'shock-wave' effect which damages the apical nerve supply. In such cases the pulp may have a normal blood supply. In all sensitivity testing always include and document the reaction of uninjured contralateral teeth for comparison. In addition, all teeth neighbouring the obviously injured teeth should be regularly assessed as they have probably suffered concussion injuries.

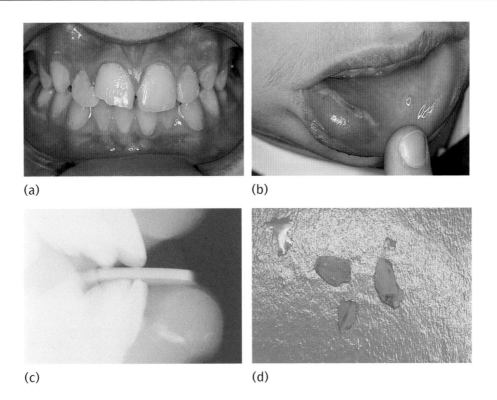

(a)   (b)

(c)   (d)

Figure 12.5 (a) A 12-year-old child presented with an enamel and dentine fracture of the upper right permanent central incisor. (b) The lower lip was swollen with a mucosal laceration. (c) A lateral radiograph confirmed the presence of tooth fragments in the lip. (d) Fragments were retrieved from the lip under local anaesthesia.

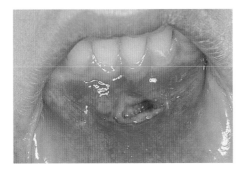

Figure 12.6 Degloving injury to the lower labial sulcus that required exploration to remove grit.

12.4.5 Radiographic examination

Periapical

Reproducible 'long-cone technique' periapicals are the best for accurate diagnosis and clinical audit. Two radiographs at different angles may be essential to detect a root fracture. However, if access and co-operation are difficult, a single anterior occlusal radiograph rarely misses a root fracture. Periapical films positioned behind the lips can be used to detect foreign bodies.

Occlusal

This view detects root fractures when used inta-orally and foreign bodies within the soft tissues when held by the patient/helper at the side of the mouth in a lateral view (Fig. 12.5(c)).

Orthopantomogram

This is essential in all trauma cases where underlying bony injury is suspected.

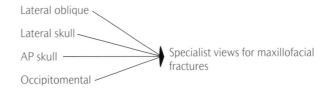

Lateral oblique

Lateral skull

AP skull → Specialist views for maxillofacial fractures

Occipitomental

Trauma stamp

In the patient's clinical notes the clinical and radiographic examinations at each visit can be combined into a simple aide-memoire in the form of a 'trauma stamp' (Fig. 12.7). Information that is collected in this standardized way is easily accessible when making clinical decisions and comparing responses at review appointments.

Tooth, e.g.	12	11	21	22
Colour				
Mobility				
TTP				
EC				
EPT				
Radiograph				

TTP, tenderness to percussion; EC, ethyl chloride; EPT, electric pulp tester

Figure 12.7 The trauma stamp.

12.4.6 Photographic records

Good clinical photographs are useful for assessing the outcome of treatment and for medico-legal purposes. Written consent must be obtained, and in the case of digital images uncropped originals must be held in an appropriately secure format and location. (See Key Point 12.1.)

Key Point 12.1

Develop a systematic approach to history and examination.

12.5 Injuries to the primary dentition

During its early development the permanent incisor is located palatally to and in close proximity with the apex of the primary incisor. With any injury to a primary tooth, there is risk of damage to the underlying permanent successor.

Most accidents in the primary dentition occur between 2 and 4 years of age. Realistically, this means that few restorative procedures will be possible and in the majority of cases the decision is between extraction or maintenance without performing extensive treatment. A primary incisor should always be removed if its maintenance will jeopardize the developing tooth bud.

A traumatized primary tooth that is retained should be assessed regularly for clinical and radiographic signs of pulpal or periodontal complications. Radiographs may even detect damage to the permanent successor. Soft tissue injuries in children should be assessed weekly until healed. Tooth injuries should be reviewed every 3–4 months for the first year and then annually until the primary tooth exfoliates and the permanent successor is in place.

Traumatic injuries that occur prior to eruption of primary teeth can also interfere with their development.

12.5.1 Uncomplicated crown fracture

Either smooth sharp edges or restore with an acid etch restoration if cooperation is satisfactory.

12.5.2 Complicated crown fracture

Extraction is normally the treatment of choice. However, pulp extirpation and canal obturation with zinc oxide cement, followed by an acid etch restoration, is possible with reasonable cooperation.

12.5.3 Crown–root fracture

The pulp is usually exposed and any restorative treatment is very difficult. It is best to extract the tooth.

12.5.4 Root fracture

If there is no displacement and only a small amount of mobility, the tooth should be kept under observation. If the coronal fragment becomes non-vital and symptomatic, it should be removed. The apical portion usually remains vital and undergoes normal resorption. Similarly, with marked displacement and mobility only the coronal portion should be removed.

12.5.5 Concussion, subluxation, and luxation injuries

Associated soft tissue damage should be cleaned by the parent twice daily with 0.2% chlorhexidine solution using cotton buds or gauze swabs until it heals.

Concussion

This is often not brought to a dentist's attention until the tooth discolours.

Subluxation

If there is slight mobility, the parents are advised to keep the child on a soft diet for 1–2 weeks and to keep the traumatized area as clean as possible. Marked mobility requires extraction.

Extrusive luxation

Marked mobility requires extraction.

Lateral luxation

If the crown is displaced palatally the apex moves buccally and hence away from the permanent tooth-germ. If the occlusion is not gagged, conservative treatment to await some spontaneous realignment is possible. If the crown is displaced buccally, the apex will be displaced towards the permanent tooth bud and extraction is indicated in order to minimize further damage to the permanent successor.

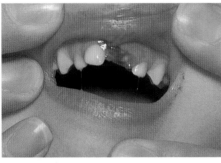

(a)

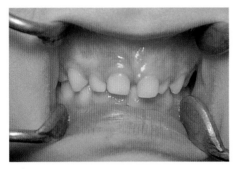

(b)

Figure 12.8 (a) A 4-year-old boy with complete intrusion of the upper right incisor. (b) Six months post-trauma, the tooth has spontaneously re-erupted.

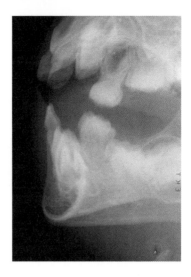

Figure 12.9 Severe intrusion of an upper primary central incisor necessitating extraction.

Intrusive luxation

This is the most common type of injury. The aim of investigation is to establish the direction of displacement by thorough radiological examination. If the root is displaced palatally towards the permanent successor, the primary tooth should be extracted to minimize the possible damage to the developing permanent successor. If the root is displaced buccally, there should be periodic review to monitor spontaneous re-eruption (Fig. 12.8). Review should be weekly for a month and then monthly for a maximum of 6 months. Most re-eruption occurs between 1 and 6 months. If this does not occur, ankylosis is likely and extraction is necessary to prevent ectopic eruption of the permanent successor (Fig. 12.9).

Exarticulation (avulsion)

Replantation of avulsed primary incisors is not recommended because of the risk of damage to the permanent tooth-germs. Space maintenance is not necessary following the loss of a primary incisor as only minor drifting of adjacent teeth occurs. The eruption of the permanent successor may be delayed for about a year as a result of abnormal thickening of connective tissue overlying the tooth-germ.

12.6 Sequelae of injuries to the primary dentition

12.6.1 Pulpal necrosis

Necrosis is the most common complication of primary trauma. Evaluation is based on colour and radiography. Teeth of a normal colour rarely develop periapical inflammation but, conversely, mildly discoloured teeth may be vital. A mild grey colour occurring soon after trauma may represent intrapulpal bleeding with a pulp that is still vital. This colour may recede, but if it persists necrosis should be suspected. Radiographic examination should be every 3 months to check for periapical inflammation (Fig. 12.10). Failure of the pulp cavity to reduce in size is an indicator of pulpal death. Teeth should be extracted whenever there is evidence of periapical inflammation to prevent possible damage to the permanent successor.

12.6.2 Pulpal obliteration

Obliteration of the pulp chamber and canal is a common reaction to trauma (Fig. 12.11). Clinically, the tooth becomes yellow/opaque. Normal exfoliation is usual, but occasionally periapical inflammation may intervene and therefore annual radiography is advisable.

12.6.3 Root resorption

Extraction is advised for all types of root resorption where there is evidence of infection (Fig. 12.12).

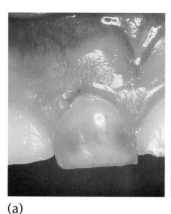
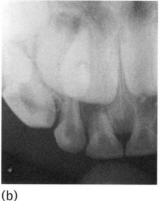

(a) (b)

Figure 12.10 (a) Severe discolouration of the upper right primary central incisor. (b) Radiographic evidence of periapical pathology. Extraction was necessary.

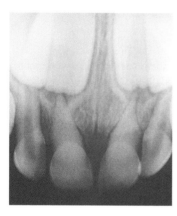

Figure 12.11 Pulp canal obliteration and external surface resorption of upper primary central incisors after a luxation injury.

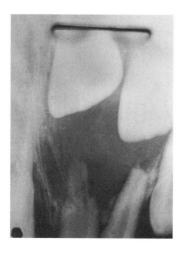

Figure 12.12 External inflammatory resorption of previously injured primary incisors.

12.6.4 Injuries to developing permanent teeth

Injuries to the permanent successor tooth can be expected in 12–69% of primary tooth trauma and 19–68% of jaw fractures. Intrusive luxation causes most disturbances, but avulsion of a primary incisor will also cause damage if the apex moved towards the permanent tooth bud before the avulsion. Most damage to the permanent tooth bud occurs under 3 years of age during its developmental stage. However, the type and severity of disturbance are closely related to the age at the time of injury. Changes in the mineralization and morphology of the crown of the permanent incisor are most common, but later injuries can cause radicular anomalies. Injuries to developing teeth can be classified as follows:

1. White or yellow-brown hypomineralization of enamel. Injury at 2–7 years (Fig. 12.13).
2. White or yellow-brown hypomineralization of enamel with circular enamel hypoplasia. Injury at 2–7 years (Fig. 12.14).
3. Crown dilaceration. Injury at about 2 years (Fig. 12.15).
4. Odontoma-like malformation. Injury at 1–3 years.
5. Root duplication. Injury at 2–5 years.
6. Vestibular or lateral root angulation and dilaceration. Injury at 2–5 years (Fig. 12.16).
7. Partial or complete arrest of root formation. Injury at 5–7 years (Fig. 12.17).
8. Sequestration of permanent tooth-germs.
9. Disturbance in eruption.

The term dilaceration describes an abrupt deviation of the long axis of the crown or root portion of the tooth. This deviation results from the traumatic displacement of hard tissue, which has already been formed, relative to developing soft tissue.

The term angulation describes a curvature of the root resulting from a gradual change in the direction of root development, without evidence of abrupt displacement of the tooth-germ during odontogenesis. This may be vestibular (i.e. labiopalatal) or lateral (i.e. mesiodistal).

Evaluation of the full extent of complications following injuries must await complete eruption of all permanent teeth involved. However, most serious sequelae (disturbances in tooth morphology) can usually be diagnosed radiographically within the first year post-trauma.

Eruption disturbances may involve delay because of thickening of connective tissue over a permanent tooth-germ, ectopic eruption due to lack of eruptive guidance, and impaction in teeth with malformations of crown or root. (See Key Points 12.2.)

Key Points 12.2

In primary tooth trauma:

- risk of damage to permanent successors is high—warn parents
- intrusive injuries carry the highest risk to the permanent successors.

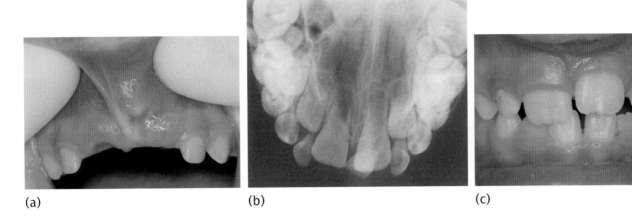

(a)   (b)   (c)

Figure 12.13 (a) Investigation of delayed eruption of the permanent upper central incisors revealed (b) an intruded upper left primary central incisor on radiograph. (c) Following removal of the retained primary incisor, the permanent successor erupted spontaneously with a white hypoplastic spot on the labial surface.

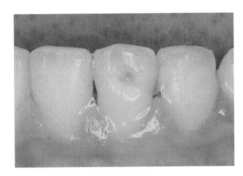

Figure 12.14 Brown hypoplastic area on the lower left permanent central incisor resulting from trauma to the primary predecessor.

12.6.5 Treatment of injuries to the permanent dentition

Yellow-brown hypomineralization of enamel with or without hypoplasia

1. Acid–pumice micro-abrasion.
2. Composite resin restoration: localized, veneer, or crown.
3. Porcelain restoration: veneer or crown (anterior); fused to metal crown (posterior). Conservative approaches are preferred whenever possible.

Crown dilaceration

1. Surgical exposure + orthodontic realignment.
2. Removal of dilacerated part of crown.
3. Temporary crown until root formation complete.
4. Semi-permanent or permanent restoration.

Vestibular root angulation

Combined surgical and orthodontic realignment.

Other malformation

Extraction is usually the treatment of choice.

Disturbance in eruption

Surgical exposure + orthodontic realignment.

Injuries to supporting bone

Most fractures of the alveolar socket in primary dentition do not require splinting because bony healing is rapid in small children. Jaw fractures are treated in the conventional manner, although stabilization after reduction may be difficult because of lack of sufficient adjacent teeth.

12.7 Injuries to the permanent dentition

Most traumatized teeth can be treated successfully. Prompt and appropriate treatment improves prognosis. The aims and principles of treatment can be broadly categorized as follows:

1. Emergency:
   (a) retain vitality of fractured or displaced tooth;
   (b) treat exposed pulp tissue;

(c) reduction and immobilization of displaced teeth;

(d) antiseptic mouthwash ± antibiotics and tetanus prophylaxis.

2. Intermediate:

(a) + pulp therapy;

(b) minimally invasive crown restoration.

3. Permanent:

(a) apexogenesis/apexification;

(b) root filling + root extrusion;

(c) + gingival and alveolar collar modification;

(d) semi-permanent or permanent coronal restoration.

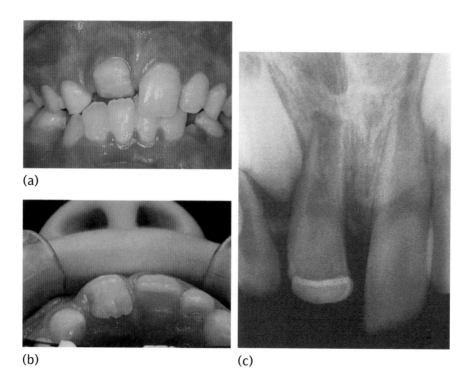

(a)

(b)

(c)

Figure 12.15 (a) Labial, (b) palatal, and (c) radiographic appearance of a severe crown dilaceration of the upper right permanent central incisor which erupted spontaneously.

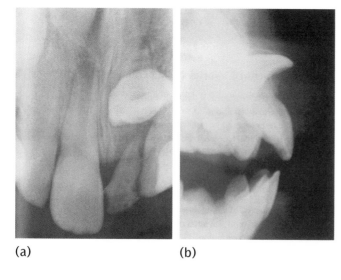

(a)

(b)

Figure 12.16 Unerupted dilacerated upper left permanent central incisor resulting from an accident sustained by a 3-year-old child.

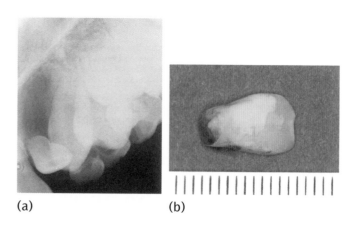

(a)

(b)

Figure 12.17 Failure of root formation of the upper left permanent lateral incisor (against a centimetre scale) in a 5-year-old child with a history of intrusive trauma to the primary predecessor.

Trauma cases require painstaking follow-up to identify any complications and institute the correct treatment. The trauma stamp is invaluable in this. In the review period the following schedule is a guide: 1 week; 1, 3, 6, and 12 months; then annually for 4–5 years.

12.7.1 Injuries to the hard dental tissues and the pulp

Enamel infraction

These incomplete fractures without loss of tooth substance and without proper illumination are easily overlooked. Review is necessary, as above, as the energy of the blow may have been transmitted to the periodontal tissues or the pulp.

Enamel fracture

No restoration is needed and treatment is limited to smoothing of any rough edges and splinting if there is associated mobility. Periodic review as above.

Enamel–dentine (uncomplicated) fracture

Immediate treatment is necessary and the pulp requires protection against thermal osmotic irritation and from bacteria via the dentinal tubules. Restoration of crown morphology also stabilizes the position of the tooth in the arch.

Emergency protection of the exposed dentine can be achieved by the following:

1. A composite resin (acid etched) or compomer bandage.

2. Glass ionomer cement within an orthodontic band or incisal end of a stainless steel crown if there is insufficient enamel available for acid-etch technique.

Intermediate restoration of most enamel–dentine fractures can be achieved by the following:

1. Acid-etched composite applied either freehand or utilizing a celluloid crown-former. The majority of these restorations can be regarded as semi-permanent/permanent. Larger fractures can utilize more available enamel surface area for bonding by employing a complete celluloid crown-former to construct a 'direct' composite crown. As the child becomes older, this could be reduced to form the core of a full- or partial-coverage porcelain crown preparation.

2. Reattachment of crown fragment. Few long-term studies have been reported and the longevity of this type of restoration is uncertain. In addition, there is a tendency for the distal fragment to become opaque or require further restorative intervention in the form of a veneer or full-coverage crown (Fig. 12.18). If the fracture line through dentine is not very close to the pulp, the fragment can be reattached immediately. However, if it runs close to the pulp, it is advisable to place a suitably protected calcium hydroxide dressing over the exposed dentine for at least a month while storing the fragment in saline, which should be renewed weekly.

Technique

1. Check the fit of the fragment and the vitality of the tooth.

2. Clean fragment and tooth with pumice–water slurry.

3. Isolate the tooth with rubber dam.

4. Attach fragment to a piece of sticky wax to facilitate handling.

5. Etch enamel for 30 seconds on both fracture surfaces and extend for 2mm from fracture line on tooth and fragment. Wash for 15 seconds and dry for 15 seconds.

6. Apply bonding agent ± dentine primer according to the manufacturer's instructions and light cure for 10 seconds.

7. Place appropriate shade of composite resin over both surfaces and position fragment. Remove gross excess and cure for 60 seconds labially and palatally.

8. Remove any excess composite resin with sandpaper discs.

9. Remove a 1mm gutter of enamel on each side of the fracture line both labially and palatally to a depth of 0.5mm using a small round or pear-shaped bur. The finishing line should be irregular in outline.

10. Etch the newly prepared enamel, wash, dry, apply composite, cure, and finish.

Enamel–dentine–pulp (complicated) crown fracture

The most important function of the pulp is to lay down dentine which forms the basic structure of teeth, defines their general morphology, and provides them with mechanical strength and toughness. Dentine deposition commences many years before permanent tooth eruption, and when a tooth erupts the pulp within still has work to do in completing root development. Newly erupted teeth have short roots, their apices are wide and often diverging, and the dentine walls of the entire tooth are thin and relatively weak (Fig. 12.19(a)). Provided that the pulp remains healthy, dentine deposition and normal root development will continue for 2–3 years after eruption in permanent teeth (Fig. 12.19(b)). Loss of pulp vitality before a tooth has reached maturity may leave the tooth vulnerable to fracture, and with an unfavourable crown–root ratio. In addition, endodontic treatment of non-vital immature teeth can present technical difficulties which may compromise the long-term prognosis of the tooth.

The major concern after pulpal exposures in immature teeth is the prevention of physical, chemical, and microbial invasion and the preservation of pulpal vitality in order to allow continued root growth. The radicular pulp has enormous capacity to remain healthy and undergo repair if all infected and inflamed coronal tissue is removed and an appropriate wound dressing and sealing coronal restoration is applied. Pulp amputation by partial pulpotomy or complete coronal pulpotomy is often the treatment of choice, but pulp capping can be considered in certain circumstances.

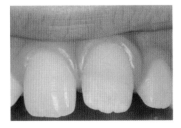

Figure 12.18 An upper left permanent central incisor 3 years after reattachment of a fractured incisal fragment.

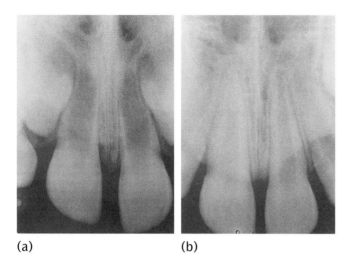

(a)   (b)

Figure 12.19 Maturation of permanent incisors. (a) Immature incisors showing short roots with incomplete wide open apices. The lateral walls of the roots are thin and structurally weak. (b) The same teeth 2 years later: the roots are now almost complete following continued dentine deposition by healthy pulp.

- Vital pulp therapy:

  – pulp capping
  – pulpotomy — partial
                  complete

- Non-vital pulp therapy:
  – pulpectomy

Vital pulp therapy: pulp capping

The procedure must be done within 24 hours of the incident. The tooth should be isolated with rubber dam and no instruments should be inserted into the exposure site. Any bleeding should be controlled with sterile cotton wool which may be moistened with saline or sodium hypochlorite, and not with a blast of air from a three-in-one syringe which may drive debris and micro-organisms into the pulp. A layer of setting calcium hydroxide cement is gently flowed onto the exposed pulp and surrounding dentine and quickly overlaid with a 'bandage' of adhesive material (e.g. compomer) pending definitive aesthetic restoration at a later date. A successful direct pulp cap will preserve the remaining pulp in health and should promote the deposition of a bridge of reparative dentine to seal off the exposure site.

   Review after a month, then 3 months, and eventually at 6-monthly intervals for up to 4 years in order to assess pulp vitality. Periodic radiographic review should also be arranged to monitor dentine bridge formation and root growth, and to exclude the development of necrosis and resorption. On the radiograph check the following:

- root is growing in length
- root canal is maturing (narrowing).

Compare with antimere. If growth is not occurring, the pulp should be assumed to be non-vital.

Vital pulp therapy: pulpotomy

In pulpotomy a portion of exposed vital pulp is removed to preserve the radicular vitality and allow completion of apical root development (apexogenesis) and further deposition of dentine on the walls of the root. This procedure is the treatment of choice following trauma where the pulp has been exposed to the mouth for more than 24 hours. The amount of pulp that is removed depends on the time since exposure, which will also determine the depth of contamination of the pulp. Attempts must be made to remove only the pulp that is deemed to be contaminated. If the patient presents within 24–48 hours of the incident, it is safe to assume that the contaminated zone is no more than 2–4mm around the exposure site and only the pulp in the immediate vicinity of the exposure is removed, in a procedure also termed partial pulpotomy (Cvek's technique). For more extensive exposures all coronal pulp can be removed down to the cervical constriction of the tooth (See Key Points 12.3). The operative procedure (Fig. 12.20) is as follows:

Key Points 12.3

Pulpotomy procedures:
- give a better prognosis than pulp capping for small exposures exposed for more than 24 hours;
- are not recommended if there are signs and symptoms of radicular pathosis.

- Under local anaesthesia and rubber dam, pulp tissue is excised with a diamond bur running at high speed under constant water cooling. This causes least injury to the underlying pulp and is preferred to hand excavation or the use of slow-speed steel burs.
- Microbial invasion of an exposed vital pulp is usually superficial and generally only 2–4mm of pulp tissue should be removed (partial pulpotomy (Cvek)).
- Excessive bleeding from the residual pulp which cannot be controlled with moist cotton wool, or indeed no bleeding at all, indicates that further excision is required to reach healthy tissue (coronal pulpotomy).
- Removal of tissue may occasionally extend more deeply into the tooth (full coronal pulpotomy) in an effort to preserve the apical portion of the pulp and safeguard apical closure.
- Gently rinse the wound with sterile saline or sodium hypochlorite (1–2%) and remove any shredded tissue. All remaining tags of tissue in the coronal portion must be removed as they may act as a nidus for re-infection and a pathway for coronal leakage.
- Apply a calcium hydroxide dressing to the pulp to destroy any remaining micro-organisms and promote calcific repair. In superficial wounds a setting calcium hydroxide cement may be gently flowed onto the pulp surface, but if the excision is deep it is often easier to prepare a

stiff mixture of calcium hydroxide powder (analytical grade) in sterile saline or local anaesthetic solution which is carried to the canal in an amalgam carrier and gently packed into place with pluggers.

- Overlay the calcium hydroxide dressing with a hard cement to prevent its forceful injection into the pulp by chewing forces and a final adhesive restoration which will seal the preparation against the re-entry of micro-organisms.

Review

- After a month.
- At 3 months.
- At 6-monthly intervals for up to 4 years in order to assess pulp vitality.

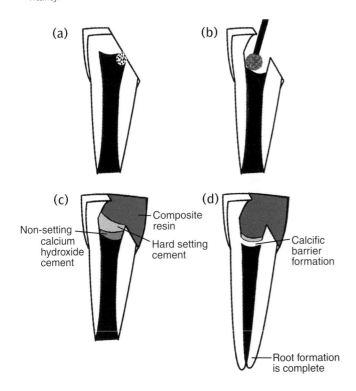

Figure 12.20 Pulp amputation (apexogenesis procedure) of a permanent incisor. (a) Complicated fracture of an immature incisor with microbial invasion of the coronal pulp. The pulp has been exposed to the mouth for more than 24 hours. (b) Access to the coronal pulp and amputation of coronal pulp tissue with a diamond bur running at high speed with constant water cooling. (c) Dressing the pulpal wound to promote calcific repair. Non-setting calcium hydroxide cement is flowed on to the pulp and then overlaid with a hard cement, and the tooth is restored with composite resin. (d) The same tooth after 12 months showing calcific barrier formation. The calcific barrier was directly inspected in this case (not always required), and a new layer of setting calcium hydroxide cement was placed on the barrier before definitive restoration. The remaining pulp has stayed healthy and deposited dentine to complete root formation.

- Periodic radiographic reviews should also be arranged to monitor dentine bridge formation and root growth, and to exclude the development of necrosis and resorption. If vitality is lost, non-vital pulp therapy should be undertaken whether or not there is a calcific bridge (see below).

Success rates for partial (Cvek) pulpotomies are quoted as 97% and for coronal pulpotomies as 75%.

Elective pulpectomy and root canal treatment of a vital pulp may be considered at a later date only if the root canal is required for restorative purposes.

Non-vital pulp therapy: pulpectomy

When there is death of the pulp in immature teeth, clinicians face a challenge. Because there is no further root development, the root has thin dentine walls liable to fracture under physiological forces and a wide open apex which is time-consuming and technically difficult to treat. The treatment first requires the elimination of bacterial infection from the root canal and the prevention of re-infection of this space. Disinfection of the root canal space is straightforward for most cases. However, there is no natural apical constriction or stop against which a suitable root filling material can be placed to prevent re-infection of this space. Traditionally the treatment has been aimed at producing a barrier against which a root canal filling material can be placed, thereby preventing the extrusion of material into the surrounding tissues (Fig. 12.21). This has usually been achieved with prolonged dressing of the root canal with calcium hydroxide to achieve 'apexification'. Although this technique has been reliable and has consistently allowed clinicians to achieve root canal obturation successfully, there have been recent concerns about the long-term use of calcium hydroxide in root canals. It is thought that, through the desiccation of dentinal proteins,

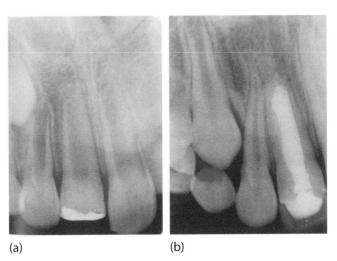

Figure 12.21 Root-end closure (apexification). (a) Immature permanent central incisor devitalized by trauma. (b) The same tooth 18 months later. Canal debridement and calcium hydroxide therapy has allowed the development of an apical calcific barrier. The canal has been densely obturated with thermoplastic GP and sealer.

calcium hydroxide might make dentine more brittle and more predisposed to root fractures. Indeed, an increased prevalence of root fractures has been reported for teeth that have been treated using this technique (Cvek 1992).

Although in this chapter we describe the technique for calcium hydroxide apexification for the sake of producing a comprehensive written text, it is the authors' opinion that clinicians should avoid the prolonged use of calcium hydroxide in the root canals. Therefore alternatives to apexification with calcium hydroxide should be explored wherever possible. Two such alternatives, the use of mineral trioxide aggregate and the regenerative endodontic technique, are described in later sections (see pages 234–6) and should be considered in preference to the prolonged use of calcium hydroxide. Traditional root-end closure with the use of calcium hydroxide may take 9–24 months before definitive canal obturation and restoration is possible.

Operative procedure (Fig. 12.22)

- Access with a high-speed medium-tapered fissure bur. In the pulp chamber use safe-ended burs to remove the entire roof without the danger of overcutting or perforation.
- Remove loose debris from the pulp chamber with hand instruments, accompanied by copious gentle irrigation with sodium hypochlorite solution (1–2%).
- Gates Glidden drills may be used to improve access to canals for instruments and irrigant. They should not be used deep in the canals of immature teeth where they may overcut and create a strip perforation.

- Canal preparation involves two processes: *cleaning* with irrigants to free the root canal system of organic debris, micro-organisms, and their toxins, and *shaping* with enlarging instruments to modify the form of the existing canal to allow placement of a well-condensed root filling. In canals which are often as wide as this, little dentine removal and shaping is needed. Sodium hypochlorite solution (1–2%) as an irrigant will continue dissolving organic debris and killing micro-organisms deep in the canal.
- Working apically, files are directed around the canal walls with a light rasping action to remove adherent debris. Instrumentation is frequently punctuated by high-volume low-pressure irrigation to flush out debris.
- Irrigant is delivered either by pre-measured 27 gauge needle and syringe or with the aid of sonic/ultrasonic energy. The latter involves flooding the canal with irrigant before inserting a small file (size 16–20) attached to a sonic/ultrasonic unit to stir the irrigant in the canal. Wall contact with the file should be avoided, as the action is liable to cause turbulence in the irrigant which scrubs the walls of debris.
- The provisional working length should be 2–3mm from the radiographic apex, estimated from an undistorted preoperative periapical film. A radiograph is then taken to establish a definitive working length 1mm short of the radiographic root apex. Further gentle filing and irrigation is then continued to the definitive working length.
- Dry the canal with pre-measured paper points to avoid inadvertent over-extension and damage to the periapical tissues.

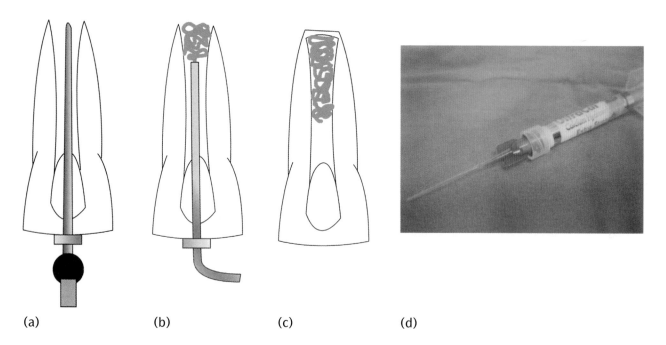

(a) (b) (c) (d)

Figure 12.22 (a) Following irrigation and gentle debridement in a crown-to-apex direction, the working length is determined. (b) Non-setting calcium hydroxide paste is syringed into the canal via a flexible tip. (c) The same tooth 18 months later. A calcific barrier is apparent, and the tooth is ready for definitive obturation and restoration. (d) The flexible tip system (Ultracal).

- Fill the canal with a relatively fluid proprietary calcium hydroxide paste such as Ultracal (Optident, UK). This can be syringed into the canal via a disposable flexible tip (Fig. 12.22(d)) or alternatively spun into the canal with a spiral paste filler. The antimicrobial and mild tissue solvent activity of non-setting calcium hydroxide will continue to cleanse the canal, and its high pH is believed to encourage calcific root-end closure.

- A radiograph may be taken to ensure a dense fill to each root terminus (Fig. 12.23).

- Seal the access cavity tightly between appointments to prevent the leaching of calcium hydroxide and, critically, the re-entry of micro-organisms from the mouth which would disturb the process of root-end closure. A 3mm thickness of glass ionomer cement or composite resin is adequate to provide a bacteria-tight seal. Cotton wool fibres should not be allowed to remain at the cavo-surface of the cavity.

Review

- Every 3 months to monitor root-end closure. At each appointment the calcium hydroxide dressing is carefully washed from the canal and the presence of a calcified barrier is assessed by gently tapping a pre-measured paper point at the working length.

- Radiographs should be taken to assess the progress of barrier formation.

- If the canal is closed, obturation can proceed. If calcific barrier formation is not complete, the canal should be re-dressed for a further 3 months. Calcific barrier formation is usually complete within 9–18 months, but could take up to 2 years. (See Key Points 12.4.)

> ### Key Points 12.4
>
> Root-end closure
> - Gives predictable results if infection is controlled and the canal is sealed bacteria tight.
> - Infection is controlled by irrigation and disinfection.
> - The canal is enlarged enough only to allow irrigant access and dense obturation.
> - Closure adds nothing to the strength of the tooth.
> - Coronal restoration is critical to long-term success.

Techniques for obturation

Obturation with GP and sealer prevent the re-entry of oral micro-organisms to the apical tissues. Cold lateral condensation of GP and sealer may provide satisfactory results in regular apically converging canals, but in irregular and diverging canals a thermoplastic GP technique is required to improve adaptation. The use of single-cone techniques cannot be recommended in any circumstances.

Manual obturation in apically divergent canal (Fig. 12.24)

- Select a master point and try into the canal. This is usually the widest point which will reach the canal terminus, and may be inverted in the widest canals.

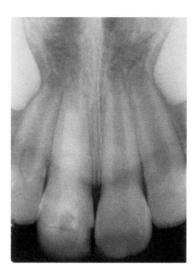

Figure 12.23 Radiograph to confirm dense obliteration of the prepared canal with non-setting calcium hydroxide paste.

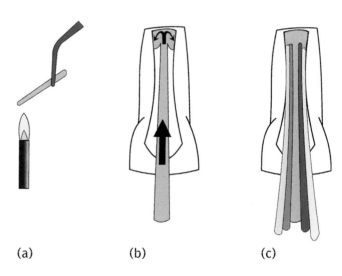

(a)   (b)   (c)

Figure 12.24 Obturation following root-end closure in an apically diverging canal. (a) The widest GP point that will reach the apical terminus of the canal is warmed by passage of its tip through a flame. (b) Without delay, the point is introduced to the canal (the canal is already lightly coated with sealer) and advanced to adapt against the apical barrier. (c) Additional points are now packed around the master point with cold or warm condensation until the canal is densely filled.

- Dry the canal and lightly coat its walls with a slow-setting sealer.

- Soften the tip of the master point by passage through a bunsen burner flame. Insert the point to the apical limit of the canal and press gently against the calcific barrier to adapt the softened GP.

- Apply cold lateral condensation with a spreader to within 1mm of the apical limit of the canal, adding accessory GP cones lightly coated with sealer. Continue condensation until the spreader can advance no more than 2 or 3mm into the canal.

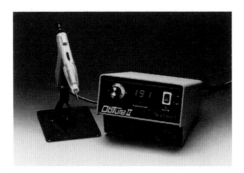

Figure 12.25 Obtura II: low-temperature injection-moulded thermoplastic GP.

- Check the radiograph to assess the quality of fill before removing excess GP with a hot instrument and vertically condensing the warm GP at the canal entrance. Further cold or warm condensation may be undertaken at this stage if required to obtain a uniformly dense obturation.

Thermoplastic obturation (Figs 12.25 and 12.26).

Warm GP techniques offer the possibility of extremely rapid and dense obturation of the most irregularly shaped spaces.

- Dry the canal and lightly coat its walls with a slow-setting sealer.
- Inject thermoplastic GP into the apical portion of the canal and condense.
- Radiograph to check apical GP is in the correct place.
- Backfill with GP and seal access cavity with an adhesive restoration.

While allowing dense and controlled canal obturation, the root-end closure procedure adds nothing to the canal wall thickness or mechanical strength of immature teeth. Therefore the final restoration should be planned to optimize the durability of the remaining tooth structure. Dentine-bonded composite resins may be particularly helpful in this regard, especially if extended several millimetres into the root canal to provide internal splinting. The advent of light-transmitting fibre posts opens new potential for rehabilitation and also provides a ready patency for canal re-entry if needed. Periodic clinical and radiographic review should be arranged.

Alternatives to apexification with calcium hydroxide

Two techniques that are now preferred over apexification are use of MTA and the regenerative endodontic technique.

Use of MTA In the last decade the introduction of mineral trioxide aggregate (MTA) has meant that dentists can create a plug which allows immediate obturation of the root canal. MTA, which is based on Portland building cement, is packed into the canal with pre-measured pluggers and sets to form a hard sealing biocompatible barrier within 30 minutes. Moist cotton wool is placed in the canal for 30 minutes to promote setting, after which a paper point or a file is used gently to check whether the MTA has set to a hard barrier. The root canal can

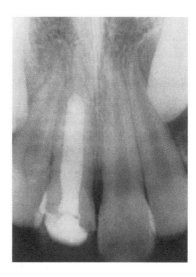

Figure 12.26 Rapid dense obturation of a wide irregularly shaped canal with injection-moulded thermoplastic GP and sealer.

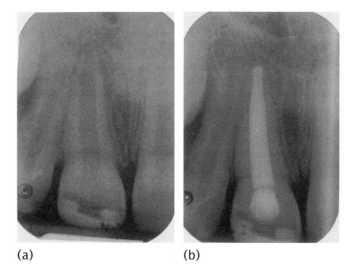

(a)   (b)

Figure 12.27 (a) Immature apex tooth 11. (b) Apical 'plug' of MTA and backfill with thermoplastic GP.

then be obturated with GP and sealer in the same visit. Many clinical studies over the last 10 years have shown that this should be the material of choice for teeth with incomplete root development that need endodontic management (Pradhan *et al.* 2006). The greatest advantage of MTA is that it allows root-end closure and obturation in one visit, which will demand less patient compliance (Fig. 12.27). However, it remains expensive but, considering the reduced number of treatment visits required, it is more cost-effective than the multiple visit procedures such as those required with calcium hydroxide.

When pulp vitality is lost in an almost fully formed tooth, it may be possible to avoid lengthy root-end closure procedures by creating an apical stop against which a root filling can be packed. Following crown-to-apex preparation as described above, endodontic hand files can be

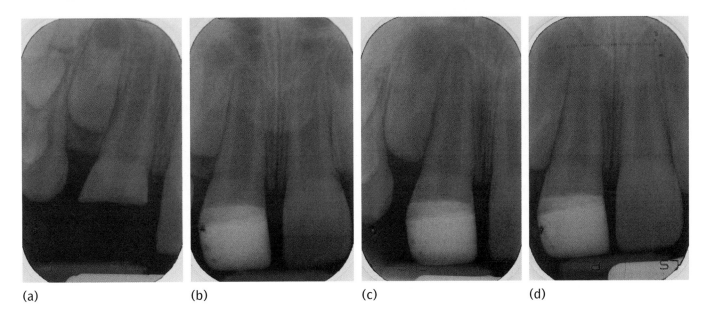

(a)   (b)   (c)   (d)

Figure 12.28 A series of sequential periapical radiographs showing continued root development and hard tissue deposition along the root canal in an upper right central incisor treated with RET. (a) Complicated fracture of right upper central incisor leading to the tooth becoming non-vital. Note the incomplete root development. (b) The tooth was restored with composite and treated with RET. (c) Periapical radiograph 6 months later showing continued root development and narrowing of the root canal. (d) Periapical radiograph a year after treatment showing root development almost complete with further development in the apical area.

used in gentle watch-winding or balanced-force motion at working length to shave an apical seat for canal obturation. Alternatively, MTA can be packed into the apical 1–2mm of the canal with pluggers to provide an immediate apical seal.

The regenerative endodontic technique Recently there has been a paradigm shift in the proposed treatment for non-vital incisors with incomplete root development. Techniques have been proposed in which the stem cells at the apical area of immature incisors would be harnessed, thereby allowing the root canal to be repopulated with vital tissue which might then allow the continued deposition of hard tissue or even further root development (Banchs and Trope 2004). This technique is widely referred to as the regenerative endodontic technique (RET).

Rationale for the use of RET With an increasing understanding of stem cell biology, it has become possible to aspire to further root development and further hard tissue deposition in non-vital teeth with incomplete root development. This will occur via repopulation of the root canal with vital tissue, and therefore it is regeneration as opposed to revascularization, which is a term usually used for the re-attachment of the blood supply in teeth which have been replanted. We now know that the apical area surrounding teeth with incomplete root development is rich in stem cells, and this region has been termed stem cells of the apical papilla (SCAP) in the literature. Recently cells in SCAP have been characterized as similar to dental pulp progenitor cells. If the right conditions are created within the root canal system with intense disinfection and the provision of a biological scaffold and signalling, the stem cells from SCAP can migrate into the scaffold in the root canal and repopulate the root canal with vital tissue. This has now been shown to occur, and the success of this procedure has been indicated in a number of case reports and medium-term studies. The advantage of this is that the vital tissue will produce further hard tissue, thereby reinforcing the root canal system and making the roots less prone to fracture in the future, as often occurs in teeth where endodontic treatment has been carried out using conventional methods (Fig. 12.28).

Clinical technique for RET There are currently no standardized protocols for RET in the treatment of non-vital immature teeth with wide open apices. Minor modifications to the procedures have been made by various groups who have carried out clinical case studies. The general outline of the technique proposed is as follows:

- All procedures are carried out under local anaesthetic and rubber dam isolation.
- Pulpal extirpation and copious irrigation of root canals with mild disinfectants is performed for 30 minutes.
- Minimal or no filing of the root canal is done to prevent further weakening of the existing dentinal walls.
- The root canal is dressed with a mixture of antibiotics. The most commonly used mixture is minocycline, ciprofloxacin, and metronidazole. Local dispensaries should be able to supply all three antibiotics in capsule form, and these can be individually opened, mixed together, and then mixed in distilled water or propylene glycol. Note that minocycline can cause discolouration and attempts are being made to substitute it. If there are concerns about this, perhaps only the two other antibiotics should be used. The paste is

introduced into the root canal with either a syringe or a spiral paste filler. To avoid discolouration, especially if minocycline is used, ensure that there is no antibiotic in the pulp chamber or the coronal part of the tooth.

- The tooth is sealed temporarily and a review is scheduled in 2 weeks. If there is no sign of periapical infection at this visit, the root canal is re-accessed and the antibiotics flushed out with saline.

- At the same appointment, a sterile 23-gauge needle with a length of 2mm beyond the working length is pushed past the confines of the root canal into the periapical tissues to intentionally induce bleeding into the root canal. The bleeding is then allowed to fill the root canal.

- When frank bleeding is evident at the cervical portion of the root canal, a cotton pellet is inserted 3–4mm into the canal below the cervical margins and held there for 7–10 minutes to allow formation of a blood clot in the apical two-thirds of the canal. This blood clot acts as a scaffold rich in growth and differentiation factors that are essential to aid in the growth of viable tissue into the pulpal space and in wound-healing processes.

- The access is then sealed with materials such as MTA or glass iono-mer cements to prevent coronal leakage, extending about 4mm into the coronal portion of the root canal. In the authors' opinion MTA should be avoided as it causes discolouration of the crown.

- Periapical radiographs are then taken as baseline record. This is essential for comparison with future 6-monthly radiographs to ascertain continued root development, hard tissue deposition in root canal, and thus success of the treatment.

Endodontic surgery with root-end filling is becoming less popular as a means of treatment in the case of non-closure. However, it may be considered for addressing problems of serious irretrievable overfill which may arise if the calcific barrier has been erroneously diagnosed as complete or broken by heavy-handed obturation. (See Key Points 12.5.)

Key Points 12.5

- Avoid prolonged use of calcium hydroxide in root canals.
- The use of mineral trioxide aggregate (MTA) to create root-end closure should be the technique of choice with current levels of evidence.
- Consider the use of the regenerative endodontic technique (RET) where the root development is so incomplete that the tooth is deemed to have poor prognosis even with use of MTA.

Uncomplicated crown–root fracture

After removal of the fractured piece of tooth these vertical fractures are commonly a few millimetres incisal to the gingival margin on the labial surface but down to the cemento-enamel junction palatally. Prior to placement of a restoration the fracture margin has to be brought supra-gingival by either gingivoplasty or extrusion (orthodontically or surgically) of the root portion.

Complicated crown–root fracture

Proceed as with uncomplicated crown–root fractures, with the addition of endodontic requirements. If extrusion is planned, the final root length must be no shorter than the final crown length otherwise the result will be unstable. Root extrusion can be successful in a motivated patient and leads to a stable periodontal condition.

Root fracture

Root fractures occur most frequently in the middle or apical third of the root. The coronal fragment may be extruded or luxated. If displacement has occurred, the coronal fragment should be repositioned as soon as possible by gentle digital manipulation and the position checked radiographically. Optimal repositioning favours healing with hard tissue and reduces the risk of pulpal necrosis. Mobile root fractures need to be splinted to encourage repair of the fracture. With the possible exception of coronal-third fractures, which may require longer splinting periods, a period of 4 weeks with a semi-rigid or functional splint appears to be sufficient to ensure healing. A functional splint includes one abutment tooth on each side of the fractured tooth. Splinting for longer periods may be required in individual cases. The splint should allow colour observations, sensitivity testing, and access to the root canal if endodontic treatment is required. The splint design and placement techniques are discussed in Section 12.7.2.

Three main categories of repair are recognized:

1. Repair with calcified tissue: invisible or hardly discernible fracture line (Fig. 12.29).

2. Repair with connective tissue: narrow radiolucent fracture line with peripheral rounding of the fracture edges (Fig. 12.30).

3. Repair with bone and connective tissue: the two fragments are separated by a bony bridge (Fig. 12.31).

In addition to these changes in the fracture area, pulp canal obliteration is commonly seen. Fractures in the cervical third of the root will repair as long as no communication exists between the fracture line and the gingival crevice. If there is communication, splinting is not recommended and an early decision must be made to extract the coronal fragment and retain the remaining root, internally splint the root fracture, or extract the two fragments.

Extraction of coronal fragment and root retention

The remaining radicular pulp should be removed and the canal temporarily dressed prior to obturating with GP. Three options are now available for the treated radicular portion of the root.

1. Post, core, and crown restoration if access is adequate.

2. Extrusion of the root either surgically or orthodontically if the fracture extends too subgingivally for adequate access. Rapid orthodontic extrusion over 4–6 weeks, aiming to move the root a maximum of 4mm, is the best option. This is achieved by cementing a J-hook made from 0.7mm stainless steel wire into the canal and using elastic traction applied over an arch wire cemented between one abutment tooth on either side of the injured tooth. Retention for a month at the end of movement is advised to prevent relapse (Fig. 12.32). If

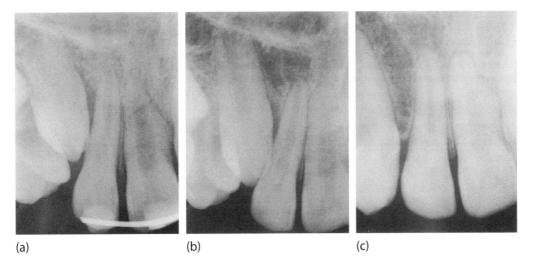

(a)   (b)   (c)

Figure 12.29 (a) An apical third root fracture of the upper right permanent central incisor with a rigid splint. (b) Appearance of the fracture 15 months later. (c) Good calcified tissue repair evident 3 years post trauma.

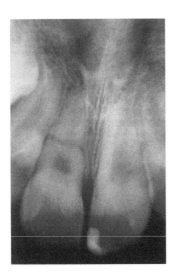

Figure 12.30 Middle third root fracture of the upper right permanent central incisor with connective tissue repair.

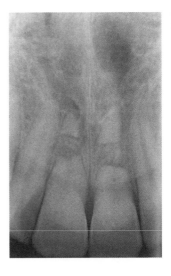

Figure 12.31 Middle third root fracture of both permanent central incisors with bony repair and sclerosis of the apical fragments.

aesthetics are a particular concern, an orthodontic bracket can be bonded to a temporary crown made over the J-hook. The temporary crown length will need to be reduced as extrusion occurs (Fig. 12.33).

3. Cover the root with a mucoperiosteal flap. This will maintain the height and width of the arch and facilitate later placement of a single tooth implant.

Internal splinting

Fractures arising in the coronal and middle third of the root often result in excessive mobility of the coronal fragment, and techniques have been described to splint the coronal and apical portions together internally with a rigid root-filling material. Internal splints have ranged from Hedstrom files to nickel–chromium points, screwed and cemented into position. These approaches are, in effect, single-cone root-filling procedures and cannot be relied upon to provide a long-term safeguard against the re-entry of oral micro-organisms to the canal and fracture line. Most are doomed to failure and other restorative options are preferred.

Pulpal necrosis in root fracture

Pulpal necrosis occurs in about 20% of root fractures and is the main obstacle to adequate repair. The initial amount of displacement of the coronal portion, rather than the level of the fracture or the presence of an open or closed apex, is the most significant factor in determining future pulpal prognosis. Most cases of necrosis are diagnosed within 3 months of a root fracture. A persistent negative response to electric stimulation is usually confirmed on radiography by radiolucencies adjacent to the fracture line. The apical fragment almost always contains viable pulp tissue and invariably scleroses. Rarely, it may require surgical removal.

In apical and middle-third fractures any endodontic treatment is usually confined to the coronal fragment only. A barrier is achieved on the coronal aspect of the fracture line by preparation of a stop with non-setting calcium hydroxide or MTA, and the coronal canal is obturated with GP. After completion of endodontic treatment, repair and union between the two fragments with connective tissue is a consistent finding.

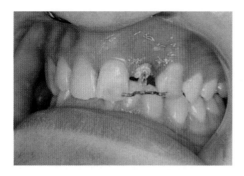

Figure 12.32 Extrusive force being applied via a J-hook cemented into the root canal of the upper left permanent lateral incisor.

In coronal-third fractures that develop necrosis the radicular portion can be retained (see above), both portions can be extracted, or the fracture can be internally splinted (see above).

12.7.2 Splinting

Trauma may loosen a tooth by damaging the periodontal ligament (PDL) or fracturing the root. Splinting immobilizes the tooth in the correct anatomical position so that further trauma is prevented and healing can occur. Different injuries require different splinting regimens. A functional splint involves one, and a rigid splint two, abutment teeth on either side of the injured tooth.

Regimens
PDL injuries

Sixty per cent of PDL healing has occurred after 10 days and it is complete within a month. The splinting period should be as short as possible, and the splint should allow some functional movement to prevent replacement root resorption (ankylosis). As a general rule, exarticulation (avulsion) injuries require 14 days and luxation injuries 2–4 weeks of functional splinting.

Root fractures

Generally apical and middle third injuries require 4 weeks of functional splinting. Coronal third injuries may require 8 weeks. Excessive mobility leads to the fracture site becoming filled with granulation tissue.

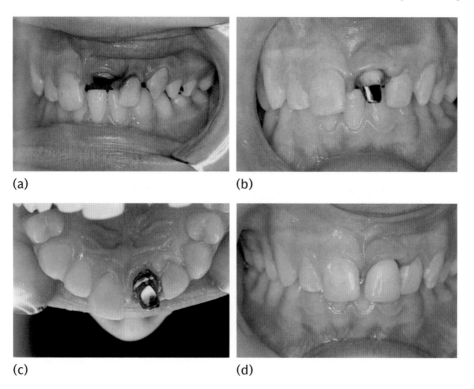

(a) (b) (c) (d)

Figure 12.33 (a) Initial presentation of a high coronal root fracture which extended palatally below alveolar bone. (b), (c) Post, core, and diaphragm after root extrusion. (d) Final ceramic crown.

Dento-alveolar fractures

These require 3–4 weeks of rigid splinting.

Types and methods of constructing splints

Composite resin/acrylic and wire splint

This method uses either a composite resin or a temporary crown material. The composite resin is easier to place, but the acrylic resin is easier to remove. Although acrylic resin does not bond as strongly to enamel as the composite resin does, it is suitable for all types of functional splinting (Fig. 12.34).

The technique for a functional resin–wire splint is as follows:

1. Bend a flexible orthodontic wire to fit the middle third of the labial surface of the injured tooth and one abutment tooth either side.

2. Stabilize the injured tooth in the correct position with soft red wax palatally.

3. Clean the labial surfaces. Isolate, dry, and etch the middle of the crown of the teeth with 37% phosphoric acid for 30 seconds, wash, and dry.

4. Apply a 3mm diameter circle of either unfilled and then filled composite resin or acrylic resin to the centre of the crowns.

5. Position the wire into the filling material and then apply more composite or acrylic resin.

6. Use a brush lubricated with unfilled composite resin to mould and smooth the composite. Acrylic resin is more difficult to handle, and smoothing and excess removal can be done with a flat plastic instrument.

7. Cure the composite for 60 seconds. Wait for the acrylic resin to cure.

8. Smooth any sharp edges with sandpaper discs.

Figure 12.35 shows an example of a functional splint. There is a newer splint, a prefabricated titanium trauma splint, available commercially as a TTS splint. This splint has a number of advantages, including ease of adaptation owing to its flexibility. It is also easy to apply with composite resin, easy to remove, and allows the tooth to retain the physiological mobility which is essential for healing the PDL.

The same technique is used for a rigid splint, but two abutment teeth are incorporated on either side of the injured tooth. These splints should not impinge on the gingiva and should allow assessment of colour change and sensitivity testing.

Orthodontic brackets and wire

These splints have the advantage of allowing a more accurate reduction of displacement injuries and exarticulations by gentle forces (Fig. 12.36).

Foil–cement splint

A temporary splint made of soft metal (cooking foil) and cemented with quick-setting zinc oxide–eugenol cement is an effective temporary measure either during the night when it is difficult to fit a composite wire splint as a single-handed operator or while awaiting construction of a laboratory-made splint.

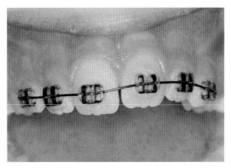

Figure 12.35 A TTS splint in place.

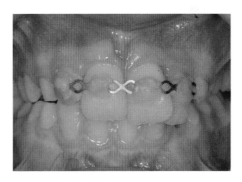

(a)

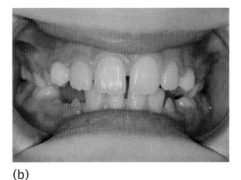

(b)

Figure 12.36 (a) Gentle reduction and splinting of luxated upper right permanent central incisor. (b) Final position.

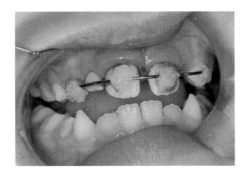

Figure 12.34 Composite resin and wire splint for a luxation injury of both upper permanent central incisors.

The technique is as follows:

1. Cut metal to size, long enough to extend over two or three teeth on each side of the injured tooth and wide enough to extend over the incisal edges and 3–4mm over the labial and palatal gingiva.

2. Place the foil over teeth and mould it over the labial and palatal surfaces. Remove any excess.

3. Cement the foil to the teeth with quick-setting zinc oxide–eugenol cement.

Laboratory splints

These are used where it is impossible to make a satisfactory splint by the direct method: for example, a 7- to 8-year-old with traumatized maxillary incisors, unerupted lateral incisors, and either carious or absent primary canines. Both methods require alginate impressions, and very loose teeth may need to be supported by wax, metal foil, or wire ligature so they are not removed with the impression.

- *Acrylic splint* There is full palatal coverage and the acrylic is extended over the incisal edges for 2–3mm of the labial surfaces of the anterior teeth. The occlusal surfaces of the posterior teeth should be covered to prevent any occlusal contact in the anterior region. This also aids retention and Adams cribs may not be required. The splint should be removed for cleaning after meals and at bedtime.

- *Thermoplastic splint* The splint is constructed from polyvinylacetate–polyethylene (PVAC–PE) copolymer in the same way as a mouth-guard with extension onto the mucosa. Like the acrylic splint, it should be removed after meals and at bedtime. However, with more severely loosened teeth it could be retained at night.

Both forms of laboratory splint allow functional movement and therefore promote normal periodontal healing. They are not suitable for root fractures as they compromise oral hygiene.

12.7.3 Injuries to the periodontal tissues

Concussion

The impact force causes oedema and haemorrhage in the PDL and the tooth is tender to percussion (TTP). There is no rupture of PDL fibres and the tooth is firm in the socket.

Subluxation

In addition to the above there is rupture of some PDL fibres and the tooth is mobile in the socket, although not displaced (Fig. 12.37). The treatment for both concussion and subluxation is as follows:

- occlusal relief;
- soft diet for 7 days;
- immobilization with a functional splint for 2 weeks if teeth have fully formed apices or if TTP is significant;
- chlorhexidine 0.2% mouthwash, twice daily.

Figures for pulpal survival 5 years after injury (Table 12.2) show that there is minimal risk of pulpal necrosis. In addition, in over 97% of cases there is no evidence of any resorption.

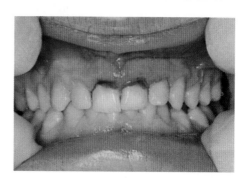

Figure 12.37 Subluxated upper permanent central incisors.

Table 12.2 Five-year pulpal survival after injuries involving the periodontal ligament

Type of injury	Open apex (%)	Closed apex (%)
Concussion	100	96
Subluxation	100	85
Extrusive luxation	95	45
Lateral luxation	95	25
Intrusive luxation	40	0

Extrusive luxation

There is a rupture of PDL and pulp. Functional splint for 2 weeks.

Lateral luxation

There is a rupture of PDL, pulp, and the alveolar plate (Fig. 12.38(a)).

The treatment for both extrusive and lateral luxation is as follows:

- atraumatic repositioning with gentle but firm digital pressure (Fig. 12.38(b));
- local anaesthetic if there is an alveolar plate injury;
- non-rigid functional splint for 4 weeks (Fig. 12.38(c));
- antibiotics, e.g. amoxycillin 250mg three times daily (<10 years old: 125mg three times daily) for 5 days;
- chlorhexidine 0.2% mouthwash twice daily while splint is in position;
- soft diet for 2–3 weeks.

There is limited evidence for the use of antibiotics in the management of luxation injuries and no evidence that antibiotics improve the outcome of root fractures. Antibiotic use remains at the discretion of the clinician. Soft tissue injuries and medical status may warrant antibiotic coverage.

After 4 weeks the teeth are radiographed. If there is no evidence of marginal breakdown, the splint can be removed. If marginal breakdown is present, it should be retained for a further 2–3 weeks.

For both these injuries the decision whether to progress to endodontic treatment depends on the combination of clinical and radiographic signs at regular review (Fig. 12.7). Five-year pulpal survival figures (Table 12.2) show that the prognosis is significantly better for open apex teeth, but nevertheless a proportion of mature closed apex teeth will retain vitality. In addition, over 4% of mature teeth involved in luxation injuries

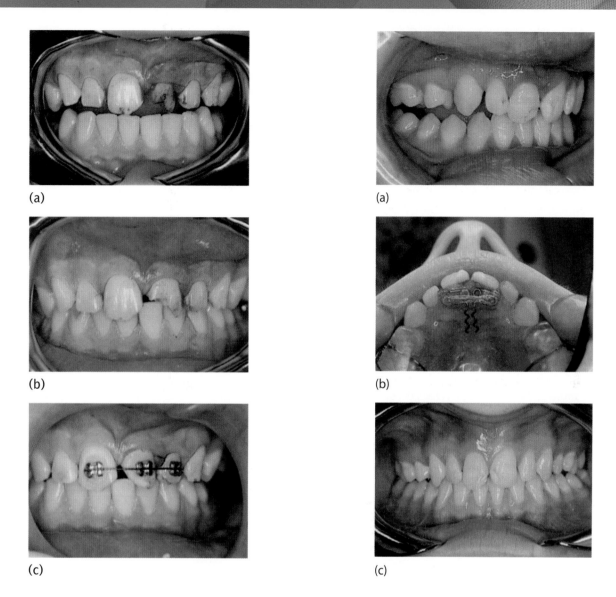

(a)

(b)

(c)

(a)

(b)

(c)

Figure 12.38 (a) Palatally luxated upper left permanent incisor with other associated injuries. (b) Upper left permanent central incisor repositioned atraumatically. (c) Non-rigid orthodontic splint in place.

Figure 12.39 (a) Delayed presentation of palatally luxated upper permanent central incisors in traumatic occlusion. (b), (c) An upper removable appliance used to procline the upper incisors over 2 months.

will exhibit on radiographs a natural healing phenomenon known as 'transient apical breakdown' (TAB) which can mimic apical inflammation. Ambivalent clinical and radiographic signs should be given the benefit of the doubt until the next review.

With more significant damage to the PDL in both extrusive and lateral luxation injuries there is an increased risk of root resorption. Thirty-five per cent of mature teeth which have undergone lateral luxation show subsequent evidence of surface resorption.

In some cases of lateral luxation the displacement cannot be reduced with gentle finger pressure. It is not advisable to use more force as this can further damage the PDL. Orthodontic appliances, either removable or sectional fixed, can be used to reduce the displacement over a period of a few weeks (Fig. 12.39).

Intrusive luxation

These injuries are the result of an axial apical impact and there is extensive damage to the PDL, pulp, and alveolar plate(s).

There are two distinct treatment categories: the open apex and the closed apex. Both categories can be discussed depending on whether the intrusive injury is <7mm or >7mm.

Open apex

- (<7mm). There is eruptive potential which may be improved by disimpaction with forceps. Treat conservatively and review. If no movement in 2–4 weeks, move orthodontically (Fig. 12.40).

- (>7mm). Orthodontic repositioning may be impossible and dis-impaction followed by surgical repositioning under local anaesthetic, local anaesthetic/sedation, or general anaesthetic is appropriate. Functional splint for 4–8 weeks.

Non-setting calcium hydroxide in the root canal does not preclude against orthodontic movement.

Closed apex

- (<7mm). Orthodontic extrusion is probably indicated straight away. The danger of a tooth ankylosing in an intruded position should always be borne in mind, and in this respect active treatment is preferable to a conservative approach.
- (>7mm). Surgical repositioning. Functional splint for 4–8 weeks (Fig. 12.41).

Monitor pulpal status clinically and radiographically at regular intervals during the first 6 months after injury, and then every 6 months, and start endodontics if necessary. Elective pulp extirpation will be necessary for all significant intrusive luxation injuries in closed apex teeth (Table 12.3) at about 10 days.

If endodontic treatment is commenced within 2 weeks after any injury to the PDL, the initial intracanal dressing could be an antibiotic–steroid. Some advocate the use of Ledermix (Lederle) paste. This may help to reduce the incidence of inflammatory resorption, but also causes severe discolouration of the teeth. Therefore the use of Ledermix should be avoided. At the initial examination patients with both

Table 12.3 Periodontal ligament healing after intrusive luxation injuries

Type of healing	Open apex (%)	Closed apex (%)
Normal	33	0
Inflammatory resorption	41	35
Replacement resorption (ankylosis)	10	31

open and closed apex teeth should receive antibiotics, chlorhexidine mouthwash, and be told to follow a soft diet.

The risk of pulpal necrosis in these injuries is high, especially in the closed apex (Table 12.2). The incidence of resorption and ankylosis sequelae is also high (Table 12.3). (See Key Points 12.6.)

Key Points 12.6

In PDL injuries:

- the incidence of pulpal necrosis is higher in closed apex teeth;
- the incidence of resorption increases with severity of injury.

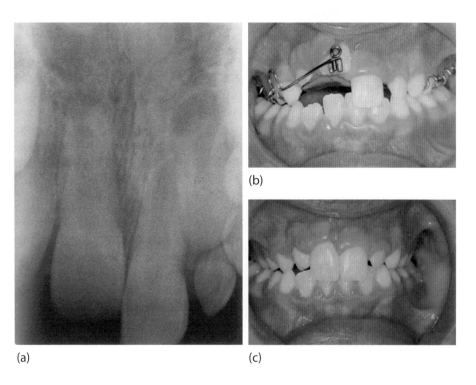

(a)

(b)

(c)

Figure 12.40 (a) A 7-year-old child with intrusion of the upper right permanent central incisor which failed to re-erupt spontaneously. (b), (c) Orthodontic extrusion of the upper right central incisor.

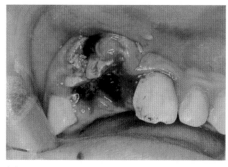

(a)

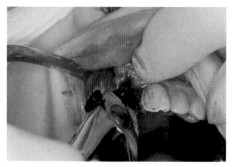

(b)

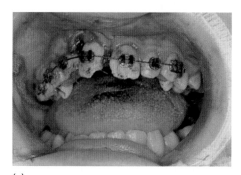

(c)

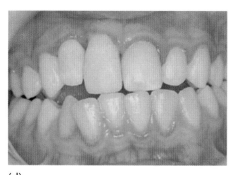

(d)

Figure 12.41 (a) A severe intrusive injury in a 15-year-old girl. (b) Surgical extrusion of the upper right permanent incisors. (c) Orthodontic splinting. (d) Completed composite restorations.

Avulsion and replantation

Replantation should nearly always be attempted even though it may offer only a temporary solution because of the frequent occurrence of external inflammatory resorption (EIR). Even when resorption occurs, the tooth may be retained for years, acting as a natural space maintainer and preserving the height and width of the alveolus to facilitate later implant placement.

Successful healing after replantation can only occur if there is minimal damage to the pulp and PDL. The extra-alveolar dry time (EADT), the type of extra-alveolar storage medium, and the total extra-alveolar time (EAT), i.e. the time that the tooth has been out of the mouth, are critical factors. The first question that must be answered is 'What is the EADT of the tooth?'

Replantation of teeth with a dry storage time less than 1 hour
Advice on phone (to teacher, parent, etc.)

1. Don't touch the root—hold by the crown.
2. If the tooth is dirty, wash briefly (10 seconds) under cold running water.
3. Replace in the socket or transport in milk to the surgery.
4. If replaced, bite gently on a handkerchief to retain it and come to the surgery.

The best transport medium is the tooth's own socket. Understandably, non-dentists may be unhappy to replant the tooth and milk is an effective iso-osmolar medium. Saliva, the patient's buccal sulcus, or normal saline are alternatives.

Immediate surgery treatment

1. Do not handle the root. If replanted, remove tooth from socket.
2. Rinse the tooth with normal saline. Note the state of root development. Store in saline.
3. Local analgesia.
4. Irrigate the socket with saline. Remove clot and any foreign material.
5. Push the tooth gently but firmly into the socket.
6. Non-rigid functional splint for 14 days.
7. Check occlusion.
8. Baseline radiographs: periapical or anterior occlusal. Any other teeth injured?
9. Systemic antibiotics, chlorhexidine mouthwash, soft diet as previously.
10. Check tetanus immunization status.

Antibiotics
Tetracycline is first choice for age >12 years at dose appropriate for age and weight for 1 week post replantation. Phenoxymethylpenicillin (Pen V) or Amoxycillin at dose appropriate for age and weight for 1 week post replantation are suitable for children <12 years.

Review

1. Radiograph prior to splint removal at 14 days.

2. Remove splint at 14 days.

3. Endodontics—commence prior to splint removal for categories (b) and (c).

   (a) Open apex, EAT <30–45 minutes. Observe.

   (b) Open apex, EAT >30–45 minutes. Endodontics:

   (i) initial intracanal dressing—antibiotic–steroid paste;

   (ii) subsequent intracanal dressings—non-setting calcium hydroxide paste;

   (iii) replace calcium hydroxide 3 monthly until apical barrier or place MTA plug;

   (iv) obturate canal with GP.

   (c) Closed apex. Endodontics:

   (i) initial intracanal dressing antibiotic–steroid paste;

   (ii) subsequent intracanal dressing with non-setting calcium hydroxide paste;

   (iii) obturate with GP as soon as possible as long as no progressive resorption.

4. Radiographic review: 1 month; 3 months; every 6 months for 2 years; then annually.

5. If resorption is progressing unhalted, keep non-setting calcium hydroxide in the tooth until exfoliation, changing it every 6 months.

The immature tooth with an EAT <30–45 minutes may undergo pulp revascularization (Table 12.2). However, these teeth require regular clinical and radiographic review because once EIR occurs it progresses rapidly.

Replantation of teeth with a dry storage time more than 1 hour

The consensus opinion is that teeth with very immature apices should not be replanted. The incidence of resorption, ankylosis, and subsequent loss is high because of the high rate of bone remodelling in this age group.

Mature teeth with a dry storage time of more than 1 hour will have a non-vital PDL. The necrotic PDL and pulp should be removed at chairside with pumice and water on a bristle brush prior to rinsing with normal saline. The root canal is then obturated with GP and the tooth replanted and splinted for 4 weeks. The aim of this treatment is to produce ankylosis, allowing the tooth to be maintained as a natural space maintainer, perhaps for a limited period only.

Pulpal and periodontal status in PDL injuries

Pulpal necrosis is the most common complication and is related to the severity of the periodontal injury (Table 12.2). Immature teeth have a better prognosis than mature teeth because of the wide apical opening where slight movements can occur without disruption of the apical neurovascular bundle. Necrosis can be diagnosed within 3 months of injury in most cases but sometimes may not be evident for at least 2 years. A combination of clinical and radiological signs is often required to diagnose necrosis.

Sensitivity testing

The majority of injured teeth test negatively to EPT immediately following trauma. Most pulps which recover test positively within months, but responses have been reported as late as 2 years after injury. Therefore a negative test alone should not be regarded as proof of necrosis. Postpone endodontics until at least one other clinical and/or radiographic sign is present.

Tooth discolouration

Initial pinkish discolouration may be due to subtotal severance of apical vessels, leading to penetration of haemoglobin from such ruptures into the dentine tubules. If the vascular system repairs, most of this discolouration will disappear. If the tooth becomes progressively grey, necrosis should be suspected. A grey colour that appears for the first time several weeks or months after trauma signifies decomposition of necrotic pulp tissue and is a decisive sign of necrosis. Colour changes are usually most apparent on the palatal surface of the injured teeth.

Tenderness to percussion

This may be the most reliable isolated indicator of pulpal necrosis.

Periapical inflammation

Radiological periapical involvement secondary to pulp necrosis and infection can be seen as early as 3 weeks after trauma. In mature teeth TAB may be mistaken for periapical inflammation and may be present up to 2–3 months after trauma. It represents the response to an ingrowth of new tissue into the pulp canal.

Arrest of root development

If necrosis involves the epithelial root sheath before root development is complete, no further root growth will occur (see Fig. 12.17). In an injured pulp necrosis may progress from the coronal to the apical portion, and hence residual apical vitality may result in formation of a calcific barrier across a wide apical foramen. Failure of the pulp chamber and root canal to mature and reduce in size on successive radiographs compared with contralateral uninjured teeth is also a reliable indicator of necrosis.

12.7.4 Resorption

Root resorption is a serious and destructive complication which may follow trauma to primary and permanent teeth. Primary teeth which develop pathological resorptive lesions are not good candidates for conservative treatment and should be extracted. However, permanent teeth may often be successfully treated provided that tissue destruction has not advanced to an unrestorable state.

Two general forms of pathological root resorption are recognized—inflammatory and replacement.

Inflammatory root resorption

Internal and external root surfaces injured as a result of trauma are rapidly colonized by multinuclear giant cells. If giant cells are continuously stimulated, most commonly by microbial products from an infected root canal or periodontal pocket, progressive inflammatory root resorption may follow, with catastrophic consequences. Inflammatory root resorption can be classified according to its site of origin as external root resorption, cervical resorption (a special form of external resorption), or internal root resorption. Inflammator resorption is now increasingly being referred to as infection-related resorption.

External inflammatory root resorption

Teeth affected by external inflammatory root resorption are invariably non-vital with infected pulp canals. Resorptive activity is initiated by damage to PDL in trauma but propagated by infected root canal contents seeping to the external root surface through patent dentinal tubules, and may be extremely aggressive. However, if the infected canal contents are removed, the propagating stimulus is lost and the lesion will predictably arrest.

Diagnosis External inflammatory root resorption is usually a chance radiographic finding, and is characterized by a change in the external contour of the root which is often surrounded by a bony lucency (Figs 12.42 and 12.43). Sometimes it may present as a radiolucency overlying the root, and can be distinguished from internal resorption by its asymmetrical shape, the superimposed contour of the intact root canal walls, and the fact that it moves in relation to the root canal on periapical films of different horizontal angle.

Treatment Provided that the tooth is still restorable, external inflammatory root resorption should be treated without delay. Following access cavity preparation, the root canal should be cleaned and shaped, taking care not to weaken the root excessively or to risk perforation into the resorbed area. It is common practice to dress the root canal with non-setting calcium hydroxide paste and to monitor the tooth for several months prior to definitive obturation to ensure that the lesion has arrested. Nevertheless, control of intracanal infection is the key determinant of success, and there is good evidence to suggest that if the canal is adequately prepared, it can be filled without protracted calcium hydroxide treatment.

Periodic clinical and radiographic review should be arranged.

Cervical resorption

Cervical resorption is an unusual form of external inflammatory root resorption initiated by damage to the root surface in the cervical region, and propagated by either infected root canal contents or the periodontal microflora. From a very small entry point, the resorptive process may extend widely before penetrating the pulp chamber (Fig. 12.44).

Diagnosis Extensive intracoronal extension may occasionally present cervical resorption as a clinically visible pink spot. More commonly, it is identified on routine radiographs as a characteristically sited radiolucency (Fig. 12.44).

Treatment If the tooth is non-vital, conventional root canal therapy should be undertaken to eliminate the propagating stimulus. Arrangements should then be made to open the resorptive defect in a similar manner to cavity preparation and to curette away all traces of inflammatory tissue before restoring the resultant defect (Fig. 12.45). Often, a flap must be raised to eliminate resorptive tissue adequately and contour the subgingival restoration.

If the tooth is vital and the pulp has not been invaded, treatment may be limited to opening and curetting the resorption lacuna before placing a setting calcium hydroxide lining and restoring the defect with an appropriate material.

Periodic clinical and radiographic review should be arranged.

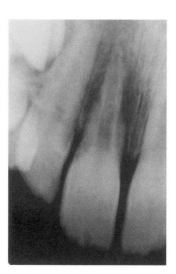

Figure 12.42 External inflammatory resorption.

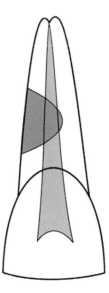

Figure 12.43 External inflammatory root resorption. Usually presents as an asymmetrical radiolucency on the lateral surface of the root. If the lesion overlies the root canal, its lateral walls are usually still visible.

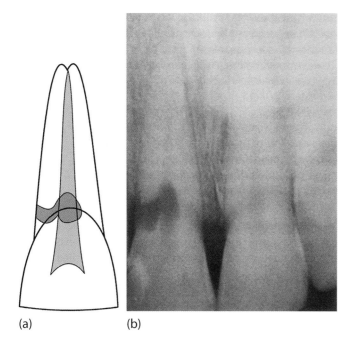

(a)   (b)

Figure 12.44 Cervical resorption. (a) Resorption commences from a small entry point below the gingival crevice and often spreads widely within the crown before the root canal is invaded. The lateral walls of the pulp chamber are often superimposed over the defect. (b) Periapical radiograph showing a typical clinical case.

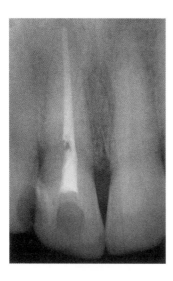

Figure 12.45 Cervical resorption following endodontic treatment of the necrotic pulp and surgical repair of the external defect.

Internal inflammatory root resorption

Internal inflammatory root resorption is seen in the canals of traumatized teeth which are undergoing progressive pulp necrosis. Infected material in the non-vital coronal part of the canal is believed to propagate

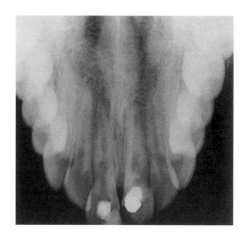

Figure 12.46 Internal inflammatory resorption of both upper central incisors.

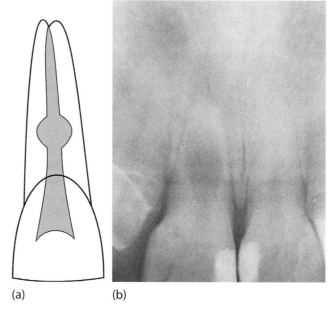

(a)   (b)

Figure 12.47 Internal inflammatory root resorption. (a) Symmetrical expansion of the root canal walls in a permanent central incisor. (b) Periapical radiograph showing a typical clinical case.

resorption by the underlying vital tissue, and rapid tissue destruction follows.

Diagnosis Large resorptive defects affecting the coronal third of the canal may present as a pink discolouration of the affected tooth. More commonly, it is detected as a chance finding on routine radiographic examination. Radiographically, internal resorption presents as a rounded symmetrical radiolucency, centred on the root canal. The contours of the root canal walls are rarely superimposed (Figs 12.46 and 12.47).

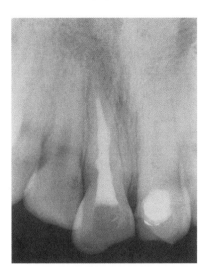

Figure 12.48 Internal inflammatory root resorption. Maxillary central incisor demonstrating internal resorptive defects at two levels. The canal was cleaned, shaped, and obturated with thermoplasticized GP and sealer.

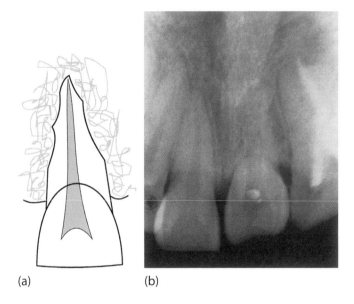

(a)　　　　　　　　(b)

Figure 12.49 Replacement resorption. (a) Roots affected by replacement resorption have ragged outlines, and merge with the surrounding bone to which they are fused. (b) Periapical radiograph showing advanced replacement resorption. Clinically, the tooth is rock solid.

Treatment Internal resorption should be considered to be a form of irreversible pulpitis and treated without delay. Following standard access cavity preparation, the pulp chamber and coronal portion of the canal is usually found to contain necrotic debris. However, deeper penetration of the canal often provokes torrential haemorrhage as the vascular resorptive tissue is entered.

Root canal preparation is undertaken in the usual manner, and following apical enlargement haemorrhage from the canal is greatly reduced as the blood supply to the resorptive tissue is severed. Instrumentation of the expanded resorbed area is difficult, and can be greatly enhanced by the use of sonic or ultrasonic devices which are able to throw irrigant into uninstrumented areas. The antimicrobial and tissue solvent actions of sodium hypochlorite make it the irrigant of choice in such cases.

As in the case of external inflammatory resorption, it is usual to dress the canal with non-setting calcium hydroxide following debridement. This may be highly advantageous in the internal resorption case where the antimicrobial and mild tissue solvent actions of calcium hydroxide can be exploited further to clean the resorbed area.

Obturation can then be undertaken with GP and sealer, usually employing a thermoplastic technique to allow satisfactory condensation and adaptation in the resorbed area (Fig. 12.48). Where internal reinforcement is indicated, dual curing composite resin and fibre posts may offer some advantages over full canal filling with GP and sealer.

Replacement resorption

Replacement resorption is a distinct form of root resorption which follows serious luxation or avulsion injury that has caused damage to the investing periodontal ligament. A classic scenario is an avulsed tooth which has been stored dry, or PDL removed before replantation with resultant death of periodontal fibroblasts on much of the root surface. If more than 20% of the periodontal ligament is damaged or lost and the tooth is subsequently reimplanted, bone cells are able to grow into contact with the root surface more quickly than the remaining periodontal fibroblasts are able to recolonize the root surface and intervene between tooth and bone. The consequence is that the root now becomes involved in the normal remodelling process of the bone in which it is implanted, and is gradually replaced by bone over the course of the following years. In young children where the rate of bone remodelling is high, the root may be entirely lost within 3–4 years. In adolescents, it may be 10 years or more before the tooth is lost.

Diagnosis

The absence of a ligamentous joint between the tooth and its supporting bone (ankylosis) means that even when root resorption is advanced, the tooth will appear rock solid. A bright metallic tone will also be noted if the tooth is percussed. Radiographically, the root will appear ragged in outline, with no obvious periodontal ligament space separating it from the surrounding bone (Fig. 12.49).

Treatment

There is no effective treatment for ankylosis but the rate of progression is relatively slow and in many cases the tooth can be maintained for 10 years or more. However, in many cases the ankylosed tooth shows severe infra-occlusion and in the growing child it may cease to 'move' or 'grow' with the rest of the jaws and cannot be moved orthodontically (Fig. 12.50) This infra-occlusion means that the alveolar bone in this region will not develop and will appear to move further and further in the apical direction. Once the discrepancy in

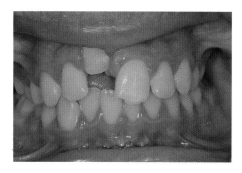

Figure 12.50 Severe infra-occlusion. Clinicians should monitor ankylosed teeth closely and not allow such a situation to develop.

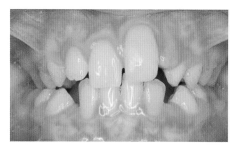

Figure 12.51 Moderate ankylosis of the left upper central incisor. Once this is detected, the ankylosed tooth should be decoronated and the ankylosed root buried in the alveolar bone.

the gingival margins of the ankylosed tooth compared with the contralateral unaffected tooth is deemed to be more than 1–2mm, clinicians should consider decoronating this tooth and removing root canal filling materials from the retained root in order to maintain the bone levels to facilitate future placement of an autotransplant (see also Chapter 15) or an implant in this region (Fig. 12.51). The root left behind is slowly resorbed, but importantly is replaced with bone, thereby maintaining the bone in that region. Failure to do this results in the bone in the region being of inadequate quantity or quality for an implant or autotransplantation procedure to be carried out, and bone augmentation would probably be necessary in the future. An example of decoronation is shown in Fig. 12.52.

From an endodontic point of view, it is important to reiterate that if pulp extirpation is undertaken within 2 weeks of reimplantation, the initial root canal dressing should not be calcium hydroxide. There is some evidence that placement of the highly alkaline calcium hydroxide in the first 2 weeks increases the risk of ankylosis because it can have an inflammatory effect on the periodontal ligament which is already inflamed. After extirpation the canal should be left empty for the first 2 weeks or an antibiotic–steroid preparation can be used, which should be replaced subsequently with non-setting calcium hydroxide, but no sooner than 2 weeks after tooth reimplantation. The antibiotic–steroid paste may help to reduce subsequent resorption, although the authors advise against the use of Ledermix which causes severe discolouration of the teeth.

If endodontic treatment is not undertaken soon after reimplantation and the tooth subsequently loses vitality, conventional root canal therapy may be used in order to address any painful periapical pathosis and to avoid the additional insult of inflammatory resorption which would lead to more rapid loss of root substance. A resorbable root filling material, such as root canal sealer alone or reinforced zinc oxide–eugenol cement, may be preferred to GP in some cases.

Where resorption is progressive, consideration should be given to autotransplantation of either an upper second premolar or a lower first or second premolar if any of these teeth are to be removed as part of an orthodontic treatment plan. If autotransplantation is completed while the root of the premolar is about two-thirds formed, there is a good chance of revascularization and further root growth (Fig. 12.53). If the autotransplanted tooth has a mature apex, revascularization is unlikely, and the tooth should be extirpated at splint removal and the canal left empty for 2 weeks and then dressed with non-setting calcium hydroxide. The tooth can be obturated with GP when there is no evidence of progressive resorption. (See Key Points 12.7.) See also Section 15.5.7 which describes the technique of autotransplantation.

Key Points 12.7

Pathological root resorption

- Inflammatory resorption: external (including cervical) and internal.
- Inflammatory resorption may arrest if cause is removed.
- Replacement resorption is not amenable to treatment.
- Maintain a resorbing tooth for as long as possible. It is the best space maintainer!
- For moderate to severe infra-occlusion decoronation should be carried out to preserve the alveolar bone in that region and to facilitate future placement of autotransplant or implant in the region.

12.7.5 Pulp canal obliteration

There is progressive hard tissue formation within the pulp cavity leading to a gradual narrowing of the pulp chamber and root canal and partial or total obliteration. There is a reduced response to vitality testing and the crown appears slightly yellow/opaque. The exact initiating factor which produces this response from the odontoblasts is unknown. It is more common in immature teeth and luxation injuries than in concussion and subluxation injuries. Although radiographs may suggest complete calcification, a minute strand of pulpal tissue usually remains. Pulpal obliteration has been described as 'nature's own root filling', and although late development of necrosis and infection in the thin thread of pulpal tissue in the sclerosed canal has been reported, it is less common than the endodontic complications that would be necessary to treat it. The obturation of an 'obliterating' canal is not justification for pre-eruptive root canal treatment in the absence of signs of pulp breakdown.

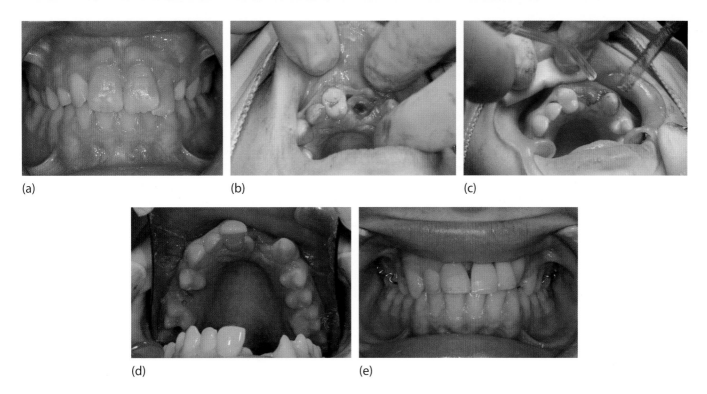

Figure 12.52 Example of decoronation. (a) Ankylosed upper central incisors. (b) The upper right central incisor was extracted and replaced with a premolar autotransplant and the left upper central incisor was decoronated below the level of the alveolar bone margin. (c) Primary closure over the root of the left upper central incisor ensures that the alveolar bone height will be maintained as the remaining root will be resorbed and replaced with bone. (d) The level of the alveolar bone is then maintained in that position. (e) The autotransplant in the position of the right upper central incisor built up and a partial denture replacing the decoronated left central incisor.

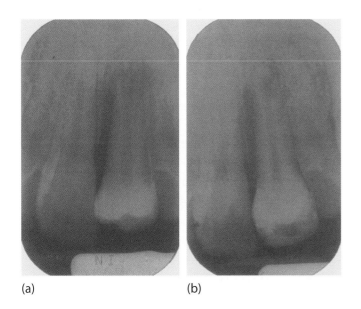

Figure 12.53 (a) Autotransplanted premolar in 21 position. (b) Continued growth and revascularization of autotransplanted premolar.

12.7.6 Injuries to the supporting bone

The extent and position of the alveolar fracture should be verified clinically and radiographically. If there is displacement of the teeth to the extent that their apices have risen up and are now positioned over the labial or lingual/palatal alveolar plates ('apical lock'), they will require extruding first to free the apices prior to repositioning. The segment of alveolus with teeth requires only 3–4 weeks of rigid splintage (composite wire type) with two abutment teeth either side of the fracture (Fig. 12.54), together with antibiotics, chlorhexidine, soft diet, and a tetanus prophylaxis check. Pulpal survival is more likely if repositioning occurs within an hour of the injury. Root resorption is rare.

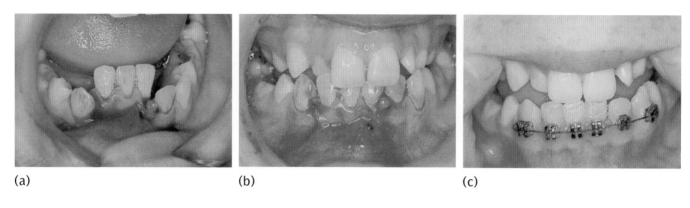

(a)   (b)   (c)

Figure 12.54 (a) Dento-alveolar fracture of the lower labial segment. (b) Fracture reduced into the correct occlusion. (c) Splint *in situ* prior to removal.

12.8 Child physical abuse

A child is considered to be abused if he/she is treated in a way that is unacceptable in a given culture at a given time (see Fig. 12.4). Child physical abuse or non-accidental injury (NAI) is now recognized as an international issue and has been reported in many countries. Each week one or two children in the UK and 80 children per month in the USA will die as a result of abuse or neglect. At least one child per 1000 in the UK suffers severe physical abuse (e.g. fractures, brain haemorrhage, severe internal injuries, or mutilation), and in the USA more than 95% of serious intracranial injuries during the first year of life are the result of abuse. Although some reports prove to be unfounded, the common experience is that proven cases of child abuse are four to five times as common as they were a decade ago. Physical abuse is not a full diagnosis; it is merely a symptom of disordered parenting. The aim of intervention is to diagnose and cure the disordered parenting. It has been estimated that 35–50% of severely abused children in the USA will receive serious re-injury and 50% will die if they are returned to their home environment without intervention. In some cases the occurrence of physical abuse may provide an opportunity for intervention. If this opportunity is missed, there may be no further opportunity for many years.

More than 50% of cases diagnosed as physical abuse have extra- and intra-oral facial trauma, and so the dental practitioner may be the first professional to see or suspect abuse. Injuries may take the form of contusions and ecchymoses (Fig. 12.55), abrasions and lacerations, burns, bites, dental trauma (Fig. 12.56), and fractures. The incidence of common orofacial injuries is shown in Table 12.4.

The following 11 points should be considered whenever doubts and suspicions are aroused about an injury:

1. Could the injury have been caused accidentally and if so how?

2. Does the explanation of the injury fit the age of the child and the clinical findings?

3. If the explanation of cause is consistent with the injury, is this itself within normally acceptable limits of behaviour?

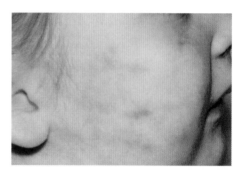

Figure 12.55 Characteristic parallel bruising of a slap mark. (Reproduced from Andreasen and Andreasen, *Textbook and Colour Atlas of Traumatic Injuries to the Teeth*, 3rd edition, with permission from John Wiley & Sons.)

4. If there has been any delay seeking advice are there good reasons for this?

5. Does the story of the accident vary?

6. The nature of the relationship between parent and child.

7. The child's reaction to other people.

8. The child's reaction to any medical/dental examinations.

9. The general demeanour of the child.

10. Any comments made by the child and/or parent that give concern about the child's upbringing or lifestyle.

11. History of previous injury.

Dental professionals should be aware of any established system in their locality which is designed to cope with these cases. Recognition of physical abuse, emotional abuse, sexual abuse, and neglect, and how to respond are discussed in greater detail in Chapter 18.

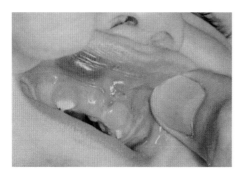

Figure 12.56 A torn labial frenum in a young child not yet learning to walk could be an indicator of a non-accidental injury. (Reproduced from Andreasen and Andreasen, *Textbook and Colour Atlas of Traumatic Injuries to the Teeth*, 3rd edition, with permission from John Wiley & Sons.)

Table 12.4 The incidence of common orofacial injuries in physical abuse

	Type of injury	Incidence (%)
Extra-oral	Contusions and ecchymoses	66
	Abrasions and lacerations	28
	Burns and bites	4
	Fractures	2
Intra-oral	Contusions and ecchymoses	43
	Abrasions and lacerations (including frenal tears)	29
	Dental trauma	29

12.9 Summary

1. Boys experience dental trauma almost twice as often as girls.
2. Maxillary central incisors are the most commonly involved teeth.
3. Regular clinical and radiographic review is necessary to limit unwanted sequelae, institute appropriate treatment, and improve prognosis.
4. Injuries to the developing permanent dentition occur in half of all trauma to the primary dentition.
5. Splinting for avulsion, luxation, and root fractures should be functional to allow physiological movement and promote normal healing of the PDL. Splinting for dento-alveolar fractures should be rigid.
6. In all luxation injuries the prognosis for pulpal healing is better with an immature apex.
7. Root resorption increases with the severity of damage to the PDL.
8. The prognosis for replantation of avulsed teeth is best if it is undertaken within an hour of the injury with a hydrated PDL.
9. Orofacial injuries are found in at least 50% of cases of physical abuse.
10. Successful endodontics demands the cooperation of a comfortable child. Effective local anaesthesia should be provided if there is any risk of pain during treatment.
11. From indirect pulp capping to non-vital pulp therapy, control of microbial infection is the key determinant of endodontic treatment success. A well-fitting rubber dam should be in place wherever possible, and all stages of all endodontic procedures should be conducted with due regard to the elimination of infection and the prevention of its recurrence.
12. Root canal systems in young teeth are cleaned principally by antimicrobial and tissue-solvent irrigants and medicaments, not by exuberant dentine removal. Dentine removal, especially in fragile primary and young permanent teeth, should be rational and restricted to that required for effective irrigation and successful obturation only.

12.10 Further reading

Andreasen, J.O. and Andreasen, F.M. (1994). *Textbook and colour atlas of traumatic injuries to the teeth* (3rd edn). Munksgaard, Copenhagen. (*An excellent reference book with colour slides of each clinical procedure.*)

Andreasen, J.O., Borum, M.K., Jacobsen, H.L., and Andreasen, F.M. (1995). Replantation of 400 avulsed permanent incisors. *Endodontics and Dental Traumatology*, **11**, 51–89. (*The largest published series on avulsed permanent incisors.*)

Andreasen, J.O., Andreasen, F.M., Mejàre, I., and Cvek, M. (2004). Healing of 400 intra-alveolar root fractures: effect of treatment factors such as treatment delay, repositioning, splinting type and period and antibiotics. *Dental Traumatology*, **20**, 203–11.

Cohen, S. and Burns, R.C. (2001). *Pathways of the pulp* (8th edn). Mosby, St Louis, MO. (*The definitive endodontic reference book.*)

European Society of Endodontology (1994). Consensus report of the European Society of Endodontology on quality guidelines for endodontic treatment. *International Endodontic Journal*, **27**, 115–24. (*A synopsis of current terminology and good practice in endodontics.*)

International Association of Dental Traumatology (2012). Guidelines for the management of traumatic dental injuries. 1. Fractures and luxations of permanent teeth. 2. Avulsion of permanent teeth. 3. Injuries to primary teeth. *Dental Traumatology*, **28**, 2–12, 88–96.

Kindelan, S.A., Day, P.F., Kindelan, J.D., Spencer, J.R., and Duggal, M.S. (2008). Dental trauma: an overview of its influence on the management of orthodontic treatment. Part 1. *Journal of Orthodontics*, **35**, 68–78.

Kinirons, M.J. (1998). Treatment of traumatically intruded permanent incisor teeth. *International Journal of Paediatric Dentistry*, **8**, 165–8. (*UK National Clinical Guideline*.)

Welbury, R.R. (2007). Child physical abuse (non-accidental injury) In *Textbook and colour atlas of traumatic injuries to the teeth* (4th edn) (eds J.O. Andreasen, F.M. Andreasen, and L. Andersson). Munksgaard, Copenhagen. (*A reference of prevalence and orofacial signs in non-accidental injury*.)

12.11 References

Banchs, F. and Trope, M. (2004). Revascularization of immature permanent teeth with apical periodontitis: new treatment protocol? *Journal of Endodontics*, **30**, 196–200.

Cvek, M. (1992). Prognosis of luxated non-vital maxillary incisors treated with calcium hydroxide and filled with gutta-percha. A retrospective clinical study. *Endodontics and Dental Traumatology*, **8**, 45–55.

Pradhan, D.P., Chawla, H.S., Gauba, K., and Goyal, A. (2006). Comparative evaluation of endodontic management of teeth with unformed apices with mineral trioxide aggregate and calcium hydroxide. *Journal of Dentistry for Children*, **73**, 79–85.

13

Anomalies of tooth formation and eruption

P.J.M. Crawford and M.J. Aldred

Chapter contents

13.1 Introduction

Both the primary and permanent dentitions may be affected by variations in the number, size, and form of the teeth, as well as the structure of the dental hard tissues. These variations may be exclusively genetically determined, brought about by either local or systemically acting environmental factors, or possibly a combination of both genetic and environmental factors acting together. The same interplay of influences may affect the eruption and exfoliation of primary teeth, as well as the eruption of permanent teeth. This chapter considers a range of conditions involving abnormalities of the number, size, form, and structure of teeth and their eruption.

It is important to be aware of the psychosocial aspect when meeting children and families affected by these conditions. We have too often heard stories of social isolation of even very young children as a result of their missing or discoloured teeth. In the case of discoloured teeth, parents have told us that they have been taken to task by other adults for not looking after their child's teeth when the discolouration was intrinsic and unavoidable. Society's preoccupation with 'the perfect smile' seems to increase and, in a world where employment opportunities are at a premium, children denied access to dental aesthetic adjustment may be genuinely disadvantaged.

While investigating inherited conditions, it is important to enquire of both sides of the family tree equally. Not only does this ensure that the investigation is complete, but also it may help to alleviate any sense of 'guilt' felt by an affected parent.

Wherever possible, we try to avoid the use of the word 'normal' in our clinical care, although the word will be used in this text. The vast majority of children with these conditions want to become 'one of the crowd'. Thus we would speak, when offering restorative treatment for example, of making a smile 'ordinary' or 'boring'. We have found this approach successful in our practices; our readers may choose this or one of many other approaches in order to further the care of these children.

We have been questioned repeatedly about the possibility of genetic treatment for some of these inherited conditions. We are not aware of any progress in this direction at present.

13.2 Missing teeth

Hypodontia is the term most often applied to a situation where a patient has missing teeth as a result of their failure of development. Anodontia describes the total lack of teeth of one or both dentitions. Oligodontia is a term used to describe a situation where multiple (usually more than six) teeth are missing.

13.2.1 Prevalence

In the primary dentition, missing teeth occur more commonly in the maxilla and typically the maxillary lateral incisor is the tooth involved. Various studies have shown the prevalence of missing primary teeth to be between 0.1% and 0.9% of Caucasian populations, with males and females affected equally. Developmentally missing permanent teeth are seen in both the maxilla and mandible (Fig. 13.1). In Caucasian populations the third molars are the most common missing teeth, followed by the mandibular second premolar, the maxillary lateral incisor, and then the maxillary second premolar. A female-to-male ratio of 4:1 has been reported. Missing third molars occur in 9–30% of individuals. If the third molars are excluded, the prevalence in the permanent dentition varies between 3.5% and 6.5% according to the study quoted. (See Key Points 13.1.)

Figure 13.1 Hypodontia, absent 41, retained 81.

13.2.2 Aetiology

The cause of an isolated developmentally missing tooth is often unclear; this is most likely to be genetic in origin. Rarely, it may be a consequence of some environmental insult during development. Missing teeth have been reported in association with multiple births, low birth weight, and increased maternal age. Rubella and thalidomide embryopathies may also be associated with missing teeth.

Single-gene disorders have been associated with missing teeth. Multiple missing teeth, as well as teeth with small crowns, may be seen in a number of syndromes including X-linked hypohidrotic ectodermal dysplasia (Fig. 13.2), autosomal dominant and autosomal recessive cases of ectodermal dysplasia, and autosomal recessive chondroectodermal dysplasia (Ellis–van Creveld syndrome). Down syndrome (trisomy 21) is also associated with hypodontia.

Hypodontia and microdontia involving the maxillary lateral incisor occur in clefts involving the lip and palate. X-linked hypohidrotic ectodermal dysplasia is characterized in males by thin sparse hair, dry skin, absence of sweating (and therefore heat intolerance), and multiple missing teeth. These children are at risk because of their inability

---

Key Points 13.1

Hypodontia
- 0.1–0.9% in the primary dentition
- 3.5–6.5% in the permanent dentition
- Missing permanent teeth are seen in 30–50% of patients who have missing primary teeth

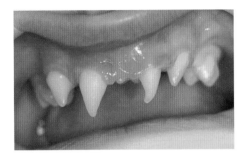

Figure 13.2 Hypohidrotic ectodermal dysplasia: erupted permanent teeth.

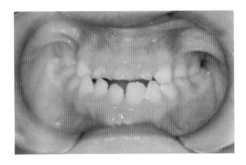

Figure 13.3 Median maxillary central incisor syndrome.

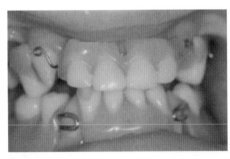

(a)

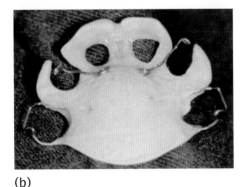

(b)

Figure 13.4 (a) Hypohidrotic ectodermal dysplasia: (b) erupted permanent teeth masked by a 'porthole' denture with canine retractors during eruption.

to cool themselves and may die of hyperthermia in infancy if undiagnosed. This condition, while rare, is of particular importance as the dental professional may be the first to come to a diagnosis, and thus introduce families to support mechanisms. In heterozygous females the changes are milder and may be restricted to the teeth, although a distinctive facial profile (slight retrusion of the maxilla) may be recognized. Most commonly, one or both maxillary lateral incisors and/or the second premolars are missing. In some patients one or both of the maxillary lateral incisors may be of peg form. The responsible gene is the *ED1* gene on the X chromosome which encodes the protein ectodysplasin-A.

Autosomal dominant inheritance of missing teeth is seen in families with mutations in the *MSX1* gene on chromosome 4. Missing third molars and second premolars are the most common finding. These families may also have clefting segregating with the missing teeth. Mutations in the *MSX1* gene are also seen in the tooth-nail (Witkop) syndrome.

A pattern of autosomally dominant inheritance of missing teeth, particularly molars, is seen as a result of mutations in the *PAX9* gene on chromosome 14.

Some patients with a solitary median maxillary central incisor in combination with other developmental defects have been found to have mutations in the sonic hedgehog (*SHH*) gene on chromosome 7 (Fig. 13.3).

13.2.3 Treatment

The care of children with multiple missing teeth can be complex and ideally requires multidisciplinary input from paediatric dentists, orthodontists, and prosthodontists, as well as genetic counselling. Active repeated preventive input and support is essential, and the general practitioner has a large part to play in the underpinning care of these children. Missing teeth and small teeth often present together, and so masking conical or similarly distinctive teeth with composite is strongly advised. This is possible from a very early age and can be made easier by using laboratory-made composite 'onlay crowns' cemented with flowable composite. In cases of anodontia, full dentures are required. These can be provided, albeit with likely limited success, from about 3 years of age, with the possibility of implant support for prostheses provided in adulthood (Fig. 13.4). Multiple missing teeth can be treated using partial dentures, with implants as part of the treatment protocol at a later age. Implant placement is best left until skeletal maturity. Dentures will need to be replaced as the jaws grow; 'holes' may have to be provided within the denture base for teeth to erupt through, thereby masking their form until an appropriate time for crown modification. Progressive provision of dentures with annual replacements during the school holidays (the long vacation), mimicking the developing dentition at the child's age, can do much to minimize the stigma of these conditions. Although, ultimately, dentures can be retained by implants, the lack of development of the alveolar bone may prove to be a limiting factor.

13.3 Extra teeth

Extra teeth (supernumerary teeth) have been reported to occur in 0.2–0.8% of Caucasians in the primary dentition and 1.5–3.5% in the permanent dentition in the same populations. There is a male-to-female ratio of approximately 2:1. Patients with supernumerary primary teeth have a 30–50% chance of these being followed by supernumerary permanent teeth. Teeth that resemble those of the normal series are referred to as supplemental teeth (Fig. 13.5) while those of less typical, often reduced, form—sometimes further described as tuberculate or conical—may be termed accessory supernumerary teeth.

Supernumerary teeth are most often located in the anterior maxilla in or immediately adjacent to the midline, and are then referred to as a mesiodens. Supernumerary teeth in the molar regions adjacent or distal to the normal sequence of teeth are referred to as paramolars or distomolars, respectively. In some cases the supernumerary teeth may be an odontome.

Supernumerary teeth are more common in the maxilla than in the mandible, with a ratio of about 5:1. Apart from those in the midline, they may be present bilaterally and symmetrically; hence the presence of a supernumerary in one part of the jaw should lead to consideration of further supernumeraries elsewhere. Supernumerary teeth may fail to erupt and may delay eruption of a permanent tooth which is developing deeper within the jaw. This commonly occurs in the case of a mesiodens (Fig. 13.6).

There is a significant association between supernumerary teeth and invaginated teeth (see Section 13.5.3). There is also an association with palatal clefts, with approximately 40% of patients with a cleft of the anterior palate having supernumerary teeth.

Multiple supernumerary teeth are seen in cleidocranial dysplasia as well as in other syndromes such as oral–facial–digital syndrome type 1 and Gardner syndrome. The management of supernumerary teeth is discussed in Chapter 14. (See Key Points 13.2.)

> **Key Points 13.2**
>
> Supernumerary teeth:
> - 0.2–0.8% of the primary dentition
> - 1.5–3.5% of the permanent dentition
> - male-to-female ratio 2:1
> - maxilla-to-mandible ratio 5:1

13.4 Abnormality of tooth size

13.4.1 Crown size

There is a degree of subjectivity regarding what constitutes normal ('ordinary') tooth size (and shape). Teeth which are obviously larger than normal are referred to as megadont or macrodont, whereas teeth which are smaller than normal are termed microdont. Crown size is often related to root size, so teeth with large crowns often have large (broad) roots, while teeth with small crowns tend to have small (slender) roots. Microdontia can be associated with hypodontia, as in the example of X-linked hypohidrotic ectodermal dysplasia where a heterozygous female might have one missing lateral incisor and a peg-shaped crown of the contralateral maxillary lateral incisor (Fig. 13.7).

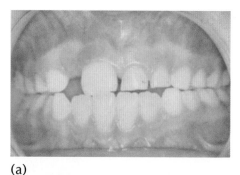

(a)

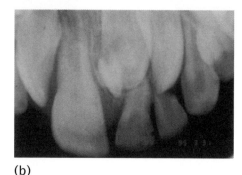

(b)

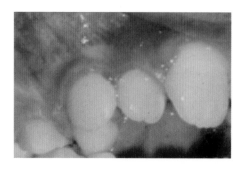

Figure 13.5 Supplemental tooth 12.

Figure 13.6 (a) Clinical and (b) radiographic views of a supernumerary tooth delaying the exfoliation of teeth 61 and 62, and the eruption of tooth 21.

Megadont teeth

Megadont maxillary incisors can occur as a result of fusion of adjacent tooth-germs or as a result of an attempt at separation of a single tooth-germ to form two separate teeth (gemination). To determine which of these possibilities has occurred, it is necessary to count the number of teeth—in fusion there will be a reduced number of teeth, and in gemination there will be a normal number with one larger tooth or an increased number if the division of the one tooth-germ into two is complete. The permanent maxillary central incisors are most often affected (Fig. 13.8) followed by the mandibular second premolars. Isolated megadontia in the permanent dentition has been estimated to occur in approximately 1% of patients. The condition may be symmetrical. Generalized megadontia has been reported in association with pituitary gigantism, unilateral facial hyperplasia, and hereditary gingival fibromatosis.

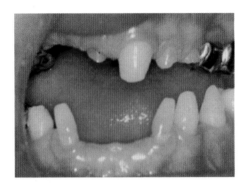

Figure 13.7 Hypodontia concurrent with microdontia.

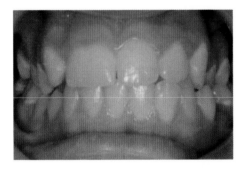

Figure 13.8 Megadont tooth 11, absent tooth 12.

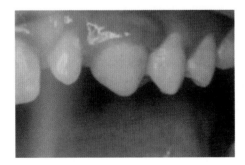

Figure 13.9 Isolated microdontia affecting 22 in a female. The gingival architecture is suggestive of occult cleft.

Microdontia

Microdont primary teeth are uncommon, with a reported prevalence of 0.2–0.5%. In the permanent dentition the prevalence is approximately 2.5% for individual teeth, with generalized microdontia occurring in approximately 0.2% of individuals. Females are more often affected than males, with the maxillary lateral incisor being most commonly affected, having a peg-shaped or conical crown (Fig. 13.9). As noted in Section 13.2, there is an association between microdontia and hypodontia.

13.4.2 Root size

Root length appears to be subject to some racial variation, with shorter roots being seen in people of Oriental background and larger roots in patients of African origin.

Large root size

Larger than normal roots are most typically seen affecting the permanent maxillary central incisors, with a population prevalence in one Swedish study of 2.3%. Males were four times more likely to be affected than females.

Small root size

Short-rooted teeth in the primary dentition may be associated with other dental abnormalities. Short roots may also be seen in a number of conditions affecting the dentine and/or pulp. These will be considered in a later section.

Short roots may be seen affecting the permanent maxillary central incisors. The shortening affects approximately 2.5% of children and some 15% of these may have shortened roots on other teeth, most often premolars and/or canines. The cause is often unknown, although it can occur as a result of orthodontic treatment.

In regional odontodysplasia (Section 13.7.1) there is typically abnormal root formation as well as abnormalities of the crowns of the teeth.

Irradiation of the jaws or chemotherapy during the period of root formation may lead to truncation of roots which were developing at the time of treatment (Fig. 13.10).

13.4.3 Treatment

As with hypodontia, the active cooperation of paediatric dentist, orthodontist, and restorative dentist should be encouraged to optimize treatment planning for young people affected by these conditions from an early age.

A megadont maxillary central incisor can be cosmetically unaesthetic and treatment decisions may need to be considered soon after (or, in some cases, before) eruption of the tooth. The options include acceptance, remodelling of the tooth, extraction of the tooth with orthodontic treatment if necessary, and subsequent masking of the space with a bridge, denture, or implant (Fig. 13.11).

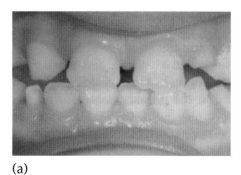

(a)

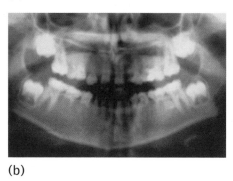

(b)

Figure 13.10 (a) Clinical and (b) radiographic views showing disturbed dental development following chemotherapy for leukaemia.

A microdont tooth, particularly if this affects the maxillary lateral incisors, can be modified by the addition of acid-etch composite material to the tooth to reproduce the typical contours of the crown (Fig. 13.12). In adult life, porcelain veneers may also be used or the tooth can be crowned. However, the continued use of composite has the benefit of minimal tooth preparation and delay of the start of the 'restorative cycle' with its ultimate end in the loss of the tooth.

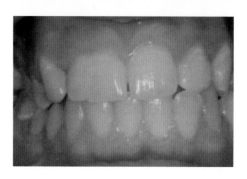

Figure 13.11 Megadont tooth 11. Minimal adjustment of tooth form 11, 13, from its original state in Fig. 13.8.

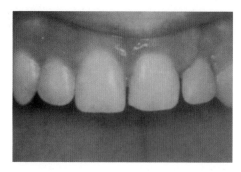

Figure 13.12 Isolated microdontia affecting 22 in a female. Restored with composite.

13.5 Abnormality of tooth form

13.5.1 Abnormality of crown form

Fusion and gemination

Some cases of megadont crowns are due to fusion of adjacent tooth-germs (fusion) or attempts at developmental separation of a single tooth-germ to produce two separate teeth (gemination), and a variety of terms have been used for such situations. The term 'double teeth' has been applied to cover both situations. It is necessary to count the number of teeth present clinically and with the aid of radiographs determine whether fusion or gemination has occurred. The prevalence of such abnormalities in the primary dentition ranges from 0.5% to 1.6% of Caucasian populations studied. The permanent dentition is less commonly affected (prevalence 0.1–0.2%). Males and females are affected equally. A genetic basis has been suggested, but not confirmed.

The clinical manifestation may vary from a minor notch on the incisal edge of an abnormally wide incisor crown to two separate crowns with a single root. The crowns and root may be in continuity along their entire length or may be almost separate; some pulp intercommunication is

often present. The most typical areas affected are the anterior segments of the arches in the primary dentition, with the mandible more commonly affected than the maxilla (Fig. 13.13). There may be an association with hypodontia, so that a larger than normal tooth of the primary series together with a missing tooth in that series may represent an intermediate stage between the presence or absence of a tooth.

Physiological root resorption of primary fused or geminated teeth may be delayed and this may lead to delayed eruption of the permanent successors.

Treatment

When this condition affects the primary dentition no treatment *per se* is required. However, it is important to consider the possibility of abnormalities of the number and/or form of the permanent dentition in the area. One problem which can occur is that caries can develop at the interface between the two crown segments (Fig. 13.14). This can be prevented by an etch-retained sealant before any decay has occurred, or a similar restoration to fill in the defect, which will also improve the cosmetic

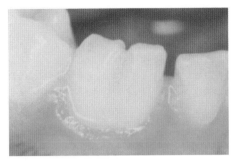

(a)

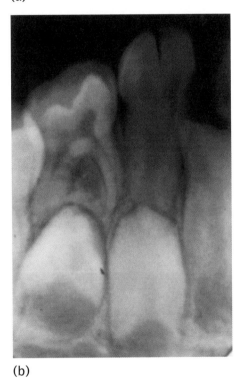

(b)

Figure 13.13 (a) Clinical and (b) radiographic appearance of geminated lower primary lateral incisor/canine.

appearance. In the permanent dentition, the final decision on whether to retain, extract, surgically divide, or otherwise treat such teeth will depend on many factors including space available within the arch, the morphology of the pulp chambers and/or root canals, and the degree of attachment between the two parts of the tooth or teeth. (See Key Points 13.3.)

Key Points 13.3

Double teeth:

- 0.5–1.6% in the primary dentition
- 0.1–0.2% in the permanent dentition
- no sex predilection
- permanent anomalies in 30–50% of primary cases

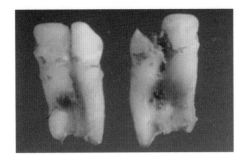

Figure 13.14 Caries in extracted geminated teeth.

13.5.2 Accessory cusps

Extra cusps are not uncommon in the human dentition and may occur in both the primary and permanent dentition, most commonly affecting molar teeth. In the primary dentition the most common accessory cusps are seen on either the mesiobuccal aspect of the maxillary first molar or the mesiopalatal aspect of the maxillary second molar, the latter being similar to the cusp of Carabelli seen on the first permanent molar. The latter is a relatively frequent finding on the mesiopalatal aspect of the crown of the maxillary first molars, is typically bilateral, and may be seen in 10–60% of various populations. Permanent incisor teeth may have an additional cusp arising from the cingulum, often referred to as a 'talon cusp'. This most commonly affects the maxillary central incisor. Talon cusps may interfere with the occlusion and may be aesthetically unpleasing (Fig. 13.15). As with double teeth, caries may occur in the groove between the cusp and the palatal surface of the incisor. Other incisor evaginations have been reported (Fig. 13.16). Permanent canines may also have a prominent lingual/palatal cusp, perhaps indicating a tendency towards a premolar tooth form. Additional cusps may uncommonly be seen on premolars.

Treatment

The talon cusp may require action for both aesthetic and occlusal reasons. Selective grinding, repeated over a period of time, will reduce the height of the cusp and allow deposition of reactionary dentine on the pulpal surface of the dentine. Single-visit sectioning of the cusp from the tooth followed by elective pulpotomy can also be considered.

13.5.3 Invaginated teeth

This term refers to the presence of an invagination in the crown of the tooth, forming an infolding lined by enamel within the crown of the tooth and sometimes extending into the root. An invagination of enamel epithelium into the dental papilla during development leads to the formation of the abnormality. The terms invaginated tooth or dens invaginatus can be used; other terms commonly applied (but not necessarily correctly) are dens in dente, gestant composite odontome, and dilated composite odontome.

The maxillary lateral incisor is the most commonly affected tooth (Fig. 13.17). The maxillary central incisors are less commonly affected, and occasionally the canines are affected. In its mildest form

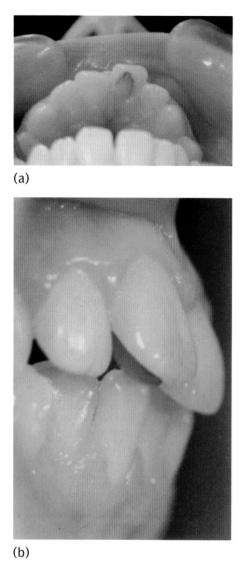

(a)

(b)

Figure 13.15 Accessory cusps—talon cusp with plaque accumulation interfering with the occlusion.

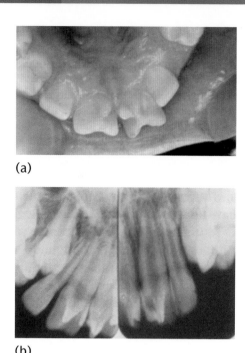

(a)

(b)

Figure 13.16 (a) Clinical and (b) radiographic appearance of accessory cusps—triform and cruciform teeth, 11, 21.

an invaginated tooth is typically a maxillary lateral incisor with a deep cingulum pit on the palatal aspect of the crown. In its more extreme form the invagination is associated with grossly abnormal crown and root forms (Fig. 13.18). In these gross examples the crown is tuberculate with the invagination appearing on the cusp (which is the modified incisal edge) of the abnormal tooth. Radiographs show the extent of the invagination chamber. Enamel, which may be extremely thin or even absent, can be seen lining this chamber. The pulp may be displaced and surround the invagination cavity, appearing radiographically as narrow slits around the dentine forming the wall of the invagination. Sometimes the root is significantly expanded.

Invagination of primary teeth is uncommon, but in the permanent dentition has been estimated to affect between 1% and 5% of different groups. Males are more commonly affected than females, with a ratio of 2:1. Invaginations may also differ in different racial groups, with people of Chinese ethnicity being reportedly more commonly affected.

Invaginated teeth may cause problems because of the development of caries and pulpal pathology. This can occur soon after tooth eruption, with the child presenting with an acute abscess or facial cellulitis. In such cases the radiograph will invariably demonstrate incomplete root formation as well as periapical rarefaction (Fig. 13.17). The presence of one invaginated tooth should lead to consideration of the contralateral tooth and/or adjacent teeth being affected. Invaginations are often bilateral, although not necessarily symmetrical. Some patients with invaginated teeth may also have supernumerary teeth, and therefore a full radiographic examination is warranted.

Treatment

If invaginations are identified at an early stage after eruption of the tooth, etch-retained resin sealants can be placed to prevent bacteria entering the invagination and the subsequent development of caries. Acute infective episodes, particularly when associated with cellulitis, should be treated with incision and drainage of any pointing abscess, as well as appropriate antibiotic therapy. The tooth should be opened, or extracted if the long-term prognosis is poor. This tends to be the case with the more gross examples where the crown and root form are abnormal. In less extreme forms endodontic treatment, firstly involving apexification, can be considered.

13.5.4 Evaginated teeth

Evagination, or dens evaginatus, most commonly affects the premolar teeth. Permanent molar teeth may also be affected. Typically there is a small tubercle on the occlusal surface of the premolar in the central

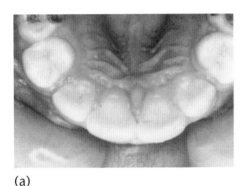

(a)

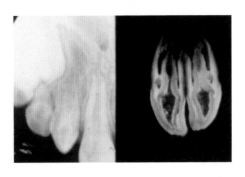

Figure 13.18 Infected invaginated odontome, tooth 12.

part of the fissure pattern. The condition is more common in patients of Chinese descent and has been estimated to occur in 1–4% of this group. The evaginations are typically fractured off or eroded by normal wear, leading to pulpal exposure, pulpal pathology, and periapical involvement.

Treatment

Careful radiographic evaluation is necessary to determine the extent of any pulpal extension into the evagination. Restricted and repeated grinding of the tubercle can be undertaken to promote reactionary dentine deposition on the pulpal aspect of the evagination. However, this approach may only be applicable in a small number of cases and, more commonly, removal of the tubercule and a limited pulpotomy are required.

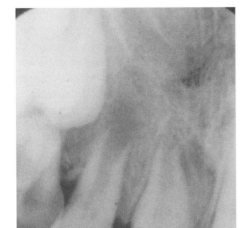

(b)

Figure 13.17 (a) Clinical and (b) radiographic appearance of an infected palatal invagination, affecting tooth 12.

13.6 Abnormality of root form

13.6.1 Taurodontism

The term taurodontism (literally, bull-like teeth) is used to describe molar teeth in which the body of the tooth is enlarged vertically at the expense of the roots. The normal constriction of a tooth at the level of the amelocemental junction is frequently reduced or absent in affected teeth. The mechanism leading to taurodontism is the late (or failed) invagination of Hertwig's root sheath which usually maps out the shape of root formation. The furcation is displaced apically. Varying degrees of taurodontism are seen, with the most extreme example being when only a single root is present rather than separate roots. Taurodont teeth may also be described as pyramidal, cuneiform, or fused. The root canal morphology may have implications when endodontic treatment or extraction is required.

Taurodontism is most commonly recognized in the permanent dentition. Although the term is traditionally applied only to molars, in some patients with taurodontism of the molar teeth the pulps of single-rooted teeth may be larger than normal. The prevalence of taurodontism varies according to the criteria used. In British schoolchildren a prevalence of 6% for mandibular first permanent molars has been reported. Higher prevalences have been recorded in certain racial groups such as the Bantu in South Africa. In some families taurodontism seems to follow an autosomal dominant pattern of inheritance. It is found in association with amelogenesis imperfecta, the tricho-dento-osseous syndrome, ectodermal dysplasias, and a number of other syndromes. Taurodontism is also more common in X-chromosomal aneudoploidy. Taurodontism has also been considered to be an atavistic trait, i.e. reverting to an ancestral form.

13.6.2 Accessory roots

Accessory roots can occur in almost any tooth. In the primary dentition this most commonly affects the molars, but the primary canines and maxillary incisors can also be affected. In the permanent dentition, accessory roots are occasionally seen in maxillary incisors, mandibular canines, premolars, and molars. These accessory roots are often situated on the distolingual/palatal aspect of the tooth, may vary in shape, and may be difficult to identify radiographically. Accessory roots have been reported to occur in 1–9% of the primary dentition and in 1–45% of the permanent dentition. There is an association between accessory roots and large cusps of Carabelli on the maxillary first permanent molar and with accessory cusps on maxillary second and third molars. In some cases the presence of accessory roots reflects macrodontia.

13.7 Abnormality of tooth structure

13.7.1 All tissues

Arrested development of tooth-germs

Arrested development of tooth-germ formation may occur following such external influences as trauma, ionizing radiation, osteomyelitis, or chemotherapy. The teeth and the particular tissues affected will depend on the nature and timing of the insult. This may result in enamel defects in teeth whose crowns are developing, and corresponding dentine defects may be seen on microscopic sections if the tooth is ultimately to be extracted (see Fig. 13.10). If roots are developing at the time of the insult these may appear stunted.

Locally, one or more permanent tooth-germs may be affected by infection from an overlying primary predecessor. Such teeth are termed Turner teeth and typically have areas of enamel hypoplasia and/or enamel hypomineralization. The mandibular premolars are most commonly affected (Fig. 13.19).

Regional odontodysplasia

This is a very uncommon developmental anomaly, typically affecting the primary teeth and corresponding permanent successors within a segment of the dentition. The anterior teeth are more commonly affected and the defect may cross the midline. The term 'ghost teeth' is sometimes applied to reflect the radiographic appearance seen. Affected patients may present with abscesses prior to the eruption of the teeth. The abnormal teeth have poorly developed crowns with enamel and dentine changes, large pulp chambers, and open apices. The permanent teeth may be less severely affected than the primary predecessors (Fig. 13.20).

Treatment

The removal of teeth affected by regional odontodysplasia is often necessary. As this often occurs in the primary dentition, consideration needs to be given to management of the affected permanent successors. While there are reports of the effective use of etch-retained restorations in these cases, the teeth are often slow to erupt, with a distinctive local gingivitis, and the pulpal morphology is such that infection is a frequent outcome. Root development may be slow but restoratively useful. A case-by-case approach to treatment planning is required. Block removal of unerupted teeth with surrounding bone is not required.

13.7.2 Enamel defects

Enamel defects may be caused by genetic or environmental factors acting alone or in combination. Where less enamel matrix than normal is

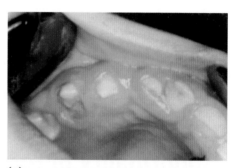

(a)

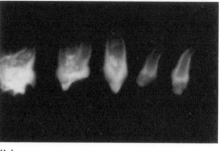

(b)

Figure 13.20 Regional odontodysplasia—(a) clinical and (b) radiographic appearance.

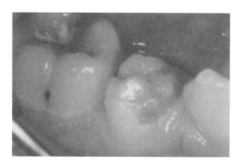

Figure 13.19 Turner tooth. Hypoplastic lower premolar—previous infection in primary tooth.

produced, the resulting enamel will be thinner (hypoplasia). If there is a defect in mineralization of the enamel matrix proteins, the result will be poorly mineralized enamel (hypomineralization—sometimes subdivided into hypocalcification for more severe defects and hypomaturation for milder changes). In many cases there will be a combination of both hypoplasia and hypomineralization, although sometimes the defect will be perceived clinically as predominantly one or the other. When enamel hypoplasia is seen the enamel may be either uniformly thin or grooved or pitted. In hypomineralization the enamel will typically be discoloured, usually a yellow-brown colour. This is particularly so where the defect is more severe (hypocalcification), whereas in a less severe presentation (hypomaturation) the enamel may be almost normal but appear mottled or even only slightly opaque rather than translucent. (See Key Points 13.4.)

> ## Key Points 13.4
>
> Enamel defects
> - Hypoplasia—deficient matrix volume
> - Hypomineralization—poor mineralization

Amelogenesis imperfecta

Amelogenesis imperfecta is the term applied to generalized enamel defects affecting all (or predominantly all) the teeth of both the primary and permanent dentitions (Fig. 13.21). It is of genetic origin, and thus there may be a history of similar defects in other family members. Although the term strictly relates to enamel defects only, in some patients there may be subtle or substantial changes in other dental tissues and craniofacial structures, or the condition may involve more widespread abnormalities as part of a syndrome. Dentally, there may be failure of eruption with resorption of the unerupted teeth. A case can be made for regular radiographic review of these patients.

Amelogenesis imperfecta is seen in single-gene mutations with autosomal dominant, autosomal recessive, and X-linked patterns of inheritance. Apparently sporadic cases are also seen—it is not clear whether these represent new mutations, or whether these will then be passed

on to future offspring (Fig. 13.22). Amelogenesis imperfecta is relatively uncommon, but there are marked population differences in prevalence. In parts of Sweden the condition is relatively common (one in approximately 700 of the population). However, in one study in the USA the prevalence was found to be approximately 1 in 14 000.

The classification of amelogenesis imperfecta has traditionally been based on the phenotype—the clinical appearance. Following this system, patients are allocated according to the perceived defect—hypoplasia, hypocalcification, or hypomaturation. Some classifications have an additional category of hypomaturation–hypoplasia with taurodontism to reflect the fact that some families show a combination of thin and/or poorly mineralized enamel as well as taurodontism. However, it is important to realize, from both a diagnostic and a classification point of view, that not all individuals within a family may show precisely the same findings. As a result, phenotype classifications become problematic when different members of the same family are grouped into different categories. Furthermore, this classification system fails when there is uncertainty as to which is the presumed predominant defect. It is possible that the inheritance pattern will be forgotten in attempting to categorize individuals.

For this reason an alternative classification system has been suggested where the mode of inheritance (autosomal dominant, autosomal recessive, X-linked, or apparently sporadic) is considered before the clinical phenotype. This classification also allows for the fact that there may be some overlap between the clinical defects in the same or different members of a family. The full classification scheme includes the genomic and biochemical identity of the defect. However, for practical purposes, a simplified use of this modern classification might, for example, define a patient's presentation as 'autosomal dominant hypoplastic amelogenesis imperfecta'.

Autosomal dominant amelogenesis imperfecta

In autosomal dominant amelogenesis imperfecta there is typically a clear pattern of inheritance with individuals in successive generations being affected (Fig. 13.23). Because the mutant gene is on one of the autosomes there is a 50% chance of an affected individual passing it on to each offspring. Males and females are equally affected. The primary and permanent dentitions are generally both involved, although the permanent dentition may be more severely affected than the primary

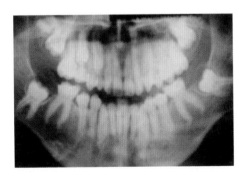

Figure 13.21 Sporadic case; amelogenesis imperfecta; hypomineralized; anterior open bite. Shows failure of eruption teeth 17, 15, 13, 27, 37, 47.

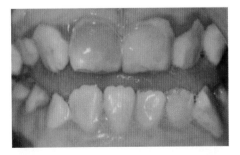

Figure 13.22 Sporadic case; amelogenesis imperfecta; hypomineralized; anterior open bite. The poor oral hygiene and staining are typical when, as here, the teeth are sensitive to thermal and mechanical stimuli.

dentition (Fig. 13.24). There is a wide range of presentations (phenotypes). The enamel may be thin and hard with normal translucency, but may be difficult to discern on radiographs because of its limited thickness. In some cases the enamel may be both hypoplastic and hypomineralized, in which case it is thin and discoloured with a loss of normal translucency. Some patients may have enamel of normal thickness which is poorly mineralized, and yet others may have enamel of normal thickness which lacks the normal translucency and is therefore regarded as showing features of hypomaturation. Occasionally, subtle enamel defects may only be identified on histopathological examination of extracted teeth. Taurodontism is seen in some families. Anterior open bite may occur in up to 50% of autosomal dominant amelogenesis imperfecta cases as well as in other inheritance patterns. The mechanism producing the sometimes associated anterior open bite has not yet been elucidated.

Aetiology

The enamelin gene on chromosome 4 has been shown to be mutated in some families with autosomal dominant amelogenesis imperfecta (and in some with autosomal recessive amelogenesis imperfecta). Other genes involved in normal enamel formation have also been implicated. Patients with tricho-dento-osseous syndrome, an autosomal dominant syndrome characterized by amelogenesis imperfecta with taurodontism as well as curly hair and bone changes, have been found to have mutations in the *DLX3* gene on chromosome 17.

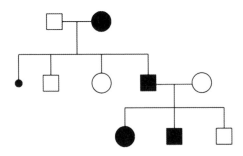

Figure 13.23 Pedigree chart. Autosomal dominant inheritance of amelogenesis imperfecta.

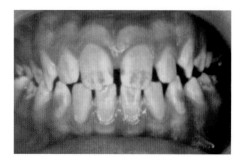

Figure 13.24 Autosomal dominant amelogenesis imperfecta. All teeth are affected similarly.

Autosomal recessive amelogenesis imperfecta

Autosomal recessive conditions are typically seen when there is parental consanguinity, for example the parents may be first cousins (Fig. 13.25). There may be cultural reasons for this or, alternatively, consanguinity may be seen in isolated communities with little outside contact where there is consequently a limited gene pool. This situation does not apply in other recessive conditions, such as cystic fibrosis, and the relative prevalence of the condition is related to the frequency of gene carriers in the population. Where the parents are close relatives, both carrier adults may be unaffected but there will be a one in four chance of offspring inheriting two copies of the mutant gene.

Autosomal recessive mutations causing amelogenesis imperfecta seem to be uncommon apart from in Polynesia, where, presumably, the mutation is relatively common. Such individuals may have enamel hypoplasia and/or enamel hypomineralization, and the designator 'pigmented enamel' has been applied. A gene on chromosome 2 has been linked to autosomal recessive amelogenesis imperfecta associated with ocular defects.

X-linked amelogenesis imperfecta

X-linked amelogenesis imperfecta is characterized by a difference in the appearance of the teeth of affected males and females. The majority of families studied to date have an alteration in the amelogenin gene on the short arm of the X chromosome. Affected males cannot pass on the condition to their sons (by virtue of passing on their Y chromosome to their sons), but their daughters (to whom they necessarily pass on their X chromosome) will all inherit the mutant gene. Such daughters will always show some dental features, although these might be subtle in some cases. These heterozygous females can pass on the mutant gene to children of either sex (Fig. 13.26).

The enamel in both sexes may be hypoplastic, hypomineralized, or show elements of both features. The appearance seen will be the result

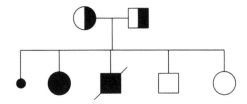

Figure 13.25 Pedigree chart. Autosomal recessive inheritance of amelogenesis imperfecta.

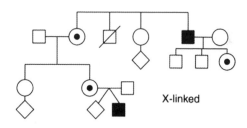

Figure 13.26 Pedigree chart. X-linked inheritance—no male-to-male transmission.

of the exact nature of the change in the amelogenin gene and the sex of the patient and the family in which it occurs.

Males, by virtue of having a single X chromosome, will be more severely and uniformly affected. The enamel may be thin (hypoplastic—reduced in quantity) or discoloured (with affected mineralization) or a combination of both (Fig. 13.27). Females within the same family who inherit the affected gene will show a vertical pattern of markings on the enamel, either vertical ridges and grooves (the equivalent of the male uniform hypoplasia), with or without discolouration, or loss of translucency of the enamel in the same vertical bands (where the mineralization is affected) (Fig. 13.28).

Aetiology

The amelogenin gene, which encodes the enamel protein amelogenin, is located on the short arm of the X chromosome. Mutations in the gene are responsible for most cases of X-linked amelogenesis imperfecta, but there also appears to be another gene on the long arm of the X chromosome which is responsible for similar clinical appearances in another family.

Genetic enamel defects associated with generalized disorders

Widespread enamel defects can be seen in a number of conditions with extra-oral manifestations, including epidermolysis bullosa, tuberous sclerosis, oculo-dento-osseus dysplasia, and amelogenesis imperfecta associated with tricho-dento-osseous syndrome. The exact genomic relationship between these and other conditions and amelogenesis imperfecta remains to be established in most cases. (See Key Points 13.5.)

Key Points 13.5

Amelogenesis imperfecta
- Inheritance
- Autosomal dominant
- Autosomal recessive
- X-linked
- Apparently sporadic

Phenotype

Hypoplastic ± hypomineralization (hypocalcification to hypomaturity). Pure hypoplasia or hypomineralization is probably rare. Profound hypomineralization leads to teeth so soft that they are reduced in size, although this reduction is, in fact, a later (post-eruptive) change.

Molar incisor hypoplasia

In recent years reports have been published of children with mineralization defects of the first permanent molars and, sometimes, the permanent incisors. This has been referred to as molar incisor hypomineralization or hypoplasia and also as 'cheese molars' because of the friable nature of the enamel of the molar tooth enamel. Although the condition appears to have a chronological distribution (Fig. 13.29), close inspection will often show that

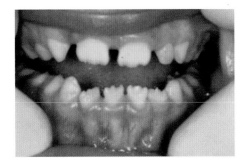

Figure 13.27 X-linked; amelogenesis imperfecta; male; thin smooth enamel.

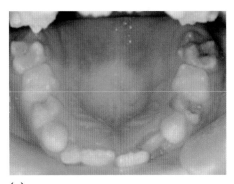

(a)

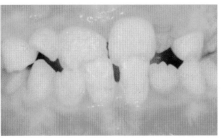

(b)

Figure 13.29 (a) Molar and (b) incisor hypomineralization with features of chronological disturbance but no relevant medical history.

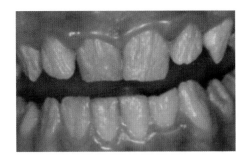

Figure 13.28 X-linked; amelogenesis imperfecta; female; ridged, predominantly hypoplastic enamel.

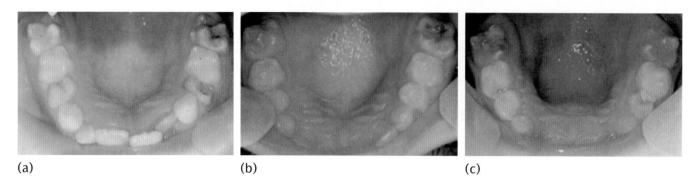

(a)   (b)   (c)

Figure 13.30 (a, b, and c) Molar incisor hypomineralization in a sister and two brothers.

'unmatched' teeth are affected, i.e. teeth that would have been form-ing at the same time do not present with symmetrical affliction. Only one molar, or perhaps three of the four, may be affected. The defects in the incisors, which are usually less severe and most likely to show demarcated isolated mottling, will likewise be irregularly distributed (Fig. 13.30). Childhood infections, specific antibiotics, and repeated fevers have all been suggested as causes (see also Chapter 10). It has been suggested that a genetic predisposition combined with an envi-ronmental insult might produce these changes, but this has yet to be substantiated.

Treatment

The condition is problematic for both patients and practitioners. The destruction of the molar teeth in particular, although probably a post-eruptive change, presents in many cases at a time when children are not acclimatized to dental treatment. Treatment options should include a careful analysis of the occlusion, since many of the molar teeth are severely compromised, and in the long term the child may benefit from their elective loss as part of a comprehensive treatment plan (see Chapter 14). The preservation 'at all costs' of first permanent molars shows considerable dental-cultural variation, with some nations firmly resistant to the very idea of their loss. Reluctance to consider the removal of first molars as part of a comprehensive treatment plan probably harks back to the time of removable orthodontic therapy when the loss of these teeth undoubtedly complicated or compromised treatment. Mod-ern orthodontic mechanics has done away with much of this difficulty, but careful treatment planning by the paediatric dentist and orthodon-tist from the first identification of the potential problem will optimize the outcome.

Maintaining compromised molars indefinitely when a guided tooth realignment is possible does the child (and the subsequent adult) no favours. Root canal therapy at the end of a course of orthodontics when healthy premolars have been removed is a failure of treatment planning.

In the 2 years between the eruption of the first permanent molar teeth and the commonly recommended time for their removal, man-agement may be difficult. It is clear that many children with this condi-tion are apprehensive patients for dental treatment. This is likely to be because, in its early stages, practitioners adopt a minimalist approach with the attempted use of fissure sealants and adhesive restorations.

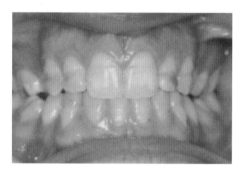

Figure 13.31 Hypoplasia in a 'chronological distribution'.

These are often applied without local anaesthesia, are painful, and are frequently unsuccessful anyway. Preformed metal crowns applied under local anaesthesia provide a useful interim measure in these cases.

The incisor defects are not noticeably uncomfortable and should be managed using the techniques described in Chapter 10.

'Environmentally determined' enamel defects

Enamel defects may arise as a result of an 'environmental' insult. Within this sense we include both a systemic upset and the result of a local factor involving a developing tooth (as discussed in Section 13.7).

Where there is a systemic insult the teeth will be affected in a chron-ological pattern, so that a band of abnormal enamel is seen in a hori-zontal distribution affecting some part on the tooth crown. Typically this results in a groove in the enamel of affected teeth. The term chron-ological hypoplasia is often used to describe such cases (Fig. 13.31). A knowledge of the timing of commencement of formation of the teeth will aid in understanding the timing of such an insult.

Systemic (chronological) enamel defects

Enamel formation *in utero* may be affected by a wide range of maternal and fetal conditions. These include endocrine disturbances (hypopara-thyroidism), infections (rubella), drugs (thalidomide), nutritional defi-ciencies, and haematological and metabolic disorders (rhesus incompatibility). In such cases, the enamel covering the incisal portions of the crowns of the primary incisors will typically be affected in the

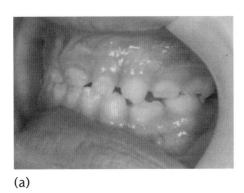

(a)

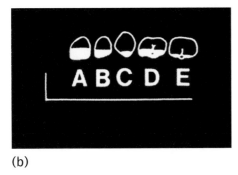

(b)

Figure 13.32 (a) Clinical and (b) diagrammatic representation of pre-term hypoplasia in the primary dentition.

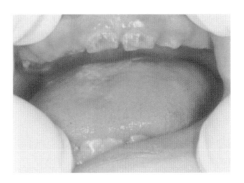

Figure 13.33 Primary teeth: both jaws affected by icterus gravis neonatorum (rhesus disease); upper teeth with super-added 'bottle caries'.

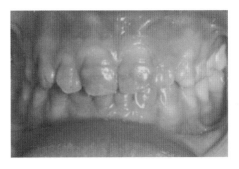

Figure 13.34 Tetracycline staining associated with horizontal hypoplastic banding representing repeated childhood illness and its treatment.

pattern shown in Fig. 13.32. Similar changes may be seen in pre-term low-birthweight infants. It is not yet clear whether this is associated with the use of intubation for these children in the neonatal period, although the latter has been identified as a local cause affecting forming incisors only.

When there is a systemic upset or marked physiological changes occur at birth or in the neonatal period, corresponding enamel defects may be seen in the primary dentition. Illness in the neonatal period may also affect the tips of the first permanent molars as these commence development at around birth.

Enamel defects may also arise as a result of acute or chronic childhood illnesses (Fig. 13.33). These include hypothyroidism and hypoparathyroidism, chronic renal disease, and gastrointestinal disorders producing malabsorption, such as coeliac disease. The use of tetracycline during pregnancy and childhood should be avoided because of deposition of the tetracycline in developing dental matrices, producing a distinctive blue-grey discolouration of the teeth, sometimes in a chronologically banded distribution (Fig. 13.34).

In the past, exanthematous fevers caused by measles and other infections were associated with a disturbance of normal enamel formation and a corresponding chronological hypoplasia affecting the crowns of developing teeth. Modern medical care has now made this uncommon, unless such changes occur in babies and infants who develop pneumonia.

Enamel formation is also sensitive to chemical agents such as fluoride. Excessive intake of fluoride, from either naturally occurring sources such as drinking water with fluoride levels over 1–2ppm or over-use of fluoride supplements or fluoride toothpastes, can cause enamel mottling. In its mildest form fluorosis appears as an opacity of the enamel. The condition is dose dependent, with increasing intake of fluoride being associated with more marked opacity, areas of discolouration of the enamel, and pitting or more extensive hypoplastic defects (Fig. 13.35(a)). Fluorosis and amelogenesis imperfecta can be confused. One distinguishing feature may be that amelogenesis imperfecta does not show a chronological distribution, whereas fluorosis, which depends on the timing of the excessive intake, does. Local fluorotic lesions may respond very well to the micro-abrasion technique (Fig. 13.35).

Local factors

As well as the possibility of damage to the forming teeth that may be caused by dental injuries (Fig. 13.36) (see Chapter 12), pressure on the premaxilla from the use of an oro-tracheal tube may cause damage to the developing primary incisor teeth. Children with a cleft lip and palate often have enamel defects of the maxillary incisors. Sometimes this may be related to surgical treatment rather than the effect of the cleft *per se*.

Treatment

The treatment of children with enamel defects requires more consideration than simply mechanical treatment of the teeth. Children with amelogenesis imperfecta, in particular, may be subject to teasing. This is a serious issue and requires the most sensitive handling by

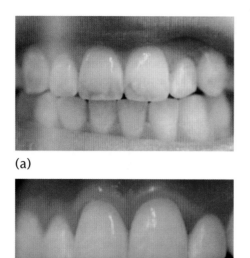

(a)

(b)

Figure 13.35 (a) Disturbed dental development, fluorotic mottling: (a) pre- and (b) post-micro-abrasion.

professionals. Affected adult family members will often describe their own childhood in lurid and painful terms. Many children will not admit to this from the outset and need to be given 'permission' (with their parent's knowledge) to contact the practitioner at a later date to revisit these issues. We have found this approach helpful; children, in the presence of their parent, are told that 'It's good that you're OK about your smile at the moment. Some children find that they change their minds about that. You can change your mind from the moment that you walk out of this door' (i.e. finish the consultation). 'If you do change your mind, then tell Mum or Dad (that's important) and send us a picture postcard of somewhere that you like, with the message "Please can I come to see you before I was next supposed to?" ' We have never felt that the children have abused this system; relatively few make use of it, but several have arrived for a recall to say that they would have sent us a postcard but knew that they were due to see us so they decided to wait.

Typically, as well as the aesthetics, there may be thermal, contact, or osmotic sensitivity of the teeth. Oral hygiene may be poor and irremediable as a result (Fig. 13.22). The occlusion may be compromised by a lack of vertical dimension as a result of thinner enamel than normal, or there may be loss of enamel because of poorly mineralized enamel matrix. Some practitioners advocate the early preventive use of full-coverage restorations in the primary dentition for these children. Localized defects are much more amenable to simple measures.

13.7.3 Dentine defects

As with enamel defects, dentine defects may be of genetic origin or caused by environmental effects.

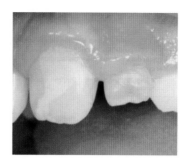

Figure 13.36 Disturbed dental development—previous primary tooth injury.

Genetically determined dentine defects

Dentinogenesis imperfecta

Dentinogenesis imperfecta is an autosomal dominant inherited condition. It may occur in isolation or in association with osteogenesis imperfecta. This represents two conditions, rather than a spectrum of effect. The term hereditary opalescent dentine is sometimes applied because of the typical opalescent hue of the teeth.

Dentinogenesis imperfecta, both the typical variant and the 'Brandywine isolate' variant in the eastern United States, has been mapped to chromosome 4 and the *DSPP* gene has been shown to be mutated in several families (some of whom have also had hearing defects). In some of the Brandywine isolate families, occasional individuals have teeth which are indistinguishable from the more typical form of dentinogenesis imperfecta; therefore it is likely that this represents an allelic variant of the same genetic condition. Similarly, the distinct diagnosis of coronal dentinal dysplasia has been proposed but this also seems likely to be a variant of dentinogenesis imperfecta.

Dentinogenesis imperfecta occurring in association with osteogenesis imperfecta is a result of mutations in one of the two collagen type 1 genes on chromosome 7 or 17. The dentine defects may be very apparent or rather subtle, in some cases requiring electron microscopy for their identification.

Dentine changes (sometimes accompanied by enamel changes) can also be seen in some types of Ehlers–Danlos syndrome involving mutations in the collagen 1 genes.

Dentinogenesis imperfecta occurring in the absence of osteogenesis imperfecta is inherited as an autosomal dominant trait. The primary and permanent dentitions are usually affected. The teeth are opalescent with a greyish or brownish colour (Figs 13.37 and 13.38). There may be some variation in the severity of the appearance in different members of the same family. Some variability may also be seen in the severity of affliction of individual teeth in any one individual (Fig. 13.39). The enamel may chip away from the dentine such that it is exposed and the crowns may suffer from attrition so that the teeth are worn down to the level of the gingivae (Fig. 13.40). This situation is most dramatically seen to affect the primary dentition. In the primary dentition the pulps may be large and hence pulpal exposure may occur early. In many cases, the pulps of the teeth tend to be obliterated; hence pulpal exposure and abscess formation tend not to occur, or to develop later than might otherwise be expected. The chipping of the

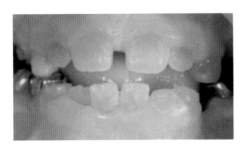

Figure 13.37 Dentinogenesis imperfecta—early mixed dentition.

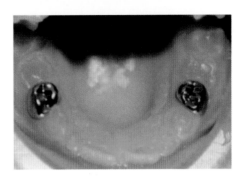

Figure 13.40 Dentinogenesis imperfecta showing tooth wear 55, 65.

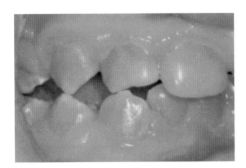

Figure 13.38 Dentinogenesis imperfecta—18-year-old-male; composite additions teeth 12, 11, 42, 41. Typical dark dentine colouration; short clinical crowns.

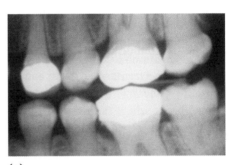

(a)

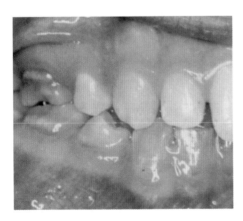

Figure 13.39 Dentinogenesis imperfecta—variable expression in one individual.

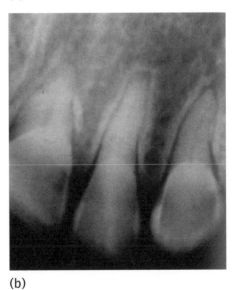

(b)

Figure 13.41 (a) Bitewing and (b) periapical radiographs of dentinogenesis imperfecta showing bulbous molar crowns and obliterated pulp chambers.

enamel has often been claimed to result from a smooth enamel–dentine junction, but some studies have demonstrated that the contour of the enamel–dentine junction is not a factor and that the weakness is within the dentine.

Radiographically the crowns appear relatively bulbous; the roots are shortened and may be thinner than normal. The pulp chambers may be large initially, particularly in the primary dentition, but more typically the pulps are obliterated as a result of deposition of dentine in a rather haphazard manner (Fig. 13.41). This can be seen in histopathological sections where the mantle dentine adjacent to the

enamel–dentine junction is essentially normal but the deeper dentine is grossly abnormal. (See Key Points 13.6.)

Osteogenesis imperfecta

Osteogenesis imperfecta arises as a result of a mutation in one of the two collagen type 1 genes. Although it used to be regarded as having

Key Point 13.6

Dentinogenesis imperfecta

- Autosomal dominant condition—isolated trait or associated with osteogenesis imperfecta or other collagen abnormalities.

autosomal dominant and autosomal recessive modes of inheritance, it is now believed that autosomal dominant mutations are the norm but that the severity varies in different individuals and families. Cases such as those previously thought to be autosomal recessive are now considered most likely to arise as a result of gonadal mosaicism.

The condition is characterized by bone fragility so that children may have a history of fractures (from such mild trauma as walking into furniture), blue sclera, deafness (although this does not usually develop until the third decade of life), and lax ligaments around joints. There may or may not be dentinal changes, or these may be so subtle that they are not apparent clinically or radiographically.

Dentinal dysplasia

Dentinal dysplasia was first described in the 1920s; 'rootless teeth' is an alternative descriptive title. The condition is an autosomal dominant trait with both dentitions being affected. The teeth may be clinically normal but root formation is abnormal to varying degrees. Some teeth may have extremely short blunt roots, while others taper markedly towards the apex (Fig. 13.42). The pulp is partially obliterated, appearing in the molar teeth as a small demilune. Under the microscope the coronal dentine is normal but the root dentine is not, with masses of abnormal dentine obliterating the pulp space. The microscopic appearance has been likened to

boulders in a flowing stream. The short roots may cause problems because of mobility and this may lead to the condition being identified.

The above condition is often referred to as dentinal dysplasia type I to distinguish it from a condition referred to by some as dentinal dysplasia type II (coronal dentinal dysplasia). As already stated, the latter is most likely to represent an allelic variant of dentinogenesis imperfecta, as genetic linkage studies have shown it to map to the same region of chromosome 4 as dentinogenesis imperfecta and a mutation in the *DSPP* gene has also been identified in one family diagnosed as having dentinal dysplasia type II. It remains to be seen whether dentinal dysplasia type I is also allelic to dentinogenesis imperfecta.

Vitamin-D-resistant rickets

Vitamin-D-resistant rickets is an X-linked inherited condition. Affected males tend to be short in stature with bowed legs and other skeletal changes. They may present dentally with abscesses forming in the absence of caries. Dentine is the most markedly affected of the dental hard tissues, with interglobular dentine being the chief histopathological finding. Radiographically the pulp spaces are larger than normal and pulpal extensions of the pulp horns may be exposed as a result of attrition of the teeth (Fig. 13.43). Heterozygous females tend to be more mildly affected and may not exhibit any dental manifestations.

Environmentally determined dentine defects

Local trauma may interfere with tooth formation. This may be permanently recorded in the dentine as a prominent incremental line. Systemic influences, including nutritional deficiencies, tetracycline administration, and chemotherapeutic agents such as anticancer therapy involving cytotoxic drugs, can also affect the formation of dentine.

Treatment

As with enamel defects, severe psychosocial problems may occur as a result of the appearance of the teeth. Many of the arguments presented in the consideration of enamel conditions also apply to dentine. In dentinogenesis imperfecta, management is focused on the prevention of tooth wear, the maintenance of the vertical dimension, and improvement of the appearance (Chapter 10). In rickets, the treatment should be similarly directed. Aggressive dental support, including cuspal coverage without tooth preparation, may be needed in order to prevent bacterial access to these extended pulps, but cases presenting late may require acute management of dental abscesses on the teeth as a result of pulp death.

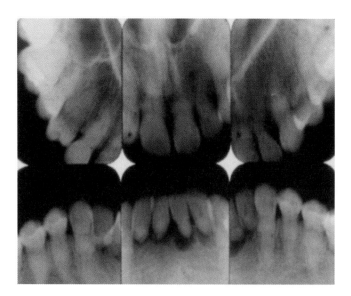

Figure 13.42 Radicular dentinal dysplasia.

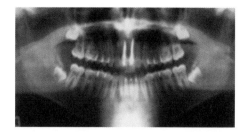

Figure 13.43 Vitamin-D-resistant rickets. Dental panoramic tomograph of male showing large pulp chambers, with less dense dentine adjacent to the enamel–dentine junction.

13.7.4 Cementum defects

The cementum can be affected in a number of genetic disorders. The consequences of alterations in cementum can have profound effects on the fate of the dentition.

There are a number of rare but significant conditions associated with the early loss of primary teeth. Any case of early or spontaneous loss of teeth is a cause for further investigation. In one of these, hypophosphatasia (both autosomal dominant and autosomal recessive inheritance are known), there may be premature exfoliation of the primary teeth or loss of the permanent teeth. The serum alkaline phosphatase level is low and phosphoethanolamine is excreted in the urine. Histopathological examination in hypophosphatasia will show aplasia or marked hypoplasia of the cementum. There may also be abnormal dentine formation with a wide predentine zone and the presence of interglobular dentine (similar to vitamin-D-resistant rickets).

Treatment

Local measures such as scrupulous oral hygiene may slow the loss of teeth in cases of hypophosphatasia, but the prime focus of treatment may need to be the replacement of teeth of the primary and permanent dentitions as they are lost.

13.8 Disturbances of eruption

There are considerable variations in the timing of eruption of the permanent dentition. There may be some racial variation, and eruption may also be influenced by environmental factors such as nutrition and illness. Eruption times of permanent teeth in females tend to be slightly ahead of the corresponding eruption times in males; this becomes a more marked difference with the later erupting teeth.

13.8.1 Premature eruption

Some families report that early tooth eruption is a family feature. Children with high birthweight have been reported to have earlier eruption of their primary teeth than children with normal or low birthweights. Early eruption of the permanent dentition may occur in children with precocious puberty and children with endocrine abnormalities, particularly those of the growth or thyroid hormones.

Natal and neonatal teeth

Teeth present at birth are known as natal teeth and those that erupt within the first month of life as neonatal teeth. Approximately one in 2000–3000 live births are so affected. The mandibular central incisor is the most common natal or neonatal tooth. Occasionally maxillary (central) incisors or the first molars may appear as natal teeth. The vast majority of cases represent premature eruption of a tooth of the normal sequence. It has been suggested that this condition is a result of an ectopic position of the tooth-germ during fetal life.

Natal or neonatal teeth may also be seen in association with some syndromes including pachyonychia congenita, Ellis–van Creveld syndrome, and Hallermann–Streiff syndrome.

Natal or neonatal teeth are often mobile because of limited root development and may be a danger to the airway if they are inhaled. The crowns may be abnormal in form and the enamel may be poorly formed or thinner than normal. The mobility of the tooth frequently causes inflammation of the surrounding gingivae. Trauma to the ventral surface of the tongue may cause ulceration (Fig. 13.44), and there may be difficulty with breastfeeding.

Treatment

Local measures such as smoothing the sharp edges of the tooth with a rubber cone in a dental handpiece may help resolve the ulceration. In a number of cases, the tooth should be extracted if it is markedly loose, as it is unlikely to form a useful part of the dentition. Firm application of Spencer–Wells forceps to the tooth crown is advised, followed by minor local curettage to remove the remains of the developing tooth-germ at that site.

13.8.2 Delayed eruption

Delayed eruption of primary teeth may arise from either systemic or local factors. It may be associated with prematurity or low birth weight.

Delayed eruption of teeth of both dentitions may occur in association with Down syndrome and Turner syndrome. It may also be associated with nutritional abnormalities or endocrine disorders such as hypothyroidism or hypopituitarism.

Cleidocranial dysplasia is an autosomal dominant condition characterized by aplasia or hypoplasia of the clavicles and widespread cranial changes. These include a brachycephalic skull (short in the anteroposterior dimension), frontal and parietal bossing, hypoplasia of the maxilla and zygomatic arches, hypertelorism, and delayed closure of the anterior fontanelle and skull sutures. Multiple Wormian bones are present in the line of the cranial sutures, particularly the lambdoid suture. With respect to the jaws, the most striking dental feature is the presence of multiple supernumerary teeth, particularly of the permanent dentition, and particularly in the anterior parts of the jaws.

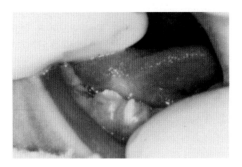

Figure 13.44 Natal teeth 71, 81. Ulceration of ventral surface of tongue.

Permanent tooth eruption is often delayed or there is failure of eruption, partly because of the number of supernumerary teeth. The primary teeth may fail to resorb. Although it has been suggested that there may be hypoplasia of cementum on the roots of the teeth, this has not been definitively established. The proportion of cellular to acellular cementum does not seem to be significant.

Hereditary gingival fibromatosis may be associated with delayed eruption, presumably because of a local effect whereby the teeth are unable to penetrate the enlarged and thickened gingivae. Other, truly localized, causes of delayed eruption include ectopic crypt position. This most often affects the maxillary or mandibular permanent canines, or may present with the impaction of the maxillary first permanent molars against the distal aspect of the adjacent primary second molar.

Local causes such as the presence of supernumeraries or odontomes may also interfere with eruption of an adjacent permanent tooth (Fig. 13.6). A delay of more than 6 months between the eruption of a tooth and its antimere requires investigation, usually radiographically.

The position of the permanent canines, particularly those in the maxilla, should be ascertained by palpation not later than the child's 10th birthday. Any uncertainty as to their presence or position should be followed by radiographic examination. The potential for palatal impaction of these teeth may be identified by this simple measure, and

simple intervention by the prompt removal of the primary canine in selected cases may prevent the need for later surgery (Chapter 14).

Delayed eruption of permanent teeth may also be due to dilaceration of developing roots and crowns as a result of trauma to the primary dentition (Chapter 12).

Early extraction of a primary tooth may be associated with delayed eruption of the permanent successor because of thickening of the overlying mucosa.

Treatment

Any systemic condition may require treatment if this is available. Local obstructions such as supernumerary teeth or odontomes need to be removed. Surgical exposure and orthodontic traction may be necessary for late-presenting permanent canines, and patients with hereditary gingival fibromatosis may require gingivectomy.

In cleidocranial dysplasia, a combined restorative, surgical, and occlusal management approach to treatment planning is required. Retained primary teeth will probably need to be extracted, together with the surgical removal of unerupted supernumerary teeth. This requires careful treatment planning, as the successful eruption of the permanent dentition cannot be guaranteed. Orthodontic treatment to guide the teeth into occlusion may be one of the treatment options, with prosthetic replacement of the teeth being considered if the teeth fail to erupt.

13.9 Disturbances of exfoliation

13.9.1 Premature exfoliation

Premature exfoliation is always a cause for further investigation. Its association with hypophosphatasia was considered in Section 13.7.4. Premature exfoliation may also be seen in cases of severe congenital neutropenia, cyclic neutropenia, Chediak–Higashi syndrome (where it is associated with gross periodontal destruction), the Langerhans' cell histiocytoses, and Papillon–Lefèvre syndrome.

13.9.2 Delayed exfoliation

Infra-occlusion

The terms infra-occlusion, submerged teeth, and ankylosed teeth are often used to describe teeth which have failed to come into normal occlusion or, more typically, have remained in their relative position in the arch while other teeth have continued to erupt. This is most commonly seen when one or more premolars fails to develop; hence the primary molars have no stimulus to become resorbed. As the adjacent permanent teeth erupt, alveolar growth occurs, but in some cases the primary molars become ankylosed within the bone and fail to alter their position (Fig. 13.45). As a result, there is an open bite in the affected area, with the occlusal plane of the primary molars being lower than that of the adjacent permanent teeth. It should be recognized that the process of physiological resorption of primary teeth is not unremitting and there are phases of resorption and repair. If there is an imbalance between the two, with the latter predominating (particularly in the absence of normal physiological stimulus for resorption), the net result is ankylosis. Genetic factors may be important, but the aetiology has not yet been resolved.

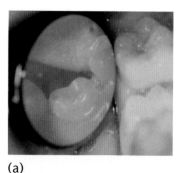

(a)

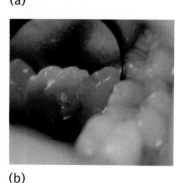

(b)

Figure 13.45 Infra-occlusion tooth 75 (a) before and (b) after restoration with a laboratory-made composite onlay.

Treatment

A substantial study has shown that removal of infra-occluded primary molars will lead to progressive space loss at that site with a potential to give rise to or focus crowding at that site, that all non-extacted infra-occluded teeth in the study were shed within the expected time limits, and that a more conservative approach to the management of these teeth may be indicated.

Where there is no permanent successor, the infra-occluded primary teeth may be retained and the crowns built up with acid-etch composite restorations or other restorative material. Onlays, either in metal or laboratory-cured composite, may be considered (Fig. 13.45(b)). If extraction is contemplated, consideration needs to be given to orthodontic alignment, a denture, a bridge, or an implant. (See Key Points 13.7.)

Other causes of delayed exfoliation

Delayed exfoliation of primary teeth may be seen in association with a number of local causes, including fused/geminated primary teeth, ectopically developing permanent teeth, and subsequent to trauma or severe infection of primary teeth.

Key Points 13.7

- There is a time range in which teeth erupt—but this range will affect the dentition as a whole.
- Dentitions falling substantially outside this range, or individually affected teeth delayed by 6 months, should be investigated.
- Premature exfoliation always demands investigation.
- There is a place for a conservative approach to the management of infra-occluded primary teeth.
- When seeking a diagnosis of a developmental dental condition please remember:
  - Common things occur commonly (rarities are rarely seen!).
  - Is this a chronological distribution?
  - Are any other members of the family affected?
  - Are all the teeth (more or less) equally affected?
  - And finally, 'When everything else has been excluded, that which remains, however improbable, must be the answer' (Sherlock Holmes—paraphrase).

13.10 Summary

1 Dental anomalies may have both a functional and a psychosocial impact on the child and their family.

2 The presence of one dental anomaly may be associated with others. Thorough clinical examination and radiographic investigations are essential.

3 An anomaly in the primary dentition may be associated with a similar anomaly in the permanent dentition.

4 All cases of missing teeth require treatment planning with multidisciplinary input.

5 Both developmental enamel defects and developmental dentine defects may be genetic or environmental in origin.

6 Both development enamel defects and developmental dentine defects may be seen in isolation or in association with extraoral features.

7 The distribution of an environmentally induced enamel defect will depend on the stage of tooth development at the time of the insult.

8 Excessive fluoride ingestion can cause enamel defects.

9 Dental professionals have an important part to play in the diagnosis and care of children with these conditions.

10 Careful monitoring of dental development, together with interception when appropriate, may reduce the impact of these conditions.

13.11 Acknowledgement

We wish to record both our personal and professional gratitude to the late Professor G.B. (Gerry) Winter. He always encouraged our work and was generous in his comments and sharing of material. Above all, he was an enthusiast and a champion of his patients. He is missed.

13.12 Further reading

Aldred, M.J. (2003). Human genetics. In *Oxford handbook of applied dental science* (ed. C. Scully), pp. 389–406. Oxford Medical Publications, Oxford.

Aldred, M.J. and Crawford, P.J.M. (1997). Molecular biology of hereditary enamel defects. In *Dental enamel* (ed. H.C. Slavkin), pp. 200–9. John Wiley, Chichester.

Aldred, M.J., Crawford, P.J.M., and Savarirayan, R. (2003). Amelogenesis imperfecta—a classification and catalogue for the 21st century. *Oral Diseases*, **9**, 19–23.

Brook, A.H. and Winter, G.B. (1970). Double teeth. A retrospective study of 'geminated' and 'fused' teeth in children. *British Dental Journal*, **129**, 123–30.

Crawford, P.J.M. and Aldred, M.J. (1989). Regional odontodysplasia: a bibliography. *Journal of Oral Pathology and Medicine*, **18**, 251–63.

Crawford, P.J.M. and Aldred, M.J. (1992). X-linked amelogenesis imperfecta. Presentation of two kindreds and a review of the literature. *Oral Surgery, Oral Medicine, and Oral Patholgy*, **73**, 449–55.

Gorlin, R.J., Cohen, M.M., Cohen, R., and Hennekam, R. (2001). *Syndromes of the head and neck*. Oxford University Press, Oxford.

Hall, R.K., Bankier, A., Aldred, M.J., Kan, K., Lucas, J.O., and Perks, A.G.B. (1997). Solitary median maxillary central incisor, short stature, choanal atresia/midnasal stenosis (SMMCI) syndrome: an analysis of the clinical features of 19 consecutive cases of the syndrome, a review of the literature and consideration of its aetiology. *Oral Surgery, Oral Medicine, and Oral Pathology*, **84**, 651–62.

Kurol, J. and Koch, G. (1985). The effect of extraction of infraoccluded deciduous primary molars: a longitudinal study. *American Journal of Orthodontics*, **87**, 46–55.

Online Mendelian Inheritance in Man, OMIM™. McKusick–Nathans Institute for Genetic Medicine, Johns Hopkins University (Baltimore, MD) and National Center for Biotechnology Information, National Library of Medicine (Bethesda, MD), 2000. Available online at:

http://www.ncbi.nlm.nih.gov/omim/

14

The paedodontic–orthodontic interface

T.J. Gillgrass

Chapter contents

14.1 Introduction

The long-term management of a child's developing occlusion often benefits greatly from a good working relationship between the paediatric dentist and the orthodontist. Typical problems range from minimizing damage to the occlusion caused by enforced extraction of poor-quality teeth, through the management of specific local abnormalities such as impacted teeth, to referral for comprehensive treatment of all aspects of the malocclusion. This chapter discusses the principles of when to refer to a specialist colleague, and looks at some common clinical situations where collaboration is often needed.

14.2 Recognition of malocclusion

14.2.1 Orthodontic assessment

From the age of 8 years all children should be screened for the presence of malocclusion when they attend for a routine dental examination. Although orthodontic treatment is usually carried out in the late mixed and early permanent dentition, some conditions benefit from treatment at an earlier stage. The screening need only be a brief clinical assessment, but it should be carried out systematically to ensure that no important findings are overlooked.

An outline of a basic orthodontic assessment is given in Table 14.1. With practice this can be carried out quite quickly to give an overall impression of the nature and severity of a malocclusion. In essence, it comprises assessments of the following elements:

- the patient's awareness of their malocclusion (the complaint, if any);
- their general level of dental awareness;
- an extra-oral examination of facial form (skeletal pattern and soft tissues);
- general oral condition—oral hygiene and tooth quality;
- the presence or absence of all teeth;
- the alignment and form of each arch;
- the teeth in occlusion.

Table 14.1 Orthodontic assessment

Complaint	Aesthetic or functional concerns about the position of the teeth
Medical history	May affect decisions about extractions, or where appliances may compromise gingival health
Dental history	Caries experience, previous extractions, dental awareness
Attitude to treatment	Of patient and parents. Likely level of cooperation with dentistry generally, orthodontic appliances, monthly adjustment visits (time off school, travelling), etc.
Extra-oral examination	
General	Height, developmental stage (pre, during, or post pubertal growth spurt)
Facial skeletal pattern	
Anteroposterior	Facial profile: skeletal class I, II, or III Mild, moderate, severe
Vertical	Steepness of mandibular plane Facial proportions: increased, normal, reduced
Transverse	Facial asymmetry Discrepancies in widths of upper and lower arches
Soft tissues	
Lips	Competent or incompetent Relationship of lower lip to upper incisors
Tongue	Tongue thrust (rare) Tongue to lower lip seal
Habits	Digit sucking or other habit
Temporomandibular joint	Pain, clicks, limitation of opening, mandibular deviation

Table 14.1 Continued

Intra-oral examination	
Dentition	Teeth present in the mouth
	Delayed eruption of teeth
	Oral hygiene
	Teeth of poor prognosis: caries, extensive restorations, trauma
Lower arch	Crowding, misplaced teeth
	Angulation of incisors and canines
Upper arch	Crowding, misplaced teeth
	Palpate for unerupted canines
	Angulation of incisors and canines
Incisor relationship	Overjet (mm)
	Overbite: increased or reduced; complete or incomplete centre-lines: coincident, correct within face?
	Anterior cross-bites
	Check for premature occlusal contact and associated displacement of mandible on closure: forward and/or lateral
Posterior occlusion	Both sides: class I, II, or III
	Check first molars and canines
	Posterior cross-bites—local, unilateral, bilateral
	Mandibular displacement?
Radiographs	Presence of permanent teeth; absent teeth, supernumerary teeth, ectopic teeth
	Pathology (skeletal assessment using cephalometric radiographs is not needed for routine screening for malocclusion)

Radiographs are not necessarily routinely used when screening for the presence of malocclusion and should only be taken when there is a clinical indication. A panoramic radiograph gives a useful general scan of the dentition and indicates the presence or absence of teeth. Some authorities advise that it should be supplemented with a naso-occlusal view as the premaxillary region, which is commonly the site of dental anomalies, is often poorly shown on panoramic views using older machines. However, provided that the panoramic view is of reasonable quality, intra-oral views of this region are not necessary unless there is a specific indication for them, such as delayed eruption of an incisor or a history of trauma. A radiographic assessment must always be made when considering any extractions.

Good-quality study models are often helpful when planning orthodontic treatment, and full orthodontic records comprising study models, relevant radiographs, and photographs should be obtained before any active treatment is started. Full-face and profile photographs are a record of facial form, including lip morphology. Intra-oral photographs are a further record of the malocclusion, give some indication of the standard of oral hygiene, and are valuable where enamel defects are present before treatment.

14.2.2 Need and demand for orthodontic treatment

The Index of Orthodontic Treatment Need (IOTN) is based upon the severity of the malocclusion, and has been developed to try to establish a consensus within the profession as to which malocclusions will gain a worthwhile benefit from orthodontic treatment (Brook and Shaw 1989). It is important to emphasize that IOTN does not indicate the difficulty or complexity of treatment, as mild malocclusions often need extensive and sophisticated treatment if any improvement is to be made at all. Other indices have been developed to assess the complexity (Index of Complexity, Outcome, and Need (ICON)) and success of treatment (Peer Assessment Rating (PAR)). The IOTN has two components.

1. The Dental Health Component categorizes malocclusion into five grades (Table 14.2) according to severity, based upon current evidence at its inception for the detrimental effects of various occlusal features. It is based on an index from the Dental Board of Sweden. A malocclusion is graded according to its worst feature, i.e. it is not cumulative. Therefore once mastered, it is quick to apply.

   Grade 1 no need

   Grade 2 little need

   Grade 3 borderline need

   Grade 4 need

   Grade 5 great need

To assess the malocclusion a ruler has been developed although this is not essential for scoring. The acronym MOCDO is used to systematically analyse each feature of the malocclusion (**M**issing, **O**verjet, **C**rossbite, **D**isplacement of contacts, **O**verbite). Each

Table 14.2 Dental Health Component of the Index of Orthodontic Treatment Need

Grade 5 (great need for treatment)	
5.i	Impeded eruption of teeth (except for third molars) due to crowding, displacement, the presence of supernumerary teeth, retained primary teeth and any pathological cause
5.h	Extensive hypodontia with restorative implications (more than one tooth missing in any quadrant) requiring pre-restorative orthodontics
5.a	Increased overjet >9mm
5.m	Reversed overjet >3.5mm with reported masticatory and speech difficulties
5.p	Defects of cleft lip and palate and other craniofacial anomalies
5.s	Submerged primary teeth
Grade 4 (need treatment)	
4.h	Less extensive hypodontia requiring pre-restorative orthodontics or orthodontic space closure to obviate the need for a prosthesis
4.a	Increased overjet >6mm but ≤9mm
4.b	Reverse overjet >3.5mm with no masticatory or speech difficulties
4.m	Reverse overjet >1mm but <3.5mm with recorded masticatory and speech difficulties
4.c	Anterior or posterior cross-bites with >2mm discrepancy between retruded contact position and intercuspal position
4.l	Posterior lingual cross-bite with no functional occlusal contact in one or both buccal segments
4.d	Severe contact point displacements >4mm
4.e	Extreme lateral or anterior open bites >4mm
4.f	Increased and complete overbite with gingival or palatal trauma
4.t	Partially erupted teeth, tipped and impacted against adjacent teeth
4.x	Presence of supernumerary teeth
Grade 3 (borderline need)	
3.a	Increased overjet >3.5mm but ≤6mm with incompetent lips
3.b	Reverse overjet >1mm but ≤3.5mm
3.c	Anterior or posterior cross-bites with >1mm but ≤2mm discrepancy between retruded contact position and intercuspal position
3.d	Contact point displacements >2mm but ≤4mm
3.e	Lateral or anterior open bites >2 mm but ≤4mm
3.f	Deep overbite complete on gingival or palatal tissues but no trauma
Grade 2 (little)	
2.a	Increased overjet >3.5mm but ≤6mm with competent lips
2.b	Reverse overjet >0mm but ≤1mm
2.c	Anterior or posterior cross-bites with ≤1mm discrepancy between retruded contact position and intercuspal position
2.d	Contact point displacements >1mm but ≤2mm
2.e	Lateral or anterior open bites >1mm but ≤2mm
2.f	Increased overbite ≥3.5mm without gingival contact
2.g	Pre- or post-normal occlusions with no other anomalies (includes up to half a unit discrepancy)
Grade 1 (none)	
1	Extremely minor malocclusions including contact point displacements <1mm

occlusion can be numerically graded with an indication for treatment and an associated alphabetical descriptor describing the feature for which it has been scored.

2. The Aesthetic Component uses a scale of 10 photographs showing different levels of dental attractiveness (Fig. 14.1). The appearance of the dentition is rated using the photographs as a guideline. Grades 1–4 indicate little or no need for treatment on aesthetic grounds, grades 5–7 are borderline, and patients in grades 8–10 would clearly benefit from orthodontic treatment. However, it is difficult to be truly objective when making judgements of this kind about an individual's appearance, although when scoring the aesthetics **the operator** should assess the aesthetic component score. Particular difficulty is found when analysing class III malocclusion and anterior open bite as this type of malocclusion does not appear within the aesthetic component. It should be emphasized that the scoring of the aesthetics using the component is based on **equivalence** rather than matching the malocclusion to one that is within the component.

Demand for orthodontic treatment is affected by many factors and not necessarily by need. Females, those in higher socio-economic groups, and those in areas with a plentiful supply of orthodontic provision appear the most likely to seek treatment. Patients vary enormously in how they perceive their own dental appearance, with some apparently being unaware of obvious malocclusions while others express dissatisfaction about very minor irregularities. Thus demand for treatment depends in part upon the severity of the malocclusion as perceived by patients, and particularly by the parents, rather than by the dentist. This is backed up by studies suggesting that malocclusion has an effect on the quality of life of the patients and the parents.

Long-term studies have questioned the long-term health and psychological benefit of orthodontic treatment, but this must be weighed against the relatively short-term psychological boost that orthodontics brings to a patient during what is, in the case of adolescents, an emotional rollercoaster.

There is little doubt that demand continues to increase, particularly in the adult population. This continues to create increasing strain where state-funded treatment is still available and inevitably leads to the use of indices (IOTN) to decide who is eligible for the treatment.

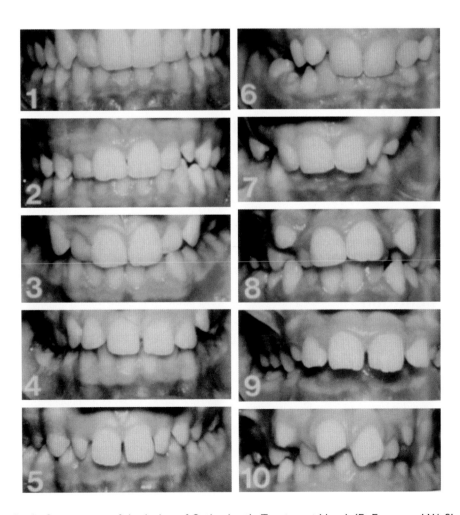

Figure 14.1 The Aesthetic Component of the Index of Orthodontic Treatment Need. (R. Evans and W. Shaw 1987. Reproduced with kind permission of the Editor of the *European Journal of Orthodontics*.)

14.2.3 Referral for orthodontic advice

Before referring a patient for orthodontic advice it is important to ensure that his/her dental health is under control and that the referring practitioner has made some assessment as to the severity of the orthodontic need. The referring dentist can give the orthodontist a lot of invaluable information.

Timing of referral

The right time for orthodontic intervention will vary according to the condition, but if specialist advice is needed it is better to refer too early than too late. Often, a good time is as the first premolar teeth are erupting. The majority of orthodontic treatments are carried out in the late mixed and early permanent dentition, but some conditions can be treated earlier (see Section 14.4) and some treatments, such as functional appliances, depend on active facial growth and should not be delayed too long before starting. It is important that prior to referral the patient's oral hygiene has reached an adequate standard for treatment and caries is under control. There may be some instances where referral is sought for extraction decisions on carious teeth where an assessment of long-term prognosis is helpful to the decision-making process. Important information to include on your referral is the patient's name, address with postcode, date of birth, and telephone number. The patient's medical practitioner should be included, particularly for hospital-based

referral, and any previous correspondence reference. Key information regarding the clinical condition includes:

- past medical and dental history;
- reason for referral;
- patient's/parents' attitude to treatment in general and likelihood of cooperation with future orthodontic treatment if required;
- radiographs where taken.

(See Key Points 14.1.)

Key Points 14.1

Screening
- All children should be screened for malocclusion from 8 years of age.
- Judge the need for treatment using the Index of Treatment Need (IOTN): dental health and aesthetics.
- Check oral hygiene and attitude to treatment.
- Refer in good time and give as much background information as possible.

14.3 Primary to mixed dentition

The dentist is responsible for noticing deviations from normal in the development of the occlusion. To do this, the practitioner must have a thorough knowledge of 'normal development' (see Chapter 1).

The primary dentition usually erupts between the ages of 6 months and 2½ years. The classic sequence of eruption is given in Chapter 1, with lower teeth erupting before uppers. However, deviation from this 'normal' sequence is not unusual (Fig. 14.2).

14.3.1 Primary dentition

The primary dentition classically presents as spaced and the molars often present with a ½ class II molar relationship or 'flush terminal plane' (Chapter 1, Fig. 1.18). It is essential for this spacing to be present, as without it crowding in the permanent dentition is likely. Malocclusion at this stage is merely noted, although it is unlikely to improve particularly in the case of a significant class III incisor relationship (Fig. 14.3), although intervention would not be considered at this stage. Habits are common and depending upon the extent of the habit, be it dummies or digits, malocclusion may exist because of it.

A supernumerary tooth may occur in the primary dentition and usually erupts. The likelihood of its being followed by a permanent successor is up to 50%, and it should be identified to parents and noted for future assessment.

14.3.2 Early mixed dentition

The permanent teeth erupt from the age of about 6 years, usually in two stages. The first stage, with eruption of the first molars and incisors, takes place up to the age of 9 years and the second stage, including premolars and canines, occurs between the ages of 10½ and 12 years. The key for the practitioner is to ensure sequence and symmetry of eruption, as a change in either may represent abnormal development and warrant radiological investigation.

As the incisors erupt it is not unusual for the lower to appear slightly crowded (Fig. 14.4) and upper to appear slightly spaced. Crowding in the lower labial segment is usually relieved through transverse expansion and when the lower deciduous canines are lost. The upper arch spacing is frequently associated with fanning of the incisor crowns and is described as the ugly duckling stage of development. This incisor spacing will usually close spontaneously as the upper permanent canines erupt.

It is important for the dentist to recognize these signs of normal development so that he/she can give some reassurance to the patient and parents if they are concerned. The spacing and diastema between the central incisors should not be mistaken for that due to other causes (see later). The early mixed dentition is a useful time for orthodontic assessment, as once the incisors have erupted there is a break in the eruption period until the upper premolars and lower canines start to appear at the age of 10½ years and this period allows simple interceptive measures.

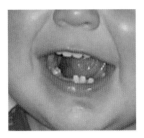

Figure 14.2 An unusual sequence of eruption in the primary dentition.

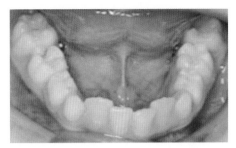

(a)

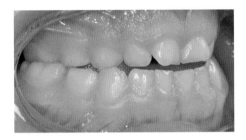

Figure 14.3 Class III incisor relationship in primary dentition.

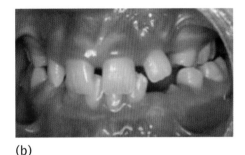

(b)

Figure 14.4 (a) Mild lower labial segment crowding and (b) fanned upper incisors on first eruption of the incisors.

Interceptive measures are often designed at this stage to reduce the severity/complexity of a malocclusion rather than eliminate it completely, and are frequently the first part of a more complex orthodontic plan.

Things to consider and possible interceptive measures include the following:

- Monitor eruption of incisors and first molars, paying attention to **sequence** and **symmetry**.
- Extract primary teeth displacing permanent successors.
- Possible balancing extractions of primary teeth to prevent centre-line deviation.
- Check long-term prognosis of first permanent molars and extract if necessary.

- Correct cross-bites (anterior or posterior) with associated mandibular displacement.
- Remove supernumeraries causing displacement or impeded eruption (central incisors and median diastema).
- Severe jaw discrepancies requiring early specialist referral (class III, class II, and bilateral cross-bites).
- Habit deterrents.
- Space maintenance.

Some or all of these may require specialist referral.

14.4 Extraction of children's teeth

The extraction of teeth in children may be needed as part of orthodontic treatment, or may be necessary because of caries, trauma, or developmental anomalies. The extraction of teeth in the mixed dentition for purely orthodontic reasons, usually crowding, can sometimes be helpful, but managing the enforced extraction of carious or poor-quality teeth is a matter of trying to minimize disruption of the developing dentition.

14.4.1 Extraction of primary teeth

In general, where a child has crowding, the extraction of primary teeth will worsen this as adjacent teeth will be able to drift into the resultant space (Fig. 14.5). Normally the resultant space loss is greater in the maxilla than the mandible. Usually, it is the teeth distal to the extraction

that migrate forwards as a result of mesial drift. This drifting is generally unhelpful where the extraction is enforced, but in some rare situations it can be harnessed to help with the management of dental crowding.

As there is an increase in the size of the arches during the mixed dentition stage, decisions about the treatment of crowding should be deferred until the permanent incisors have erupted for at least a year, usually at about 8½–9 years of age. Historically where severe crowding existed, the extraction of primary teeth might have been considered at this point as part of a programme of serial extractions. However, this is unusual with modern orthodontic techniques other than for children where cooperation with orthodontic treatment is unlikely. Where the crowding is mild or moderate, the decision should be delayed until the permanent canines and premolars are erupting.

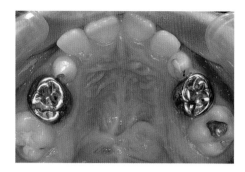

Figure 14.5 Complete space loss in the upper arch after early extraction of carious upper first primary molars.

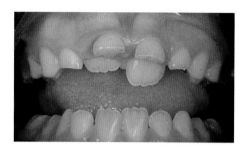

Figure 14.6 Retention of upper primary central incisors and deflection of the permanent successors.

The term **balancing extraction** refers to the contralateral tooth in the same arch. This is usually carried out to prevent centre-line shift. **Compensating extraction** refers to the equivalent tooth in the opposite arch. The rationale for this is based on the assumption that such an extraction will maintain the occlusal relationship.

Extraction of retained primary teeth

Suspicions should be raised where the difference between the exfoliation of contralateral teeth is greater than 6 months. Primary teeth should also be removed where they are partially exfoliated but causing deflection of a permanent successor (Fig. 14.6). If this is done early it will lead to normalization of the permanent tooth position.

14.4.2 Serial extraction

Serial extraction is a form of interceptive orthodontic treatment which aims to relieve crowding at an early stage so that the permanent teeth can erupt into good alignment, thus reducing or avoiding the need for later appliance therapy. It consists of a planned sequence of extractions.

1. *Primary canines*—extracted as the permanent lateral incisors erupt to allow them space to align.
2. *First primary molars*—about 1 year later, or when the roots of the first primary molars are at least half resorbed, to encourage eruption of the first premolars. In the lower arch these often tend to erupt after the canines.
3. *First premolars*—on eruption to make space for the eruption of the permanent canines into alignment.

In effect, the extraction of primary canines transfers the crowding from the incisors to the canine regions where it is more easily treated by extracting the first premolars. It is essential to carry out a full orthodontic assessment before embarking on a course of serial extractions. The intended advantage of serial extraction is to minimize or eliminate the need for appliances to align the arches after the permanent teeth have erupted. Sometimes this is very successful (Fig. 14.7), but the results can be disappointing. The great disadvantage of serial extraction is the multiple episodes of extractions, starting when the child is quite young. The primary canine extractions should usually be balanced by removing the

contralateral canine to prevent a centre-line shift, but it is not necessary to compensate by extracting the canines in the opposite arch. (See Key Points 14.2.)

Key Points 14.2

Indications of serial extractions.
- Class I occlusion
- Crowding of the lateral incisors
- 8½- to 9-year-old patient
- All teeth present
- Permanent molars of good prognosis

14.4.3 Enforced extraction of primary teeth

The main complication of the enforced extraction of poor-quality primary teeth is mesial drift of the teeth distal to the extraction space, causing crowding of the permanent successors. The extent to which this occurs is determined by:

- the tooth that is extracted
- the age of the patient
- the arch from which it is extracted
- the amount of pre-existing crowding present at the time of extraction.

In general terms the younger the patient the greater the pre-existing crowding, and the more distal the tooth the greater the space loss by mesial migration. Space loss also tends to be greater in the maxilla than the mandible where unerupted posterior teeth have a distal inclination and tend to tip and rotate mesially. In this section we shall use the terminology **balancing** and **compensating**. It should be borne in mind that many of the original 'rules' for balancing and compensating are from an era where correction of centre-lines and molar–canine relationships was challenging because of the limitation of appliances and provision of orthodontic care. Well-managed modern orthodontic techniques make such corrections possible, although not

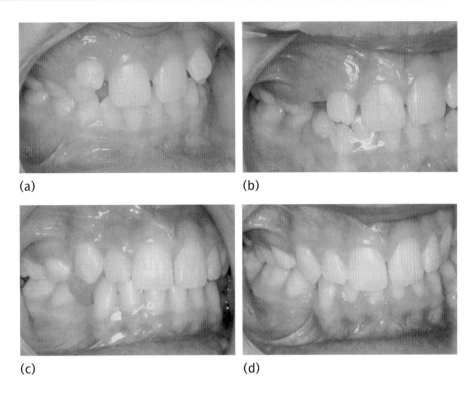

(a)   (b)

(c)   (d)

Figure 14.7 (a) Before extraction of primary canines. (b) Aged 10½: 6 months before extraction of first premolars. Upper canines palpable in buccal sulcus, lower canines crowded buccally. (c) Aged 13: excess space in lower arch. (d) Aged 15: upper spaces closed and lower spaces reducing. (Courtesy of Mr T.G. Bennett.)

necessarily straightforward. As such, any decision as to whether to extract a sound deciduous tooth for balancing and compensating reasons should be weighed against the trauma of such a procedure to the child.

1. *Primary incisors* Premature loss usually causes virtually no drifting of other teeth, but if done very early may delay the eruption of the permanent incisors. Loss of a permanent incisor is a very different matter.

2. *Primary canine* Loss causes some mesial drift of the buccal segment, depending upon the degree of crowding. There is also drift of the incisors into the space, which causes a centre-line shift towards the extraction site (Fig. 14.8). Ideally this should be prevented by balancing the extraction with loss of the contralateral canine, particularly as this is to be completed under general anaesthetic.

3. *Primary first molar* Loss of a primary first molar allows more mesial drift of the teeth distal to it than with the loss of a canine. There may also be some effect on the centre-line (Fig. 14.9), although this is likely to be less pronounced than that with loss of a canine. Balancing of a sound first primary molar would not necessarily be indicated unless general anaesthetic is considered. Where the distribution of caries indicates loss of a primary canine on one side and a primary first molar on the other, these extractions can be regarded as balancing each other reasonably well and the contralateral teeth can be retained.

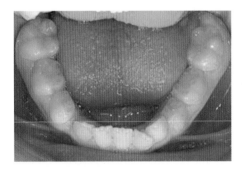

Figure 14.8 Early mixed dentition where early loss of the lower right primary canine has resulted in mesial drift of the buccal segment and loss of space. There also appears to be a centre-line shift to the right.

4. *Primary second molar* Loss allows significant mesial migration of the first permanent molar in that quadrant, causing potentially severe local crowding with displacement or impaction of the second premolar, especially in the upper arch where mesial drift is greatest (Fig. 14.10). In principle, however, the loss of a primary second molar should be avoided if at all possible, especially in the upper arch. A space maintainer, either removable or fixed, can be

considered unless the patient's caries rate is high or the oral hygiene is poor, which is frequently the case in patients requiring early extraction of primary second molars. Primary second molar extractions should never be balanced on the contralateral side as there is very little effect on the centre-line and the potential crowding becomes even more complicated.

In general, there is no need to compensate primary tooth extractions with extractions in the opposing arch. (See Key Points 14.3.)

Key Points 14.3

Mixed dentition extractions

- Early loss of primary teeth generally worsens crowding.
- Extraction of primary canines should be balanced. Benefit of this must be balanced against the trauma of extractions.
- Primary second molars should be preserved if at all possible.

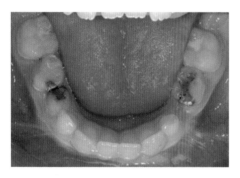

Figure 14.9 The lower left first molar has been extracted in the mixed dentition. There has been some space loss but the effect on the centre-line has been minimal.

14.4.4 Enforced extraction of first permanent molars

First permanent molars are very rarely the teeth of choice for extraction for orthodontic reasons—in practice, their removal often makes treatment more difficult.

- The space they provide is remote from the labial segments and is poorly placed for either the relief of anterior crowding or overjet reduction.
- Depending on the timing of the extractions, much of the space is lost to mesial migration of the second molars, especially in the upper arch.
- The behaviour of the lower second molars following loss of the lower first permanent molars is fairly unpredictable and is greatly influenced by the timing of the extractions.

In general, therefore, first permanent molars are only extracted if their long-term prognosis is felt to be poor because of caries or increasingly hypoplasia. In an ideal world where the loss of one or more first molars is necessary in the mixed dentition, the management of the extractions would depend on whether or not the patient is likely to have active treatment with orthodontic appliances in the future—often a difficult judgement to make. However, owing to caries and the nature of compliance in patients who present with extensive caries, the decision is frequently enforced (Fig. 14.11).

A panoramic radiograph must be taken to confirm the presence of all permanent teeth (except third molars) before finalizing the extractions. Where optimal space closure (Fig. 14.12) is the goal, particularly in the lower arch, the radiographic examination should show:

- a 15–30° angle between the long axes of the first and second molars;
- overlap between the crypt of the second molar and the mesial root of the first molar;
- formation of the bifurcation of the second molars.

In the following discussion the presence of all permanent teeth is assumed—if a premolar is congenitally absent, the first molar in that quadrant should be saved if possible.

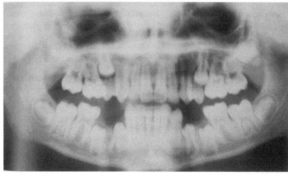

(a)

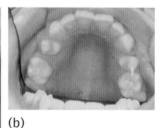

(b)

Figure 14.10 Localized crowding of upper second premolars on (a) OPG and (b) clinically due to the early loss of primary upper second molars. (Courtesy of Professor J.H. Nunn.)

Extractions where no orthodontics is planned

The objective is to minimize disruption of the occlusion. Following the extraction of a first molar, the paths of eruption of adjacent unerupted teeth alter, and erupted adjacent and opposing teeth also start to drift. Many of these changes are unhelpful, but some can be used to advantage with careful planning.

1. *Lower arch* In general, the most obvious change is mesial drift of the second molar. However, some distal movement of premolars and canines may also be expected in the lower arch. The extraction of first molars can be a convenient way of relieving premolar crowding, especially in the lower arch. In the lower arch the timing of the extraction is important. If it is carried out very early the unerupted lower second premolar migrates distally, sometimes leaving a space

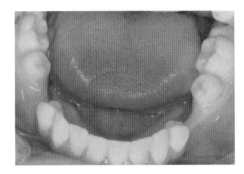

(a)

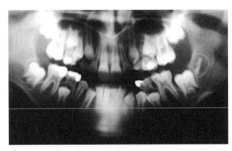

Figure 14.11 Spaces between the lower first and second premolars resulting from very early extraction of the lower first molars.

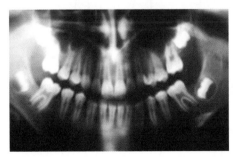

(b)

Figure 14.12 (a) Pre-extraction and (b) good space closure following loss of all four first permanent molars.

between the first and second premolars if the arch is uncrowded (Fig. 14.11). If it is carried out late, as or after the lower second molars erupt, that tooth tilts mesially under occlusal forces and can cause an occlusal interference, especially if the opposing upper first molar over-erupts into the lower extraction space (Fig. 14.13). There is often residual space mesial to the tilted second molar and this poor relationship with the second premolar may cause a stagnation area. These unwanted effects can be minimized in two ways:

(i) extraction of the upper first molar—this eliminates the problem of over-eruption of the opposing first molar and removes the occlusal contact which exaggerates mesial tilting of the lower second molar (Fig. 14.14);

(ii) optimal timing of the extractions—usually at about 8½–9½ years of age (Fig. 14.15).

2. *Upper arch* The behaviour of the second molar is more predictable in the upper arch, although timing is still important. The tendency to mesial drift is much greater than in the lower arch, and there is almost no distal drift of the upper premolars. If the upper first molar is extracted early, the unerupted second molar migrates mesially so that it erupts into the position of the first molar (Fig. 14.10). If the second molar has erupted before the extraction, it still migrates forward, taking up most or all of the space depending on the degree of crowding, and it usually tilts mesially and rotates mesiopalatally about the palatal root. However, compensating extraction of the lower first molar is **not** indicated (Fig. 14.16).

Balancing extractions of the contralateral first permanent molars are not routinely necessary unless they are also in poor condition. Where the arch is crowded, an extraction on the opposite side is usually needed to relieve crowding. If the first permanent molars are in good condition, extraction of first premolars may well be more appropriate. A balancing extraction may prevent any shift of the centre-line, although this is likely to be minimal and is not an indication for extraction by itself. (See Key Points 14.4.)

Key Points 14.4

First permanent molar extractions

- These are never the teeth of choice for orthodontic extraction.
- The best age for loss is 8½–9½ years.
- Extraction of the upper first molar may reduce occlusal disturbance where the lower first molar has to be extracted.
- There is no need to extract the lower first molar if the upper first molar has to be extracted.

Extraction where orthodontic treatment is planned

Where future appliance treatment is anticipated, the objective is to try to avoid complicating it and a specialist orthodontic opinion is often beneficial. Historical guidelines have to some extent been superseded

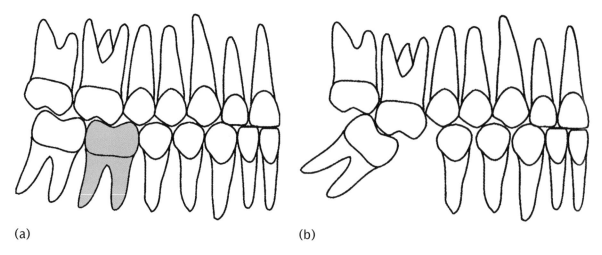

(a)

(b)

Figure 14.13 (a) Loss of the lower first molar after eruption of the second molar causes (b) severe tipping of the lower second molar and over-eruption of the upper first molar.

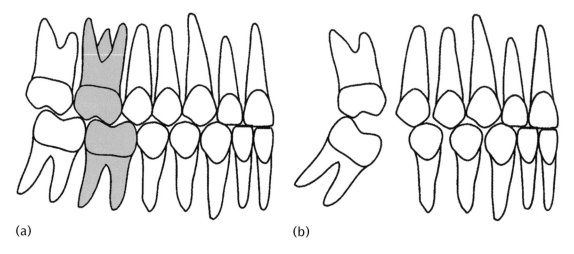

(a)

(b)

Figure 14.14 (a) Extraction of the upper first molar as well as the lower (b) prevents over-eruption of the opposing first molar and reduces the mesial tilting of the lower second molar.

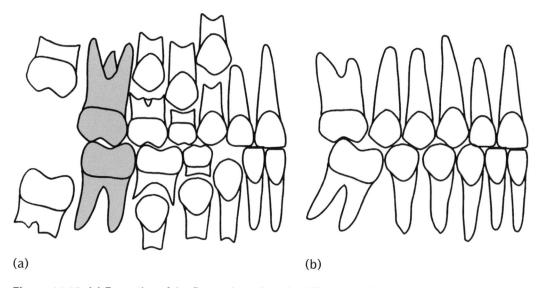

(a)

(b)

Figure 14.15 (a) Extraction of the first molars when the bifurcation of the roots of the lower second molar is starting to calcify, usually at 8½–9½ years of age, gives (b) the best chance of a good result.

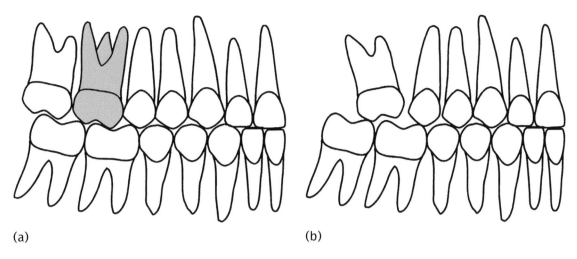

(a)   (b)

Figure 14.16 (a) Extraction of the upper first molar does not need (b) to be compensated by extraction of the lower first molar.

by modern anchorage methods including functional appliances, mini-screws, and implants. Where there is any doubt about the long-term prognosis of the first molar, it is often better to remove it sooner rather than later. It is difficult to give hard and fast rules as the management strategy will differ for each patient, but the main factor to consider is the amount of space that will be needed. Where the extraction space is to be used to relieve crowding or reduce an increased overjet, unwanted mesial drift of the second permanent molars must be minimized. This is best achieved by waiting for the second molars to erupt and then a controlling mesial movement of the second molar after extraction of the first molar (Fig. 14.17). On the other hand, where there will be excess space, mesial drift of the second permanent molars should be encouraged.

In the **lower arch** the extractions are managed according to severity of crowding. Where there is little or no crowding the extraction should, if possible, be carried out at the 'ideal' age of about 8½–9½ years so as to encourage mesial migration of the second molar. Where there is significant crowding it is better to delay the extraction, if possible, until after the lower second molar has erupted, so that the space is available for alignment of the arch.

The **upper arch** is also managed according to space requirements, but these are determined not only by the amount of crowding but also by the class of malocclusion. Where there is significant crowding, the upper first molars should be preserved, if possible, until after the upper second molars have erupted and can be included in an appliance. Similarly, in a class II malocclusion space will be useful to reduce an increased overjet and, again, where possible the extractions should be delayed. Conversely, excess upper arch space in a class III malocclusion complicates treatment, as proclining the upper incisors is a form of expansion which itself creates more space.

Clearly, where active orthodontic treatment is planned the loss of a lower first molar is not automatically compensated by the extraction of the opposing upper first molar.

The broad principles of the management of enforced extraction of first molars are summarized in Table 14.3.

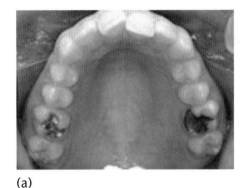

(a)

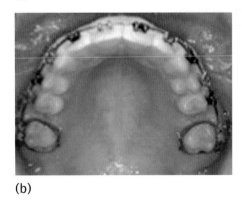

(b)

Figure 14.17 (a) To correct the class II incisor relationship there has been a delay in extraction of the upper first molars until the upper second molars have erupted. (b) The space from the extraction is then utilized to relieve crowding and reduce the overjet using fixed appliances.

Table 14.3 Management of enforced extraction of first permanent molars in the mixed dentition*

Malocclusion	Minimal/uncrowded	Crowding	General comment
Class I	**Lower arch** Compensate unless upper erupted with occlusal contact **Upper arch** Do not compensate	**Buccal segment** If bilateral consider balance **Labial segment** Little spontaneous improvement in crowding likely	Aim to extract for both crowded and uncrowded at the optimal time unless space from extraction is to be utilized for relief of labial segment crowding
Class II	**Lower arch** Remove at optimal time **Upper arch** Where temporization is possible maintain and utilize for overjet reduction or functional appliance retention	**Lower arch** Remove at optimal time **Upper arch** Where temporization is possible maintain and utilize for overjet reduction or functional appliance retention and relief of crowding	More difficult to plan as space is often required for reduction of overjet and in crowded cases the relief of crowding Where an upper first molar is left temporized and unopposed there is a risk of over-eruption and its extraction may be considered Any residual overjet and crowding would be considered on its own merits in permanent dentition
Class III			Difficult to plan If teeth have to be extracted, remove at optimal time Generally extraction in upper arch should be avoided

*These guidelines are very broad and their application will vary greatly between individual patients. They assume that only one first molar is of poor prognosis, and with crowding their application should be modified where more than one first molar is of poor prognosis.

14.5 **Correction of cross-bites**

The great majority of orthodontic treatments are carried out during the late mixed and early permanent dentitions to avoid prolonged appliance wear while permanent teeth erupt. However, a few conditions can benefit from earlier intervention. Where early intervention is planned it is important to:

- set clear objectives;
- keep it simple;
- ideally complete within 6 months so as to not waste compliance.

14.5.1 **Anterior cross-bite**

Although it may be a sign of a developing class III problem, a local anterior cross-bite involving one or two incisors is often simply due to the positions of the developing tooth-germs causing the teeth to erupt into cross-bite. Possible complications of a localized anterior cross-bite are as follows: premature contact with the tooth in cross-bite causes the mandible to displace forwards as the teeth come into maximum intercuspal position; one lower incisor in cross-bite may be driven labially through the supporting tissues, causing localized gingival recession (Fig. 14.18).

Early correction encourages development of a class I occlusion, and treatment in the mixed dentition is often straightforward provided that the following criteria are met:

- *Normal skeletal pattern*. Check for anterior displacement of the mandible. Beware of class III growth.

- *Adequate space in the arch*. Primary canines may need to be extracted to accommodate labial movement of upper incisors.
- *Adequate overbite*. Stable correction of the cross-bite depends on there being positive overbite after treatment.

There are many designs of removable appliance to correct anterior cross-bites, and a typical example is shown in Fig. 14.19. Its essential features are:

- an *active component* such as a Z-spring or a screw palatal to the tooth to be moved;
- *retention* as far anteriorly as possible to resist the tendency of the spring to displace the front of the appliance;

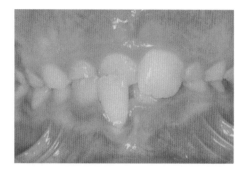

Figure 14.18 Localized gingival recession associated with incisor cross-bite.

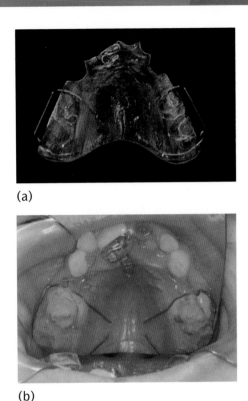

(a)

(b)

Figure 14.19 (a) Appliance to procline upper incisor. (b) Note posterior capping to disengage occlusion and retention anterior to 6 6 to resist the displacing force generated by the Z-spring.

- *posterior capping* to open the occlusion while the upper incisor moves labially over the lower incisors.

Where these features do not exist specialist advice should be sought. An example of treatment is shown in Fig. 14.20.

14.5.2 Posterior cross-bite with displacement

Where the upper arch is slightly narrow, the buccal teeth may initially occlude cusp to cusp and only achieve full intercuspation when the mandible displaces laterally (Fig. 14.21), causing a unilateral posterior cross-bite. This can be difficult to detect if the patient cannot relax the jaw muscles fully during examination, but it is important to determine whether or not there is a lateral displacement. A unilateral posterior cross-bite with a displacement is easily corrected during the mixed dentition. Where no displacement is visible, the displacement is usually skeletal in origin and as with bilateral cross-bites correction should not be attempted without specialist advice.

A unilateral posterior cross-bite with a displacement is treated by expansion of the upper arch to remove the initial cusp-to-cusp contact, using an appliance such as that shown in Fig. 14.21(c). It has a mid-line expansion screw which is turned by the parent once or twice a week, and double Adams clasps on 6e|e6. The d|d are usually unsuitable for

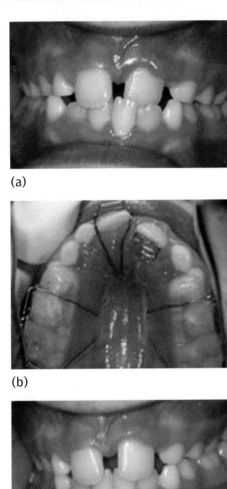

(a)

(b)

(c)

Figure 14.20 (a) A patient with UL1 in cross-bite with small anterior displacement and LL1 labially displaced. (b) A patient wearing a removable appliance. (c) UL1 in correct position. Note overbite and improved gingival condition of LL1.

clasping as they have little or no undercut. The appliance should contact c|c as these usually need to be expanded, but need not contact the incisors unless a bite plane is required.

14.5.3 Increased overjet

The incidence of trauma to the upper incisors is greater where the overjet is increased to the extent that twice as many 13-year-olds with overjets of 10mm or more have traumatized upper incisors compared with children with overjets of less than 5mm. Therefore it would seem sensible to reduce overjets as early as possible to prevent the occurrence of this trauma. However, clinical trials have found that reduction in overjet in the mixed dentition has little if any effect overall on the

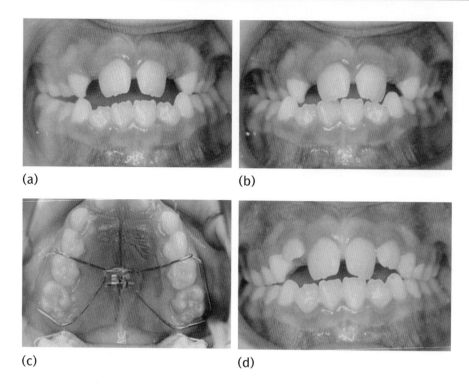

(a)

(b)

(c)

(d)

Figure 14.21 Unilateral posterior cross-bite with lateral mandibular displacement. (a) Initial contact on closure. (b) Lateral displacement of the mandible on closure into maximum intercuspal position causing unilateral posterior cross-bite. (c) Upper expansion appliance. (d) Displacement has been eliminated after upper arch displacement.

incidence of trauma. This observation is probably because trauma tends to occur at an age younger than that of the timing for conventional orthodontic intervention for increased overjets.

Orthodontic intervention to reduce overjets is usually done with a functional appliance. Details of the management and effects of these appliances can be found in orthodontic texts—they induce correction of the incisor and molar relationships by a combination of dento-alveolar and skeletal changes. This is not done by active components such as springs, but instead the appliances harness forces generated by the masticatory and facial musculature. They achieve this by holding the mandible in a forward postured position. All designs of functional appliance are similar in that they engage both dental arches and cause mandibular posturing and displacement of the condyles within the glenoid fossae (Fig. 14.22). In the UK the most commonly used type of functional appliance is the twin block appliance which is composed of two parts, one worn in the lower and one in the upper arch. The blocks on each of the two parts occlude to posture the mandible forwards. Their advantage over many of the other types of functional appliances is that they can be worn full time, which allows rapid correction of the overjet.

Functional appliances work most efficiently when the child is growing. Greater skeletal effect and shorter overall treatment times have been shown for those children treated in the late mixed/early

adult dentition than those treated earlier. However, this fact does not preclude earlier treatment in those with a significant overjet and/or those where it is having a negative psychological impact on the child.

Although functional appliances will correct an overjet, they will have little effect on tooth irregularity. Therefore they are frequently the first part of a two-part orthodontic plan comprising a first phase of overjet correction and a second phase of fixed appliances to improve alignment and detail the occlusion.

14.5.4 Space maintenance

Historically, much has been written about space maintenance where deciduous teeth have been extracted. In the author's experience patients who have deciduous teeth extracted are rarely ideal candidates for any type of appliance that will collect plaque and increase the chances of decay. The only exception is where oral hygiene is acceptable and the space maintenance may lead to the prevention of any further treatment.

Space maintenance is often important so that drifting of teeth into an extraction space is prevented, for example, following loss of a primary molar or an upper incisor, or where the crowding is so severe that

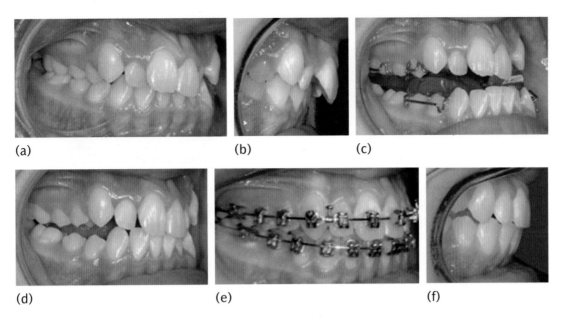

Figure 14.22 (a) Class II, division I malocclusion. (b) Increased overjet. (c) Twin block functional appliance in place showing posturing of the mandible. (d) Post functional appliance occlusion showing an edge-to-edge incisor relationship and lateral open bites, a common feature on post twin block occlusions. (e) Fixed appliances in place to align and detail the occlusion. (f) Post fixed appliance occlusion with overjet within normal limits.

extractions give only just enough space. As a general rule of thumb, where a tooth is extracted for crowding and more than half of its width is required for tooth alignment, some form of space maintenance would be prudent (Fig. 14.23).

14.5.5 Digit-sucking habits

Sucking habits in the form of dummies or pacifiers or finger/thumb-sucking are common in children in the primary dentition. Generally speaking, dummies or pacifiers have little effect on the dentition other than mild symmetrical anterior open bites, particularly if orthodontic dummies or teats, which have a flatter cross-section and collapse in the mouth, are used. Intervention is unnecessary unless cross-bites start to develop (Fig. 14.24), although after the age of 2 years there may be a detrimental effect on speech development.

Thumb- and finger-sucking habits tend to be more detrimental to the dentition and more persistent where they continue into the mixed dentition. It has been suggested that where a digit habit exists in a young child, the digit should be swapped for a dummy.

The effect of the thumb or fingers depends upon the duration and method of sucking. Classically they cause:

- asymmetric anterior open bite;
- increased overjet with proclined upper incisors and retroclined lower incisors;
- class II buccal segment relationship;
- unilateral posterior cross-bite with displacement.

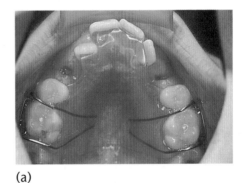

(a)

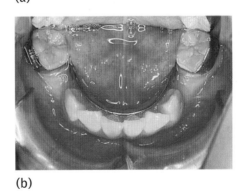

(b)

Figure 14.23 (a) Upper first premolars have been extracted for relief of crowding and alignment of upper canines and incisors. More than 50% of the width of the canine is required for alignment and so a space maintainer has been fitted. (b)Lower lingual arch serving as a space maintainer

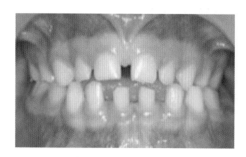

Figure 14.24 Symmetrical anterior open bite in primary dentition. Note the unilateral cross-bite and deviation in the centre-line associated with mandibular displacement. The habit should be discouraged.

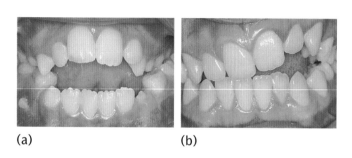

(a)   (b)

Figure 14.25 A 9-year-old child with an anterior open bite associated with thumb-sucking. (b) A 16-year-old girl with a continuing digit-sucking habit causing a localized open bite.

The unilateral posterior cross-bite can occur because the tongue position is low during digit-sucking, allowing activity of the buccal musculature to narrow the upper arch slightly.

Although a few children continue the habit into their teenage years, nearly all grow out of it by about 10 years of age. It is important to start gentle discouragement before the permanent incisors start to erupt. An anterior open bite caused by a sucking habit (Fig. 14.25) will usually resolve if the habit is broken early enough and the incisors still have significant eruption potential (<10 years) although the class II buccal segment relationship will not. If the anterior open bite persists it is often because the tongue has adapted to the open bite by contacting the lower lip to make an anterior seal during swallowing. This is known as an 'adaptive tongue position'.

Habit deterrents in the form of removable appliances with a simple goal-post design (Fig. 14.26) have a place if non-physical methods fail. Their success depends upon whether the child wishes to stop. If the child derives some support from the habit and does not wish to stop, their success is less predictable. Orthodontic treatment to correct the resulting malocclusion should not be started until the habit is broken, and it has been noted that patients with a history of a habit are more prone to root resorption with treatment.

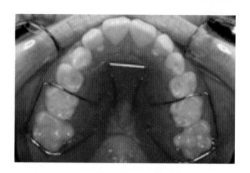

Figure 14.26 Habit-breaker appliance: double Adams clasps on first molars and second deciduous molars and a goal-post to prevent digit access.

14.5.6 Incisor spacing—midline diastema

This is mentioned only to point out that treatment just for spacing is rarely indicated in the mixed dentition stage. Parents are often concerned about spacing of the upper incisors, and they can usually be reassured that it is part of normal development and will often reduce or close as the permanent upper canines erupt if less than 2.5mm. Other possible causes of a midline diastema are:

- familial or racial characteristics
- diminutive teeth
- absence of upper lateral incisors
- palatally placed lateral incisors
- midline supernumerary (Section 14.7.1).

There is some disagreement about the role of frenectomy in the treatment of diastema, but it is very rarely indicated in the mixed dentition stage and is probably best carried out during active orthodontic treatment if the frenum is felt to be a contributory factor. (See Key Points 14.5.)

Key Points 14.5

- Cross-bites with significant displacement should be treated in the mixed dentition.
- An increased overjet is treated in the late mixed dentition unless it is very large or there is psychological impact suggesting earlier intervention.
- Patients with enforced extractions for caries in the deciduous dentition are rarely good candidates for space maintainers.
- Start discouraging patients with persistent digit-sucking habits before permanent incisors erupt.
- Upper incisor spacing usually reduces as the permanent canines erupt, but check for other anomalies.

14.6 Anomalies of eruption—the ectopic maxillary canine

The path of eruption of any tooth can become disturbed. Sometimes the reason is obvious, such as a supernumerary tooth impeding an upper incisor (see Section 14.7.1), but often it is obscure. In clinical orthodontics, the most common problem of aberrant eruption is the impacted maxillary canine (Fig. 14.27), which is second only to the third molar in frequency of impaction.

14.6.1 Prevalence of impacted maxillary canines

Ectopic maxillary canines occur in about 2% of the population; 85% of these canines are palatal and 15% buccal to the line of the upper arch. The risk of impaction of the upper canine is greater where the lateral incisor is diminutive or absent—the lateral incisor root is known to guide the erupting canine. An impacted canine can frequently resorb adjacent incisor roots and this risk may be as high as 48% (Fig. 14.28), although it has been suggested that the chances of resorption decrease after the age of 14 years.

14.6.2 Clinical assessment

During the mixed dentition stage the normal path of eruption of the maxillary canines is slightly buccal to the line of the arch, and from about 10 years of age the crowns should be palpable as bulges on the buccal aspect of the alveolus, slightly distal to the lateral incisor. From this position the canine is likely to erupt. If a hollow or asymmetry is noted on palpation, this should be considered suspicious and further investigation or close monitoring is warranted.

Unerupted maxillary canines should be palpated routinely on all children from the age of 10 years until eruption.

14.6.3 Radiographic assessment

Where the canine is not palpable it should be assessed radiographically. A panoramic radiograph gives a great deal of valuable information including the position of the canine and asymmetries in the path of eruption. If the apex of the primary canine is not resorbing normally, with either no root resorption or only lateral resorption, the path of eruption of the permanent canine may be abnormal. When the canine appears enlarged on a panoramic radiograph compared with the normally erupting side, it is suggestive of a palatal position. However, to assess the canine position more accurately using plain radiography two views are needed at right angles to each other (parallax technique). Parallax can be considered in the vertical plane using a panoramic radiograph and an anterior occlusal or periapical radiograph, or more accurately in the horizontal plane using two periapical radiographs. Alternatively, modern three-dimensional positional assessment using cone beam computed tomography (CT) can be used, although the radiation dose for the patient is higher than that with plain radiographs.

Parallax technique

This method, also known as the tube-shift method, compares two views of the area taken with the X-ray tube in two different positions. Figure 14.29 shows an image of a palatal canine on a periapical film taken with the tube positioned forward or mesially. A second film taken with the tube positioned further distally gives an image that apparently shows the canine crown in a different position relative to the adjacent roots. In this case the image of the canine appears to have shifted distally compared with the first film, i.e. in the same direction as the tube was moved, which indicates that the canine is palatal to the other teeth. An apparent shift in the opposite direction to the tube shift would indicate that the tooth is lying buccally to the other teeth. Parallax in the vertical direction may be slightly more difficult to assess (Fig. 14.30). When performed using a panoramic radiograph the tube is in a horizontal or lower position, but when an anterior occlusal or periapical radiograph is taken the tube moves into a higher or more vertical position. The cephalometric radiograph used in full orthodontic assessment will also give an indication of buccal or canine tooth position.

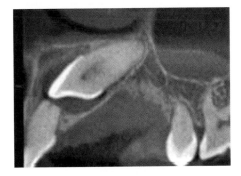

Figure 14.27 Cone beam CT showing resorption of a permanent incisor by an impacted canine.

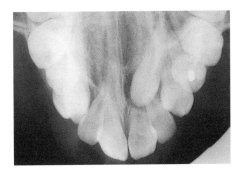

Figure 14.28 An impacted upper left canine causing root resorption of upper left central and lateral incisors.

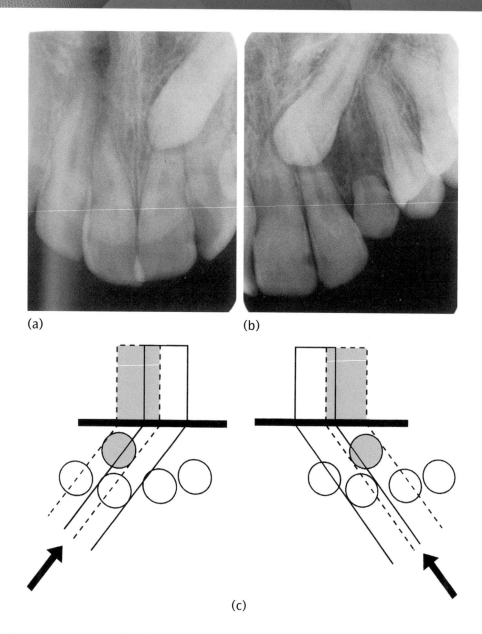

Figure 14.29 Parallax location of 23. (a) Radiograph taken with the tube positioned forward shows that the image of the canine crown is slightly mesial to the image of 21. (b) Radiograph taken with the tube positioned further distally shows that the image of 23 is located further distally. The image of 23 has shifted in the same direction as the tube shift. Therefore 23 is nearer to the film than 21, i.e. it is palatal to the line of the arch. (c) Diagrammatic representation of how a palatally positioned tooth moves 'with' the tube from left to right.

14.6.4 Early treatment

During the later mixed dentition, if an upper canine is not palpable and is found to be ectopic, extraction of the primary canine gives a >70% chance of correcting or improving the path of eruption of the permanent canine provided that there is adequate space for its eruption (Fig. 14.31). Specialist advice should usually be sought before considering this procedure.

The success of deciduous canine extraction is improved by:

- early detection (<12 years)
- adequate space for the canine to erupt
- mild/moderate canine displacements.

Once the deciduous canine has been extracted, the tooth position should be reassessed at 1 year. If no improvement is noted, other treatment options should be considered.

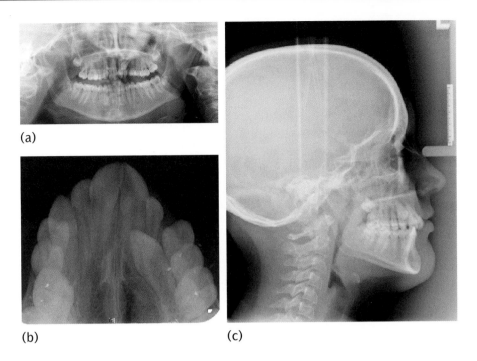

(a)

(b)

(c)

Figure 14.30 (a) A panoramic radiograph showing a child in permanent dentition with an ectopically placed upper left canine. (b) Anterior occlusal view showing the canine appearing more apical to the upper left central incisor, i.e. moving with the tube (therefore palatal). (c) A lateral cephalometric radiograph of the same patient confirming that the misplaced canine is palatal to the roots of the central incisors.

14.6.5 Later treatment

Treatment options in the permanent dentition are:

- leave *in situ* and monitor;
- remove impacted canine ± space closure with orthodontic appliances;
- expose the canine and align it with orthodontic appliances;
- transplant the canine.

Table 14.4 gives a simplified review of the later treatment options for an impacted canine with some indications and general comment for each. Before the final decision is made, an assessment should be made of the patient's motivation and appearance, the presence of crowding and malocclusion, canine position, and probable longevity of the deciduous canine.

In relation to the position of the unerupted canine the following should be noted:

- Vertically, its relationship to the apex of the adjacent incisor—the more apical the canine crown, the poorer the prognosis.

- The tooth angulation to the occlusal plane—the more horizontal the tooth, the poorer the prognosis.

- The relationship to the midline—the more mesial, the worse the prognosis.

- The position of the apex—the more distal to the first premolar, the poorer the prognosis.

(See Key Points 14.6.)

Key Points 14.6

Ectopic canines

- About 2% of children have ectopic upper canines, of which 85% are palatal.
- Ectopic canines frequently cause incisor resorption.
- Always palpate for upper canines from the age of 10 years until eruption.
- Non-palpable upper canines should be located radiographically or referred for investigation.
- Consider extraction of a primary canine if uncrowded and patient is <13 years old.
- Orthodontic alignment of ectopic canines requires prolonged orthodontic treatment.

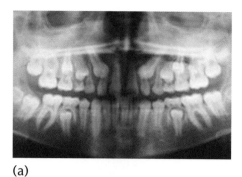

(a)

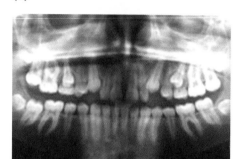

(b)

Figure 14.31 (a) A panoramic radiograph of a patient in the mixed dentition with unerupted palatally positioned maxillary canines. (b) One year after extraction of the maxillary deciduous canines, the canine eruption path has normalized.

14.6.6 Other anomalies of eruption

Three other anomalies of eruption are fairly common in the mixed dentition.

1. *Infraoccluded primary teeth* (Chapter 13) usually exfoliate, provided that the permanent successors are present, within a year of the contralateral tooth and therefore should be kept under review. If they are not shed, the infra-occlusion becomes more marked, or the adjacent teeth start to tip, the tooth should be removed.

2. *Impaction of the upper first permanent molar* into the distal of the upper second primary molar causing resorption (Fig. 14.32). It is possible to disimpact the tooth with an appliance, but in 66% of cases the problem usually resolves spontaneously or when the primary molar is shed. The resorption may cause pain if it involves the pulp, in which case the primary molar should be removed. This allows the permanent molar to move rapidly mesially, and a space maintainer or active appliance to move it distally should be considered.

3. *Second premolars* in unfavourable positions are sometimes seen as incidental findings on panoramic radiographs, but fortunately they usually correct spontaneously and eventually erupt satisfactorily. Very occasionally this does not happen, and a few cases have been reported of a lower second premolar migrating towards the mandibular ramus. Upper or lower second premolars that are blocked from the arch because of crowding usually erupt, but are displaced lingually.

Table 14.4 Later treatment options for impacted canines

Treatment option	Possible indications	General comment
Leave *in situ* and monitor	Significant displacement	Despite being left *in situ* the tooth will require occasional monitoring to check for pathology
	Patient unwilling to consider orthodontics/surgery	
	Removal presents significant risks to adjacent structures	
Surgical removal (± orthodontic treatment)	Associated pathology	Best aesthetic results are achieved where there is close approximation between the first premolar and lateral incisor
	Poor position for alignment	
	Orthodontic treatment but extraction of sound teeth required for alignment	
Expose canine and align with orthodontic treatment	Patient willing and motivated to undergo orthodontic treatment	Orthodontic treatment to align palatally placed canines can be prolonged (>2 years)
	Canine position favourable: <50% past midpoint of the central apex in line of arch no higher than apex of lateral incisor	Complications include canine discolouration, associated resorption of adjacent teeth, and significant relapse potential
	Space available for alignment, preferably without extraction	
Transplant	Poor prognosis for alignment	Very technique sensitive
	Adequate space for transplant	Method may be superseded by implant with retention of primary canine until late teens

14.7 Anomalies of tooth size and number

These anomalies are discussed in Chapter 13, but their clinical management often has orthodontic implications.

14.7.1 Supernumerary teeth

Supernumerary teeth are very common in the pre-maxilla, occurring in approximately 2% of the population but less than 1% in the primary dentition. They can interfere with the eruption of normal teeth (Figs 14.33, 14.34, 14.35, and 14.36) or cause localized crowding if they erupt. The most common description of supernumerary teeth is in terms of their morphology:

- conical
- tuberculate
- supplemental
- odontomes.

Table 14.5 describes supernumerary teeth in terms of their location and effects, and comments on their management.

For a successful outcome, the key to management is early detection and removal if they are causing physical obstruction.

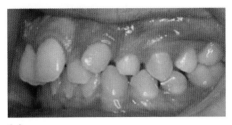

(a)

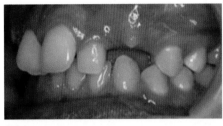

(b)

Figure 14.34 (a) Supplemental lateral incisor in the mixed dentition. (b) A year after extraction of the lateral incisor, resulting in relief of crowding in that quadrant.

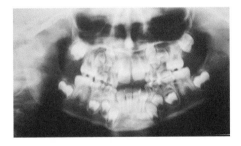

Figure 14.32 Impaction of 26 causing distal resorption of the upper left second primary molar (65).

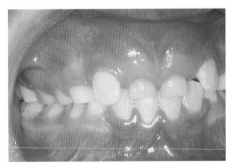

(a)

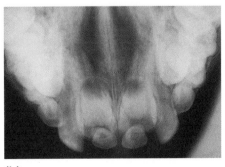

(b)

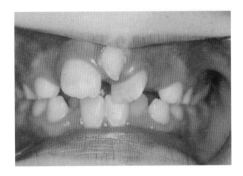

Figure 14.33 An erupted conical midline supernumerary which has not prevented eruption of 11, 21, but has displaced ⌐1.

Figure 14.35 (a) Failure of eruption of 11, 21 because of (b) the presence of two tuberculate supernumerary teeth. (Photos courtesy of Mr T.G. Bennett.)

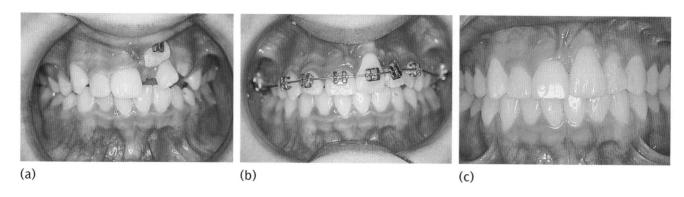

(a)   (b)   (c)

Figure 14.36 (a) Surgical exposure of unerupted 21. (b) Orthodontic alignment of 21 (note the poor gingival contour as a result of open exposure). (c) The poor gingival contour persists for several years after treatment.

Table 14.5 Supernumerary teeth: location, effect, and management

Type	Location	Effects	Comment
Conical	Most common, conical/triangular with root formation Close to midline between central incisors (mesiodens) Sometimes inverted	Usually does not prevent eruption but may cause displacement (median diastema)	If causing displacement should be extracted If high leave *in situ* unless closely associated with roots of teeth and orthodontics is planned
Tuberculate	Barrel-shaped with incomplete or absent roots Rarely erupt Usually palatal and often paired	Most common cause of eruption failure of central incisors Early detection is key to good outcome with unerupted central incisors	Management principles: remove primary tooth create sufficient room for eruption remove supernumerary ± closed exposure with attachment bonded palatal of incisal to prevent fenestration 50–75% erupt in 18 months
Supplemental	Normal morphology, most commonly lateral incisor In the deciduous dentition the majority of supernumeraries are supplemental	Localized crowding	Extraction of one of the two lateral incisors taking into account displacement and alignment difficulties
Odontomes	Described as complex (irregular mass of dental tissue) or compound small separate tooth-like structure Located in anterior maxilla or lower molar regions	As tuberculate Tend to cause physical obstruction	As tuberculate

14.7.2 Hypodontia

Any tooth in the arch can be congenitally absent but, apart from third molars, the teeth most commonly affected are lower second premolars and upper lateral incisors (Chapter 13). Where one or two teeth are absent, the orthodontic options are to open, maintain, or close the space. Where multiple teeth are absent, orthodontic treatment may be able to give a more favourable basis for restorative replacement. In general, missing teeth are best managed in a multidisciplinary environment with input from oral surgeons, restorative and paediatric dentists, and orthodontists.

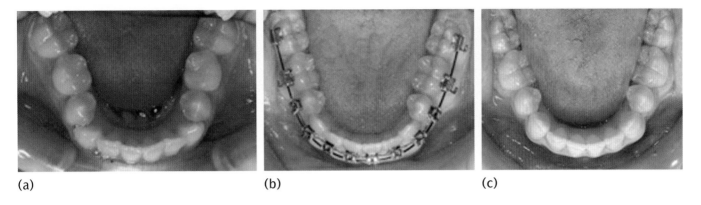

(a)　　　　　　　　　　　(b)　　　　　　　　　　　(c)

Figure 14.37 (a) Lower arch with moderate incisor crowding and retained lower second primary molars with absent lower second premolars. (b) Fixed appliances in place after removal of lower second primary molars. (c) After fixed-appliance treatment with crowding relieved and residual space closed.

Second premolars

Where the arch is aligned or spaced the primary second molar should be left *in situ*, but where there is crowding the space can be used for arch alignment (Fig. 14.37). In the upper arch and in a significantly crowded lower arch, the primary second molar should be retained until the start of orthodontic treatment. Where there is mild lower arch crowding which is to be treated, the primary second molar can be extracted earlier to allow some of the space to be lost to mesial drifting of the first molar. This occurs most favourably when the teeth are extracted as the permanent lateral incisors are erupting.

Upper lateral incisors

Upper lateral incisors are congenitally absent in approximately 2% of the Caucasian population. If one tooth is absent, the contralateral tooth is often small or peg-shaped. Patients with absent lateral incisors often have other dental anomalies present including ectopic canine teeth. Where one or both upper lateral incisors are absent in an uncrowded arch, the excess space is often distributed as generalized anterior spacing. The spacing is often accentuated as it is not uncommon to find that the remaining teeth are also small and some have unusual morphology (Fig. 14.38).

In general terms the treatment options for absent lateral incisors are space opening followed by prosthetic replacement (bridge or implant) or space closure (with or without extensive canine modification and bleaching). Orthodontic treatment is utilized to obtain optimal aesthetic results. The options chosen are driven by a number factors:

- patient's wishes and likely cooperation;
- skeletal relationship;
- smile aesthetics, particularly the upper lip line;
- the teeth that are absent, anterior or posterior;
- colour and form of adjacent teeth, particularly canine;
- existing malocclusion and buccal segment relationship.

Irrespective of the decision made, a trial set-up (Kesling) is often utilized as a method of informing patient and clinician of the options. This is

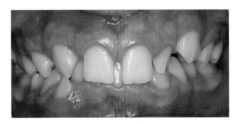

Figure 14.38 Absent upper right lateral incisor, diminutive peg-shaped upper left lateral incisor, and small chisel-shaped central incisors.

particularly relevant where there are a number of missing dental units or where space needs to be reconfigured to allow build-up of small teeth (Fig. 14.39).

Indications and general management of either space closure or space opening are shown in Table 14.6. Irrespective of the plan, retention is critical on completion as both methods of treatment have a high relapse potential. In the case of space closure, long-term bonded retention between the upper anterior teeth is the usual method of choice with an upper removable retainer for a minimum of 1 year (Fig. 14.40). In relation to space opening, the method of retention depends on the type of prosthesis employed to replace the missing tooth. Where a single-wing resin-retained bridge is employed, a bonded retainer between the upper central incisors can be utilized (Fig. 14.41). If a fixed-fixed design is used, this is not required. Irrespective of the prosthesis, a removable retainer (usually a pressure-formed type) made after prosthetic replacement would usually be required long-term.

Where the definitive prosthesis is considered to be an implant, it may be prudent to delay definitive orthodontic treatment until later adolescence. While it may be possible to treat earlier, it has been suggested that retention of root position and prevention of their convergence are problematic. (See Key Points 14.7.)

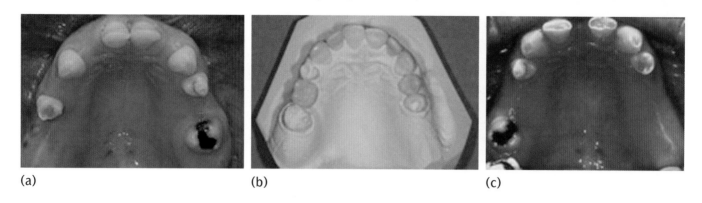

(a) (b) (c)

Figure 14.39 (a) Prior to treatment. (b) Kesling set-up showing the ideal tooth positioning for replacement. (c) After orthodontic space redistribution.

Table 14.6 Treatment options for absent upper lateral incisors

Treatment option	Indications	General comment
Space opening with prosthetic replacement	High lip line	The definitive size of the missing lateral incisor is based on the central incisor in the ratio 1.6:1
	Class I/III incisor relationship	
	Spaced upper arch with class I buccal segment	Retention is usually for 3–6 months post-orthodontics prior to replacement with resin-retained bridge
	Dark/large canines	If replacement with an implant is planned it may be better to delay treatment until the end of growth as there are issues of prolonged retention with relapse of root positions
Space closure	Low lip line	Canine modification to improve the appearance is usually carried out progressively throughout orthodontic treatment
	Class II malocclusion or class I with crowded lower arch	Selective bleaching can improve canine colour post-orthodontics
	Small rounded light canines	Bonded retention is required long term to maintain space closure

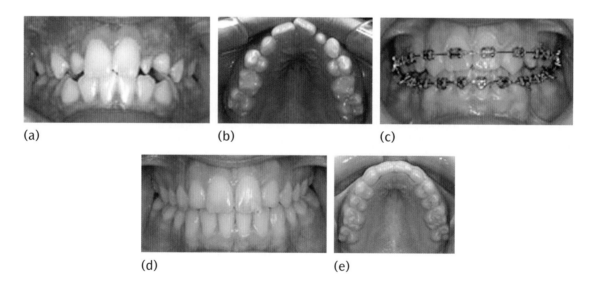

(a) (b) (c)

(d) (e)

Figure 14.40 (a), (b) Missing upper right lateral and peg upper left lateral. (c) Peg extracted and fixed appliances to close spaces and align. (d) Upper canines masked to look like laterals. (e) Long-term bonded palatal retainer. (Courtesy of Mr I.B. Buchanan.)

Key Points 14.7

Supernumerary teeth

- Variations from the normal eruption sequence and symmetry should be investigated.
- Supernumerary teeth that interfere with the eruption of permanent teeth should be removed. Closed exposure is often beneficial at the same time. Early diagnosis is important.
- The space for the permanent tooth should be created or maintained while it erupts.
- The majority of the unerupted teeth will erupt within 18 months.
- Spacing due to congenitally absent teeth is best managed in a multidisciplinary setting.
- Irrespective of the type of orthodontic treatment performed, long-term retention is critical.

More severe hypodontia with multiple missing teeth

This often needs complex treatment. Preliminary orthodontic treatment can often help restoration by making the space distribution more favourable, uprighting tilted teeth, and reducing the overbite. Fixed appliances are usually needed and orthodontic retention requires careful management.

14.7.3 Anomalies of tooth size

Anomalies of tooth size are discussed in Chapter 13. Any tooth may be affected, but the upper lateral incisor is most commonly involved.

Megadontia

If the upper and lower teeth do not match for size it is impossible for them to be both aligned and in normal occlusion. An abnormally large upper incisor is associated with crowding or increased overjet, or both. A grossly oversized tooth may have to be extracted and replaced with a pontic after completion of any orthodontic treatment. In milder cases it is possible to narrow the tooth by reducing the enamel interdentally. Up to 1mm can be removed after the teeth have been aligned but before appliances are removed, so that the resulting spaces can be closed.

Microdontia

Upper lateral incisors are most commonly affected. Any orthodontic treatment should precede the restoration of a diminutive tooth, and should leave adequate space for it to be enlarged. Build-up of the tooth can occur during the orthodontic treatment or at its completion. Build-up during treatment relies on the space being created, and brackets and archwire may need to be removed and replaced after the build-up (Fig. 14.42). Mid-treatment build-up has the benefit to the orthodontist of allowing easier detailing of the occlusion. If the decision is made to build the tooth up at the completion of treatment, a Hawley type retainer should carry interdental spurs to prevent adjacent teeth from drifting into the space, and it should be worn for at least 3 months before the tooth is built up. If a pressure-formed retainer is used, it will need replacement after restoration of the diminutive tooth.

Where the upper arch is inherently crowded but the lateral incisors are diminutive on one side and congenitally absent on the other, it may be appropriate to extract the diminutive tooth and close the spaces (see Fig. 14.40).

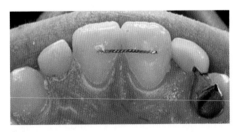

(a)

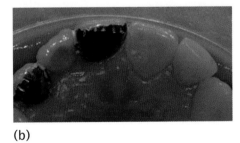

(b)

Figure 14.41 (a) Upper left lateral incisor replaced with a resin-retained bridge utilizing a cantilever design. A bonded retainer has been placed between the central incisors to prevent diastema relapse. (b) Upper left lateral incisor replaced utilizing a fixed-fixed design resin-retained bridge

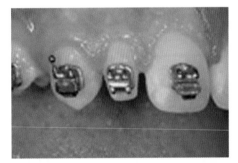

(a)

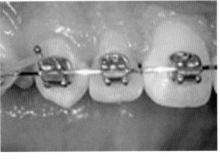

(b)

Figure 14.42 (a) Pre build up and (b) composite build-up of a microdont lateral followed by bracket and archwire replacement.

14.8 Orthodontics and dental trauma

Orthodontic brackets are often used as an immediate measure after trauma to stabilize loosened or reimplanted teeth, to realign displaced teeth, or to extrude teeth that have been intruded (Chapter 12). Teeth that have been fractured at the gingival level may require extrusion later to facilitate restoration.

14.8.1 Orthodontic movement of traumatized teeth and non-vital teeth

In general, root-filled teeth can be moved orthodontically quite normally, with no increased risk of external root resorption compared with normal teeth. The risk factors associated with root resorption during orthodontic treatment are discussed in Section 14.8.3. However, traumatized teeth are already at an increased risk of root resorption, especially those which have been displaced or reimplanted, and those that already show signs of resorption are at risk of further resorption with orthodontic treatment. Pre-treatment radiographs should be compared with those taken 6–9 months into treatment to check for changes in resorption levels. Where resorption is increasing, a 3-month break or 'rest' from active movement is considered appropriate, followed by re-evaluation of the treatment objectives.

The present recommendations on non-vital teeth and orthodontics are that, ideally, the definitive gutta percha root filling is completed prior to commencement. The exceptions are where non-setting calcium hydroxide is being used for apexification of an immature root or resorption is considered to be inflammatory and progressive.

When the definitive root treatment has been completed, a period of observation is considered prudent. The duration of this is determined by the reason for the loss of vitality. Where the cause is caries, orthodontic treatment can be carried out immediately after root treatment completion. Where there has been extensive bone loss it is advisable to wait for a year for signs of healing and, in the case of trauma, the absence of ankylosis. If a previously traumatized tooth fails to move as expected with orthodontics, there should be a high suspicion of ankylosis.

A summary of recommended observation periods prior to orthodontic movement with regard to dental trauma is given in Table 14.7. (See Key Points 14.8.)

Key Points 14.8

Trauma

- Traumatized teeth with signs of resorption are prone to further resorption with orthodontic treatment.
- Definitive endodontic treatment with gutta percha root filling is considered preferable prior to commencing orthodontic treatment.
- However, the orthodontic treatment should be preceded by a period of observation, determined by the cause of loss of vitality of the tooth.

14.9 Complications of orthodontic treatment

The complications or hazards of orthodontic treatment can be divided into:

- tissue damage
- treatment failure and relapse
- predisposition to dental-related disorders.

14.9.1 Tissue damage

Tissue damage in relation to orthodontics and its prevention is summarized in Table 14.8.

The most common and aesthetically distressing type of damage for the patient is decalcification. Orthodontic patients in general are usually well motivated because of use of careful selection criteria prior to commencement. However, by placing appliances the operator is converting them from essentially low-caries-risk patients to patients with high caries risk because of plaque collection and hygiene difficulties (Fig. 14.43). In common with all high-caries-risk patients the following methods of prevention should be mandatory:

- oral hygiene instruction;
- dietary advice;

- fluoride in the form of a toothpaste (≥1400ppm F), a mouthwash (250ppm F taken daily at a different time to brushing), and the addition of a varnish (22 600ppm F three times a year if necessary).

Where areas of decalcification are noted during appliance therapy (Fig. 14.44) the patient should be informed and the treatment aims re-evaluated. Once the appliances are removed, the lesions will probably improve, particularly if a high-dose fluoride regime is instigated. Those that remain unsightly will usually respond to the acid–pumice micro-abrasion technique described in Chapter 10, although severe lesions may require localized composite restoration.

Root resorption as a consequence of orthodontic treatment is common. Most teeth will undergo root shortening of approximately 1–2mm during active treatment. Fortunately significant reduction in root length is relatively rare (<10%) and usually involves the upper incisors and lower first molars (Fig. 14.45). Prediction prior to treatment commencement can be difficult although root shape may give an indication.

14.9.2 Treatment failure and relapse

Failure of orthodontic treatment is most commonly due to poor patient compliance, but may also be due to poor diagnosis and therefore poor

Table 14.7 Summary of recommended observation periods prior to orthodontic tooth movement

Type of dental injury	Observation period
Crown and crown–root fractures without pulpal involvement.	3 months.
Crown and crown–root fractures with pulpal involvement.	After coronal pulpotomy and radiographic signs of establishment of a hard tissue barrier (~3 months).
Root fractures.	1–2 years; shorter period if asymptomatic. If healing is by connective tissue, the coronal fragment must be treated as a tooth with a short root. If granulation tissue is interposed, teeth should not be moved until successful endodontic treatment and connective tissue healing of the coronal fragment has occurred.

Minor damage to periodontium
 	
    Concussion
 	
    Subluxation
 	
    Extrusion
 	
    Lateral luxation (minor displacement).
	3 months.

Moderate/severe injury to periodontium
 	
    Lateral luxation (moderate/severe displacement)
 	
    Intrusion
 	
    Avulsion and replantation.
	1 year if no ankylosis can be detected.
	
	Orthodontic tooth movement is not recommended before complete periodontal healing has occurred (6 months). If teeth are orthodontically moved between 6 and 12 months keep a strong suspicion that the tooth is ankylosed where tooth movement is not as expected.

Immature traumatized teeth.	Await radiographic evidence of continued root development. Clinical and radiographic controls should be carried out after 6 months, 1 year, and 2 years.
Teeth requiring endodontic treatment due to caries.	Immediate orthodontic movement provided no periapical pathosis is evident. We would recommend definitive obturation with gutta percha rather than maintenance of calcium hydroxide in the root canal.
Teeth requiring endodontic treatment due to inflammatory resorption.	Await radiographic evidence of healing and allow at least 1 year to elapse before commencement of orthodontic tooth movement. Teeth with evidence of root resorption appear to be more liable to further resorption during orthodontic tooth movement.
Teeth requiring endodontic treatment due to trauma.	In a mature closed apex tooth, following an initial dressing of calcium hydroxide, a definitive gutta percha root filling should be placed. This contradicts previous advice given by others. The observation period depends on the nature of the original traumatic injury.
Autotransplanted teeth.	3–9 months, i.e. after PDL healing (8 weeks) and before complete alveolar bone repair. Extrusion may be commenced earlier than rotation or bodily tooth movement. Ankylosis must be excluded when tooth movement does not occur as expected.

Reproduced by kind permission of the *Journal of Orthodontics*.

treatment planning or poor operator management of the treatment itself. It is important that the consent process fully explains to the patient what is required of them during treatment. It is important that patients realize that teeth continue to move throughout life, and therefore any movement after active treatment is completed may not be due to relapse.

Relapse is described as the return, following correction, of the features of the original malocclusion, but it can sometimes be difficult to differentiate from normal physiological or age changes. Four broad areas have been suggested as factors in relapse.

- **Gingival/periodontal**, due to stretched and unremodelled fibres in periodontal ligament and gingival cuff.
- **Occlusal**, due to interdigitation and unstable tooth position.

- **Soft tissue**, i.e. teeth moved out of the neutral zone where they are in balance within the soft tissue environment, or in the case of the incisors outside the control of the lower lip.
- **Growth**, where correction is achieved during pubertal growth but this unfavourable pattern continues after active treatment.

Studies suggest this process continues long term and is unpredictable. Although the role of the clinician should be to place the teeth in as stable a position as possible, patients should be warned that the likelihood of relapse is high. As a consequence, retention should be continued indefinitely if the tooth position at the end of treatment is to be maintained.

Retainers are either fixed or removable. Oral hygiene is certainly easier with **removable retainers** although they are compliance

Table 14.8 Damage related to orthodontic treatment and its prevention

Tissue type	Effects	Prevention
Enamel	Decalcification (Fig. 14.44). Incidence variously reported as 15–85% related to method of observation).	Careful patient selection. Oral hygiene/diet instruction. Fluoride (patient compliance and non-compliance methods).
	Fracture (rare).	Careful debonding method particularly with ceramic brackets.
Periodontium	Gingivitis (Fig. 14.43) (common).	Careful patient selection. Oral hygiene/diet instruction.
	Periodontitis.	Removal of active sites prior to commencement. Where predisposed, scale and polish every 3 months.
	Recession.	Avoid excessive expansion or labial segment proclination. Free graft prior to treatment in sites of recession.
Root	Resorption (Fig. 14.45). Variable but inevitable. Particularly noted on upper incisors and lower first molars.	Careful history and radiographic assessment of root morphology prior to commencement. High risk: Blunt/pipette-shaped roots Signs of resorption
		Avoid excessive torquing forces, intrusion, and prolonged treatment duration.
Pulp	Loss of vitality.	Avoid excessive force on heavily restored teeth or teeth with a history of trauma.
Soft tissue	Fixed appliance iatrogenic damage.	Check archwire ends not sticking out. Methods to prevent archwire rotation particularly with self-ligating brackets.
	Removable appliance iatrogenic damage (Fig. 14.32).	Oral hygiene instruction including appliance hygiene. Consider part time wear.

dependent. The most popular removable retainer historically is the Hawley retainer which is robust and to which components (e.g. a prosthetic tooth) can be added relatively easily. Because it has limited occlusal coverage it allows some vertical eruption of the dentition or settling. Its main drawbacks are the palatal coverage, and therefore its effects on speech, and the labial bow anteriorly which is unsightly (Fig. 14.46). The pressure-formed retainer is now the most popular method of removable retention. It is more aesthetic and cheaper than the Hawley retainer, and has been shown to hold the tooth position more accurately. However, it has the drawback of not allowing vertical settling, suffers wear-through if worn long term, and is contraindicated in patients with poor oral hygiene. The retention regime for pressure-formed retainer varies between clinicians. Part-time wear (nights only) is usually preceded by a short period of full-time wear (except eating) immediately after debond.

Fixed retainers bonded to the teeth require meticulous oral hygiene and regular monitoring. Therefore they are usually reserved for teeth where the orthodontic result is relatively unstable (derotations, diastema closure, lower incisor proclination). Because of their long-term nature the patient should be instructed in hygiene maintenance. The bonding area should be checked on a regular basis to make sure that there is no localized area of debond and tooth movement (Fig. 14.47).

14.9.3 Predisposition to dental-related disorders

Temporomandibular joint disorder (TMD)

The most common clinical symptoms in children and adolescents are clicking (10–30%) and muscle tenderness on palpation (20–60%). Clinical signs such as reduced opening, pain on movement, and tenderness of the joints on palpation are less frequent than in adults. There seems to be no consistent pattern in the development of either subjective symptoms or clinical signs during growth. Headache is common in children (girls more than boys) and its prevalence increases with age. The connection between headache, bruxism, hyperactivity of jaw muscles, and mandibular dysfunction is well recognized and should not be missed.

In general, the presence of malocclusion is not associated with an increased prevalence of TMDs. There is a slightly greater prevalence in subjects with malocclusions of the type that often have associated occlusal interferences, including class III cases, cross-bites, and open bites, but the correlation is weak. Patients who present with TMDs should be advised that orthodontics will not cure their symptoms. It has been claimed that many forms of orthodontic treatment cause

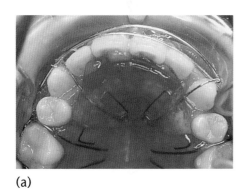

(a)

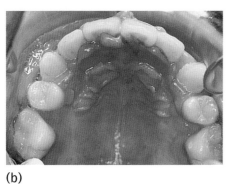

(b)

Figure 14.43 (a) Upper removable appliance for retraction of the upper incisors. (b) Severe gingival inflammation resulting from compression of the gingival tissues under the appliance during incisor retraction.

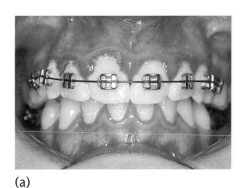

(a)

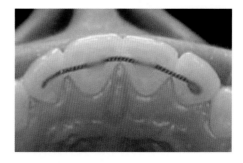

(b)

Figure 14.44 (a) Neglected fixed appliance with associated gingival inflammation and decalcification. (b) The decalcification is obvious following bracket removal.

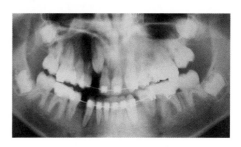

Figure 14.45 Panoramic radiograph showing widespread root resorption during fixed appliance orthodontic treatment.

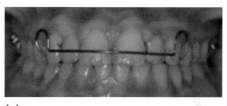

(a)

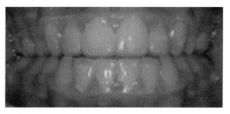

(b)

Figure 14.46 (a) Upper Hawley retainer with two pontics replacing the upper lateral incisors and an unsightly labial bow. (b) Upper and lower pressure-formed retainer.

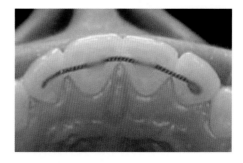

Figure 14.47 Fixed multistrand retainer bonded to the upper incisor teeth.

TMDs, with premolar extractions coming under the greatest attack. However, extensive studies have found no evidence of an increased prevalence of TMDs in subjects who have had orthodontic treatment, including extractions, compared with untreated controls.

Periodontal disease

Although it has been suggested that orthodontic treatment may lead to periodontal disease, plaque is the most important contributory factor. Teeth can be moved without any further loss of attachment where plaque control is excellent. (See Key Points 14.9.)

> **Key Points 14.9**
>
> - Orthodontic treatment moves patients from low caries risk to high caries risk.
> - Good oral hygiene and diet control are especially important during orthodontic treatment.
> - Careful radiological assessment of root form should be carried out prior to commencement of orthodontic treatment.
> - Retention is an essential part of orthodontic treatment.
> - To maintain tooth alignment long-term retention should be indefinite.
> - There is little evidence that malocclusion or orthodontic treatment are associated with temporomandibular joint disorders.
> - There is no evidence of significant long-term periodontal disease associated with orthodontic treatment.

14.10 Cleft lip and palate

Orofacial clefting is the most common craniofacial anomaly, with an incidence of one in 700 live births in the UK. However, there is a variation in incidence between different racial groups. Cleft palate (CP) and cleft lip and palate (CLP) (Fig. 14.48) represent different clinical entities with different incidence, gender bias, and genetic predisposition. However, there is substantial variation in their presentation.

The aetiology of orofacial clefting is complex and is described as multifactorial. Although many known syndromes with clear genetic aetiology are described, including clefts of the oral region, the majority of isolated orofacial clefts show no obvious aetiology and are likely to represent a complex environmental–genetic interaction in a period of intricate and coordinated processes during facial and/or palate formation.

Patients with orofacial clefting commonly need extensive and specialized treatment, which is provided by a multidisciplinary team of specialists including a specialist cleft nurse, a cleft surgeon, a psychologist, a geneticist, a speech and language therapist, an ear, nose, and throat (ENT) surgeon, and members of a specialized cleft dental team. To prevent this care from being fragmented, the key multidisciplinary players have in recent years been incorporated into specialized cleft multidisciplinary teams. The advantage of this incorporation, and in some cases centralization, of services is that they encourage high-volume operators, a full range of facilities, and clinical expertise in their particular discipline. Perhaps the most important aspect of care centralization or centres of expertise is that worthwhile audits of outcomes and processes are possible because of the increased numbers of patients treated. The reason for and role of each specialist within the multidisciplinary team are summarized in Table 14.9.

14.10.1 Dental care for patients with cleft lip and palate

Clefts involving the palate have minimal effect on the developing dentition. In general, patients with a cleft palate tend to have small dental arches. Therefore the dentition is often crowded and a deep overbite is common. Clefts of the lip may or may not have some underlying effect on the alveolus. The growth of the maxilla in a forward direction in these patients tends to be normal. Although the alveolus at birth may show little signs of being affected, the teeth associated with the cleft (most commonly the cleft-side lateral incisor) may be affected. In some instances the defect in the alveolus associated with the cleft of the lip may be significant enough to require alveolar bone grafting (Fig. 14.49).

Clefts involving the alveolus have a greater dental effect and therefore are of more significance to the dental practitioner. Associated dental anomalies include:

- delayed dental development (usually on the cleft side);
- impacted first permanent molars (associated with shortened dental arch);
- hypodontia (most commonly the lateral incisor (50%) associated with the cleft but also teeth distant to the cleft site);
- microdontia/hypoplasia (particularly the central incisor associated with the cleft);
- supernumeraries (associated with the cleft site in both primary and secondary dentitions);
- impacted cleft canine;
- rotated tooth positions.

Owing to the varied nature of these anomalies, the dental team includes a cleft orthodontist, a paediatric dentist, a restorative dentist, and an oral surgeon. It is the role of the dental team to coordinate any specialized dental care through them, whilst encouraging regular dental care through their local dental practitioner.

While these anomalies obviously have an impact on the dental health of the child, it is worth noting that children with cleft lip and

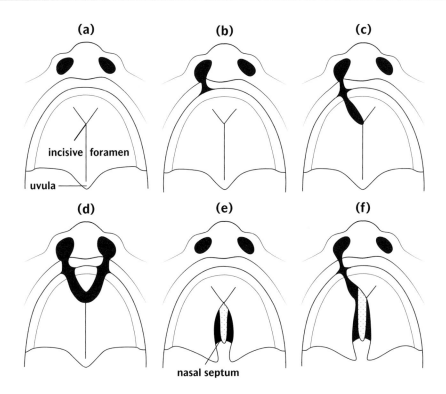

Figure 14.48 Diagrammatic representation of some of the different types of clefts of the lip and palate. (a) Normal; (b) unilateral cleft lip; (c) unilateral cleft lip and anterior palate; (d) bilateral cleft lip and anterior alveolus; (e) cleft of posterior palate (hard and soft); (f) unilateral cleft of the lip and anterior and posterior palate. (Reproduced from Johnson and Moore, *Anatomy for Dental Students*, 1997, with permission of Oxford University Press.)

Table 14.9 Members of the multidisciplinary cleft team and their duties

Team member	Reason for involvement	Role and timing
Cleft specialist nurse	Difficult adjustment for parents of a child with CLP Early feeding issues Anxiety over surgery Continued requirement for support throughout child development.	Role of support and counselling throughout life and often the first point of contact within the team at diagnosis. Expertise in early feeding management.

Paediatrician	Issues over child development (failure to thrive), and contact with community support.
	
	Medical-related issues with regard to educational needs and requirements (abnormal behaviour, bullying.)
		Early input from first diagnosis.
		
		Expertise in:
		
		    assessment of other abnormalities and child's ability to thrive
		
		    assessment of whole-child perspective.
		
		Liaison with social and community services.
		
		Monitoring child's psychological well-being and family functioning.

Cleft surgeon	Significant aesthetic impact due to facial cleft Functional issue due to CP and its effect on speech Secondary defects related to cleft and iatrogenic effects of surgery (nasal/lip asymmetry, lack of maxillary development.)	Primary surgery to close lip (3–6 months) and palate (6–12 months). Further preschool palatal surgery and lip revision if there are issues with speech or aesthetics. Alveolar bone grafting (9–11 years) to allow canine eruption. Nasal revision (mid to late teens) and maxillary advancement surgery (end of growth unless psychological issues.)

Table 14.9 Continued

Team member	Reason for involvement	Role and timing
ENT/paediatric audiology	CP affects the ability of the Eustachian tubes to ventilate the middle ear; this may result in middle ear effusion, middle ear disease (otitis media (OME)) and some hearing loss; hearing loss is likely to lead to problems and delay in speech and language development	Developmental milestones with normal hearing: 4 months—child responds to parent's voice 6 months—child will turn head to sound 9 months—child copies sounds 12 months—child babbles Delays in these milestones may be due to OME and hearing difficulties and should be treated promptly
Speech and language therapist	CP and unusual palatal and dental anatomy as a result of clefting may have a significant impact on speech production and language development	Early input to advise and stimulate normal speech and language development Close monitoring throughout early development, particularly through preschool to monitor milestones and language development Liaise with local speech and language therapists, school, and the team as required
Psychologist	Issues for the child as they grow: coping with the fact they may look and sound different struggling to cope with social relationships low self-esteem	Regular child assessment as they are developing Advise those treating and offer psychological intervention as necessary Help with coping strategies and encourage self-worth
Geneticist	In the majority of cases of CLP it will be the only defect; however, there are a number of cases where the clefting occurs with other anomalies and as part of a syndrome	Parents frequently wish to know soon after birth of their child with a cleft the risk of having another child with the same condition. Before giving occurrence risks the geneticist must be confident that there is no syndromic base. In non-syndromic clefts the risk for siblings born with unaffected parents is 4%; with two affected siblings it is 10%. If one parent is affected, the risk is also 10%
Dental	Majority of dental effects related to CLP rather than CP: delayed dental development supernumeraries hypodontia impacted upper first permanent molars impacted cleft canine alveolar defect hypoplastic teeth crowding restricted maxillary growth.	Multiple and complex dental problems are associated with clefts involving the alveolus; this requires a multidisciplinary dental approach to patient management Input from the dental team should start soon after birth with preventive and dental advice to parents from a paediatric dentist and assessment by the orthodontist of the requirements for pre-surgical orthopaedics Regular dental care should be provided through the local dental practitioner and the dental team with close coordination and a personally tailored preventive regime for these high-risk patients

palate also have a higher incidence of dental decay than the general population. Therefore these children should be considered high risk for caries, and personal, practical, and positive preventive regimes and monitoring should be instigated.

Dental care in general for cleft patients has been transformed with the advent of alveolar bone grafting, which has allowed orthodontic intervention around the cleft site and in many cases eliminated the need for prosthetic replacement of teeth.

14.10.2 Orthodontist within the cleft team

The orthodontist tends to have a pivotal role within the cleft team and the dental team. He/she tends to be the specialist who has the most frequent appointments with the child and therefore the greatest burden of care of that child and their parents. The orthodontist should be mindful of this, and when treatment is instigated it should

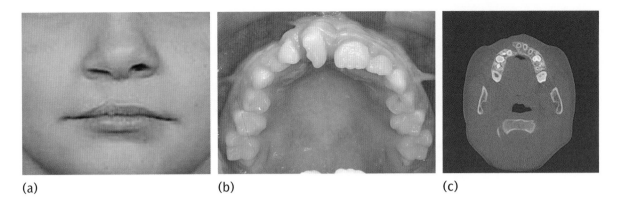

(a)   (b)   (c)

Figure 14.49 (a) Excellent lip repair but slight nasal symmetry suggesting an underlying bony defect. (b) Rotated central incisor, a supplemental deciduous lateral incisor, and a possible labial defect in the region of the deciduous lateral incisor. (c) Cone beam CT confirming the alveolar defect.

be kept to the minimum duration but gain the maximum benefit for the patient.

There are four key stages of orthodontic input:

- presurgical orthopaedics
- alveolar bone grafting
- definitive orthodontic alignment
- orthodontic treatment for orthognathic surgery.

As well as the key stages the orthodontist also has a significant role in audit. Once the permanent teeth have erupted, patients with clefts involving the alveolus are often keen for improved dental alignment. In considering the orthodontic plan it is important to realize that growth in a class III direction is likely and therefore the orthodontist should be wary of incisor correction. Data collection, including photographs, radiographs, and study models, acts as a basis for assessment of cleft lip and palate patient outcome.

Presurgical orthopaedics

The principal aim is to realign the bone segments prior to primary surgery to ease surgical correction. This was done using active or passive acrylic plates constructed on plaster models from impressions taken of the infant's maxilla and stabilized in the patient's mouth externally. Numerous benefits including improved feeding, better growth, and speech development have been put forward as reasons for their use. However, recent studies of their use in unilateral CLPs have found that they confer little benefit in relation to surgical outcomes and produce a significantly greater burden of care for the parents of these children.

Alveolar bone grafting

Alveolar bone grafting has transformed the orthodontic and prosthetic management of patients with CLP. Grafting is performed in the mixed dentition prior to permanent canine eruption. Medullary, and in some cases cortical, bone from a distant site (usually the ileac crest) is grafted into the alveolar defect. The timing of the graft is critical to the success and is determined radiographically at the age 7–8 years. The optimal

timing is when the canine root is half-formed (9–11 years), although earlier grafting may occur if a viable cleft lateral incisor is present.

The aims of grafting are as follows:

- it allows eruption of the cleft canine/lateral incisor;
- it provides bony support for teeth on either side of the cleft;
- it allows orthodontic intervention in the cleft region;
- it provides stability between the cleft segments;
- it may improve the alar base contour.

The role of the orthodontist is not only to assess the need and timing of the graft, but also in some cases to provide presurgical orthodontics to improve access to the cleft site for the surgeon and to correct incisors in cross-bite and collapsed lateral segments (Figs 14.50 and 14.51). This treatment should be completed within 6 months. In the case of bilateral CLP cases, the orthodontist also provides stabilization of the mobile pre-maxilla during the healing phase.

Fixed appliances in the form of a quad-helix are most frequently utilized to complete the treatment. Some form of retention is kept in place until postoperative radiographs are taken 3–6 months postsurgery. Once both surgeon and orthodontist are happy that the bone graft has been successful, the appliances are removed and the patient is monitored until full dental eruption.

Definitive orthodontic alignment

The introduction of alveolar bone grafting has allowed the orthodontist to close any residual spacing in the cleft region. Once the permanent teeth have erupted, patients with clefts involving the alveolus are often keen for improved dental alignment. In considering the orthodontic plan, it is important to realize that growth in a class III direction is likely and therefore the orthodontist should be wary of incisor correction. This means that incisor correction is neither possible nor desirable in a significant minority of patients (as they may consider later orthognathic treatment) However, this does not make dental alignment any less worthwhile (Fig. 14.52). Microdontia, hypodontia, and hypoplasia can make symmetry and good occlusal fit difficult to achieve.

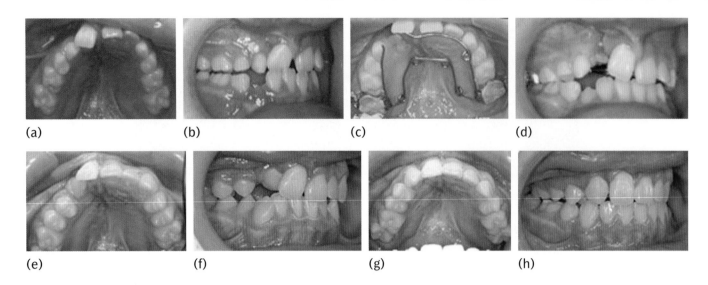

(a)   (b)   (c)   (d)

(e)   (f)   (g)   (h)

Figure 14.50 (a, b) Pre- and (c) post-orthodontic expansion using a quad-helix appliance. (d) Note the improved access to the cleft site, maxillary arch form, and incisor cross-bite correction. (e, f) On full dental eruption, note the continued cross-bite correction anteriorly with positive overbite and collapse of the lateral segment, but canine eruption through the graft site. (g, h) After orthodontic alignment, note space closure, cross-bite correction, and bonded retainer in the upper labial segment.

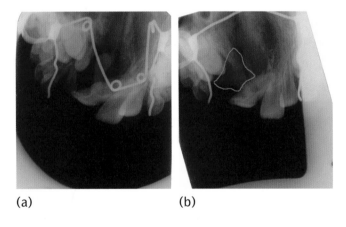

(a)   (b)

Figure 14.51 (a) Pre- and (b) postoperative radiographs of a patient who has had an alveolar bone graft. Note in the pre-treatment, two supernumeraries in the cleft site and the cleft-side canine root that are 50% formed. The postoperative opacity in the cleft site shows bony infill (the supernumeraries and the primary incisor and canine have been removed).

Because of the complex nature of tooth movement required for alignment, orthodontics is usually carried out with fixed appliances. Scarring and the frequently rotated positions of the teeth within the labial segment associated with the cleft mean that fixed retention is essential to maintain tooth position.

Orthodontics for orthognathic surgery

Class III correction with orthodontics is not possible for a significant minority of patients, and in these cases dental alignment alone is considered. This will not preclude further orthodontics prior to surgery once the most active growth has been completed.

It is obvious that the success of all this treatment depends on the maintenance of sound dentition over many years, and that loss of teeth due to caries greatly complicates and hinders treatment. Thus the dentist has a vitally important role in maintaining continuity of routine preventive and restorative care. It is well recognized that patient compliance with long and complex treatments dwindles, and unfortunately many patients with clefts, and their families, do not give routine dentistry a high enough priority compared with other aspects of their treatment, such as surgery. Therefore an enthusiastic and supportive dental team must play a central part in the multidisciplinary management of clefts of the lip and palate.

14.10.3 Paediatric dentist within the cleft team

The role of the paediatric dentist is to work closely with the orthodontist:

- giving preventive advice and treatment from the time teeth first erupt;
- providing restorative treatment if that cannot be obtained in the general dental services;
- maintaining a mouth free of active disease;
- delivering to the orthodontist a child who is not nervous about dental care and has no history of tooth loss.

Assessments should take place at 1, 3, 5, 7, 10, and 14 years. Like the orthodontist, the paediatric dentist has a role in audit.

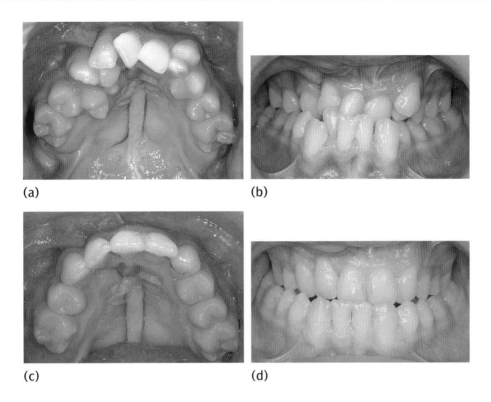

(a) (b) (c) (d)

Figure 14.52 (a, b) Pre- and (c, d) post-orthodontic treatment where the reverse overjet is accepted in a patient with a right unilateral cleft lip and palate. Note multiple rotations, crowding, and retained primary teeth. Post-operatively note the bonded retainer, extracted upper left and lower lateral incisors to relieve crowding, and space closure to maintain symmetry with the reverse overjet accepted.

14.11 Summary

1 All children should be screened for malocclusion from the age of 8 years.

2 Unerupted maxillary canines should be palpated routinely on all children from the age of 10 years until eruption. A maxillary canine that is not palpable should be investigated.

3 Significant variation from the normal sequence of eruption should be investigated (e.g. upper lateral incisor erupting before the upper central incisor).

4 Consider the orthodontic aspects when extractions in the mixed dentition are necessary.

5 A space maintainer should be fitted immediately if a traumatized upper incisor is lost.

6 Cross-bites with displacement can be treated in the mixed dentition.

7 Treatment of increased overjet in the mixed dentition can become lengthy, although it may be indicated in those with a significant overjet and those where it is having a negative psychological impact.

8 Good oral hygiene and cooperation are essential for successful orthodontic treatment with appliances.

9 Orthodontic treatment with appliances moves patients from low caries risk to high caries risk.

10 To maintain tooth alignment long-term retention should be indefinite.

11 Patients with cleft lip and palate are treated within a multidisciplinary environment. However, the dentist plays an essential role within this in maintaining dental heath.

14.12 Further reading

Andreasen, J.O. and Andreasen, F.M. (1994). *Textbook and colour atlas of traumatic injuries to the teeth* (3rd edn). Munksgaard, Copenhagen. (*Comprehensive coverage of the management of dental trauma, including the role of orthodontics.*)

Houston, W.J.B., Stephens, C.D., and Tulley, W.J. (1992). *A textbook of orthodontics* (2nd edn). Butterworth–Heinemann, Oxford. (*An excellent introductory textbook.*)

Isaacson, K.G., Reed, R.T., and Stephens, C.D. (1990). *Functional orthodontic appliances*. Blackwell Scientific, Oxford. (*A clear and thorough review of the role, management, and effects of functional appliances.*)

Okeson, J.P. (1989). Temporomandibular disorders in children. *Pediatric Dentistry*, **11**, 325–9. (*A useful short summary of the subject.*)

Proffitt, W.R. (1993). *Contemporary orthodontics* (2nd edn). Mosby, St Louis, MO. (*A superb comprehensive orthodontic textbook.*)

Richardson, A. (1989). *Interceptive orthodontics* (2nd edn). British Dental Journal Publications, London. (*A concise handbook of the role of orthodontics in the mixed dentition.*)

Royal College of Surgeons of England (1997, updated 2010). Clinical Guidelines. 1. Management of palatally ectopic maxillary canine. Available online at:
 www.rcseng.ac.uk

Royal College of Surgeons of England (1997, updated 2010). Clinical Guidelines. 2. Management of unerupted maxillary Incisors. Available online at:
www.rcseng.ac.uk

Royal College of Surgeons of England (2004, revised 2009). Clinical Guidelines. 3. A guideline for first permanent molar extraction in children. Available online at:
www.rcseng.ac.uk

Royal College of Surgeons of England (2001, revised 2006). Clinical Guidelines. 4. Extraction of primary teeth—balance and compensation.
www.rcseng.ac.uk

Shaw, W.C. (ed.) (1993). *Orthodontics and occlusal management*. Butterworth–Heinemann, London. (*An authoritative orthodontic textbook, including cleft lip and palate, and risk–benefit of treatment.*)

14.13 References

Brook, P. and Shaw, W. (1989). The development of an index of orthodontic treatment priority. *European Journal of Orthodontics*, **11**, 309–20.

Evans, R. and Shaw, W. (1987). Preliminary evaluation of an illustrated scale for raising dental attractiveness. *European Journal of Orthodontics*, **9**, 314–18.

15

Oral pathology and oral surgery

J.G. Meechan

Chapter contents

15.1 Introduction

The incidence of pathological conditions of the mouth and perioral structures varies between children and adults. For example, mucocoeles are more common in the young, whereas squamous cell carcinomas occur more frequently in older individuals. The management of pathology in the child differs from that in the adult. Growth and development may be affected by the disease or by its treatment. On a more practical basis, anaesthetic considerations for surgical treatment of simple pathological conditions can make management more complex in the young patient. This chapter deals with those conditions that occur exclusively or more commonly in children. It is not an exhaustive guide to paediatric oral pathology, for which readers should refer to oral pathology textbooks. Surgical treatment of the simpler conditions is discussed in the oral surgery section of this chapter (Section 15.5).

15.2 Lesions of the oral soft tissues

Conditions affecting the oral mucosa and associated soft tissues can be classified as follows: infections, ulcers, vesiculobullous lesions, white lesions, cysts, and tumours.

15.2.1 Infections

Viruses, bacteria, fungi, or protozoa may cause infections of the oral mucosa. Odontogenic infections will be discussed in Section 15.5.6.

Viral infections
Herpetic infections

Primary herpes simplex infection This condition usually occurs in children between the ages of 6 months and 5 years. Circulating maternal antibodies usually protect young babies. The symptoms, signs, and treatment are covered in Chapter 11.

Secondary herpes simplex infection Secondary infection with herpes simplex usually occurs at the labial mucocutaneous junction and presents as a vesicular lesion that ruptures and produces crusting (see Chapter 11).

Herpes varicella-zoster Shingles, which is caused by the varicella-zoster virus, is much more common in adults than in children. The vesicular lesion develops within the peripheral distribution of a branch of the trigeminal nerve.

Chickenpox, a more common presentation of varicella-zoster in children, produces a vesicular rash on the skin. The intra-oral lesions of chickenpox resemble those of primary herpetic infection. The condition is highly contagious.

Mumps

Mumps produces a painful enlargement of the parotid glands. It is usually bilateral. The causative agent is a myxovirus. Associated complaints include headache, vomiting, and fever. Symptoms last for about a week and the condition is contagious.

Measles

The intra-oral manifestation of measles occurs on the buccal mucosa. The lesions appear as white speckling surrounded by a red margin and are known as Koplick's spots. The oral signs usually precede the skin lesions and disappear early in the course of the disease. The skin rash of measles normally appears as a red maculopapular lesion. Fever is present and the disease is contagious.

Rubella

Rubella (German measles) does not usually produce signs in the oral mucosa; however, the tonsils may be affected. Protection against the diseases of mumps, measles, and rubella can be achieved by vaccinating children with MMR vaccine in their early years.

Herpangina

This is a Coxsackie virus A infection. It can be differentiated from primary herpetic infection by the different location of the vesicles, which are found in the tonsillar or pharyngeal region. Herpangina lesions do not coalesce to form large areas of ulceration. The condition is short-lived.

Hand, foot, and mouth disease

This Coxsackie virus A infection produces a maculopapular rash on the hands and feet. The intra-oral vesicles rupture to produce painful ulceration. The condition lasts for 10–14 days.

Infectious mononucleosis

The Epstein–Barr virus causes this condition. It is not uncommon amongst teenagers. The usual form of transmission is by kissing. Oral ulceration and petechial haemorrhage at the hard–soft palate junction may occur. There is lymph node enlargement and associated fever. There is no specific treatment. It should be noted that prescription of ampicillin and amoxicillin (amoxycillin) can cause a rash in those suffering from infectious mononucleosis. These antibiotics should be avoided during the course of the disease. Treatment of the above viral illnesses is symptomatic and relies on analgesia and maintenance of fluid intake. It must be remembered that aspirin should be avoided in children under 12 years of age (see later).

Human papillomavirus

This is associated with a number of tumour-like lesions of the oral mucosa, which are discussed in Section 15.2.6.

Bacterial infections
Staphylococcal infections

Staphylococci and streptococci may cause impetigo. This can affect the angles of the mouth and the lips (Fig. 15.1). It presents as crusting vesiculobullous lesions. The vesicles coalesce to produce ulceration over a wide area. Pigmentation may occur during healing. The condition is self-limiting, although antibiotics may be prescribed in some cases. Staphylococcal organisms can cause osteomyelitis of the jaws in children. Although the introduction of antibiotics has reduced the incidence of severe forms of the condition, it can still be devastating. In addition to aggressive antibiotic therapy, surgical intervention is required to remove bony sequestrae.

Streptococcal infection

Streptococcal infections in childhood vary from a mucopurulent nasal discharge to tonsillitis, pharyngitis, and gingivitis. Scarlet fever is a β-haemolytic streptococcal infection consisting of a skin rash with maculopapular lesions of the oral mucosa. It is associated with tonsillitis and pharyngitis. The tongue shows characteristic changes from a strawberry appearance in the early stages to a raspberry-like form in the later stages.

Congenital syphilis

Congenital syphilis is transmitted from an infected mother to the fetus. Oral mucosal changes such as rhagades, which is a pattern of scarring at the angle of the mouth, may occur. In addition, this disease may cause characteristic dental changes in the permanent dentition. These include Hutchinson's incisors (the teeth taper towards the incisal edge

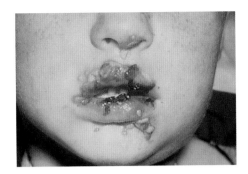

Figure 15.1 Bacterial infection on the lips of an immunocompromised child. (Reproduced from *Dental Update* (ISSN 0305-5000), by permission of George Warman Publications (UK) Ltd.)

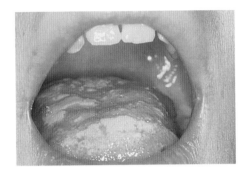

Figure 15.2 Oral candidiasis in an immunocompromised child undergoing chemotherapy for acute lymphoblastic leukaemia. (Reproduced from *Dental Update* (ISSN 0305-5000), by permission of George Warman Publications (UK) Ltd.)

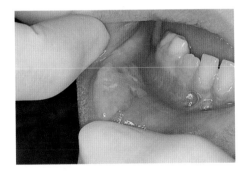

Figure 15.3 Ulceration of the lower lip produced by biting while still anaesthetized from an inferior block.

rather than the cervical margin) and mulberry molars (globular masses of enamel over the occlusal surface).

Tuberculosis

Tuberculous lesions of the oral cavity are rare. However, tuberculous lymphadenitis affecting submandibular and cervical lymph nodes is occasionally seen. These present as tender enlarged nodes, which may progress to abscess formation with discharge through the skin. Surgical removal of infected glands produces a much neater scar than that caused by spontaneous rupture through the skin if the disease is allowed to progress.

Cat-scratch disease

This is a self-limiting disease which presents as an enlargement of regional lymph nodes. The nodes are painful and enlargement occurs up to 3 weeks following a cat scratch. The nodes become suppurative and may perforate the skin. Treatment often involves incision and drainage.

Fungal infections

Candida

Neonatal acute candidiasis (thrush) contracted during birth is not uncommon. Young children may develop the condition when resistance is lowered or after antibiotic therapy (Fig. 15.2). Easily removed white patches on an erythematous or bleeding base are found. Treatment with nystatin or miconazole is effective (those under 2 years of age should receive 2.5mL of a miconazole gel (24mg/mL) twice daily; 5mL twice daily is prescribed for those under 6 years of age, and 5mL four times daily for those over 6 years of age).

Actinomycosis

Actinomycosis can occur in children. It may follow intra-oral trauma including dental extractions. The organisms spread through the tissues and can cause dysphagia if the submandibular region is involved. Abscesses may rupture onto the skin and long-term antibiotic therapy is required. Penicillin should be prescribed and maintained for at least 2 weeks following clinical cure.

Protozoal infections

Infection by *Toxoplasma gondii* may occasionally occur in children, with the principal reservoir of infection being cats. Glandular toxoplasmosis is similar in presentation to infectious mononucleosis and is found mainly in children and young adults. There may be a granulomatous reaction in the oral mucosa and there can be parotid gland enlargement. The disease is self-limiting, although an antiprotozoal such as pyrimethamine may be used in cases of severe infection.

15.2.2 Ulcers

Traumatic ulceration of the tongue, lips, and cheek may occur in children, especially after local anaesthesia has been administered (Fig. 15.3).

Recurrent aphthous oral ulceration not associated with systemic disease is often found in children (Fig. 15.4). One or more small ulcers in the non-attached gingiva may occur at frequent intervals. In the young child the symptoms may be mistaken for toothache by a parent. The majority of aphthous ulcers in children are of the minor variety (less than 5mm in diameter). These usually heal within 10–14 days. Treatment other than reassurance is often unnecessary; however, topical steroids may be prescribed in severe cases. Older children may benefit from the use of antiseptic rinses to prevent secondary infection. In the absence of a history of major aphthous

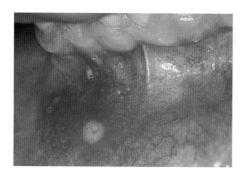

Figure 15.4 Minor aphthous ulceration. (Reproduced by kind permission of Informa Healthcare.)

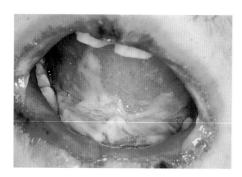

Figure 15.5 Erythema multiforme in a teenager.

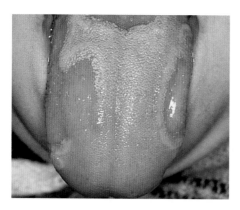

Figure 15.6 Geographic tongue. (Reproduced by kind permission of Informa Healthcare.)

ulceration any ulcer lasting for longer than 2 weeks should be regarded with suspicion and biopsied.

15.2.3 Vesiculobullous lesions

Vesiculobullous lesions cause ulcers in the later stages of such conditions. Viral causes have been mentioned above. Similarly, conditions such as epidermolysis bullosa and erythema multiforme can produce oral ulceration in children. The major vesiculobullous conditions, such as pemphigus and pemphigoid, are rare in young patients. Epidermolysis bullosa is a term that covers a number of syndromes, some of which are incompatible with life. The skin is extremely fragile and mucosal involvement may occur. The act of suckling may induce bullae formation in babies. In older children effective oral hygiene may be difficult as even mild trauma can produce painful lesions.

The oral lesions of erythema multiforme usually affect the lips and anterior oral mucosa (Fig. 15.5). There is initial erythema followed by bullae formation and ulceration. The pathogenesis of the condition is still unclear; however, precipitating factors include drug therapy and infection. Treatment involves the use of steroids and oral antiseptic and analgesic rinses to ease the pain.

15.2.4 White lesions

Trauma of either a chemical or physical nature (e.g. burns and occlusal trauma) can cause white patches intra-orally.

White spongy naevus

White spongy naevus (also known as oral epithelial naevus) is a rough folded lesion that can affect any part of the oral mucosa. It often appears in infancy. It is benign.

Leucoedema

This is a folded white translucent appearance found in children of races who exhibit pigmentation of the oral mucosa. It is considered a variation of normal.

Candidiasis

The white patches of acute fungal candidiasis mentioned above are readily removed, in contrast to the white lesions discussed here.

Geographic tongue

This condition may be seen in children. It is normally symptomless, although some patients complain of discomfort with spicy foods. Areas of the tongue appear shiny and red as a result of loss of filiform papillae (Fig. 15.6). These red patches are surrounded by white margins. These areas disappear before reappearing in other regions of the tongue. The condition is benign and requires no treatment apart from reassurance to the child and parent.

15.2.5 Cysts

Mucocoeles

The peak incidence of mucocoeles is in the second decade of life; however, they are not uncommon in younger children (Fig. 15.7) including neonates. Mucocoeles are caused by trauma to minor salivary glands or ducts and are often located on the lower lip. They are the most common non-infective cause of salivary gland swelling in children. Salivary tumours are rare in this age group.

Ranula

This appears a bluish swelling of the floor of the mouth (Fig. 15.8). It is essentially a large mucocoele. It may arise from part of the sublingual salivary gland.

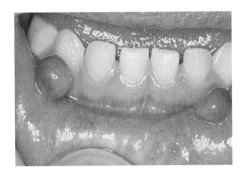

Figure 15.7 Bilateral mucocoeles in a 3-year-old girl. (By kind permission of the *Journal of Dentistry for Children*.)

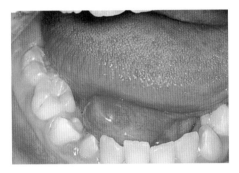

Figure 15.8 A ranula in a 14-year-old girl.

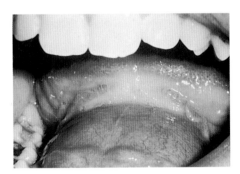

Figure 15.9 A dermoid cyst.

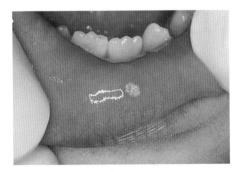

Figure 15.10 Squamous cell papilloma in a 9-year-old girl. (Reproduced from *Dental Update* (ISSN 0305-5000) by permission of George Warman Publications (UK) Ltd.)

Bohn's nodules

These gingival cysts arise from remnants of the dental lamina. They are found in neonates and usually disappear spontaneously in the early months of life.

Epstein's pearls

These small cystic lesions are located along the palatal midline. They are thought to arise from trapped epithelium in the palatal raphe. They are present in about 80% of neonates and disappear within a few weeks of birth.

Dermoid cysts

These are rare lesions of the floor of the mouth. They appear as intra-oral and submental swellings (Fig. 15.9). They are derived from epithelial remnants remaining after fusion of the mandibular processes.

Lymphoepithelial cyst

In the past this was termed branchial arch cyst as it was thought to arise from epithelial remnants of a branchial arch. Lymphoepithelial cysts are normally found in the sternomastoid region, although they can present in the floor of the mouth. Histologically, the cyst wall contains lymph tissue. The tissue of origin is thought to be salivary epithelium.

Thyroglossal cyst

This cyst, which arises from the thyroglossal duct epithelium, may present intra-orally. However, the mouth is a rare site. Most arise in the region of the hyoid bone.

15.2.6 Tumours

Congenital epulis

This is a rare lesion that occurs in neonates. It normally presents in the anterior maxilla. It consists of granular cells covered by epithelium and is thought to be reactive in nature. This is a benign lesion and simple excision is curative.

Melanotic neuroectodermal tumour

This rare tumour occurs in the early months of life, usually in the maxilla. The lesion consists of epithelial cells containing melanin with a fibrous stroma. Some localized bone expansion may occur. The condition is benign and simple excision is curative.

Squamous cell papilloma

This is a benign condition which occurs in children. The small pedunculated cauliflower-like growths, which vary in colour from pink to white (Fig. 15.10), are usually solitary lesions. They are caused by the human papillomavirus.

Verruca vulgaris

This condition, also known as the common wart, may present as solitary or multiple intra-oral lesions. These may be associated with skin warts. They are caused by the human papillomavirus.

Focal epithelial hyperplasia

This is a rare condition also known as Heck's disease. It is associated with human papillomavirus. It presents as multiple small elevations of the oral mucosa, especially in the lower lip.

Fibroepithelial polyp

This is a fairly common lesion that presents as a firm pink lump. It normally affects the buccal mucosa at the occlusal level. These lesions are caused by trauma. They are usually symptomless unless further traumatized and are easily removed.

Fibrous epulis

This presents as a mass on the gingiva. The colour varies from pink to red depending on the degree of vascularity of the lesion (Fig. 15.11). It consists of an inflammatory cell infiltrate and mature fibrous tissue; occasionally a calcified variant is found. Surgical excision is curative.

Pyogenic granuloma

These commonly occur on the gingiva, usually in the anterior maxilla. They are probably a reaction to chronic trauma, especially from subgingival calculus. As a result of their aetiology they have a tendency to recur after removal.

Peripheral giant cell granuloma

This dark-red swelling of the gingiva can occur in children. It often arises interdentally. Radiographs may reveal some loss of the interdental crest. The central giant cell granuloma (see Section 15.3.4) shows much greater bone destruction. This condition is thought to be a reactive hyperplasia. Unless excision is complete the granuloma will recur.

Haemangiomas

Haemangiomas are relatively common in children. They are malformations of blood vessels. They are divided into cavernous and capillary variants, although some lesions contain elements of both. Capillary haemangiomas may present as facial birthmarks. The cavernous haemangioma is a hazard during surgery if involved within the surgical site. It is a large blood-filled sinus that will bleed profusely if damaged (Fig. 15.12). The extent of a cavernous haemangioma can be established prior to surgery using either angiography or MRI scanning. Small haemangiomas are readily treated by excision or cryotherapy. Larger lesions are amenable to laser therapy.

Sturge–Weber syndrome

Sturge–Weber angiomatosis is a syndrome consisting of a haemangioma of the leptomeninges with an epithelial facial haemangioma closely related to the distribution of branches of the trigeminal nerve. Mental deficiency, hemiplegia, and occular defects can occur. Intra-oral involvement may interfere with the timing of eruption of the teeth (both early and delayed eruption have been reported).

Lymphangiomas

Lymphangiomas are benign tumours of the lymphatics. The vast majority are found in children. The head and neck region is a common site (Fig. 15.13). The cystic hygroma is a variant that appears as a large neck swelling which may extend intra-orally to involve the floor of the mouth and tongue.

Neurofibromas

These may present as solitary or multiple lesions. They are considered to be hamartomas (a haphazard arrangement of tissue). They present intra-orally as mucosal swellings on the tongue or gingivae. Multiple oral neuromas are a feature of multiple endocrine neoplasia

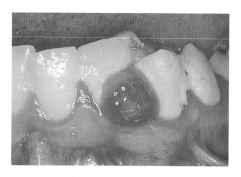

Figure 15.11 A fibrous epulis in a 10-year-old girl (a pyogenic granuloma appears similar).

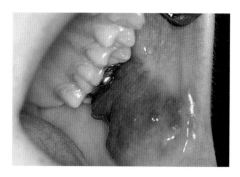

Figure 15.12 Cavernous haemangioma of the buccal mucosa. (Reproduced by kind permission of Informa Healthcare.)

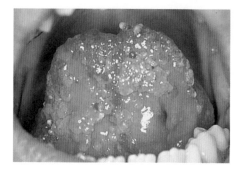

Figure 15.13 Lymphangioma of the tongue and floor of the mouth. (By kind permission of Professor C. Scully.)

syndrome. As the oral signs may precede the development of more serious aspects of this condition (such as carcinoma of the thyroid), children presenting with multiple lesions should be referred to an endocrinologist.

Orofacial granulomatosis (OFG)

OFG is not a tumour in the true sense, nor a distinct disease entity, but describes a clinical appearance. Typically, there is diffuse swelling of one or both lips and cheeks, cobble-stoning and tags of the buccal reflected mucosa, full width gingivitis, and oral ulceration (Fig. 15.14). This may represent a localized disturbance as a manifestation of an allergic reaction to foodstuffs, toothpaste, or even dental materials. Alternatively, the appearance may be due to an underlying systemic condition such as sarcoidosis or Crohn's disease.

Melkersson–Rossenthal syndrome

This condition generally begins during childhood. It consists of chronic facial swelling (usually the lips), facial nerve paralysis, and a fissured (scrotal) tongue.

Malignant tumours of the oral soft tissues

Epithelial tumours

Malignant tumours of the oral epithelium, such as squamous cell carcinoma, are rare in children. Malignant salivary neoplasms are also uncommon, although muco-epidermoid carcinomas have been reported in young patients.

Lymphomas

Hodgkin's and non-Hodgkin's lymphomas can occur in children, but they are relatively rare in the paediatric age group. An exception is Burkitt's lymphoma, which is endemic in parts of Africa and affects those under 14 years of age. Indeed, in these areas the condition accounts for almost half of all malignancies in children. Burkitt's lymphoma is multifocal, but a jaw tumour (more often in the maxilla) is

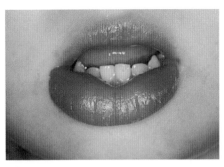

(a)

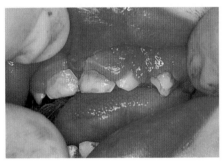

(b)

Figure 15.14 (a) Swelling of the lower lip and (b) attached mucosa and gingiva in a 3-year-old girl with orofacial granulomatosis.

often the presenting symptom. Burkitt's lymphoma is strongly linked to the Epstein–Barr virus as a causal agent.

Rhabdomyosarcomas

These malignant tumours of skeletal muscle present in patients around 9–12 years of age. The usual site is the tongue. Metastases are common and the prognosis is poor.

15.3 Lesions of the jaws

These can be divided into cysts, developmental conditions, osteodystrophies, and tumours.

15.3.1 Cysts

Eruption

Eruption cysts are really dentigerous cysts, which present as swellings of the alveolar mucosa. They may precede the eruption of both primary and permanent teeth (Fig. 15.15). When filled with blood they are often called eruption haematomas. The treatment of eruption cysts is discussed in Section 15.5.5.

Dentigerous

This is the most common jaw cyst in children (Fig. 15.16). Its origin is the reduced enamel epithelium, and attachment to the tooth occurs at

the amelocemental junction. There are often no symptoms, but eruption of the affected tooth will be prevented. The treatment of dentigerous cysts is discussed in Section 15.5.5.

Radicular

These cysts, which are related to the apex of a non-vital tooth, do occur in children although they are rare in the primary dentition. They are often symptomless and are discovered radiographically. Extraction, apicectomy, or conventional endodontics will effect a cure. Lateral periodontal cysts are very rare in children.

Keratinizing odontogenic tumour

This lesion, which was formerly known as the odontogenic keratocyst, is the most aggressive of the jaw cysts. Rates of recurrence of around 60% have been reported because fragments remaining after

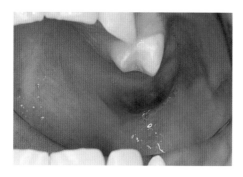

Figure 15.15 Eruption cyst prior to the appearance of the upper permanent molar.

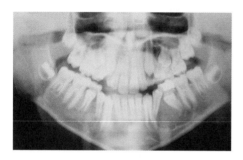

Figure 15.16 Radiographic appearance of a dentigerous cyst associated with a lower second premolar. (Reproduced from *Dental Update* (ISSN 0305-5000), by permission of George Warman Publications (UK) Ltd.)

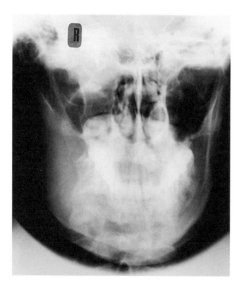

Figure 15.17 Monostotic fibrous dysplasia of right mandibular angle and ascending ramus in a 15-year-old boy.

subtotal removal will regenerate. These cysts may be found in children and may be associated with the basal cell naevus (Gorlin–Goltz) syndrome. The odontogenic tumours associated with this syndrome appear in the first decade of life, whereas the syndromic

basal cell carcinomas are rare before puberty. Other signs and symptoms include multiple basal cell carcinomas, bifid ribs, calcification of the falx cerebri, hypertelorism, and frontal and temporal bossing.

Non-odontogenic

These include the nasopalatine duct cyst, which may occur clinically as a swelling in the anterior midline of the hard palate. The radiographic appearance is a radiolucency >6mm in diameter in the position of the nasopalatine duct. The anterior teeth have vital pulps. Surgical excision is curative. The so-called globulomaxillary cyst, which occurs between the lateral incisor and canine teeth, is now thought to be odontogenic in origin. It is either a radicular cyst or a keratinizing odontogenic tumour. The haemorrhagic bone cyst is a condition that may be found in children and adolescents. It occurs most commonly in the mandible in the premolar/molar region. It is often a chance radiographic finding and normally asymptomatic. Radiographically it appears as a scalloped radiolucency between the roots of the teeth. It regresses spontaneously or after surgical investigation.

15.3.2 Developmental conditions

Numerous developmental conditions may affect the oral and perioral structures. These range from minor problems (e.g. tongue-tie) that are readily treated under local anaesthesia, to severe craniofacial disorders (e.g. Crouzon's syndrome) requiring a combined interdisciplinary approach between maxillofacial surgery and neurosurgery. Readers should refer to specialized texts for a full description of congenital jaw abnormalities. It is important to remember that patients with developmental orofacial abnormalities may have other congenital disorders that may impact on the provision of dental care.

15.3.3 Osteodystrophies

Fibrous dysplasia

This can occur as one of three variants—monostotic, polyostotic, or part of Allbright's syndrome (where associated conditions include skin pigmentation and precocious puberty in females). The monostotic type is the most common affecting the jaws, especially the maxilla. The disease presents as a slow-growing bony expansion which produces facial asymmetry and malalignment of teeth. Radiographically there is a fine granular radiopacity (Fig. 15.17). Surgery can correct the asymmetry.

Cherubism

In this rare condition there is a characteristic fullness of the cheeks and jaws. Initial presentation is commonly between 2 and 4 years of age. Size increases during growth. It is self-limiting and regression occurs in adulthood. Cosmetic surgery may be employed after active growth has finished. Multilocular radiographic radiolucencies occur at the angles of the mandible (Fig. 15.18) and the maxillary tuberosities. Histologically, the lesion is similar to the giant cell granuloma.

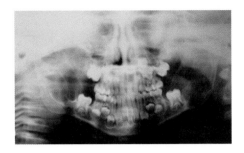

Figure 15.18 Bilateral multilocular radiolucencies affecting the angles of the mandible in a 5-year-old child with cherubism.

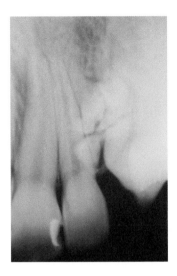

Figure 15.19 Compound odontome in the upper left canine region.

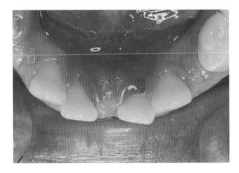

Figure 15.20 Central giant cell granuloma in a 9-year-old girl.

15.3.4 Tumours of the jaws

Odontomes

Odontomes are hamartomas that contain dental calcified tissue. They are classified as compound (a collection of discrete tooth-like structures) or complex (a haphazard arrangement of dental tissue). Compound odontomes are most commonly found in the anterior maxilla (Fig. 15.19). The complex type are usually located in the premolar/molar regions of both jaws. Odontomes are usually symptomless and are diagnosed radiographically. The mean age of patients at diagnosis is 15 years. Occasionally an odontome will become infected when partially erupted, and surgical excision is required. Similarly, removal is indicated if an odontome is interfering with the eruption of a neighbouring tooth or is needed as part of an orthodontic treatment plan.

Juvenile ossifying fibroma

This benign lesion differs from the adult ossifying (or cemento-ossifying) fibroma in that growth is rapid. It consists of fibrous tissue with a varying amount of mineralized material. It usually affects the mandible. Radiographs show a well-circumscribed radiolucency with 'speckling'. Surgical excision is required.

Central giant cell granuloma

This swelling of bone usually affects the mandible (Fig. 15.20). Radiographically, there is a well-defined radiolucency with occasional resorption of associated teeth. Histologically, there are large numbers of osteoclast-like cells in a vascular stroma. Surgical curettage is curative.

Histiocytoses

Langerhans' cell histiocytosis, formerly known as histiocytosis X, is a condition that predominantly affects children (Chapter 11). The term covers a spectrum of conditions. Lesions can be solitary (unifocal eosinophilic granuloma) or multiple sites can be affected (multifocal eosinophilic granuloma) as occurs in Hand–Schuller–Christian syndrome and Letterer–Siwe disease. Bone is replaced by Langerhans' cells, thus producing sharply defined radiographic radiolucencies that may be associated with loosening of the teeth.

Ameloblastoma

Although more commonly found in adults, this locally invasive neoplasm can occur in children. It is usually found in the mandible. It is slow growing and is often symptomless in the early stages. As it progresses it causes a bony swelling, which appears as a multilocular radiolucency in the jaw. Surgical resection to sound bone is necessary for a cure.

Ameloblastic fibroma

This rare lesion usually affects a younger age group than the ameloblastoma. The average age of patients at diagnosis is 14 years. It is a benign tumour. A related lesion is the ameloblastic fibro-odontoma. This lesion contains dentine and enamel, and occurs in children under 10 years of age.

Primary intra-osseous carcinoma

This is a very rare tumour, but when it occurs it is usually in children. It is thought to arise from odontogenic epithelium and shows rapid growth.

Sarcomas

Sarcomas of the jaws are rare. However, the highly malignant Ewing's sarcoma occurs in children between the ages of 5 and 15. The mandible is usually the bone affected and the prognosis is poor.

15.4 Oral manifestations of systemic disease

In addition to specific pathological conditions in the mouth, diseases that affect other systems of the body can produce oral manifestations (e.g. Crohn's disease). In addition, disorders such as chronic renal failure and diabetes can predispose to periodontal disease, and there may be poor resistance to the spread of odontogenic infection. It is not only the oral soft tissues that are affected by systemic conditions.

The temporomandibular joint can be involved in juvenile rheumatoid arthritis and the jaws can be affected in hyperparathyroidism (giant cell tumours). In some cases an oral condition may be the presenting feature of a systemic disease, and dental practitioners should not hesitate to refer children with abnormal oral signs for further investigation.

15.5 Oral surgery

This section deals with dental extractions and minor oral surgical procedures for children. The procedures described are those that can be performed under local anaesthesia with or without sedation (normally inhalational) or day-case general anaesthesia in healthy children. Oral surgery procedures that require inpatient facilities, other than the treatment of severe infection, will not be considered in this text.

15.5.1 Exodontia

Differences between primary and permanent teeth

1. *Size.* Primary teeth are smaller in every dimension compared with their permanent counterparts. Although the roots of primary teeth are smaller than those of the permanent dentition, they form a proportionately greater part of the tooth.

2. *Shape.* The crowns of primary teeth are more bulbous than the crowns of permanent teeth. The roots of primary molars are more splayed than the roots of permanent molar teeth. The furcation of primary molar roots is positioned more cervically than in the corresponding permanent teeth.

3. *Physiology.* The roots of primary teeth resorb naturally, whereas in the permanent dentition resorption is normally a sign of pathology.

4. *Support.* The bone of the alveolus is much more elastic in the younger patient.

These differences mean that there are some modifications to extraction techniques in children. The types of forceps employed for the removal of primary teeth differ from those used for the removal of permanent teeth. The beaks and handles are smaller. In addition, to accommodate the more bulbous crown, the beaks are more curved in forceps designed for the removal of primary teeth. The wide splaying of primary molar roots means that more expansion of the socket is required for the extraction of primary teeth. The more elastic alveolus of the younger patient allows this to be achieved. As a result of the relatively cervical position of the bifurcation in primary molars, it is injudicious to use forceps with deeply plunging beaks (such as the adult cowhorn design) as these could damage the underlying permanent successors. This is especially important with the lower primary molars. As primary roots are resorbed, it is often preferable to leave small fragments *in situ* if the root fractures. When a proportion of the root fractures and is visible, it should be removed. Blind investigation of primary sockets should not

be performed as there is a danger of damaging the underlying permanent successor. Similarly, blind investigation of the distal root socket of first permanent molar teeth must not be carried out in children with unerupted second molars, as unintentional elevation of the second molar can occur.

Problems peculiar to the child patient

A number of problems peculiar to the child patient will affect the way in which extractions are carried out. The following should be considered:

- natal and neonatal teeth
- infra-occlusion of teeth
- fusion/gemination of two teeth
- damage to the permanent successor
- dislocation of the mandible.

Natal and neonatal teeth

Most neonatal teeth (85%) are found in the mandible. About 5% of these are supernumeraries. Their management is discussed in Chapter 13.

Infra-occlusion

Surgical division is sometimes necessary to remove these teeth (Chapter 13).

Fusion/gemination (connation)

Such teeth may not lend themselves to forceps extraction because of their unusual coronal shape. Elevators are usually employed, with or without tooth division and bone removal, to effect extraction.

Damage to permanent successor

This may occur if forceps with large beaks are used or during root elevation.

Dislocation of the mandible

It is very easy to dislocate a child's mandible during extractions under general anaesthesia (when the muscles are relaxed) unless adequate support is provided by the 'non-working' hand. This is because the articular eminence is not as pronounced in young patients as in adults. It is essential to verify that dislocation has not occurred before the patient is allowed to regain consciousness.

15.5.2 Extraction techniques

Patient position

The child should be seated in a dental chair reclined at about 30° to the vertical for extractions under local anaesthesia. Under general anaesthesia the patient is usually supine. When removing upper teeth under local anaesthesia, the operator stands in front of the patient with a straight back and the patient's mouth at a level just below the operator's shoulder.

A right-handed operator removes lower left teeth from a similar position in front of the patient, except that the patient's mouth is at a height just below the operator's elbow. When removing teeth from the lower right, the right-handed operator stands behind the patient with the chair as low as possible to allow good vision. When performing extractions in the supine patient under general anaesthesia, the patient's mouth is usually at a level just below the operator's elbow. Once again, lower right teeth are removed from behind, with all the others being extracted by the operator standing in front of the patient. It saves time during general anaesthesia if teeth can be removed ambidextrously, as all teeth can be extracted with the operator standing in front of the patient. The removal of primary teeth with the non-dominant hand is not difficult to master and is a useful skill to acquire.

The non-working hand

The sections below describe the instruments and technique used by the operator's working hand. The non-working hand also has important roles to play (Fig. 15.21):

- it retracts soft tissues to allow visibility and access;
- it protects the tissues if the instrument slips;
- it provides resistance to the extraction force on the mandible to prevent dislocation;
- it provides 'feel' to the operator during the extraction and gives information about resistance to removal.

Order of extraction

When performing multiple extractions in all quadrants of the mouth (especially if under general anaesthesia) the order of extraction is as follows.

1. Symptomatic teeth are extracted before 'balancing extractions' on the opposite side.

2. Lower teeth are extracted before upper teeth (to eliminate bleeding interfering with the surgical field).

3. If there are symptomatic teeth in all quadrants, right-handed operators should begin with lower right extractions. This minimizes the number of changes of position of the surgeon, which will reduce general anaesthetic time.

Upper primary and permanent anteriors

Before applying forceps to any permanent tooth, it is useful to help loosen the attachment of the tooth to the bone by the insertion of a luxator buccally and lingually. This instrument can normally be inserted to a greater apical position compared with the beaks of forceps. In addition, further loosening and the beginning of movement can be achieved by using straight elevators, such as the Coupland design, if these are advanced along the buccal and lingual periodontium as described below. When maxillary anterior teeth are in a normal position in the dental arch, they should be removed by applying the forceps beaks to the root and then using clockwise and anticlockwise rotations about the long axis (the action one would employ when using a screwdriver). In older children, some additional buccal expansion may be required for the removal of the permanent upper canine. Upper primary anterior or upper primary root forceps are used when removing primary upper anteriors; upper straight forceps are employed for the permanent maxillary anteriors. Malpositioned permanent upper anteriors are frequently encountered, and modifications to technique must be employed. Labially placed upper lateral incisors and canines have very little buccal support and are easily removed either by using straight forceps applied mesially and distally and using a slight rotatory movement as described earlier or by the use of elevators. The most useful elevators under these circumstances are the straight and curved Warwick James and Coupland designs. The straight elevators are applied along the length of the mesial and distal surfaces of the root and directed in a rotatory manner towards the apex (Fig. 15.22). The mesiobuccal and distobuccal surfaces are used

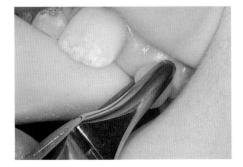

Figure 15.21 The non-working hand supports the tooth for extraction and reflects soft tissues.

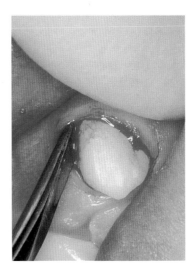

Figure 15.22 Use of a Coupland elevator to deliver a buccally placed upper canine.

alternately, although in many instances the tooth will be elevated after application to only one of these surfaces. When the curved Warwick James elevators are used, the right-sided Warwick James is positioned on the mesiobuccal surface of the upper right teeth and the distobuccal surface of the upper left teeth and then rotated towards the midline of the tooth. The left-sided instrument is used on the opposite root surface in a similar fashion. Palatally positioned lateral incisors and canines are not usually accessible with forceps and thus elevators are used as described above, with the exception that they are applied on the palatomesial and palatodistal surfaces. When the curved elevators are used, the right-sided instrument is applied distally on the right side and mesially on the left side.

Upper primary molars

These teeth display the most widely splayed roots found in either dentition, and thus considerable expansion of the socket is required. Upper primary molar forceps are used and applied to the roots. The initial movement after application of the forceps is palatal, to expand the socket in this direction. The tooth is then subjected to a continuous bucally directed force, which results in delivery. Occasionally, buccal movement is not adequately obtained because of gross caries on the palatal aspect, causing slippage of the forceps beak on the palatal side during buccal expansion. This can be overcome by completing the extraction by continued palatal expansion, as the elastic bone of younger patients allows this to be performed.

Upper premolars

The two-rooted upper first premolar is best removed by buccal expansion using upper premolar forceps. The upper second premolar is often single-rooted and, although buccal expansion with premolar forceps should be attempted in the first instance, this tooth can also be subjected to a rotation about its long axis to effect delivery. Palatally displaced upper premolars are difficult to remove with forceps. The use of elevators in a manner similar to that described for palatally placed canines is preferred.

Upper permanent molars

These teeth are removed using left and right upper molar forceps. Following application of the forceps to the roots of the tooth (the pointed beak is driven towards the buccal root bifurcation), it is delivered by expanding the socket in a buccal direction. The use of palatal expansion is not as successful in the removal of permanent molars, but it may be worth attempting if buccal expansion fails to deliver the tooth. The problem with palatal expansion when extracting permanent molars is that it can cause fracture of the palatal root, which is usually the most closely associated with the maxillary antrum.

Lower primary anteriors

These teeth are extracted in the same manner as their upper counterparts, employing rotation about the long axis using lower primary anterior or root forceps.

Lower permanent anteriors

Permanent lower incisors are not readily removed by rotation as their roots are thin mesiodistally and rotation is likely to cause root fracture. The most effective method of removal is to apply lower root forceps and expand the socket labially. Permanent lower canines can be delivered by a rotatory movement about the long axis or by buccal expansion. Labially displaced lower canines are removed in a manner similar to that described for buccally placed upper anteriors. Mesial and distal application of forceps or straight elevators are used. Straight elevators are used on lower incisors that are labially placed. The position of lingually placed lower anteriors normally precludes the use of forceps, and straight elevators applied mesially and distally should be employed.

Lower primary molars

These teeth are removed by buccolingual expansion of the socket. They can be extracted using either lower primary molar or lower primary root forceps. Lower primary molar forceps are similar in design to the permanent molar forceps. They have two pointed beaks which engage the bifurcation. Lower primary root forceps are used by applying the beaks to the mesial root of the primary molar. Lower first primary molars are usually more easily removed with lower primary root forceps. After application of the forceps, a small lingual movement is followed by a continuous buccal force which delivers the tooth.

Lower premolars

When these teeth are fully erupted in the arch of the young patient they are usually simply removed by a rotatory movement around the long axis of the root using lower premolar forceps. Malpositioned lower second premolars are normally lingually positioned and can be difficult to remove with lower forceps. When lingually placed, lower premolars can be extracted using straight elevators applied mesially, lingually, and distally. Alternatively, it is often possible to apply the beaks of upper fine root forceps mesially and distally to the crown of the lingually placed tooth when the forceps are directed from the opposite side of the jaw. Gentle rotation of the tooth with the forceps can then effect removal.

Lower permanent molars

Two designs of forceps are used to extract lower molar teeth. The lower molar forceps have two pointed beaks that are applied in the region of the bifurcation buccally and lingually. Once applied, the forceps are used to move the tooth in a buccal direction to expand the buccal cortical plate. When buccal expansion is not sufficient to deliver the tooth, the forceps should be moved in a figure-of-eight fashion to expand the socket lingually as well as buccally, and this is generally successful.

A different technique is used with forceps of the cowhorn design. These forceps have two beaks that taper to a point. The points are applied to the bifurcation of the lower molar in a manner identical to that described above. The next movement is to squeeze the forceps handles together, which results in the beaks approaching one another at the base of the bifurcation. The only way the beaks can approach each other is by displacing the tooth in an occlusal direction, resulting in extraction of the tooth.

Both the above methods are successful in removing permanent molar teeth in children, and the choice of technique depends mainly on the preference of the operator.

Management of buried teeth

Buried teeth (including supernumeraries) are treated in children for several reasons:

- symptomatic (e.g. pain);
- radiographic signs of pathology (e.g. dentigerous cyst formation or resorption of another tooth);
- part of an orthodontic treatment plan.

If buried teeth are symptomless, have no associated pathology, and are not causing orthodontic problems (either by their absence or in preventing the orthodontic movement of erupted teeth), they should be left alone. Such teeth should be kept under clinical and radiographic review so that any developing pathology can be detected and treated. In cases where unerupted teeth are to be removed, the first step in management is to localize the buried tooth by clinical examination and radiographic techniques. A number of radiographic views can be used:

- parallax periapicals
- orthopantomogram
- occlusal views
- true lateral facial bones
- cone beam CT scanning.

If cone beam facilities are available, the buccolingual position of the buried tooth is obvious from the scan produced. If standard radiography is used, two views at different angles are required to localize the tooth in the buccolingual plane using parallax. Either two periapical films or a sectional pantomogram and occlusal film are used. The latter combination is preferred by many as the orthopantomogram will also supply information concerning the overall shape of the tooth, its relationship to neighbouring structures (such as the antrum, the inferior alveolar nerve canal, and other unerupted teeth), and the extent of any associated pathology. Once the tooth has been located and the difficulty of removal and patient cooperation assessed, the method of anaesthesia should be determined.

Extraction of buried teeth

When removing buried dental tissue in children it is imperative to have an excellent view of the operative field. This is especially important when removing unerupted teeth or supernumeraries closely associated with other unerupted teeth that are to be retained. In these circumstances the tooth of interest and its unerupted neighbours must be clearly identified.

Flap design

Flaps should:

- be mucoperiosteal
- be cut at 90° to bone
- have a good blood supply
- avoid damage to important structures
- allow atraumatic reflection
- provide adequate access and visibility
- permit reapposition of the wound margins over sound bone.

Flaps for buccally placed teeth

Two flap designs can be used for the removal of buccally placed teeth. The first includes the gingival margin as the horizontal component and a vertical relief incision into the depth of the buccal sulcus (Fig. 15.23). It allows good exposure and easy orientation, it can be readily extended, and for the most part the wound edge will be replaced over sound bone at the end of the procedure. If this design is used in the mandible in the region of the mental foramen, care must be taken to ensure that the vertical relief is at least one tooth in front of the foramen (which will have been localized from the orthopantomogram). The only problem with this type of flap is that it may disrupt the gingival contour, but this is not a major long-term problem in children. The second design of flap for buccally placed teeth is a semilunar incision. At least 5mm of attached gingiva should be maintained at the narrowest point to ensure a good blood supply to the marginal gingivae. This flap does not provide such good exposure or orientation as the previous design, and at the end of surgery it is possible to be left with a large part of the wound margin over a bony defect. This can lead to wound breakdown.

Flaps for palatally/lingually placed teeth

Palatally positioned teeth are best removed via an incision that follows the palatal gingival margin (Fig. 15.24). Such an incision maintains the integrity of the greater palatine nerves and blood vessels. It is often possible to raise this flap without sacrificing the neurovascular bundle that leaves the incisive foramen. This bundle will stretch to a certain degree, but if access demands it should be cut. This rarely results in any postoperative complications. The extent of the palatal gingival incision depends upon the surgery involved. A flap extending between the mesial aspect of both first permanent molars is not unusual for the removal of bilateral impacted maxillary canines. Smaller flaps may be sufficient to remove palatally placed teeth or supernumeraries near the midline. In the lower jaw adequate access to the lingual side is usually obtained by raising the lingual gingiva and reflected mucosa via an incision run around the lingual gingival margin.

Bone removal

When working close to buried teeth that are to be retained it is essential that bone is removed with care. This can be carried out using a handpiece and bur very slowly. The use of chisels with hand pressure (mallets are not used unless working under general anaesthesia and are seldom required in children) is much safer because this is unlikely to damage coronal tissue.

Tooth removal

Once sufficient bone has been removed to allow identification of the tooth to be extracted and exposure of the greatest diameter of its crown, the tooth should be elevated. If this is likely to produce undue pressure on neighbouring erupted or buried teeth, the tooth should be divided using a handpiece and bur and removed in parts. Mandibular teeth that are impacted within the line of the arch are best removed by the so-called broken instrument technique, in which pressure is applied from one side of the tooth (e.g. using a straight Warwick James elevator) to force it out of the other side.

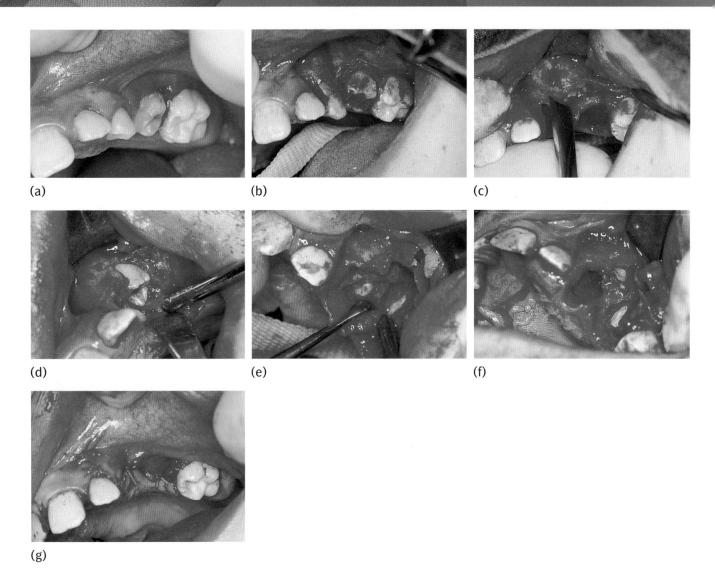

(a)　(b)　(c)

(d)　(e)　(f)

(g)

Figure 15.23 (a) Use of a buccal flap to remove erupted 63, totally submerged 64, infra-occluded 65, and unerupted 24. (b) The buccal flap is raised. (c) Bone is removed with a chisel following removal of 63, 65. (d) Totally submerged 64 is identified by occlusal amalgam. (f) 24 is removed. (g) Flap repositioned and sutured. (Reproduced from *Dental Update* (ISSN 0305-5000), by permission of George Warman Publications (UK) Ltd.)

Suturing

Resorbable sutures should be used in children whenever possible; 3/0 or 4/0 Vicryl® is ideal.

Discharge

Any bleeding should be arrested before the patient is allowed to leave the surgery. The patient and parent should receive instructions on simple methods of haemorrhage control. The patient should be encouraged to maintain good oral hygiene and may be given an antiseptic mouthwash. The problem of self-inflicted trauma in anaesthetized areas is stressed at this stage.

Pain relief

Simple analgesics are usually required, but aspirin must be avoided in those under 12 years of age because of its association with Reye's syndrome. Paracetamol elixir (120–250mg/5mL four times daily for those under 6 years of age; 250–500mg/5mL four times daily for children aged 6–12 years) is ideal. The patient is given a review appointment but should return sooner if there are any problems with bleeding, excessive pain, or swelling. A telephone number for contact in an emergency must be provided.

Review

At the review visit the surgical site should be examined for undue swelling, the area of local anaesthesia examined for evidence of self-inflicted trauma, and the patient questioned about any residual altered sensation. Any remaining sutures can be removed at this stage or allowed to resorb themselves depending on the patient's wishes. It is often necessary to reinforce good oral hygiene at this stage.

Post-extraction problems

Fortunately, post-extraction problems are rare in children. Dry socket does not seem to occur after the removal of primary teeth but it can

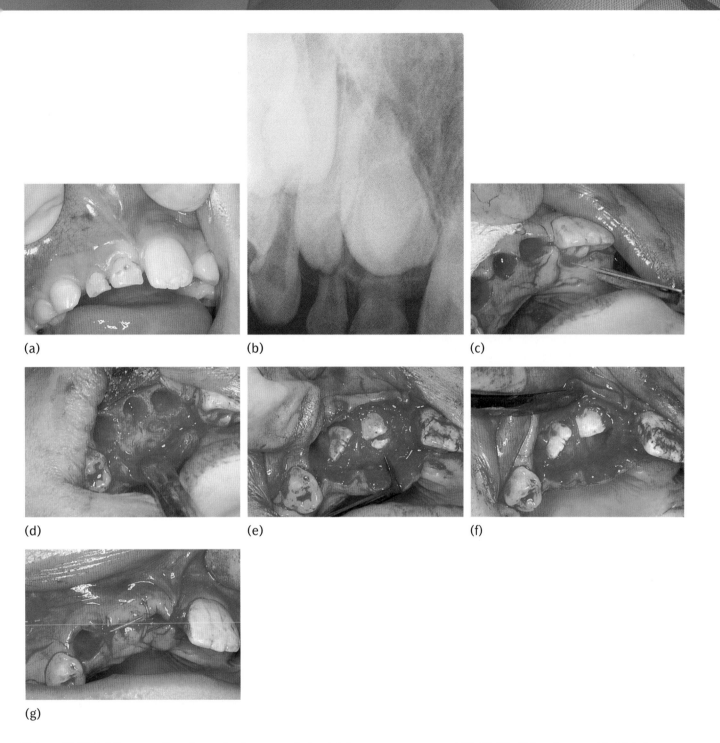

Figure 15.24 (a) Preoperative view prior to removal of palatal supernumerary and 53, 52, 51, 63 in a 9-year-old child via a small palatal flap. (b) Unerupted 11 and supernumerary obvious on radiograph. (c) Erupted teeth extracted and palatal gingival margin being incised. (d) Small palatal flap raised. (e) Supernumerary identified after bone removed. (f) 12, 11 remain. (g) Wound closure. (Reproduced from *Dental Update* (ISSN 0305-5000), by permission of George Warman Publications (UK) Ltd.)

affect older children following permanent molar extractions, although the incidence is not as great as in adults. Local measures such as irrigation and dressing with a sedative pack plus the prescription of an analgesic are sufficient. Postoperative haemorrhage is an occasional problem with children and can be impressive following multiple extractions under general anaesthesia. Pressure applied with gauze or a handkerchief is usually effective. If not, sutures with or without haemostatic gauze must be used. Severe blood loss is very rare, but if this occurs it is important to exclude a systemic cause to ensure that subsequent treatment can be performed safely.

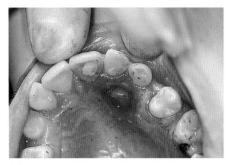

(a)

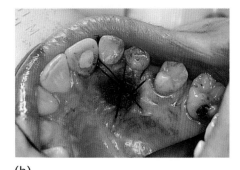

(b)

Figure 15.25 (a) Exposure of palatal canine by tissue sacrifice. (b) Ribbon gauze pack sutured in defect. (Reproduced from *Dental Update* (ISSN 0305-5000), by permission of George Warman Publications (UK) Ltd.)

15.5.3 Surgical aids to orthodontics

Surgical exposure of teeth

The exposure of buried teeth may involve either the extraction of erupted teeth or the removal of buried dental elements, but in some cases all that is required is excision of overlying soft tissue (Meechan *et al.* 2003). If the tooth can be exposed adequately through a collar of attached gingiva, the procedure is quite simple.

1. Erupted primary predecessors may be extracted.

2. A flap is raised in the manner described above.

3. Any unerupted supernumeraries or buried teeth are extracted.

4. The bony impaction is relieved and the widest diameter of the crown exposed. At this stage it may be possible to place an orthodontic appliance to aid eruption, although this is by no means essential.

5. A pack (e.g. a periodontal dressing such as Coe-Pak®), is placed around the tooth and the flap is replaced around the pack. It is not always necessary to sacrifice soft tissue if the tooth is exposed, and the pack can be placed via primary tooth sockets. Alternatively, it is possible in some cases (such as the exposure of a palatally placed canine) to incorporate the pack onto the acrylic of an upper removable orthodontic appliance to maintain exposure during healing.

6. In cases in which the removal of soft tissue from the palate or crest of the ridge is all that is required to expose a tooth it is unnecessary to raise a full flap. All that is needed is to sacrifice the overlying

tissue and pack the wound (Fig. 15.25). Occasionally this can cause excessive bleeding in the palate. This is controlled by passing a non-resorbable suture across the full thickness of the palatal mucoperi-osteum just posterior to the wound edge to ligate the greater palatine artery.

7. When an unerupted tooth, classically a canine, is palpable high in the buccal sulcus under reflected mucosa, it should not be exposed by sacrificing the overlying soft tissue. This would result in the cervical collar of the tooth being surrounded by non-keratinized mucosa. To overcome this problem a flap containing keratinized gingiva must be raised coronal to the impacted tooth, bone removed if necessary, and the flap replaced in a more apical position to allow a collar of attached gingiva around the tooth at eruption.

8. The pack and any remaining non-resorbable sutures should be removed after about 10 days.

Bonding of orthodontic appliances to unerupted teeth

When it is impossible to reposition a flap apically around an unerupted tooth, an alternative is to bond either a gold chain or a magnet (Cole *et al.* 2003) to the buried tooth (Fig. 15.26). When performing this technique the tooth is localized as described above and the gold chain or magnet is attached to the tooth using composite resin and a bonding agent. When a gold chain has been attached (Fig. 15.26(a)) it is brought through the edges of the wound in the area of natural eruption of the tooth. The free end of the chain is then either bonded to an erupted tooth or sutured to the mucosa during the healing period before orthodontic activation. When a magnet is used (Fig. 15.26(b)) the soft tissues are relocated in their original position and sutured. A magnet with the opposite polarity is incorporated within a removable appliance and this is placed over the wound to apply the magnetic force.

Surgical anchorage

Occasionally there is insufficient erupted dentition to allow orthodontic anchorage. This is especially the case for the patient with hypodontia (Chapter 13). Extra-oral anchorage can be employed in such cases. Another technique is to provide anchorage by the provision of bone screws or implants. Standard dental implants are not normally used in children as they act as ankylosed teeth and may disturb the growth of the jaws (see below). However, orthodontic implants may be placed, for example in the midline of the palate (Fig. 15.27). Orthodontic appliances can then be attached to these implants, and are removed at the end of treatment.

15.5.4 Apical surgery

Apicectomy is rarely performed in children. As with adult patients, the best treatment for pulpal pathology is normally conventional endodontic therapy. There are some indications for the technique, most commonly teeth with intransigent open apices. A number of different flap designs can be used. The best is the triangular flap involving the gingival margin and vertical relief incision described above for the removal of buccally placed buried teeth. Principally this is because the extent of apical pathology is often more extensive in children than is suggested

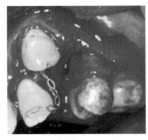

(a)

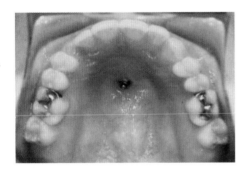

(b)

Figure 15.26 (a) Gold chain bonded to unerupted maxillary permanent canine. The free end of the chain will be bonded to the erupted maxillary permanent incisor following flap replacement. (b) Magnet bonded to unerupted lower second premolar tooth following bone removal. Following flap replacement an acrylic splint containing the magnet with the opposite pole will be positioned over the mucosa.

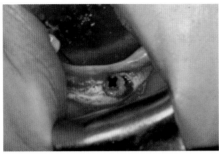

Figure 15.27 An orthodontic implant placed in the midline of the palate and used to provide anchorage. (Image kindly supplied by Straumann Ltd.)

radiographically, and use of the semilunar flap can lead to parts of the incision being left over a bony defect at the end of surgery.

Technique

The surgical technique is identical to that used in adults but there are a number of points of difference when placing the apical seal. In teeth with immature open apices through-and-through root fillings are unsatisfactory as the apex may be wider than the bulk of the canal. Therefore, some form of retrograde restoration is required. It is often difficult to secure undercuts at the apex when dealing with a tooth that has an open apex, but this can be overcome by placing a large retrograde filling and relying on multiple microscopic undercuts to secure it.

15.5.5 Cysts interfering with eruption

Eruption and dentigerous cysts can interfere with the eruption of teeth. Eruption cysts in the young child are simply incised (when occluding teeth are present this can be achieved by the patient themselves on biting). Dentigerous cysts can be marsupialized to the oral mucosal lining following the removal of any overlying primary predecessor and the permanent tooth allowed to erupt. Some authorities advocate more aggressive treatment involving enucleation of the cyst (with or without removal of the tooth) to ensure that epithelial remnants are not left behind. Fissural cysts (such as the nasopalatine cyst) are rare in children; when found they should be enucleated.

15.5.6 Treatment of acute orofacial infection

At this point it is relevant to discuss the treatment of orofacial infection. The major cause of this condition is dental in origin. The minor oral surgical treatments discussed above may all be employed to definitively treat the source of an orofacial infection. Alternatively, conservative treatments such as endodontic therapy may be appropriate. However, a rapidly spreading extra-oral infection is a surgical emergency that merits immediate treatment and may require admission for inpatient management. Two areas of extra-oral spread are of special importance. These are the submandibular region and the angle between the eye and the nose. Swelling in the submandibular region arising from posterior mandibular teeth can result in the floor of the mouth being raised. This can cause a physical obstruction to breathing, and spread from this region to the parapharyngeal spaces may further obstruct the airway. The advance from dysphagia to dyspnoea can be rapid. A submandibular swelling should be decompressed as a matter of urgency in children. A child with raising of the floor of the mouth requires immediate admission to hospital. The fact that trismus is invariably an associated feature makes expert anaesthetic help essential for safe management. Infection involving the angle between the eye and the nose has the potential to spread intracranially and produce a cavernous sinus thrombosis. This is a potentially life-threatening complication. The angular veins of the orbit (which have no valves) connect the cavernous sinus to the face, and if the normal extracranial flow is obstructed as a result of pressure from the extra-oral infection, infected material can enter the sinus by reverse flow. To prevent this complication, infection in this area (which arises from upper anterior teeth, especially the canines) must be treated expeditiously.

The principles of the treatment of acute infection are:

- remove the cause
- institute drainage
- prevent spread
- restore function.

In addition, analgesia and adequate hydration must be maintained. Removal of the cause is essential to cure an orofacial infection arising from a dental source. This usually means extraction or endodontic therapy.

Institution of drainage and prevention of spread are supportive treatments—they are not definitive cures. Drainage may be obtained during the removal of the cause (e.g. a dental extraction) or may precede definitive treatment if this makes management easier (e.g. incision and drainage of a submandibular abscess). Drainage may be intra- or extra-oral. When an extra-oral incision is made, it is created in a skin crease parallel to the direction of the facial nerve. In the submandibular region the incision is made more than one finger's breadth below the angle of the mandible to avoid the mandibular branch. Once the skin has been incised, the dissection is carried out bluntly until the infection has been located. Locules of infection are then ruptured using blunt dissection and a drain to the external surface is secured. Depending on the amount of drainage, the drain is secured for 24–48 hours. Any pus should be sent to the microbiology laboratory for culture and sensitivity testing. Prevention of spread can be achieved surgically or by the use of antibiotics. In severe cases intravenous antibiotics will be used. The antibiotic of choice in children is a penicillin such as amoxicillin.

It is important to remember that acute infections are painful and that analgesics, as well as antibiotics, should be prescribed. The use of paracetamol elixir is usually sufficient. Similarly, it is important that a child suffering from an acute infection is adequately hydrated. If the infection has restricted the intake of oral fluids because of dysphagia, admission to hospital for intravenous fluid replacement is required.

15.5.7 Autotransplantation of teeth

Replantation of a tooth which has been avulsed due to trauma was discussed in Chapter 12. In this section autotransplantation of teeth is discussed. Autotransplantation of teeth in children can be considered as a treatment for the following:

- repositioning of an ectopic tooth;
- replacement of an unrestorable tooth with a redundant member of the dentition.

The ectopic tooth most commonly repositioned by surgical means is the unerupted, palatally placed, upper permanent canine. An example of using autotransplantation as a means of tooth replacement is the substitution of an upper incisor that is undergoing resorption with a premolar tooth scheduled for extraction as part of an orthodontic treatment plan (Fig. 15.28). The management regimen for both treatments is similar and is as follows:

1. Assessment of the donor tooth and recipient site.
2. Atraumatic extraction of the donor tooth.
3. Preparation of the recipient site.
4. Transplantation.
5. Splinting of the transplanted tooth.
6. Root treatment of the transplanted tooth (if required).

In addition, some coronal preparation and orthodontic movement of the donor tooth may be required. Transplantation surgery is usually performed under antibiotic prophylaxis (either oral or intravenous amoxicillin) as the use of systemic antibiotics has been shown to decrease the incidence of root resorption.

Assessment of the donor tooth and recipient site

The tooth to be transplanted has to be appraised clinically and radiographically prior to surgery. The crown of an erupted tooth can be assessed for caries and its dimensions measured. Root status and shape will be determined using periapical radiographs. Ideally, donor teeth should have an open apex with at least three-quarters of the root formed. The morphology of unerupted teeth for transplantation can only be determined radiographically. Teeth with severe root curvature are unsuitable for transplantation as it is unlikely that they can be removed intact without trauma. In addition, a donor site suitable for a dilacerated tooth may be difficult to achieve without damaging neighbouring vital teeth. It is important to evaluate the recipient site both clinically and radiographically. The space available for the transplanted tooth must be assessed in both the horizontal and vertical dimensions. It may be necessary to create sufficient space using preoperative orthodontics. Periapical radiographs will alert the clinician to the presence of any bony pathology or retained dental remnants at the recipient site. The exact morphology and production of a 'surgical drilling template tooth' for the donor tooth can be achieved by cone beam computerized tomography (CBCT) and computer-aided prototyping.

Atraumatic extraction of the donor tooth

It is essential to remove the donor tooth using minimal trauma and avoiding contact with the root surface. Damage to the root surface will lead to resorption or ankylosis. Thus, when removing an erupted tooth for transplantation the usual rules concerning the application of forceps beaks to the root surface do not apply. The beaks are positioned on the crown. Prior to the application of the forceps a scalpel should be run around the gingival margin to the crest of the ridge to sever gingival attachments. When an unerupted tooth is being used as a donor, great care must be exercised during its removal. The entire crown must be exposed. As mentioned earlier, bone removal with hand chisels is less likely to damage the donor than the use of a bur. Once the crown has been exposed, elevators or forceps (again confined to the crown) are used to extract the tooth as gently as possible. When the tooth has been extracted it should be gently replaced into its socket and maintained there until the recipient site is prepared. This is to ensure that a satisfactory tooth is obtained before recipient site surgery is performed.

Preparation of the recipient site

The recipient site may or may not contain a tooth and is prepared using the 'drilling template tooth'. Following extraction of the tooth at the recipient site, the socket is enlarged, if necessary, using either a chisel or a bur (an implant bur is ideal). Some operators recommend that the socket is enlarged following flap raising by removing the buccal plate of bone which is stored in saline prior to being replaced with the cortical surface against the root. It is thought that this might decrease the incidence of ankylosis.

Transplantation

Once the socket has been prepared the donor tooth is gently placed in its new position. The occlusion is assessed to ensure that it is not traumatic to the transplanted tooth, and the gingival margin is held around the tooth with a horizontal mattress suture.

Splinting the transplanted tooth

The donor tooth should be splinted at the time of transplantation. It is important to stress that rigid splinting should not be employed as this may lead to ankylosis. A simple splint using orthodontic wire bonded to the tooth and its neighbours with composite resin is sufficient. It is essential that splinting is not maintained for too long a period as this may also lead to ankylosis. Three weeks is the maximum length of time; indeed in some cases the splint can be removed at 1 week.

Root treatment of transplanted tooth

Ideally immature transplanted teeth will undergo revascularization and continued root growth. The pulp of mature transplanted teeth is extirpated after 2–3 weeks and the root canal is filled with non-setting calcium hydroxide. The calcium hydroxide is replaced with gutta percha as soon as possible post-transplant provided that there is no evidence of root resorption.

Follow-up of transplanted teeth

At the time of discharge the patient should be given an antiseptic mouthwash to maintain good hygiene in the surgical site. The first review is at 1 week, at which stage sutures can be removed. It may be possible to remove the splint at this stage. The next review is at 2–3 weeks for splint removal and possible endodontic treatment. A periapical film should be taken at this stage. Further reviews should be undertaken at 3 and 6 months and then annually. Coronal reshaping can be performed at any stage.

Orthodontic movement of transplanted teeth

Transplanted teeth can be moved orthodontically. This should begin 3 months after transplantation and be completed within 9 months of the transplant.

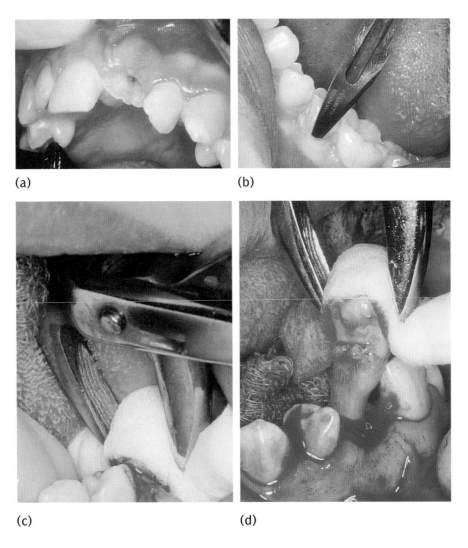

(a)　　(b)　　(c)　　(d)

Figure 15.28 (a) 21 for extraction to be replaced by 35 which is to be removed as part of an orthodontic treatment plan. (b) Incision of 35 gingival attachment. (c), (d) Extraction of 35 using cotton roll to protect root.

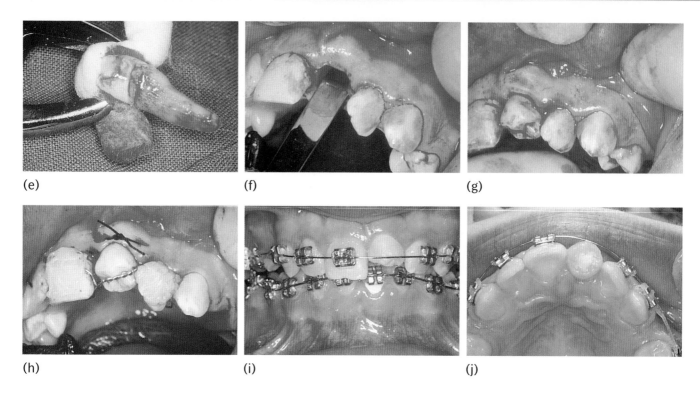

Figure 15.28 (*Continued*) (e) Extracted 35. (f) Widening of 21 socket with chisel. (g) Transplantation of 35 to 21 socket. (h) Suturing and splinting of 35. (i), (j) Labial and occlusal views of 35 at 3 months. Reproduced from *Dental Update* (ISSN 0305–5000), by permission of George Warman Publications (UK) Ltd.

15.6 Implantology

The use of implants for orthodontic anchorage was mentioned above. The use of dental implants as prostheses in children is contraindicated except under circumstances where severe psychological stress merits such treatment. There are three reasons for avoiding implants in young patients.

1. The implant does not move with the growing alveolus—it acts as an ankylosed tooth. Thus implants should not be placed until vertical growth of the jaws is virtually complete (around 18 years of age). The exception to this rule is the lower intercanine region which can receive implants earlier in exceptional cases of hypodontia (e.g. X-linked ectodermal dysplasia).

2. Implants can interfere with normal growth of the jaws.

3. Young bone does not behave in the same way as mature bone. As a result of squashing and crushing, the axis of an inserted implant may deviate widely from the axis of tap. In addition, the use of teeth for autotransplantation is often a viable alternative in young patients.

15.7 Soft tissue surgery

The following short synopsis covers the important functional and orthodontic problems in the child and adolescent.

15.7.1 Labial fraena

A prominent midline frenum in the maxilla may be present in association with a diastema. Whether or not the frenum is the cause of the diastema is open to question as a fleshy frenum does not always produce an aesthetic defect. Nevertheless, the excision of a midline maxillary frenum is often requested as part of an orthodontic treatment plan.

This procedure is very simply performed under local anaesthesia (Fig. 15.29). Before surgery a radiograph of the upper incisor area should be taken to eliminate other possible causes of a midline diastema, such as a mesiodens. A midline maxillary frenum should not be removed before the permanent canines have erupted, as the space may close spontaneously when these teeth appear.

Surgical removal is achieved by dissecting the midline tissue via incisions parallel to the frenum from the labial mucosa, at a point beyond the prominent fibrous tissue, through the interdental space to palatal mucosa. The part of the incision in attached gingiva is mucoperiosteal. The surface

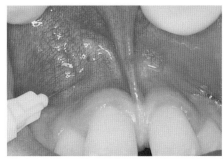

(a)

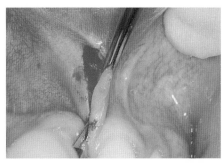

(b)

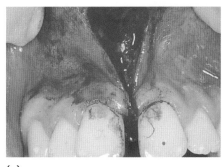

(c)

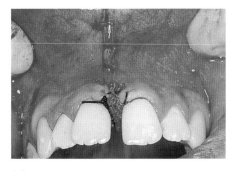

(d)

Figure 15.29 (a) Patient for upper midline labial fraenectomy. (b) Incisions parallel to the frenum. (c) Defect at the end of removal. (d) Wound closure with resorbable sutures in reflected mucosa and silk suture holding pack interdentally.

of the exposed bone in the interdental space should be curetted or gently bured to remove residual fibrous attachments. Primary closure of the labial part of the incision is achieved by suturing, and the defect in attached gingiva is covered by a pack such as Coe-Pak®, which is held in place by sutures. The pack is removed 7–10 days after surgery.

15.7.2 Lingual fraena

A prominent lingual frenum should be excised if it is interfering with speech or oral hygiene. This is simply performed under local anaesthesia. The frenum is held by a pair of haemostatic forceps and an incision is made at 90° to the fibrous band until adequate release is obtained; then the wound ends are sutured.

15.7.3 Mucocoeles

Mucocoeles are common in the second decade of life, although they occasionally occur in younger children including the newborn. If these lesions cause functional or emotional problems they should be excised, but if there is no disturbance removal can be delayed until the child is older.

An incision is made next to the lesion, which is removed by a blunt dissection under the epithelium. Invariably a number of minor salivary glands are obvious during surgery (they often appear like a bunch of grapes around the mucocoele). These should be removed in view of the fact that mucocoeles are produced as a result of trauma. Any obvious dental cause of trauma (e.g. a sharp tooth) should be remedied. One type of mucocoele that is best referred for specialist treatment is that found in the floor of the mouth, the so-called ranula (see Fig. 15.8). This lesion is often more extensive than is at first apparent and complete cure occasionally involves removing the sublingual gland.

15.7.4 Incisional biopsy

Incisional biopsies are performed to confirm a diagnosis by removing part of a lesion. It is preferable that the surgeon who is going to treat the lesion performs the incisional biopsy and therefore this procedure is best performed by a specialist surgeon.

15.7.5 Excision biopsy of non-attached mucosa

Small lesions of the oral mucosa are removed by excisional biopsy, which involves the removal of an ellipse of tissue including the lesion. The long axis of the ellipse is made parallel to the direction of muscle pull, and it is best to hold the specimen with a suture passed under it to avoid crushing which could render the specimen useless for histological examination (Fig. 15.30). All tissue surgically removed should be placed in a solution of 10% formal saline (not in water) and transported to the laboratory for histological examination. Lesions that are obviously benign and are not interfering with function or causing emotional distress can be left in the young child and removed at a later date if necessary (Fig. 15.31).

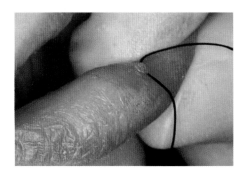

Figure 15.30 Lip lesion held by a suture. (Reproduced from *Dental Update* (ISSN 0305-5000), by permission of George Warman Publications (UK) Ltd.)

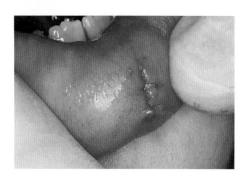

Figure 15.32 Same patient as in Fig. 15.30 showing buried knots with soft-gut sutures. (Reproduced from *Dental Update* (ISSN 0305-5000), by permission of George Warman Publications (UK) Ltd.)

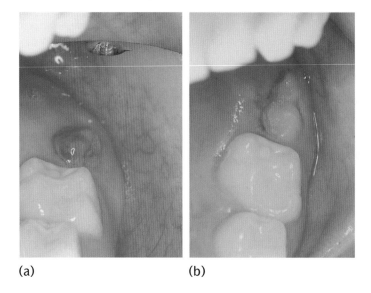

(a)　　　　　　　　　　(b)

Figure 15.31 (a) Lump related to erupting 7 and (b) view a week later—the lump has disappeared and the 7 has erupted. No treatment was given. (Reproduced from *Dental Update* (ISSN 0305-5000), by permission of George Warman Publications (UK) Ltd.)

15.7.6 Excision biopsy of attached gingiva/palate

These procedures leave a defect that is not readily treated by primary closure. Following the biopsy it is useful to lay a haemostatic material over the defect to arrest bleeding and then to cover the area with a periodontal dressing.

15.7.7 Suturing

Resorbable sutures should be used to close soft tissue wounds in children whenever possible; however, in mobile structures such as the tongue and lip these may be lost shortly after surgery as their knots may be less secure than those obtained with black silk. To overcome this problem it is useful to bury knots by taking the first bite of tissue from within the wound rather than from the mucosal surface. The second bite begins on the mucosal surface of the opposite wound edge. This ensures that the knot disappears into the wound when it is tied (Fig. 15.32).

15.8 Summary

The following have been considered in this chapter:

1 Pathological conditions of the oral and perioral structures in children.

2 Dental extractions in children.

3 Minor oral surgical procedures that can be performed without inpatient anaesthetic facilities in healthy children.

4 The management of acute spreading infection from a dental focus in children.

15.9 Further reading

Andersson, L., Kahnberg, K.-E., and Pogrel, M.A. (2010). *Oral and maxillofacial surgery*. Wiley-Blackwell, Oxford (*Everything you need to know about oral and maxillofacial surgery.*)

Meechan, J.G., Greenwood, M., Moore, U.J., Thomson, P.J., Brook, I.M., and Smith, K.G. (2006). *Minor oral surgery in dental practice*. Quintessence, London. (*A guide to minor oral surgery.*)

Scully, C.M. and Welbury, R.R. (1994). *Colour atlas of oral disease in children and adolescents*. Wolfe, London.

Soames, J.V. and Southam, J.C. (2005). *Oral pathology* (4th edn). Oxford University Press, Oxford. (*A comprehensive oral pathology text.*)

15.10 References

Cole, B.O.I., Shaw, A.J., Hobson, R.S., *et al.* (2003). The role of magnets in the management of unerupted teeth in children and adolescents. *International Journal of Paediatric Dentistry*, **13**, 204–7.

Meechan, J.G., Carter, N.E., Gilgrass, T., *et al.* (2003) Interdisciplinary management of hypodontia: oral surgery management. *British Dental Journal*, **194**, 423–7.

16
Medical disability

M.T. Hosey and R. Welbury

Chapter contents

16.1 Introduction

There are many general medical conditions that can directly affect the provision of dental care and some where the consequences of dental disease, or even dental treatment, can be life-threatening. The increasing number of children who now survive with complex medical problems because of improvements in medical care present difficulties in oral management. Dental disease can have grave consequences and so rigorous prevention is paramount. The decline in childhood mortality has led to increasing emphasis on maintaining and enhancing the quality of the child's life and ensuring that children reach adult life as physically, intellectually, and emotionally healthy as possible. Dental care can play an important part in enhancing this quality of life. Indeed, management within the primary dental services helps to 'normalize' life for these children who appreciate attending along with their family even though sometimes they might still require specialist expertise.

Even though infant mortality rates (deaths under 1 year of age) have declined dramatically in the UK, death rates are still higher in the first year of life than in any other single year below the ages of 55 in males and 60 in females. The rates are highest for the very young. The main causes of death in the neonatal period (the first 4 weeks of life) are associated with prematurity (over 40%) and congenital malformations (30%). However, in the remainder of the first year the main causes of death occur at home and often nothing abnormal or suspicious is found (SUDI (sudden unexpected death in infancy) and SIDS (sudden infant death syndrome)). Although the unexpected death of a child over 1 year of age is rare, a few infants still succumb to respiratory and other infective diseases (e.g. meningitis), congenital malformations, and accidents. (See Key Points 16.1.)

Key Points 16.1

- All children with medical illness should be classified 'at high caries risk' and receive aggressive prevention regimes.
- Infection arising from dental disease may interrupt/interfere with the medical control of their condition.
- Dental treatment for these children may require inpatient facilities because of their medical condition.

16.1.1 The medical history

All patients should have an accurate medical history taken before any dental treatment is undertaken. This is important for several reasons.

1. To identify any medical problems that might require modification of dental treatment.

2. To prioritize children who require intensive preventive dental care.

3. To identify those requiring prophylactic antibiotic cover for potentially septic dental procedures.

4. To check whether the child is receiving any medication that could result in adverse interaction(s) with drugs or treatment administered by the dentist. This would include past medication that could have had an effect on dental development.

5. To identify systemic disease that could affect other patients or dental personnel. This is usually related to cross-infection potential.

6. To establish good rapport and effective communication with the child and their parents.

7. To determine the family and social circumstances, whether other siblings are affected by the same or similar condition, and the ability of the parents to cope with attendance for dental appointments given the added burden of medical appointments and their wish to ensure adequate continued schooling.

8. To facilitate communication with medical colleagues.

9. To satisfy medico-legal requirements.

Many dental practitioners use standard questionnaires to obtain a medical history. It has been found that one of the most effective methods is to use a questionnaire followed by a pertinent personal interview with the child and their parent or guardian. (See Key Points 16.2.)

Key Points 16.2

Key medical questions—ask about:

- cardiovascular disorders
- bleeding disorders
- respiratory/chest problems
- epilepsy
- hepatitis/jaundice
- diabetes
- hospitalization or hospital investigation for any reason
- previous general anaesthetic experience/any further general anaesthetic procedures planned
- allergies
- illness in other family members
- medication.

16.1.2 The general examination

General observation of the child is invaluable and can provide vital information. The child's demeanour is important in assessing their potential cooperation for dental treatment, but assessment of general outward appearance can also be helpful in determining their state of health. An impression of height (are they as tall as their peers?) and weight (undernourished or obese?) can give clues about not only nutrition but also somatic growth and dental development. Visually accessible areas, such as skin and nails, can reveal cyanosis, jaundice, and petechiae from bleeding disorders. The hands are particularly worthy of inspection, and can show alterations in the fingernails such as finger-clubbing from chronic cardiopulmonary disorders as well as infections and splinter haemorrhages. Overall shape and symmetry of the face may be significant, and there may be characteristic faces that are diagnostic of some congenital abnormalities and syndromes.

16.2 Cardiovascular disorders

These can be divided into two main groups: congenital heart disease (existing before or at birth), and those disorders that are acquired after birth. Congenital heart disease occurs in approximately eight children in every 1000 live births. There is a wide spectrum of severity, but two or three of these children will be symptomatic in the first year of life.

16.2.1 Congenital heart disease

The cause is rarely known in individual cases but multifactorial inheritance patterns are mainly responsible. Several chromosomal abnormalities, such as Down syndrome, are associated with severe congenital heart disease, but these represent fewer than 5% of the total. The main types of congenital condition are shown in Table 16.1. In most instances there is a combination of genetic and environmental influences, including infections, during the second month of pregnancy.

Many defects are slight and cause little disability, but a child with more severe defects may present with breathlessness on exertion, tire easily, and suffer from recurrent respiratory infections. Those children with severe defects such as tetralogy of Fallot and valvular defects, including pulmonary atresia and tricuspid atresia, will have cyanosis and finger-clubbing, and may have delayed growth and development (Figs 16.1–16.3). Characteristically, these children will assume a squatting position to relieve their dyspnoea (breathlessness) on exertion.

Heart murmurs

The incidence of congenital heart disease is falling, affecting 7–8 infants per 1000. Many parents will report that their child either has, or had, a 'heart murmur'. These may only be discovered at a routine examination, although they occur in over 30% of all children. Most of these murmurs are functional or innocent, and are not associated with significant abnormalities but are the result of normal blood turbulence within the heart. Innocent murmurs are heard most frequently from 3

Table 16.1 Prevalence of congenital cardiac disease

Defect	Percentage
Ventricular septal defect	28
Atrial septal defect	10
Pulmonary stenosis	10
Patent ductus arteriosus	10
Tetralogy of Fallot	10
Aortic stenosis	7
Coarctation of the aorta	5
Transposition of great arteries	5
Rare/diverse	15

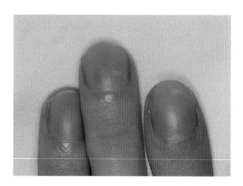

Figure 16.1 The fingers of a boy with Down syndrome and tetralogy of Fallot. The cyanosis and finger-clubbing associated with his severe cardiac disease are obvious.

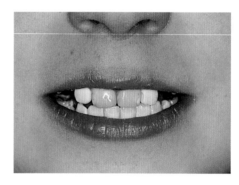

Figure 16.2 Cyanosis affecting the lips in a boy with tetralogy of Fallot. The mucous membranes appear bluish.

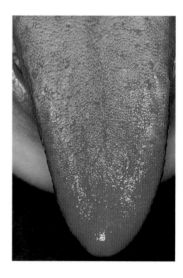

Figure 16.3 Central cyanosis affecting the tongue of the boy shown in Fig. 16.2.

to 7 years of age. In a small minority of cases a heart murmur indicates the presence of a cardiac abnormality causing the turbulence. If the dentist is in any doubt about the significance of a murmur, a cardiological opinion should be sought. Normally, contact with the child's medical practitioner will clarify the situation. Innocent murmurs do not require any special precautions or treatment.

Ventricular septal defects (VSDs)

VSDs are the most common of the cardiac malformations. Small defects are asymptomatic and may be found during a routine physical examination. Large defects with excessive pulmonary blood flow are responsible for symptoms of breathlessness, feeding difficulties, and poor growth. Between 30% and 50% of the small defects close spontaneously, usually within the first year of life. Larger defects are usually closed surgically in the second year of life, but defects involving other cardiac structures may require complex surgery or even transplantation.

Atrial septal defects (ASDs)

ASDs are not as common as VSDs in children, but are proportionately more significant in adults and more frequent in females. An isolated patent foramen ovale is of no clinical significance and is not considered to be an ASD. Even an extremely large ASD rarely produces heart failure in children, but symptoms usually appear in the third decade. Surgery is usually carried out before school age.

Pulmonary stenosis

There are usually no symptoms with mild to moderate stenosis of the pulmonary valve, but exercise intolerance and cyanosis may occur if this is severe. Treatment is required for the moderate to severe forms; in the majority of children relief of this obstruction is now carried out by balloon dilatation rather than surgery.

Patent ductus arteriosus

During fetal life most of the pulmonary arterial blood is shunted through the ductus arteriosus into the aorta, thus bypassing the lungs. Functional closure of the ductus arteriosus usually occurs at birth. Virtually all preterm babies weighing less than 1.75kg have a patent ductus arteriosus in the first 24 hours of life, but this usually closes spontaneously. Ductus arteriosus patency is mediated by prostaglandins, and the administration of inhibitors of prostaglandin synthesis, such as indometacin, is effective in closing the ductus in a significant number of babies. However, surgical ligation is a safe and effective back-up if indometacin is contraindicated or has not been successful.

Tetralogy of Fallot

This classically consists of a combination of:

- an obstruction of right ventricular outflow (pulmonary stenosis)
- VSD
- dextroposition of the aorta (its origin may be overlying the VSD)
- right ventricular hypertrophy.

Cyanosis is one of the most obvious signs of this condition, but it may not be present at birth. However, as the child grows, the obstruction to

blood flow is further exaggerated. The oral mucous membranes and nailbeds are often the first places to show signs of cyanosis. Growth and development may be markedly delayed in severe untreated tetralogy of Fallot, and puberty is delayed. Early medical management involves the use of prostaglandins so that adequate pulmonary blood flow can occur until surgical intervention can be carried out. Initially, a shunt procedure (usually the Blalock–Taussig shunt) is performed to anastomose the subclavian artery to the homolateral branch of the pulmonary artery. Later in childhood, total surgical correction is undertaken, but the mortality rate from this procedure is 5–10%.

16.2.2 Acquired cardiovascular disease

Rheumatic fever

Rheumatic fever follows a group A streptococcal infection of the upper respiratory tract, especially in developing countries, and may occur at all ages but usually between 5 and 15 years. Environmental factors, such as overcrowding, promote the transmission of streptococcal infections, and the incidence of rheumatic fever is higher among lower socio-economic groups. The clinical onset is usually acute and occurs 2–3 weeks after a sore throat. Joint pains are common and of a characteristic migratory polyarthralgia or polyarthritis. Carditis is the most serious manifestation, occurring in 40–50% of initial attacks, especially in young children. Fever is usually present, but in an insidious onset of the condition it may be low grade. Most of the carditis resolves, except the lesions on the cusps of the heart valves which become fibrosed and stenotic. Rheumatic heart disease is the most important manifestation of rheumatic fever and may affect the mitral, aortic, tricuspid, and pulmonary valves.

Diseases of the myocardium and pericardium

Major diseases involving the myocardium and pericardium include bacterial infections such as diphtheria and typhoid, tuberculous, fungal, and parasitic infections, rheumatoid arthritis, systemic lupus erythematosus, uraemia, thalassaemia, hyperthyroidism, neuromuscular diseases such as muscular dystrophy, and glycogen storage diseases. They are relatively rare in children in developed countries.

Other cardiovascular problems

There are several other important conditions that are common in adults but not in children. These include coronary artery disease (ischaemic heart disease), cardiac arrhythmias, and hypertension. In children, secondary hypertension is more common than essential hypertension and is associated with renal abnormalities in 75–80% of those affected.

16.2.3 Dental care for children with cardiovascular disorders

The most important consideration in planning dental care for children with cardiovascular disorders is the prevention of dental disease. As soon as a child is diagnosed as having a significant cardiac problem, they should be referred for dental evaluation and an aggressive preventive regimen, including dietary counselling, fluoride therapy, fissure sealants, and oral hygiene instruction, should be commenced. Regular monitoring, both clinical and radiographic, with reinforcement of the preventive advice is essential. Active dental disease should be treated before cardiac surgery is undertaken.

Antibiotic prophylaxis

Guidance from the National Institute for Health and Clinical Excellence (NICE) in the UK (NICE 2008) has shown that antibiotic prophylaxis is not effective in preventing infective endocarditis and there is no clear association between episodes of infective endocarditis and interventional procedures. Any benefits from prophylaxis need to be weighed against the risks of adverse effects for the patient and the development of antibiotic resistance. As a result, NICE recommends that antibiotic prophylaxis is no longer routinely offered for defined dental interventional procedures.

Adults and children with the following structural cardiac conditions are considered to be at risk of infective endocarditis:

- aquired valvular heart disease with stenosis or regurgitation;
- valve replacement;
- structural congenital heart disease, including surgically corrected or palliated structural conditions, but excluding isolated ASD, fully repaired VSD, or fully repaired ductus arteriosus, and closure devices that are judged to be endothelialized;
- hypertrophic cardiomyopathy;
- previous infective endocarditis.

NICE makes the following recommendations:

Advice

Offer people at risk of infective endocarditis clear and consistent information about prevention, including:

- the benefits and risks of antibiotic prophylaxis, and an explanation of why antibiotic prophylaxis is no longer routinely recommended;
- the importance of maintaining good oral health;
- symptoms that may indicate infective endocarditis and when to seek expert advice;

- the risks of undergoing invasive procedures, including non-medical procedures such as body piercing or tattooing.

When to offer prophylaxis

- Do not offer antibiotic prophylaxis against infective endocarditis to people undergoing dental procedures.
- Do not offer chlorhexidine mouthwash as prophylaxis against infective endocarditis to people at risk undergoing dental procedures.

Managing infection

- Investigate and treat promptly any episodes of infection in people at risk of infective endocarditis to reduce the risk of endocarditis developing.
- Favour more radical treatments to avoid potential sources of infection (e.g. extraction rather than pulp therapy).

Treatment planning

If the child and parent(s) are seen in infancy and effective preventive dental procedures are instituted, in theory operative dentistry should be unnecessary. In practice, the situation may be very different. Ideally, treatment in children should be carried out during short appointments so that cooperation is maximized. Other problems in these children may include prolonged bleeding following scaling or surgical procedures due to thrombocytopenia and anticoagulant medication. It is essential to check the platelet count and prothrombin time if dental extractions are planned. The patient's prothrombin time is compared with the normal value, and the ratio is called the international normalized ratio (INR). No child with symptomatic cardiac problems should have any routine dental procedures until details of the condition have been obtained and the patient's physician consulted.

Antibacterial prophylaxis recommendations are constantly updated and current guidance is based on NICE recommendations and revised as new scientific evidence and drugs become available. The latest British Cardiac Society guidelines and the *British National Formulary* should be checked.

16.3 Disorders of the blood

16.3.1 Bleeding disorders

The blood is in a dynamic equilibrium between fluidity and coagulation, but the haemostatic mechanism is more complex than just alterations in this equilibrium. It involves local reactions of the blood vessels, platelet activities, and the interaction of specific coagulation factors that circulate in the blood. In early childhood many of the bleeding disorders have a genetic background, but with increasing age more become iatrogenic—usually due to anticoagulant medication. Patients who have had cardiac surgery for some congenital abnormality, those who have had a recent myocardial infarction, and those who have had cerebrovascular accidents may all be receiving long-term anticoagulant therapy. Table 16.2 gives a classification of bleeding disorders based on disorders of coagulation, bleeding problems due to decreased numbers of platelets, and disorders of bleeding where there are normal numbers of platelets. Many of these conditions are very rare and will not be considered further.

Haemophilia

Haemophilia A is an X-linked recessively inherited condition caused by a deficiency of factor VIII. The degree of severity is very varied but tends to be consistent within the same family. Children with over 25% of normal levels of circulating factor VIII can lead normal lives, those with between 1% and 5% are moderately to severely affected by minor trauma, etc., while those with under 1% have multiple bleeds into joints (haemarthroses) and may be severely physically handicapped as a result. Obviously, prevention of trauma to those who have this condition is extremely important, but the availability of factor VIII concentrates has revolutionized the quality of life of haemophiliacs. Unfortunately, in the past some of these blood replacement products have been contaminated with hepatitis, human immunodeficiency virus (HIV) and Creutzfeldt–Jakob disease (CJD), and therefore cross-infection control is a high priority. It was found that a number of patients who were thought to be haemophiliacs did not respond to

Table 16.2 Classification of bleeding disorders

1. Coagulation defects
(a) Inherited
(i) Haemophilia A: factor VIII deficiency
(ii) Haemophilia B: factor IX deficiency (Christmas disease)
(b) Acquired
(i) Liver disease
(ii) Vitamin deficiency
(iii) Anticoagulant drugs (heparin, warfarin)
(iv) Disseminated intravascular coagulation (DIC)
2. Thrombocytopenic purpuras
(a) Primary
(i) Idiopathic thrombocytopenic purpura (ITP)
(ii) Pancytopenia, Fanconi syndrome
(b) Secondary
(i) Systemic disease—leukaemia
(ii) Drug-induced
(iii) Physical agents—radiation
3. Non-thrombocytopenic purpuras
(a) Vascular wall alteration
(i) Scurvy
(ii) Infections
(iii) Allergy
(b) Disorders of platelet function
(i) Inherited: von Willebrand's disease
(ii) Drugs: aspirin, non-steroidal anti-inflammatories, alcohol, penicillin
(iii) Allergy
(iv) Autoimmune disease
(v) Uraemia

von Willebrand's disease

This is a dominantly inherited, complex, and variable condition characterized by a vascular abnormality of large irregular capillaries, defective platelets that do not adhere to each other, and decreased levels of factor VIII. Common clinical manifestations are nosebleeds and spontaneous gingival haemorrhage. von Willebrand's disease is the most common inherited bleeding disorder, affecting one in every 1000 individuals in the USA and the UK.

Thrombocytopenia

Thrombocytopenia is caused by a reduction in the number of circulating platelets in the bloodstream. Normal levels are $150–400 \times 10^9$/L. The platelet count should be at least 50×10^9/L before surgery is attempted and continuous infusion of platelets may be required. Clinical signs are petechial haemorrhages into the skin and mucous membranes, with haematemesis (blood in the vomit), haematuria (blood in the urine), and melaena (blood in the faeces).

The usual causes of thrombocytopenia in children are idiopathic, with an acute immune response usually following an upper respiratory tract infection, leukaemic infiltration of the bone marrow, or following the administration of various drugs. (See Key Points 16.4.)

Key Points 16.4

- Genetic coagulation disorders:
  - haemophilia A (factor VIII)—80%
  - haemophilia B (factor IX)—13%
  - factor XI—6%
- Bleeding disorders:
  - haemophilia A—1 in 20,000
  - von Willebrand's disease—1 in 1000

16.3.2 Dental management of bleeding disorders

A good history is the best screening device, but a bleeding tendency may only become manifest after a surgical procedure or trauma. Effective communication with the child's physician or haematologist is important, not only to establish the aetiology of any bleeding tendency but also to liaise over any necessary medical treatment that is required to replace reduced levels of clotting factors. The cornerstone of dental care is prevention and regular review so that if disease does occur it can be treated at an early stage. Local anaesthetic infiltrations or intra-ligamentous injections are unlikely to cause problems if given carefully. Regional anaesthesia, such as an inferior dental block, is contraindicated as bleeding in the pterygo-mandibular region may result in asphyxia. Pulp treatment of primary molar teeth may be required to avoid extractions. Most primary teeth exfoliate spontaneously with little haemorrhage, but occasionally, when they are very mobile, the soft tissues develop an inflammatory hyperplastic response and bleeding may be a problem. In these situations

replacement with factor VIII (anti-haemophiliac globulin) but were deficient in another factor—factor IX. This is known as Christmas disease or haemophilia B. This is also transmitted as an X-linked recessive trait with a wide range of clinical severity, but female carriers of this condition also have a tendency to bleed. (See Key Points 16.3.)

Key Points 16.3

Factor VIII level:

- >25%—mild
- 1–5%—moderate to severe
- <1%—severe.

extraction may be necessary with the appropriate haematological replacement therapy. However, if dental extractions or surgery do become necessary, patients are usually best managed in the hospital situation.

Haemophilia

Adequate replacement and careful monitoring of factor VIII and factor IX levels are required. This is usually done with fresh-frozen plasma or freeze-dried concentrate. Patients with mild to moderate haemophilia A can often be managed on an outpatient basis using replacement therapy or DDAVP® (1-desamino-8-D-arginine vasopressin, also known as desmopressin) which stimulates the release of factor VIII. Antifibrinolytic agents, such as EACA (epsilon-aminocaproic acid), and tranexamic acid are given to prevent lysis of the clot. They also significantly reduce the requirement for replacement of factor VIII. Medications containing non-steroidal anti-inflammatory drugs (NSAIDs) or aspirin should not be given (in any case, aspirin should not be given to a child under 12 years because of the risk of developing Reye's syndrome).

von Willebrand's disease

Factor VIII concentrates are not usually effective, but DDAVP® is used in combination with EACA or tranexamic acid. Patients with more severe types of von Willebrand's disease will require fresh-frozen plasma or a cryoprecipitate replacement.

Thrombocytopenia

The platelet count should be at least 50×10^9/L before surgery is attempted and continuous infusion of platelets may be required. In children with the idiopathic form of this condition, prednisolone (4mg/kg per day for 1 week, given orally) will increase the platelet count to over 50×10^9/L within 48 hours in about 90% of cases. The necessary treatment can then be carried out.

16.3.3 Blood dyscrasias

There are several relatively common disorders of the red and white blood cells that may influence dental care in the child. Many of these conditions also give rise to abnormal bleeding, but in addition may lead to delayed healing, infection, or mucosal ulceration. An outline classification is given in Table 16.3.

Red blood cell disorders: anaemia

When there is a reduction in the red blood cell volume or haemoglobin concentration, the oxygen-carrying capacity of the blood is lowered. Anaemia is not a specific disease but a symptom of an underlying disorder. Children with anaemia may be very pale (examine the nailbeds, conjunctiva, and oral mucous membranes). They may also be tired, listless, and breathless.

Iron-deficiency anaemia

This may result from chronic blood loss, possibly as a result of haemorrhagic disorders, but in children it is more commonly due to dietary deficiency or malabsorption. Vitamin B$_{12}$ and folic acid are also needed for the maturation of red blood cells in the bone marrow.

Table 16.3 Classification of blood dyscrasias

1. Red blood cell disorders
(a) Anaemia
(i) Iron deficiency
(ii) G6PD deficiency
(iii) Sickle cell
(iv) Thalassaemia
(b) Polycythaemia
2. White blood cell disorders
(a) Leucocytosis
(i) Infectious mononucleosis (glandular fever)
(ii) Neoplasia
(b) Leucopenia:
(i) Neutropenia: congenital and drug-induced
(c) Leukaemias
(i) Acute lymphocytic leukaemia (ALL)
(ii) Acute myeloid leukaemia (AML)
(iii) Chronic leukaemia
(d) Lymphomas
(i) Hodgkin's lymphoma
(ii) Non-Hodgkin's lymphoma
(iii) Burkitt's lymphoma

Glucose-6-phosphate dehydrogenase (G6PD) deficiency

This enzyme is needed in the hexose monophosphate shunt pathway. In deficiency, the accumulation of oxidants in the red blood cells causes their haemolysis and may result in jaundice, palpitations, dyspnoea, and dizziness. Drugs such as aspirin, phenacetin, and ascorbic acid, as well as infections, may precipitate haemolysis. As the gene for G6PD is located on the X-chromosome it is inherited as a sex-linked condition. There are many variants of the condition and it is common in certain ethnic groups; for example, type A is found in 11% of African Americans and G6PD MED is relatively common in ethnic groups of Mediterranean origin.

Sickle cell anaemia

This is an inherited autosomal recessive disorder that results in the substitution of a single amino acid in the haemoglobin chain. Sickle-cell **trait** is the heterozygous state in which the affected individual carries one gene for haemoglobin S. Approximately 10% of American Black children and up to 25% of Central African Black children carry the trait. Sickle cell **anaemia** is the homozygous state, with affected genes from both parents. The red blood cells containing haemoglobin S have a life of only 30–60 days and become clumped together under certain conditions, thus blocking small blood vessels and leading to pain and necrosis. Affected children may be pale, tired, weak, and breathless. They may complain of painful joints and swelling of the hands and feet. There tends to be a failure to thrive and growth retardation with an increased susceptibility to infection. Later problems include renal function impairment and retinal and conjunctival damage. A sickle cell crisis can be brought on by hypoxia (low oxygen) or even cold. Children who need dental treatment under general anaesthesia need to be admitted as in-patients.

Thalassaemia

This is another inherited disorder of haemoglobin synthesis and may occur as a heterozygous trait or homozygous thalassaemia major. It occurs particularly in Mediterranean countries and the Middle Eastern Arab countries. Like sickle cell anaemia, it results in a severe progressive haemolytic anaemia. Regular blood transfusions are necessary to maintain the haemoglobin level above 10g/dL. If treatment is inadequate, hypertrophy of erythropoietic tissue occurs and this results in massive expansion of the marrow of the facial and skull bones, producing maxillary hyperplasia and protrusion of the middle third of the face.

Dental management of anaemia

All anaemic children have a greater tendency to bleed after invasive dental procedures. Therefore any signs or symptoms suggestive of anaemia should be investigated. The haemoglobin level and haematocrit are simple tests used for screening, and a white blood cell and platelet count should also be obtained. If these reveal any abnormalities, further more complex tests may need to be undertaken. Ideally, the underlying defect should be corrected before embarking on a course of routine dental care.

A family history of conditions such as sickle cell anaemia and thalassaemia is significant, and all patients of African origin should be tested routinely for sickle cell disease prior to a general anaesthetic. Sickle cell crises are caused by inadequate oxygenation, and if possible general anaesthetics should be avoided in preference to the use of local anaesthesia. (See Key Point 16.5.)

> ### Key Point 16.5
>
> Sickle cell disease:
> - all patients of African origin should be screened prior to general anaesthesia.

White blood cell disorders: leukaemia

Leukaemia is a malignant proliferation of white blood cells. It is the most common form of childhood cancer, accounting for about one-third of new cancer cases diagnosed each year. Acute lymphocytic leukaemia (ALL) accounts for 75% of cases, with a peak incidence at 4 years of age. The general clinical features of all types of leukaemia are similar as all involve severe disruption of bone marrow functions. However, specific clinical and laboratory features differ, and there are considerable differences in response to therapy and long-term prognosis.

Acute leukaemia has a sudden onset, but the initial symptoms are usually non-specific with anorexia, irritability, and lethargy. Progressive failure of the bone marrow leads to pallor, bleeding, and fever, which are usually the symptoms that lead to diagnostic investigation. The bleeding tendency is often shown in the oral mucosa (Fig. 16.4) and there may also be infective lesions of the mouth and throat. Therefore the dental practitioner may be the first to diagnose the condition (Fig. 16.5). Bone

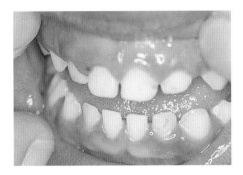

Figure 16.4 This 3-year-old child was brought to the dental surgery with spontaneous bleeding from his gums. He had recently had several nosebleeds and had become very lethargic. His skin and mucosa were very pale. Haematological investigation showed acute lymphocytic leukaemia.

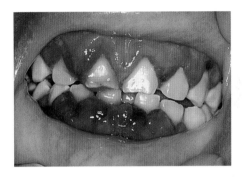

Figure 16.5 Oral appearance of a patient with acute myeloid leukaemia, with infiltration of the gingivae and spontaneous bleeding. This oral presentation and type of leukaemia is less common than the lymphocytic type shown in Fig. 16.4. (Courtesy of Dr Linda Shaw.)

pain and arthralgia are also important presenting complaints in about a quarter of children. On initial haematological examination most patients will have anaemia and thrombocytopenia. A significant proportion will have white blood cell counts of less than 3000/mm^3 and about 20% will have counts greater than 50 000/mm^3. The diagnosis of leukaemia can be suspected on seeing blast cells on the blood smear confirmed on bone marrow biopsy, which will show replacement by leukaemic lymphoblasts. The treatment varies with the clinical risk features; children under 2 years and over 10 years with an initial white blood cell count of over 100 000/mm^3 and central nervous system involvement (leukaemic cells in the cerebrospinal fluid) have the worst prognosis.

The basic components of treatment are as follows:

1. *Induction of remission* to remove abnormal cells from the blood and bone marrow. Drugs used: vincristine and prednisone.

2. *Prophylactic treatment to central nervous system.* Drugs used: intrathecal methotrexate plus irradiation of central nervous system.

3. *Consolidation.* Drugs used: cytosine arabinoside plus asparaginase.

4. *Maintenance*. Drugs used: methotrexate plus mercaptopurine for approximately 2 years.

5. *Relapse*. If relapse occurs, bone marrow transplantation can be considered.

Over 70% of affected children now survive on this regimen and can be regarded as cured. (See Key Points 16.6.)

Key Points 16.6

Childhood leukaemia:

- 75% is acute lymphocytic leukaemia;
- peak incidence at 4 years of age;
- dentists can help early diagnosis, alerted by mucosal haemorrhage and mouth and throat infections.

Dental management of leukaemia

In common with other medically compromising conditions, children with leukaemia are categorized as having a high risk of dental caries. Therefore prevention is essential. Unless there is a dental emergency no elective operative dental treatment should be carried out until the child is in remission. The drug regimen used to induce remission has numerous side-effects, including nausea and vomiting, reversible alopecia (hair loss), neuropathy, and, most importantly from a dental point of view, oral ulceration (mucositis). It can be extremely difficult to carry out normal mouth care for children at this stage and many have difficulty with toothbrushing because of acute nausea. Swabbing the mouth with chlorhexidine mouthwash and the routine use of antifungal agents are essential. Local anaesthesia preparations such as 5% lidocaine ointment, 20% flavoured benzocaine, or benzydamine hydrochloride (Difflam) applied before mealtimes can help to reduce the pain from ulceration or mucositis. The use of antibiotic paste or pastilles and ice chips can also be helpful. Gelclair®, a more recent product, is a prescription mouth gel that is designed and approved for the management and relief of pain caused by oral mucositis. It works by forming a barrier that protects the exposed mucosa. Once the leukaemia is in remission, and after consultation with the child's physician, routine dental care can be undertaken with the following adjustments:

1. If invasive procedures are planned, current haematological information is required to assess bleeding risks.

2. Prophylactic antibiotic therapy to prevent postoperative infection should be considered. This is given if the functional neutrophil count is depressed.

3. Children who are immunosuppressed are also at risk of fungal and viral infections. Fungal infections should be treated aggressively with amphotericin B, nystatin, or fluconazole, and herpetic infections with topical and/or systemic aciclovir.

4. Regional block anaesthesia may be contraindicated because of the risk of deep haemorrhage.

5. Oral preventive care is important. A typical protocol might be as follows:

- While in hospital (paediatric dentistry specialist):
  - relief of mucositis—Difflam mouthwash, topical anaesthesia, antibiotic pastilles, ice chips, Gelclair®;
  - elimination of bacterial plaque—chlorhexidine mouthwash 0.12%; povidone iodine topical application;
  - nystatin 500 000 units 'swish and swallow';
  - topical fluoride therapy;
  - manual plaque removal—toothbrushing instruction if platelet count $>20\times10^9$/L; 'foam on a stick' with chlorhexidine if platelet count $<20\times10^9$/L.

- At home (primary care provider):
  - oral surveillance;
  - topical fluoride therapy;
  - fissure sealants;
  - diet advice;
  - toothbrushing instruction;
  - prescription of antifungals if required.

(See Key Points 16.7.)

Key Points 16.7

- Oral side-effects of chemotherapy:
  - mucositis, oral ulceration;
  - infection (leucopenia);
  - haemorrhage (thrombocytopenia).
- Oral prophylaxis during chemotherapy:
  - oral hygiene;
  - pain relief for mucositis;
  - fluorides;
  - chlorhexidine;
  - antifungals.

16.4 Respiratory disorders

There are age-related disease patterns as far as the respiratory system is concerned; these patterns are also affected by sex, race, season of the year, geography, and environmental and socio-economic conditions. For example, the relatively short Eustachian tube in infants and young children allows easy access to ascending infections from the pharynx. Cystic fibrosis largely affects Caucasians, whereas lung infections and infarctions associated with sickle cell disease occur almost exclusively in children of African origin. Seasonal variation in the incidence of respiratory tract infections and asthma are quite marked, and certain infections have a well-defined geographical distribution. The frequency of bronchitis may not be very different between socio-economic groups, but the severity may reflect differences in nutritional status and perhaps the availability of medical care.

16.4.1 Asthma

Asthma is a diffuse obstructive lung disease which causes breathlessness, coughing, and wheezing. It is associated with hyper-reactivity of the airways to a variety of stimuli and a high degree of reversibility of the obstructive process. Asthma is a leading cause of chronic illness in childhood. Prevalence data are conflicting, but at least 10% of children will, at some time, have signs and symptoms compatible with a diagnosis of asthma. There is mounting recent evidence to suggest that the prevalence is increasing. Before puberty, approximately twice as many boys as girls suffer from asthma; thereafter, the sex incidence is similar. About half the children who are affected will be virtually free of symptoms by the time they become adults. The aetiology is poorly understood, but it is a complex disorder involving immunological, infectious, biochemical, genetic, and psychological factors. Acute episodes of coughing and wheezing are often precipitated by exposure to allergens and irritants, such as cold air or noxious fumes, and emotional stress. Drug therapy is now the mainstay of treatment both prophylactically and during acute exacerbations.

Dental management of asthma

Dental treatment itself can cause emotional stress, which may precipitate an attack. Routine dental care with local anaesthesia is not usually a problem; if in doubt, invite the child to take a puff of their inhaler before commencing. Steroid inhalers for asthma can cause adrenal suppression and insufficiency. Inhaling more than the following doses of steroids can cause adrenal suppression:

- beclomethasone 1000 micrograms daily
- fluticasone 500 micrograms daily
- budesonide 800 micrograms daily.

If in doubt contact the child's physician. (See Key Point 16.8.)

Key Point 16.8

- Inhaled steroids can cause adrenal insufficiency.

General anaesthesia for severe asthmatics usually requires inpatient hospital admission.

A study has been published linking dental erosion with asthma. This may be due to an increased likelihood of gastro-oesophageal reflux in people with asthma or acidic long-term medication, or the increased consumption of erosive beverages to combat 'drying' of the oral mucosa by inhalers. (See Key Points 16.9.)

Key Points 16.9

Relevant to the dental management of asthma:
- Erosion may be due to:
  - reflux
  - increased consumption of acidic beverages.
- General anaesthesia may require inpatient admission.
- Steroid inhalers may cause adrenal suppression.

16.4.2 Cystic fibrosis

Cystic fibrosis is an autosomal recessive multisystem disorder predominantly of the exocrine glands. Thick viscid mucus is produced, particularly in the lungs, which leads to chronic obstruction and infection of the airways and to malabsorption. It is the most common genetic condition in Caucasians, with approximately 5% of the population being carriers and one in 2000 of live births affected. The abnormal gene has been located on the long arm of chromosome 7.

The clinical manifestations of the condition are variable and some patients remain asymptomatic for long periods. Coughing is the most constant symptom of pulmonary involvement, and this may lead to recurrent respiratory infections and bronchiolitis. Sufferers often undergo regular physiotherapy to clear chest secretions. Lung disease progresses, leading to exercise intolerance and shortness of breath (Fig. 16.6). More than 85% of affected children show evidence of malabsorption due to exocrine pancreatic insufficiency. Symptoms include frequent bulky and greasy stools and a failure to thrive despite a large food intake.

Dental management of cystic fibrosis

There are reports of decreased caries prevalence attributable not only to the long-term use of antibiotics and pancreatic enzyme supplements but also to increased salivary buffering. Nevertheless, these children suffer from delayed dental development; more commonly they have enamel opacities and are more prone to calculus. Moreover, they need

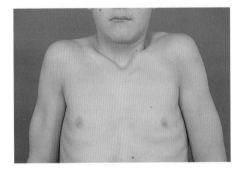

Figure 16.6 This boy has cystic fibrosis and shows a 'barrel chest' deformity due to respiratory infections. Coincidentally, he also has a deformity of the clavicles. (Courtesy of Dr Linda Shaw.)

to have a very high calorific intake and may have frequent refined carbohydrate snacks. As such, children with cystic fibrosis are still an important priority group for dental health education and care. General anaesthetics should be avoided in view of the pulmonary involvement. A significant proportion of affected children also have cirrhosis of the liver, with resultant clotting defects and a liability to haemorrhage following surgical procedures. Because of the development of multiple antibiotic sensitivities, children with cystic fibrosis may sometimes be prescribed tetracycline to prevent chest infections even though it causes intrinsic dental staining (Fig. 16.7).

Improvements in the management of people with cystic fibrosis have meant that an increasing number are not maintained on long-term antibiotic prophylaxis.

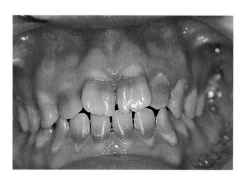

Figure 16.7 Tetracycline was administered over a prolonged period to this patient who has cystic fibrosis. This has resulted in its incorporation into the mineral matrix with marked discolouration.

16.5 Convulsive disorders

16.5.1 Febrile convulsions

Convulsions are common; about 5% of children have had one or more convulsions and accurate diagnosis of the aetiology is very important. The vast majority of these are febrile convulsions associated with illnesses that cause high fever late in infancy such as otitis media. The seizures are usually tonic–clonic with loss of consciousness followed by sustained muscle contractions. Respiration may be impaired, which may lead to cyanosis. The teeth are often firmly clenched with possible tongue- and lip-biting. There may also be a loss of bladder and bowel control. This tonic phase is followed by the clonic phase of intermittent muscular contraction. The duration is always less than 15 minutes. These convulsions usually occur early in the illness during the period of rapid temperature rise, and may be the first indication that the child is ill. It is most important to eliminate the possibility of central nervous system infection; therefore examination of the cerebrospinal fluid is essential if there is persistent drowsiness following the attack.

16.5.2 Epilepsy

It may be difficult to differentiate these simple febrile convulsions from epilepsy, but it is essential that this diagnosis is made as the therapy, prognosis, and implications differ enormously. Table 16.4 gives a list of conditions that are commonly associated with recurrent seizures. Epilepsy is not a disease in itself, but a term applied to recurrent seizures either of unknown origin (idiopathic epilepsy) or due to congenital or acquired brain lesions (secondary epilepsy). It affects about 0.5–2% of the population. Medical management usually consists of long-term anticonvulsant drug therapy. The choice of drug depends on the seizure type, but the dosage needs to control the seizures with minimal side-effects. New generation anti-epileptic drugs have become available (e.g. lamotrigine, gabapentin, oxcarbazepine, tiagabine, and topiramate) but even these are not without problems such as hyperexcitability, dizziness, depression, weight loss, and abdominal problems. The most familiar anti-epileptic drugs are sodium valproate, phenytoin, and carbamazepine.

Dental management of epilepsy

If possible, any liquid anti-epileptic medication should be sugar free (Fig. 16.8). Sodium valproate is not associated with gingival enlargement and, like carbamazepine, lamotrigine, and oxcarbazepine, is available as a sugar-free liquid. Phenytoin results in gingival enlargement in about half of patients. The child with good control of seizures needs a minimum of restrictions, although the possibility of an attack

Table 16.4 Conditions commonly associated with seizures

Febrile convulsions
Idiopathic epilepsy: often genetic predisposition
Secondary epilepsy
Cerebral neoplasms
Cerebral vascular disorders, e.g. subdural haemorrhage, especially seen in child abuse
Cerebral malformation, e.g. Down syndrome, hydrocephalus
Neurocutaneous syndromes, e.g. tuberous sclerosis, neurofibromatosis, Sturge–Weber disease
Nutritional disorders, e.g. pyridoxine deficiency, lead encephalopathy, drug intoxication
Metabolic disorders, e.g. hypoglycaemia, renal failure, phenylketonuria
Atrophic cerebral lesions, e.g. post-anoxic, post-traumatic, and post-infectious
Degenerative cerebral disease, e.g. Batten's disease
Central nervous system infection, e.g. meningitis, encephalitis, brain abscess

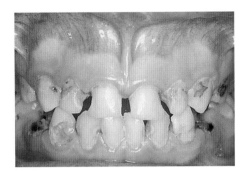

Figure 16.8 This 3-year-old child with epilepsy has rampant caries of the primary dentition, with a somewhat unusual distribution of approximal lesions in both the upper and lower incisors as well as in the molars. The child had been on long-term sucrose-based medication, but has now changed to sugar-free sodium valproate liquid. (Courtesy of Dr Linda Shaw.)

occurring in the dental chair should be considered. A very high standard of oral hygiene is required to minimize the development of gingival enlargement, and gingival surgery should never be contemplated unless the oral hygiene is good. Trauma to anterior teeth is often encountered in people with epilepsy, who may have frequent unpredictable falls. Reimplantation of avulsed teeth is usually contraindicated in those with severe learning difficulties. If prostheses are required, they should be well retained with clasps and unlikely to break or be inhaled during subsequent attacks. (See Key Points 16.10.)

Key Points 16.10

Epilepsy:

- affects 0.5–1% of the population.
- results in gingival enlargement with phenytoin.
- check that any liquid medication is sugar free.

16.6 Metabolic and endocrine disorders

16.6.1 Diabetes mellitus

Incidence of diabetes is on the rise worldwide, and consequently so is diabetes amongst children. Approximately 90% of young people with diabetes suffer from type 1, and the number of child patients varies from place to place. As metabolic syndrome, obesity, bad diet, and a sedentary lifestyle without exercise has spread, so too has the incidence of type 2 diabetes in children.

Diabetes is the most common endocrine/metabolic disorder of childhood and is due to a deficiency of insulin and abnormal metabolism of carbohydrate, protein, and fat. Type I diabetes mellitus is insulin-dependent (IDDM) and usually of juvenile onset. It is age-related with peaks of presentation between 5 and 7 years and at puberty. The prevalence of diabetes in school-age children is approximately 2 per 1000. Although there is a genetic predisposition, there may well be a triggering effect from viral infections in the aetiology of diabetes. The clinical manifestations are polydipsia (increased thirst), polyuria (increased urination), polyphagia (increased appetite), and weight loss. There may be an insidious onset of lethargy, weakness, and weight loss. The diagnosis depends on the demonstration of hyperglycaemia in association with glucosuria. The aims of treatment are to control the symptoms, prevent acute metabolic crises of hypo- and hyperglycaemia, and maintain normal growth and body weight with an active lifestyle. If there is good control of blood sugar levels with insulin therapy and nutritional management, diabetic complications are minimized. One of the major hazards of insulin treatment is the development of hypoglycaemia. It is usually of rapid onset (unlike hyperglycaemia), with sweating, palpitations, apprehension, and trembling. This progresses to mental confusion, drowsiness, and coma. Hypoglycaemia in a diabetic child indicates too much insulin relative to food intake and energy expenditure. For an acute episode a carbohydrate-containing snack or drink should be given. Another problem, particularly in adolescents, is psychological adjustment to the condition; the

rebellious teenage years may lead to non-compliance with insulin therapy and nutritional management. Many of these problems can be averted by suitable education and counselling.

Dental management of diabetes

The well-controlled diabetic child with no serious complications can have any dental treatment but should receive preventive care as a priority. Uncontrolled diabetes can result in varied problems, which mainly relate to fluid imbalance, an altered response to infection, possible increased glucose concentrations in saliva, and microvascular changes. There may be decreased salivary flow, and an increased incidence of dental caries has been reported in uncontrolled young diabetics. There is also well-documented evidence of increased periodontal problems and susceptibility to infections, particularly with *Candida* species. Dental appointments should be arranged at times when the blood sugar levels are well controlled; usually a good time is in the morning immediately following the child's insulin injection and a normal breakfast. General anaesthetics are a problem because of the pre-anaesthetic fasting that is required, and so these are normally carried out on an inpatient basis to enable the insulin and carbohydrate balance to be stabilized intravenously.

16.6.2 Adrenal insufficiency

A number of syndromes are associated with adrenal insufficiency, such as Addison's disease and Cushing's syndrome. However, problems in the dental management of patients with steroid insufficiency are more likely to occur in children who are being prescribed steroid therapy for other medical conditions, for example in the suppression of inflammatory and allergic disorders, acute leukaemia, and to prevent acute transplant rejection. The risks of taking corticosteroids are greater in children than in adults, and they should only be used when specifically indicated, in minimal dosage, and for the shortest possible time. If a child has adrenal insufficiency and/or is receiving steroid therapy, any infection or stress may precipitate an adrenal crisis. Usually, no additional steroid supplementation is necessary for routine restorative treatment. However, if extractions under local anaesthesia or more extensive procedures are planned and/or the patient is particularly apprehensive, the oral steroid dosage should be increased. General anaesthesia should not be carried out on an outpatient basis. Consultation with the child's physician is necessary before prescribing steroids, and anaesthetists must be aware of such medication in order to avoid a precipitous fall in blood pressure during anaesthesia or in the immediate postoperative period.

16.6.3 Other disorders

Many other metabolic and endocrine disorders occur in children but these are rare events.

Thyroid disease

Thyroid disease may present in early adolescence, although it is generally more common in adults. Dental management should present no problems if the thyrotoxic patient is medically well controlled. However, liaison with the physicians is important.

16.7 Neoplastic disorders

There are approximately 1200 new cases of childhood cancer each year in the UK. Child cancer patients largely reflect the child population in general and, as such, represent a cross-section of the population. Cancer causes more childhood deaths between the ages of 1 and 15 years than any other disease, but is still considerably behind trauma as the most common reason for mortality. The incidence of malignant tumours in children under 15 years of age in developed countries is estimated to be in the region of one in 10 000 children per year, but the mortality rate is high at 30–40%. Although leukaemia is the most common form of childhood cancer, tumours of the central nervous system and neural crest cells and lymphomas also form a significant proportion (Table 16.5). Prognosis varies with the type of tumour, the stage at which it was diagnosed, and the adequacy of treatment. Major advances have been made in the treatment of childhood malignancy in the last few decades, largely as a result of advances in chemotherapy and bone marrow transplantation.

Table 16.5 The major types of childhood cancer

Leukaemia	48%
Central nervous system	16%
Lymphoma	8%
Neuroblastoma	7%
Nephroblastoma	5%
Others	16%

Renal disorders

Nephrotic syndrome is a condition where protein leaks from the blood into urine via the glomeruli of the kidney, resulting in hypoproteinaemia and generalized oedema. Left untreated, sufferers would die of infections, but fortunately the majority respond to treatment using corticosteroids, usually prednisolone.

The kidney undergoes a complex developmental and migratory process leading to a high frequency of congenital anomalies, such as polycystic disease and unilocular cysts. Acute pyelonephritis is more common when a congenital abnormality is present and so, even though it is simply treated with antibiotics, children often undergo further medical investigations to rule out congenital abnormality. Therefore children with renal problems are likely to be, or have been, under specialist medical care. From a dental viewpoint, children with reduced renal function, or more importantly progressive renal failure, need extra consideration when prescribing drugs. Such children may fail to excrete a drug or its metabolites, be more sensitive to the drug's effect, or be less tolerant of side-effects, and some drugs may even be less effective. Examples of drugs where caution should be exercised by the dentist are midazolam and other benzodiazepines, chloral hydrate, NSAIDs, fluconazole, and co-trimoxazole. The *British National Formulary* should always be consulted.

16.7.1 Dental management of children with cancer

The children may have untreated caries, since many are under 5 years of age and may not have had a previous dental examination. The oral side-effects of cancer treatment (Table 16.6) can be categorized into immediate and long term. The immediate problems include mucositis (oral ulceration) and exacerbations of common oral diseases that may become life-threatening and are usually managed by paediatric dentistry specialists in liaison with their medical colleagues. Child cancer survivors present later with long-term problems relating to growth, puberty and reproduction, cardiac and thyroid function, and cognitive deficit. Oral and dental development can also be impeded, and specialist advice might again be required. Despite this, the introduction of a shared-care arrangement between the primary dental practitioner and the paediatric specialist when the child is in remission is vital to ensure continued preventive therapy and good oral health, while at the same time 'normalizing' care. (See Key Points 16.11.)

> **Key Points 16.11**
>
> - Children with cancer need the combined care of primary and specialist dental services.
> - There are immediate and long-term effects of cancer treatment.
> - Disease prevention is vital.

16.8 Organ transplantation

Kidney, heart, bone marrow, liver, and pancreas transplantations are now routine procedures. Most liver transplants in children occur because of biliary atresia. Bone marrow transplants are the treatment of choice for children with aplastic anaemia, those who fail conventional therapy for leukaemia, and for some immune deficiency disorders. Although children with end-stage renal disease can be kept alive by haemodialysis, their quality of life is considerably improved by kidney transplantation. Children who require organ transplantation are considered to be at a high caries risk and so prevention is important.

16.8.1 Pre-transplant treatment planning

Any candidate for organ transplantation should be referred for specialist dental evaluation. Whenever possible, active dental disease should be treated before the transplant procedure and any teeth with

Table 16.6 Summary of oral problems associated with cancer therapy

Mucositis
Acute inflammation of the mucosa
White/yellow fibrous slough, often with ulceration
Painful to eat/speak/swallow
Portal for microbial entry
Blood changes
Spontaneous gingival/mucosal bleeding
Crusting of lips
Immunosuppression
Non-vital primary teeth can become a medical emergency
Acute herpetic gingivostomatitis and candidal infection can rapidly progress to systemic involvement in children
Changes in saliva
Saliva becomes thick, viscous, and acidic
Acute ascending sialadenitis can occur as a complication
Loss/alteration of taste (may be difficult to persuade the child to eat, so enticed by sugary snacks)
Dysphagia (difficulty in swallowing)
Changes in oral flora
Increase in cariogenic organisms
Increased susceptibility to candidal infection
Rapid progression of periodontal disease
Dental pain and trismus
Leukaemic infiltration of dental pulp tissue or direct infiltration of jaws
Jaw pain and trismus as a direct complication of drug therapy or fibrosis following radiotherapy

doubtful prognoses extracted. This may present difficulties as many pre-transplant patients can be seriously ill and have various associated medical problems. Moreover, some children will be placed on a high-carbohydrate (cariogenic) diet (e.g. Maxijul®) to 'build them up' in preparation for surgery, and so the dental team will need to adopt a pragmatic approach to advice relating to sugar intake and frequency during this period as the child's medical well-being must take priority. Children undergoing bone marrow transplantation are prone to infection, bleeding, and delayed healing because of leucopenia and thrombocytopenia. However, the majority of children awaiting liver transplantation because of biliary atresia are very young and have not experienced dental caries, although their teeth may have intrinsic green staining due to biliverdin deposition in the developing dental tissues. This is a time when intensive oral hygiene instruction and preventive advice and therapy are of paramount importance in helping to minimize later potential oral problems. Before any invasive dental procedures are undertaken, consultation with the child's physician is vital in order to establish the extent of the organ dysfunction and its repercussions. Prophylactic antibiotics will probably be required in patients with cardiac problems and depressed white blood cell counts. Any significant alterations in bleeding times and/or coagulation status must be checked. Certain drugs should also be avoided in patients with end-stage liver or kidney disease.

16.8.2 Immediate post-transplant period

Drugs prescribed to prevent graft rejection have several side-effects. Azathioprine results in leucopenia, thrombocytopenia, and anaemia; hence, children in this immediate post-transplant phase may be even more prone to infections and haemorrhage than before. Ciclosporin (Neoral) and tacrolimus are largely replacing azathioprine, but these may cause severe kidney and liver changes leading to hypertension and bleeding problems. Ciclosporin is also associated with gingival enlargement. Steroids are prescribed at this time with the risk of adrenal suppression. Full supportive dental care is required and children complain of nausea and may develop severe oral ulceration. Routine oral hygiene procedures can become difficult, but the use of chlorhexidine as a mouthwash or spray, or on a disposable sponge, together with local anaesthetic preparations is helpful.

16.8.3 Stable post-transplant period

Once healing has occurred and any acute graft rejection has been brought under control, routine dental treatment can be undertaken. Reinforcement of all preventive advice and liaison with the child's dietitian may be helpful as many patients are still on high-carbohydrate supplementation. Steroid therapy is discontinued in children with liver transplants after 3 months, but may be continued for longer periods than this in those with other organ transplants. Antifungal prophylaxis is usually given in the first few months after transplantation to prevent oral candidal infections. Dental problems, apart from oral ulceration and those associated with immunosuppression and bleeding tendencies, include delayed eruption and exfoliation of primary teeth and ectopic eruption of permanent teeth. These are related to the gingival overgrowth associated with ciclosporin and nifedipine medication (Fig. 16.9). (See Key Points 16.12.)

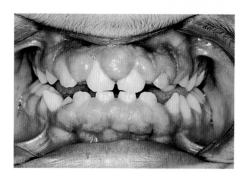

Figure 16.9 These grossly hyperplastic gingivae are associated with ciclosporin and nifedipine medication in an 11-year-old boy who has had a kidney transplant. This combination of drugs is required to prevent rejection and to control his blood pressure.

Key Points 16.12

Transplant immunosuppression:

- leucopenia
- thrombocytopenia
- gingival enlargement.

16.9 Medical emergencies

Medical emergencies can happen at any time in dental practice, and a paediatric practice is no different. Two trained people should always be available to deal with medical emergencies when dental treatment is planned to take place. Every member of staff should be trained and aware of their role if a young patient or their parents or older carers collapse.

Staff training should include the preparation and use of emergency drugs, where appropriate, and resuscitation routines in a simulated emergency. This training should occur at least annually. In the UK, the General Dental Council expects dentists and dental care professionals to complete 10 hours continuing professional development in medical emergencies in each 5-year cycle. Detailed information on medical emergencies and resuscitation has been produced by the UK Resuscitation Council (2011).

There is no statutory list of emergency drugs or equipment required for dental practices. Each practice must consider what treatments they provide, and the patients who attend, and decide accordingly. However, the Resuscitation Council recommends that drugs should be available to manage the more common medical emergencies encountered and these are shown in Table 16.7 and Fig. 16.10.

Oxygen cylinders should be easily portable but large enough for adequate flow rates (e.g. 10L/min) until the arrival of an ambulance or the patient (or carer) fully recovers. A full D-size cylinder contains 340L of oxygen and should allow a flow rate of 10L/min for up to 30 minutes.

Table 16.7 Recommended minimal emergency drugs

Emergency	Drugs required	Adult dose	Paediatric dose
Anaphylaxis	Epinephrine (adrenaline) 1:1000, 1mg/mL	0.5mL (500 micrograms) IM	<6 years 0.15mL (150 micrograms) 6–12 years 0.3mL (300 micrograms)
Hypoglycaemia	Oral glucose solution/tablets/gel/powder Glucagon injection (1mg)	1mg IM	0.5mg IM if <8 years or <25kg
Asthma	Salbutamol	100 micrograms	100 micrograms
Status epilepticus	Midazolam (buccal or intranasal)	10mg	1–5 years 5mg 5–10 years 7.5mg
Angina	Glyceryl trinitrate sublingual tablet/spray	0.3–1.0mg	
Myocardial infarct	Aspirin dispersable 300mg	300mg	
Steroid (adrenal) crisis	Corticosteroid injection (hydrocortisone sodium succinate/phosphate)	100–200mg	
All the above	Oxygen	As required	As required

IM, intramuscular.

Two such cylinders may be needed to ensure that the supply of oxygen does not fail when it is used in a medical emergency.

In addition to medical oxygen, practices should have the recommended minimum equipment (Table 16.8). If defibrillators are included as emergency treatment, it is essential that all staff are fully trained in their use and the equipment is properly maintained (Fig. 16.13). (See Key Points 16.13.)

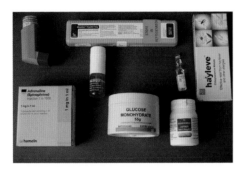

Figure 16.10 Selection of minimal emergency drugs. (Courtesy of Dr Alex Keightley.)

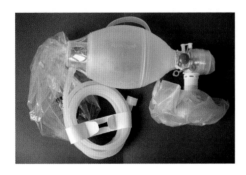

Figure 16.11 Pocket mask with oxygen port. (Courtesy of Dr Alex Keightley.)

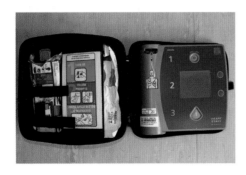

Figure 16.12 Self-inflating bag-and-mask apparatus. (Courtesy of Dr Alex Keightley.)

Key Points 16.13

- Training of staff should include the preparation and use of emergency drugs where appropriate, and resuscitation routines in a simulated emergency.
- Training should occur annually.
- Every member of staff should be trained and aware of their role if a young patient or their parents or older carers collapse.
- Medical emergencies can occur at any time.

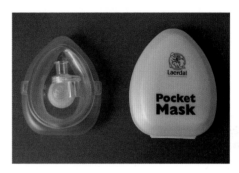

Figure 16.13 Defibrillator. (Courtesy of Dr Triona Fahey.)

Table 16.8 Recommended minimum emergency equipment

Oxygen mask with tubing
Basic set of oropharyngeal airways (sizes 1, 2, 3, and 4)
Pocket mask with oxygen port (Fig. 16.11).
Self-inflating bag-and-mask apparatus with oxygen reservoir and tubing (1L bag) (Fig. 16.12)
Variety of well-fitting adult and child facemasks for attaching to self-inflating bag
Portable suction with appropriate suction catheters and tubing (e.g. Yankauer sucker)
Single-use syringes and needles
Spacer device for inhaled bronchodilators
Automated blood glucose measurement device
Automated external defibrillator (Fig. 16.13)

16.10 Summary

In all children who are medically compromised the dental team can play a vital part not only in the overall medical management but also in helping these children and their parents adjust to normal life following recovery. Oral care is extremely important in enhancing the quality of life by reducing the morbidity and mortality of oral conditions, and by allowing the child to eat without pain and so gain optimal nutrient intake. Preventive care should be the cornerstone of any oral care programme. Since many children travel long distances to regional and supra-regional units, shared care between the hospital paediatric dentistry specialist and the primary care provider can facilitate the child's reintegration into their local community and avoid lost schooling.

1 An increasing number of children with complex medical problems now survive owing to improvements in medical care, and present difficulties in oral management.

2 An accurate detailed medical history must be obtained for all children before any dental treatment is undertaken.

3 An aggressive preventive regimen is required for all children with significant medical problems. This must encompass dietary counselling, suitable fluoride therapy, fissure sealant applications, and oral hygiene instruction.

4 Congenital heart disease is more common than acquired conditions in children. The more severe malformations may require prophylactic antibiotics prior to carrying out any invasive dental procedures. Liaison with cardiology colleagues is essential.

5 Children with bleeding disorders, such as haemophilia, thrombocytopenic purpura, and von Willebrand's disease, must be haematologically investigated prior to dental treatment. Haematological replacement therapy may be required before operative treatment.

6 Children with anaemia, whether due to iron deficiency or inherited conditions such as sickle cell anaemia or thalassaemia, represent general anaesthetic risks in particular.

7 Leukaemia is the most common form of childhood cancer and the first disseminated cancer to respond completely to chemotherapy in a significant number of children. The dental management of affected children needs to consider their haematological status as well as their immunocompromised condition.

8 Asthma is a leading cause of chronic illness in childhood. Severe asthmatics may be on systemic steroid therapy, which has implications for dental care.

9 Convulsions are common in children, occurring in approximately 5%, but many of these are associated with episodes of high fever in the child and not with epilepsy.

10 Diabetes mellitus is the most common endocrine/metabolic disorder of childhood. If there is good control of blood sugar levels with insulin therapy and nutritional management, diabetic complications are minimized and dental care should be routine.

11 Organ transplantation in children is being increasingly undertaken, and there are many side-effects of drug control of immunosuppression that affect treatment planning and oral care.

12 The participation of the dental team in the overall management of children with medical problems can significantly help to enhance their quality of life. Preventive care should be the cornerstone of dental management.

16.11 Further reading

Behrman, R.E. and Vaughan, V.C. (2003). *Nelson textbook of pediatrics* (17th edn). W.B. Saunders, Philadelphia, PA. (*One of the standard paediatric texts containing a huge amount of information about all types of medical problems in children.*)

Gorlin, R.J., Cohen, M.M., and Levin, L.S. (2001). *Syndromes of the head and neck* (4th edn). Oxford University Press, Oxford. (*The authoritative publication on this subject with erudite lists of references.*)

Little, J.W. and Falace, D.A. (2002). *Dental management of the medically compromised patient* (6th edn). Mosby Year Book, St Louis, MO.

(*Comprehensive information but with very helpful summaries on potential problems related to dental care.*)

Scully, C. and Cawson, R.A. (2005). *Medical problems in dentistry* (5th edn). Churchill Livingstone, Edinburgh. (*The most comprehensive dental textbook of medical problems and how medical issues impact on the delivery of dental treatment. It also has an excellent appendix on how to deal with medical emergencies.*)

16.12 References

NICE (2008). *Prophylaxis against infective endocarditis*. Available online at:

http://www.nice.org.uk/nicemedia/live/11938/40014/40014. pdf

UK Resuscitation Council (2011). *Medical emergencies and resuscitation— standards for clinical practice and training for general dental practitioners and dental care professionals in general dental practice* (revised and updated). Available online at:

http://www.resus.org.uk/pages/MEdental.htm

17

Childhood impairment and disability

J.H. Nunn

Chapter contents

17.1 Introduction

An impairment becomes a disability for a child only if he/she is unable to carry out the normal activities of his/her peer group. For example, a child who has broken an arm is temporarily 'disabled' by not being able to eat and write in the normal way. However, impairment is a permanent feature in the lives of some children, although it may become a disability only if they are unable to take part in everyday activities, such as communicating with others, climbing stairs, and toothbrushing.

A more contemporary view is one that moves away from the medicalization of impairment to a consideration of ability and functioning, enshrined in the World Health Organization's International Classification of Functioning, Disability, and Impairment. In this definition, a number of domains are classified from body, individual, and societal perspectives. This approach is less stigmatizing, and more enabling of children with impairments.

There are a number of reasons why children with impairments merit special consideration for dental care.

1. The oral health of some children with disabilities is different from that of their healthy peers—for example, the greater prevalence of periodontal disease in people with Down syndrome and of tooth-wear in those with cerebral palsy.

2. The prevention of dental disease in disabled children needs to be a higher priority than for so-called normal peers because dental disease, its sequelae, or its treatment may be life-threatening—for example, the risk of infective endocarditis from oral organisms in children with significant congenital heart defects (Fig. 17.1).

3. Treatment planning and the provision of dental care may need to be modified in view of the patient's capabilities, likely future cooperation, and home care—for example, the feasibility of providing a resin-bonded bridge for a teenager with cerebral palsy, poorly controlled epilepsy, and inadequate home oral care.

In the light of these considerations, do such children need special dental care? Most of the studies which have been undertaken on disabled children have indicated that the majority can in fact be treated in a dental surgery in the normal way, together with the rest of their family. However, recognizing that the complex needs of some people with special health care requirements may need targeted services, the public dental service in the UK uses a tool that identifies the particular aspects of an individual's needs which make access to specialist care a priority and, importantly, identifies that additional resources will be required to meet the needs and demands of such patients (British Dental Association 2010). (See Key Points 17.1.)

Figure 17.1 A 13-year-old boy with Down syndrome and gross caries, who was prevented from going on a combined heart and lung transplant register, as well as a renal transplant register, because of his dental disease.

Key Points 17.1

The need for special dental care arises because:

- there are differences in oral/dental presentation;
- there are differences in oral and dental disease prevalence;
- dental disease and/or its treatment may be life-threatening;
- modifications to treatment plans are required;
- there is a need for special facilities;
- treatment may be time-consuming.

Normality is desirable, provided that the disabled person actually receives good dental care. The evidence from many studies is that,

although the overall caries experience is similar between disabled children and their so-called normal contemporaries, the type of treatment they have experienced is different. Disabled children have similar levels of untreated decay, but more missing teeth and fewer restored teeth. A minority of children with complex disabilities need special facilities, usually only available in dental or general hospitals, or from specialized community dental clinics. What *is* needed by all patients with disabilities is a very aggressive approach to the prevention of dental disease. Because of the potential for dental disease, or its treatment, to disable an impaired child, priority must be given to preventive dental care for such individuals from a very young age.

Children with a significant degree of impairment are termed 'children with special educational needs' or 'children with learning difficulties'. These terms, used synonymously, encompass a wide variety of impairments, but three main areas—intellectual, physical, and sensory impairments—predominate and will now be considered in more detail. However, it is important to stress that impairment does not always present as a discrete entity; in any population of affected children, at least a quarter of the group will be multiply impaired, making it difficult to assign a 'label' to that child's overall impairment. Medical compromise, considered in more detail in Chapter 16, may also be imposed on these impairments. The ways in which some of these conditions present to a dentist are given below, together with the dental management issues relevant to each. Many of the issues raised are, of course, common to a number of impairments.

17.2 Intellectual impairment

The causes of intellectual impairment are numerous, and for many children a cause for their disability may never be identified. Approximately 25 per 1000 of the child population are affected and, as with other impairments, the majority will be males. Children with intellectual impairment can be divided broadly into those who are mentally

retarded and those who have a learning difficulty. These are broad groups, often without a well-defined aetiology or consistent presenting features, but there are two distinct subgroups where the cause is known and the features are well described, namely Down syndrome and fragile X syndrome. Intellectual impairment may be present in some children with cerebral palsy and those who have suffered birth anoxia and severe infections (e.g. meningitis and rubella). Intellectual impairment is also a feature of autism, microcephaly, and metabolic disorders (e.g. phenylketonuria), and may also be acquired after significant trauma. Not every condition will have specific dental features like Down syndrome, but an understanding of the underlying impairment will help the dentist plan treatment more effectively.

Mental retardation, pervasive developmental disorders (autism and schizophrenia), learning disabilities, dyslexia, attention-deficit disorders, and hyperactivity are all controversial categories whose definition and processes of assessment are not universally agreed. (See Key Points 17.2.)

Key Points 17.2

Classification of children with impairments:
- intellectually impaired—mentally retarded, learning difficulties;
- physically impaired—developmental, degenerative;
- sensorially impaired;
- medically compromised;
- combination of impairments.

Mental retardation

This is sometimes called mental handicap, mental subnormality, or mental deficiency. It is a general category characterized by low intelligence, failure of adaptation, and early age of onset. Low general intelligence is the main characteristic. Affected children are slow in their general mental development, and they may have difficulties in attention, perception, memory, and thinking. They may be stronger in some skills than others (e.g. music and computing), but generally they are of low intellectual attainment. Children with low intelligence are not called mentally retarded unless they also have some problem in adaptation, i.e. they are unlikely to be able to live independently and will always depend on others as a source of income and support for daily living. According to IQ levels, five levels are traditionally described. The simplicity of the classification is somewhat illusory with great individual differences among people with mental retardation. (See Key Points 17.3.)

Key Points 17.3

Intellectual impairment may be associated with:
- cerebral palsy
- birth anoxia
- severe infections
- autism
- microcephaly
- metabolic disorders
- major trauma
- some syndromes.

Down syndrome

Down syndrome is a chromosomal disorder, trisomy 21, with distinct clinical features. The prevalence is approximately 1 in 600 births, but there is variation with maternal age, so that at 40 years of age the incidence is about 1 in 40 births. However, the numbers seen in any one country will vary depending on the prevailing attitude towards prenatal screening and termination. The general physical features associated with Down syndrome are a greater predisposition to cardiac defects, myeloid leukaemia, and infective hepatitis (especially in institutionalized males), although most children will have been vaccinated against viral forms. Coeliac disease and thyroid disorders are also clinical features of this condition. Increasingly, a form of early dementia, entitled disintegrative disorder, is being recognized in adolescents with Down syndrome. The features seen are a progressive loss of skills, both cognitive and physical, and this has obvious relevance in dentistry because of the impact on personal oral care.

Varying degrees of intellectual impairment occur, and upper respiratory tract infections and an inability to withstand infections generally are common. Physically, predominant features are a small rounded face with an underdeveloped mid-face (Fig. 17.2), especially of the nasal bridge, an upward slant of the eyes with prominent epicanthic folds, squints, cataracts, and Brushfield spots on the iris. The hands of children with Down syndrome are stubby, with a pronounced transverse palmar crease. Intra-orally the tongue is large, protruding, and sometimes heavily fissured (Fig. 17.3). The palate may be high-vaulted and narrow. There is usually a delay in the exfoliation of primary teeth and the eruption of permanent teeth, while some teeth may be congenitally missing. Teeth that erupt are often microdont and/or hypoplastic (Fig. 17.4). There is a high prevalence of periodontal disease in the anterior alveolar segments, especially in the mandible. This is probably due to impaired phagocyte function in neutrophils and monocytes combined with poor oral hygiene. Other factors implicated in the pathophysiology of the extensive inflammation seen in Down syndrome patients are enhanced prostaglandin $E_2(PGE_2)$ production and increased activity of plasminogen activators, and thus collagenase activity. (See Key Points 17.4.)

Key Points 17.4

Oral and dental features in Down syndrome:
- mid-face hypoplasia
- large fissured tongue
- narrow high-vaulted palate
- delay in exfoliation/eruption
- congenitally absent teeth
- microdont/hypoplastic teeth.

Fragile X syndrome

Next to Down syndrome, this is the most common cause of intellectual impairment. This disorder is largely under-diagnosed; and people who have been classified as having 'mental handicap of unknown origin', especially if they are male, probably have fragile X syndrome. The

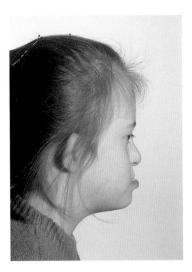

Figure 17.2 Lateral view of a Down syndrome child, showing mid-face hypoplasia.

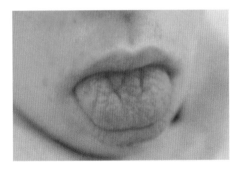

Figure 17.3 The protruberant fissured tongue of an adolescent with Down syndrome.

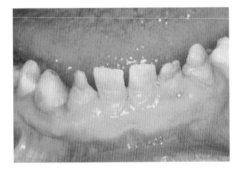

Figure 17.4 A Down syndrome patient with marked dental hypoplasia, conical teeth, and hypodontia.

condition is of particular significance because a high proportion of affected individuals have congenital heart defects, usually mitral valve prolapse, which may require antibiotic prophylaxis. Although males are predominantly affected, milder versions of the disability may be seen in females.

Pervasive developmental disorders

This group encompasses autism and childhood schizophrenia. The former is characterized by its early onset, usually before 30 months of age, whereas childhood schizophrenia presents later. They are conditions that represent profound adaptive problems in thinking, language, and social relationships. Autism in particular has the distinctive feature of restricted and stereotypical behaviour patterns. Most children score below normal on IQ testing and thus experience significant developmental delay. The more severely delayed children seem oblivious to their parents or carers, express themselves minimally, show a low level of interest in exploring objects, avoid sounds, and engage in ritualistic behaviour. Children with Asperger's syndrome display some of the features of autism but may also possess a level of skill in some areas that is well above the average for their peers. These features need to be taken into consideration when attempting dental care, and underline the particular importance of acclimatization and familiarity of routine (rituals) as part of that process.

The causes of autism are unknown but are thought to be prenatal and not social in origin. Much interest was generated in a possible link with MMR vaccine as a possible aetiological factor, but this evidence has since been discredited. A major malformation in the cerebellum has recently been implicated as a possible causative factor. The prevalence of autism ranges from 0.03% to 0.1% with fluctuations that may point to an environmental cause.

Learning difficulties

Learning difficulty is associated with dyslexia, minimal brain damage, attention-deficit disorder, and hyperactivity. All these categories are controversial, mainly because they have been over-extended.

Historically, a child with a learning difficulty has been defined as one whose performance in one academic area is more than 2 years behind that age group's ability. Thus the impairment is restricted in its range and there is a discrepancy between academic performance and tested general ability. In these two ways a learning difficulty differs from mental retardation because the latter is characterized by *general* delay and academic performance is usually at the level expected from ability. In practice, learning difficulty has been used to characterize any child with a learning problem who cannot be labelled mentally retarded, no matter how broad the range of impairment or the discrepancy from the tested ability level. This over-extension of the definition has not only increased the apparent prevalence of learning disability but also made the whole area rather confusing.

In general, the prevalence of learning difficulties is estimated on average to be about 4.5%. There is overlap between learning difficulties and other problems, for example higher levels of classroom behavioural problems and an increased risk of delinquency. In part, this accounts for the greater predominance of males in groups with intellectual impairment, as they are more likely than females to be disruptive at school and thus be referred for assessment by educational psychologists.

Dyslexia

This widely discussed form of learning disability is a specific problem with cognition. The broadest definition of dyslexia includes those children whose reading skills are delayed for any reason, and it is usually associated with a number of cognitive deficits. Prevalence varies from 3% to 16% depending on the breadth of the definition and the country. For example, prevalence rates are higher in the USA than they are in Italy, perhaps because of the complexity of the English language compared with Italian!

Minimal brain damage

This category of impairment is used to describe the child who has minor neurological signs, which are often transitory. They are not reliable predictors of future behavioural and educational problems.

Attention-deficit disorder and hyperactivity

These disorders are often confused with one another. Children who cannot sit still are thought to be inattentive in school. A child who does not pay attention often fails to finish activities, acts prematurely or redundantly, infrequently reacts to requests and questions, has difficulties with tasks that require fine discrimination, sustained vigilance, or complex organization, and improves markedly when supervised intensively. A child who is hyperactive engages in excessive standing up, walking, running, and climbing, does not remain seated for long during tasks, frequently makes redundant movements, shifts excessively from one activity to another, and/or often starts talking, asking questions, or making requests. This elevated activity level expresses itself differently at different ages. Inattentive hyperactive children are disturbing to their parents, other children, and professionals such as teachers, doctors, and dentists. They are often judged to be behaviourally disturbed. The variation in definition, age, sex, source of the data, and cultural factors produces prevalence estimates of up to 35%. However, most estimates are under 9% for boys and even less for girls. The aetiology of attention-deficit hyperactivity disorder (ADHD) is unclear, but may be related to pre-term birth, in which circumstances the prevalence may be as high as 60%.

Emotional and behavioural disorders

There are many manifestations of emotional disorder: fear, anxiety, shyness, aggressive, destructive, or chronically disobedient behaviour, theft, associating with bad companions, and truancy. When parents or teachers believe that these problems interfere with the child's socialization, they are often referred for professional help. In considering the prevalence of emotional or behavioural disorders, account has to be taken of the very common, seemingly identical, behaviour of healthy children. Eating disorders, which may be of concern to dentists because of self-injurious behaviour as well as dental erosion, are important in the preschool period and, in different ways, in adolescence.

17.2.1 General considerations

Access to care

Segregated special education and institutions, especially in rural areas, were characteristic of services for disabled children until after the Second World War. During the 1950s there was a move towards **normalizing** the lives of 'handicapped' children. This movement set about making major changes in the lives of affected children and adults, but cannot yet be considered as completely successful in many countries. The move to normalization came about largely for ideological, legal, and, probably in some countries, financial reasons.

The philosophy of this movement, which originated in Sweden, centred on the idea that an impaired person should live in an environment as near normal as possible. This involved residing in home-like residences and attending schools, workplaces, and recreational programmes that were part of the community. On the basis of this ideology, many mildly impaired people were moved out of long-stay institutions into community homes. This movement was fostered by the belief that institutionalization retarded emotional and cognitive growth. De-institutionalization would also reduce the state's expense in maintaining people with impairments, and the onus would be shifted to parents, private charities, and local authorities. Contemporary concepts within this movement are embodied in social role valorization, i.e. the concept of social devaluation of which social exclusion, for whatever reason, is just one aspect.

While most people would agree with the principle of normalization, inadequate funding has produced a less than satisfactory alternative in community care and disastrous consequences for some mentally ill people and those with whom they interact. When many children and adults with impairments were resident in long-stay institutions, the provision of dental services was relatively efficient. With the move to normalization, children were often returned to parents/guardians or housed by social services in homes in the local community, thereby placing an additional burden on these families or carers to organize dental care.

Alongside this programme has been the move to integrate as many children as possible into mainstream education. This may mean that these children are not as readily identifiable as was the case when they attended 'special schools' and thus may miss out on the opportunity to receive the prioritized dental care they need. For teenagers, it has become apparent that some managers of the adult training centres that they attend feel that, as part of normalization, their clients should receive 'normal' dental care, i.e. from a general dental practitioner. This would be desirable, provided that general dental practitioners were happy to provide this service. The evidence to date is that this is not generally the case. In the meantime, teenagers and young adults could lose out by not continuing to receive the special dental services that the publicly funded service has been able to offer, simply because it is felt by their advocates that this runs contrary to the philosophy of 'normalization'. In the UK, the genesis of the specialty of Special Care Dentistry has highlighted the potential for greater provision of special healthcare services for such often marginalized groups who, although well cared for as children, often lose out on vital services as adults.

Consent for dental care

A treatment plan for a child (less than 16 years of age in most jurisdictions) requires the consent of a parent before embarking upon active treatment. This is often by implied consent; that is, the parent brings the child to the surgery and the child sits in the chair, the implication being that the parent has consented to treatment. This is no different to the scenario with an impaired child. The United Nations Convention on the Rights of the Child requires that children's rights are protected, and in this context that cognizance is taken of the child's views on whether they wish treatment to be carried out. As with any patient, best interests must be protected. Difficulty arises in adolescents with an intellectual impairment who are over the age of consent. In this situation parents or carers are unable to give a valid consent on their charge's behalf; that is, an adult cannot consent for treatment on behalf of another adult. Dentists would be well advised to obtain a second opinion on their treatment plan before embarking on dental care for an impaired young person who is judged to be incapable of giving their own valid, i.e. informed, consent. This is particularly the case where dental care under general anaesthesia is being contemplated. It is also prudent to discuss the proposed treatment plan and to obtain the agreement for the care that is being suggested from those who have an interest in the patient.

There will be occasions when it will not be possible to easily undertake an examination of a child or adolescent with a profound learning disability. In those circumstances, a decision has to be made as to whether some form of physical intervention, previously termed restraint, may need to be used. The clinician must decide, on the basis of a number of factors, what is the best way forward. At all times, as part of the dentist's duty of care, he/she must act in the patient's best interest in reaching a decision as to whether to use some form of physical intervention. This decision must be taken in the light of a number of factors, as listed in Key Points 17.5 (modified after Shuman and Bebeau (1996)).

Key Points 17.5

Physical interventions:
- minimum to be effective
- clearly documented —type/reason
- only employed by trained staff
- beneficial for the individual to complete treatment
- not seen as punishment/for convenience
- not likely to cause physical trauma
- not likely to cause more than minimal psychological trauma
- a means of avoiding more severe restraint (e.g. general anaesthesia)
- to control involuntary movements
- to avoid injury to self or others
- agreed with others close to patient.

17.2.2 Oral health

Dental caries

In the absence of targeted preventive and treatment programmes, children with impairments fare less well than their normal peers. While overall disease experience as measured using the DMF index (decayed, missing, filled primary/permanent teeth) is similar, there is often more untreated decay, more missing teeth, and fewer filled teeth for the child with impairments. Early studies point to a reduced prevalence of dental caries in children with Down syndrome, but this feature may be attributable more to the later eruption of teeth relative to a control group of unaffected children so that the teeth are 'at risk' in the mouth for a shorter period. The relative microdontia/ spacing seen in young people with Down syndrome may also be a contributory factor in this supposed reduction in dental disease prevalence.

Periodontal disease

The periodontal status of children who are intellectually impaired may be compromised by their inability to comprehend and thus comply with oral hygiene measures. Periodontal disease is more prevalent in these children, possibly as a result of an altered immune state (Chapter 11.). Almost universally, scores for plaque and gingivitis indices are higher in children with impairments.

Malocclusion

There are no studies dealing specifically with the problems of malocclusion in intellectually impaired children. However, in published data on general dental health, the number of orthodontic anomalies is frequently higher because many remain untreated. In Down syndrome, the relative mid-face hypoplasia contributes to the pseudoskeletal class III relationship and this, in combination with the narrow high-vaulted palate, produces buccal cross-bites (see Fig. 17.2).

Other oral defects

One feature of note is the prevalence of enamel defects often caused by the aetiological agent that produced the impairment. It is possible that dentists could play a part not only in the diagnosis of some disabilities, for example coeliac disease (Fig. 17.5), but also in the timing of the insult that led to the impairment. Teeth provide a good chronological record of the timing of severe systemic upsets (Chapter 13).

17.2.3 Dental care

Children who are intellectually impaired may be able to cooperate for dental treatment, but their ability to accept specific procedures such as the use of local anaesthetic and high-speed instruments will depend on their degree of understanding and level of maturity. Isolation may be difficult because of a large tongue and poor control of movement, and in these situations it may be necessary to compromise on the treatment

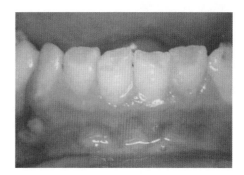

Figure 17.5 Chronological hypoplasia in a child with coeliac disease.

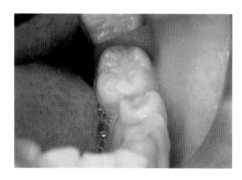

Figure 17.6 Glass ionomer cement as a fissure sealant.

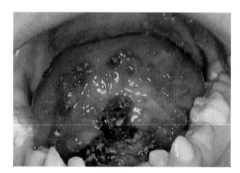

Figure 17.7 Fluoride varnish on the primary molars in a child with a mixed lymphoma–haemangioma and a learning disability.

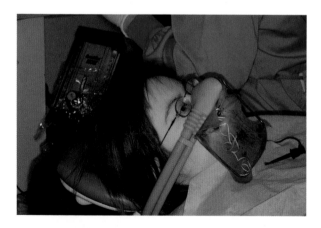

Figure 17.8 A girl with Down syndrome having endodontic treatment with the aid of inhalation sedation.

approach. In fissure sealing it may be more practicable to use a glass ionomer cement, protected by occlusal adjustment wax or a gloved finger during the setting phase, rather than to struggle with all the stages of applying a conventional resin sealant (Fig. 17.6).

Preventive care must be delivered in an evidence-based way. In the UK, the Department of Health has published guidelines to support decision-making in relation to delivering better oral health for all, children and adults (Department of Health 2009). Whilst the guidelines and supporting evidence distinguish between children and adults, they are not based on a risk assessment although there are sections for consideration of high-risk individuals or those who may have 'special needs'. However, similar evidence-based guidelines, specifically targeting children, published by a consortium of universities, the UK Cochrane group, public dental services, and research organizations in Ireland do incorporate a risk assessment into the decision-making process (Oral Health Services Research Centre 2010).

Human clinical trials investigating the use of intra-oral fluoride-releasing devices have been conducted in both the UK and the USA. These are small-diameter glass beads that are attached by composite resin to the buccal surface of a tooth (see Chapter 6). The device dissolves slowly in saliva, releasing fluoride as it does so. Data from clinical trials have indicated that there has been a sustained elevation of salivary fluoride levels for up to 2 years. Whether the released fluoride is equitably distributed around the mouth is not yet known. The placement of the glass beads in such children, and their retention *in situ*, may be a challenge.

Duraphat® fluoride varnish (2.6% sodium fluoride = 22 600ppm fluoride) is an almost ideal preventive agent for children with poor tolerance of dental procedures. The amber-coloured polyurethane-based material is applied to the tooth surfaces, preferably dry although the varnish is water tolerant, and the resulting adherent film slowly releases fluoride (Fig. 17.7). The exercise should be repeated up to four times a year depending on caries risk. A reduction of 30–62% in caries in permanent teeth has been reported using Duraphat® varnish (2.26% F; 22 600ppm F). The application of fluoride varnish by dental nurses with appropriate training is underway in the UK and means that, on a public health level, this preventive measure is now even more cost-effective.

Recourse to one or other forms of conscious sedation may be indicated for a child with impairments who finds it difficult to cooperate for dental care. However, a degree of compliance is necessary in order to retain the nasal hood for the delivery of nitrous oxide–oxygen mixture for inhalation sedation (Fig. 17.8), as it is for the insertion of a cannula for intravenous sedation. However, intravenous sedation is not usually indicated for young children. Midazolam, the drug used most commonly in the UK, can be given orally although, again, the outcome may not be predictable. (See Key Points 17.6.)

Key Points 17.6

Pre-anaesthetic assessment—important features:
- accurate medical history
- previous anaesthetic history
- significant airway difficulties
- need for premedication
- transport arrangements
- home care.

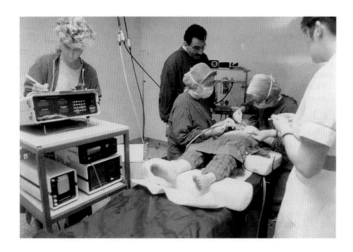

Figure 17.9 Dental treatment under day-case general anaesthesia for a child with impairments.

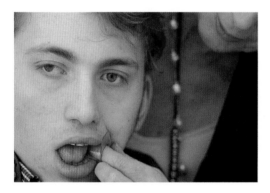

Figure 17.10 A mouth prop in use to aid toothbrushing in a patient with Angleman syndrome.

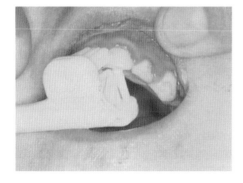

Figure 17.11 A 'superbrush' in use in a child with cerebral palsy.

General anaesthesia will be necessary to provide adequate dental care for some patients (Fig. 17.9). This facility is not widely available and often means considerable disruption for the family because of the distance involved in travelling to specialist centres. Additionally, the child may be unsettled by the whole process of being starved, looked after by strange personnel, being anaesthetized, and then waking up with a sore throat and perhaps a mouth full of blood. There is evidence that this experience only remains in the short-term memory, as many parents comment on how much better their child is in terms of behaviour, sleeping patterns, and eating after the immediate postoperative period.

Treatment planning for dental care under general anaesthesia has to be more radical. The opportunity to reduce a 'high' restoration or to review a doubtful tooth is not necessarily available without recourse to another general anaesthetic. Radiography is an important aid in theatre, especially for the patient who is totally uncooperative in the dental chair. It is particularly important for detecting otherwise hidden pathology and for early enamel lesions. The latter cannot normally be left in the hope that they will remineralize by preventive means. Similarly, the chances of restoration failure can be reduced by the use of pulpotomy techniques and preformed metal crowns. Most forms of treatment can be carried out under general anaesthesia provided that there is sufficient operating time and the patient's general condition permits it.

Success depends upon careful pre-anaesthetic assessment by dentist and anaesthetist. Appropriate perioperative care in theatre (e.g. steroid or antibiotic cover) and the back-up of inpatient facilities, where medically or socially indicated, are vital to a successful outcome. Patients with Down syndrome may have atlanto-axial joint instability and will need extra care in moving from trolley to theatre table as well as during the recovery phase.

17.2.4 Home care

Oral hygiene

There is little to be gained in embarking on elaborate treatment plans including advanced restorative work when it will not be maintained by regular oral hygiene measures at home. Parents or carers need specific advice and practical help in the best way to care for their child's mouth. Thus great reliance is placed on the parent or carer who must be actively involved in oral hygiene instruction and given positive suggestions for modifications to the standard techniques. Examples include advice on the way to position a child (a beanbag can be helpful) in order to clean their mouth more efficiently and less traumatically. Another aid is the use of a prop to gain access to tooth surfaces on the other side of the mouth (Fig. 17.10). Modification of existing toothbrushes, which often have very narrow handles, or the use of specially modified brush heads can be helpful (Fig. 17.11). Carers may be concerned about being bitten when they attempt to clean a child's mouth in situations when toothbrushing is a battle. In these circumstances, use of a finger brush (Fig. 17.12) with bristles incorporated onto the end of a plastic-type material that fits over the end of a finger, similar to a finger-stall, can overcome these problems and ensure adequate tooth cleaning.

For some children, the mechanical removal of plaque can be more readily accomplished using a powered toothbrush. Once the child has become accustomed to the sensation, results can be better than by conventional toothbrushing. Chemical agents are effective in reducing plaque in the short term, but not enough is known about the effects of their long-term usage. Many children find the taste of 0.2% chlorhexidine gluconate, as either a gel or a solution, unpalatable and parents or carers are unhappy about the extrinsic brown staining. A newer chlorhexidine-containing

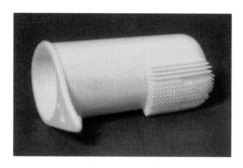

Figure 17.12 A finger brush for use with a patient who is uncooperative during oral hygiene measures.

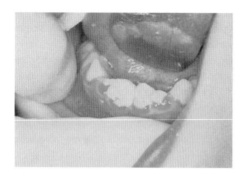

Figure 17.13 Loose calculus deposits in a child with chromosome 4p syndrome.

range of products (Kin©), including mouthwash, toothpaste, and gel, is available. The gel, which contains 0.2% chlorhexidine, is more palatable than chlorhexidine products that have been in use for many years. Kin toothpaste also contains 900ppm fluoride, and is appropriate for patients in whom caries is also a risk and who are over 7 years of age.

Many patients with impairments may be unable to use a mouthwash correctly and either swallow or spit out anything distasteful. An alternative technique is to opt for chairside application of 1% chlorhexidine as a varnish. Originally intended for treating dentine hypersensitivity, the varnish has been shown to reduce the incidence of both gingivitis and dental caries. A 40% chlorhexidine varnish (EC40©) is available but the taste is unacceptable to many users.

Some schools for children with special educational needs provide toothbrushes for their pupils during their learning of personal hygiene skills. However, supervising staff may be unaware of the best method of mouth cleaning, and their approach may depend more on their own perceptions of oral health and the perceived difficulty than any other factor.

Toothbrushing can be taught in the same way as other skills, but it requires time for the individual as well as commitment on the part of the regular carer to ensure that all areas of the mouth are being cleaned each time. However, many disabled children are intolerant not only of toothbrushing but also of toothpaste, and they may gag when toothpaste, which they cannot swallow because of poor reflexes, is introduced into the mouth. Toothpaste also obscures the view for the carer during toothbrushing and they cannot always be sure that the tooth surfaces are clean. In these circumstances, where toothpaste is unacceptable to the child, parents or carers should attempt to clean around the mouth with a piece of gauze moistened in a 0.2% chlorhexidine gluconate solution or a toothbrush dipped in fluoride mouth rinse (0.05% sodium fluoride if used on a daily basis). Alternatively, chlorhexidine in gel form or fluoride toothpaste can be rubbed as vigorously as possible around the tooth surfaces using a finger. Since chlorhexidine is inactivated by the traditional foaming agents in toothpastes, the former should be used at a different time of the day to the latter.

Children who are tube-fed, or who have had a feeding tube inserted directly into their stomach (percutaneous endoscopic gastrostomy—PEG) for some or their entire nutrient intake, still need oral care. They will frequently accumulate significant quantities of calculus which, if detached, might be inhaled. Regular mouth cleaning and the use of a 'tartar control' toothpaste are necessary (Fig. 17.13).

Diet

More severely impaired children may have well-regulated eating times and a reduced likelihood of snacking. The food consumed may be semi-solid or even liquidized, but those foods which are easily reduced to this form are often dentally undesirable. In these circumstances the dentist should offer advice on limiting the number of intakes of food, provided that it conforms to the child's general nutritional and dietary needs.

Establishing a normal eating routine while 'growing up' becomes a battlefield for some children, and impaired children are no exception to this. It is often easier for parents to 'give in' to a child and allow them to eat a limited variety of unsuitable foods frequently. This will be justified by parents saying that they are desperate to get the child to eat something, and so biscuits and other snacks high in non-milk extrinsic sugars become the norm. This pattern is further endorsed in some children with impairments where weight gain is paramount and the dental implications are secondary, if indeed they are even considered. Drinks can also be an issue, particularly the use of sweetened bottles for an extended period in a child's life. It is not uncommon for children of 2 years of age or older still to be using a bottle containing milk, often for naps, last thing at night before going to bed, and even during the night. This is an extremely difficult habit to break, but the most successful approach has been to advise the parent to gradually dilute the contents with water over a period of weeks, until eventually the child is drinking water only. This not only eliminates the undesirable habit but also gives the parent of the child, who is able to be toilet trained, some prospect of getting the child dry and out of nappies overnight. Frequent intakes of nutrient-enriched drinks may be required by some children who fail to gain weight. The dental team needs to undertake regular, often frequent, dental risk assessments and organize appropriate preventive protocols for such children.

For a number of children with impairments, the use of sweetened medication has led to an increase in dental caries (Fig. 17.14). In the past this has arisen because of a lack of sugar-free alternatives. However, with the pharmaceutical industry's greater awareness, it is often only because of ignorance among the medical profession that such outmoded prescribing continues. Some children will be taking medication as dispersible tablets or in an effervescent form, some of which, with chronic use, may predispose to dental erosion.

Another consideration is spoiling. The birth of a child who is impaired in some way is a shock for any parent. Months of eager anticipation are

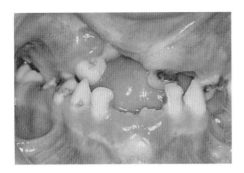

Figure 17.14 The dental effects of frequent sugared medication in a child with a cleft of the lip and palate.

followed by disbelief, anger, denial, frustration, and guilt. Parents have to grieve for the healthy child they will never have, before coming to terms with their new responsibilities. Parents continue to feel guilty; maybe their child has an impairment because of something they have done, or something they should not have done. Either way, they may attempt to assuage that guilt by spoiling the child. This may take the form of easy to eat sweet foods, which are thought to be pleasurable and are welcomed by the child with a poor appetite, thus compounding the problem of poor eating. Poor eating habits resulting in oral disease need to be tackled together with the paediatrician and dietician, as well as the parents or caregivers. (See Key Points 17.7.)

Key Points 17.7

General dietary advice

- Restrict sweet foods/drinks to meal times where practicable.
- Limit sweetened foods/drinks to three times a day.
- Keep food and drinks clear of bedtime by about an hour.
- Remember that carbonated drinks and some medicines erode teeth.
- Ask for sugar-free medicines.

Fluorides

Many special milk formulas and food supplements, as well as containing non-milk extrinsic sugars to boost the child's calorie intake, also contain quite substantial amounts of fluoride. Therefore it is wise to check the diet carefully before advocating the use of fluoride supplements for such children. Where dental caries is potentially a real problem and in the absence of any other form of systemic fluorides, the daily fluoride supplement regimen of 0.25mg from 6 months of age, followed by an increase to 0.5mg at 3 years of age, and then 1.0mg from 6 to 16 years of age is to be advocated. Once the concentration of fluoride in the local water supply is known from the water company, fluoride supplements can be prescribed by the general dental practitioner, if indicated, as either drops for the younger child or tablets for

the preschool child. It is likely that some children with impairments will never cope with fluoride tablets and have to remain on drops. As long as the parent is given written instructions to overrule the prescribing schedule given for younger children on the label of the bottle, there is no reason why older children should not be prescribed fluoride drops.

The dentist should also advise on the appropriate fluoride toothpaste to be used in conjunction with fluoride supplementation or water fluoridation. Each case should be considered individually, taking into account the relative risks and benefits that may occur. Paramount is consideration of the risk of developing dental caries versus the potential for enamel opacities in the permanent dentition. As a guideline, if the risk of caries is minimal, the diet is reasonably well controlled, and home oral care is generally good, it is sensible to suggest the use of a pea-sized amount of toothpaste containing approximately 500–600ppm fluoride for a child under 6 years of age, provided that toothpaste can be used successfully. Older children in the same risk category should use a toothpaste containing 1000–1500ppm fluoride, as the risk of enamel opacities on anterior teeth is non-existent and this formulation will provide optimal protection against caries. In the child where the development of dental disease would pose a real hazard to their general health and home care in terms of oral hygiene and diet is poorly controlled, it is advisable to confer maximum protection by recommending the use of a toothpaste containing 1000–1500ppm fluoride, even during the preschool years. For children and adolescents at high risk for dental caries, higher-concentration toothpastes (2800ppm fluoride and 5000ppm fluoride for those over 12 years and 16 years, respectively) can be prescribed.

Because many children with impairments are unable to hold solutions in their mouths or to expectorate, fluoride mouthwashes are contraindicated. However, they can be used on a toothbrush (dipped), where toothpaste is not well tolerated, to replicate the amount of topical fluoride received from toothpaste. For children where a dry mouth is an issue and caries protection is required, a commercial mousse formulation containing CPP-ACP with fluoride (900ppm) has been shown *in vitro* to have the potential to remineralize decalcified areas. (See Key Points 17.8.)

Key Points 17.8

Fluoride advice

- Supplements to give optimal caries protection.
- Fluoride mouthwash on a toothbrush instead of paste in cases of paste intolerance.
- Low caries risk: paste containing 500–600ppm fluoride (up to 6 years) or 1000–1500ppm fluoride (6 years onwards).
- Higher caries risk: paste containing 1000–1500ppm fluoride paste (pea-sized amount) from the time of tooth eruption onwards.
- High caries risk: paste containing 2800ppm fluoride (from 12 years) and 5000ppm fluoride (16 years onwards)

17.3 Physical impairment—cerebral palsy

The common physical impairments that the dentist will encounter are **developmental** neuromuscular disorders (e.g. cerebral palsy, spina bifida, scoliosis, and osteogenesis imperfecta) and **degenerative** neuromuscular disorders (e.g. muscular dystrophy and juvenile forms of arthritis). Included in this general category of physical impairment are children with clefts of the lip and/or palate (Chapter 14) where there may be an associated syndrome in up to 19% of cases.

17.3.1 General considerations

Cerebral palsy occurs in 1–2 per 1000 school-age children, a figure that has remained relatively stable because of the improved quality of survival of premature babies. The term cerebral palsy describes a group of non-progressive neuromuscular disorders caused by brain damage, which can be pre-, peri-, or postnatal in origin, and are classified according to the type of motor defect:

1. *Spasticity*—impaired ability to control voluntary movements. There is the appearance of severe muscle stiffness and the planned movement of an affected limb results in a hypotonic tendon reflex, especially with rapid movements. Spasticity occurs in about 50% of cases of cerebral palsy.

2. *Athetosis*—uncontrolled slow twisting and writhing movements, which are frequent and involuntary and occur in over 16% of cases.

3. *Rigidity*—resistance to passive movement, which may be overcome by sudden action. It is uncommon and the majority of these children are intellectually impaired.

4. *Ataxia*—disturbance of equilibrium as well as difficulty in grasping objects. It is also uncommon.

5. *Hypotonia*—all muscles are flaccid with decreased function.

6. *Mixed*—a combination of the above.

There has been a change in the proportion of the different subtypes in the last 30 years. For example, with the decrease in kernicterus (neonatal jaundice), there has been a fall in the athetoid form, but the spastic form, associated with prematurity, has increased. An affected child may be monoplegic with only one limb affected (Fig. 17.15) or have all four limbs affected (quadriplegia). In addition, the child may be disabled by other impairments such as convulsions, intellectual impairment, sensory disorders, emotional disorders, speech and communication defects, and a poorly developed swallowing and cough reflex.

17.3.2 Oral health

The following oral and dental features may be seen in children with cerebral palsy:

- poor oral hygiene, increased periodontal disease, and drug-induced gingival enlargement;
- malocclusion (increased prevalence of skeletal class II with anterior open-bite);
- a tendency to bruxism;
- tongue thrust and mouth breathing;
- an increase in caries prevalence;
- increased prevalence of anterior trauma;
- enamel hypoplasia;
- heightened gag reflex and perioral sensitivity;
- drooling;
- decreased parotid flow rate.

Although not confined to children with cerebral palsy, gastric reflux is relatively common (Fig. 17.16). There may be an obvious aetiology (e.g. a hiatus hernia), but quite often a cause for the associated erosion cannot be identified (Chapter 10).

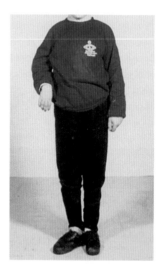

Figure 17.15 Monoplegia of the right arm in a child with cerebral palsy and a congenital heart defect.

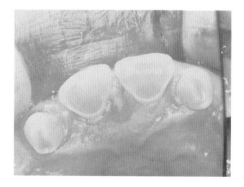

Figure 17.16 Palatal erosion due to gastric reflux on maxillary incisors in a child with cerebral palsy.

17.3.3 Dental care

Children who are severely physically impaired will probably be brought to the dental surgery in a wheelchair or will be carried. Care is required in the handling of such patients (see Section 17.4.1).

Altered gag and cough reflexes may complicate the delivery of dental care or the provision of prostheses, as well as adding to the patient's anxiety. Plentiful reassurance, efficient suction, and skilled assistance are vital to success in these situations. Impaired ventilation may accompany scoliosis and becomes an even more important consideration if procedures involving a general anaesthetic are contemplated. Children who spend long periods in one position may be predisposed to pressure sores; therefore lengthy procedures in the dental chair without a break are best avoided.

Hypoplastic teeth can be very sensitive, particularly to extreme cold. Patients can experience acute discomfort during tooth preparation or ultrasonic scaling (even when the affected teeth are distant from the operating site) merely because of the cold produced by high-volume aspiration. The use of a desensitizing agent such as Duraphat® fluoride varnish or fissure-sealing the symptomatic surface can be helpful if a restoration is not indicated. Hypoplastic enamel does not have the same ordered prism structure as normal enamel and, despite acid etching, may not provide optimum retention for conventional resins. In this situation, glass ionomer cements may be a more suitable alternative.

Some less severely disabled children will have little or no intellectual impairment, but will have a degree of spasticity or rigidity. This may prevent them from cooperating fully with dental procedures, despite their willingness to do so, and they may be helped by nitrous oxide sedation (Chapter 4). Such sedation may also help diminish an exaggerated gag reflex. In adolescents, intravenous sedation is also an option in these circumstances if nitrous oxide does not provide the degree of sedation required for the procedure. (See Key Points 17.9.)

Key Points 17.9

Oral features in cerebral palsy:

- gingival hyperplasia
- increased caries prevalence
- malocclusion
- dental trauma
- enamel hypoplasia
- heightened gag reflex
- dental erosion and attrition (bruxism).

17.3.4 Home care

Oral hygiene

Physical impairment may hinder oral hygiene procedures, and the problem may be compounded for the child who has gingival enlargement. Most children require help with brushing until they are aged 7 years or older, when they have acquired sufficient manual dexterity. For the child with physical limitations, assistance with mouth cleaning may be a permanent commitment on the part of carers. Limited or bizarre muscle movements prevent normal mouth clearing, and food is often left impacted in the vault of the palate. This is readily removed with the end of a toothbrush handle or a spoon handle, but carers need to be aware of the potential for this, otherwise food residues may be left in the oral cavity for days. Powered toothbrushes may be helpful for a child with limited dexterity, not only because of the relative efficiency of cleaning but also because of the larger handle size of most of these brushes.

When normal limb movement is impaired or absent and/or normal speech is impossible, the mouth assumes an even greater importance as a means of holding mouthsticks to grasp pens or to operate a variety of equipment. It is vital that the dentition is maintained to the highest standard as the successful use of such mouthsticks is reliant on having a good occlusal table for balanced contact (Fig. 17.17).

Children with cerebral palsy, especially where there is accompanying intellectual impairment, will occasionally adopt a habit of self-mutilation by chewing soft tissues around the mouth (Fig. 17.18). This can be triggered by teething, although often no cause can be found. It is distressing for the parents as the child is obviously in pain from the ulcerated areas and may refuse all food and drink, but there is little they can do to break the habit. It may be helpful to discuss the child's medication with their physician, as the prescription of a drug to reduce muscle tone, which can be an exacerbating factor in this situation, may be considered.

There are a number of solutions to the problem depending on the cause and severity of the condition. In a child who is erupting primary

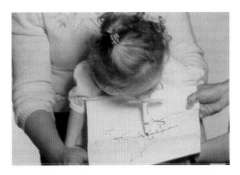

Figure 17.17 A modified pen-holder for a child with arthrogryposis.

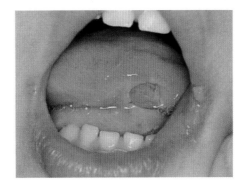

Figure 17.18 Self-mutilation in a child with cerebral palsy.

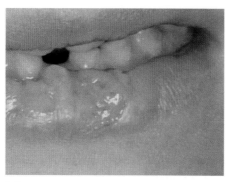

(a)

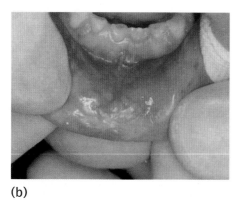

(b)

Figure 17.19 Traumatic self-mutilation in a boy with cerebral palsy: (a) before and (b) after the use of a composition 'splint' to protect the traumatized area.

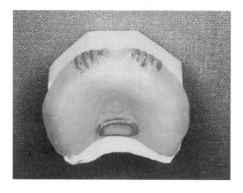

Figure 17.20 A palatal training plate designed to improve lip and tongue posture.

teeth it may be possible to fit an occlusal splint, provided that sufficient teeth are available for retention. Fabrication of the splint may necessitate

a short general anaesthetic for impression-taking. Alternatively, addition of glass ionomer cement to the occlusal surfaces of the primary molars, to open the occlusion and prevent the teeth from contacting the soft tissues, may be successful. If only anterior primary teeth are present, composition moulded over the offending tooth surfaces as a temporary splint may break the habit and allow healing (Fig. 17.19). If the problem is more severe and a splint is not feasible, it is sensible to extract the primary teeth involved. In the permanent dentition, rounding-off the pointed or sharp tooth surfaces and/or fitting a splint is usually successful. During the acute phase the use of a topical analgesic such as 0.15% benzydamine hydrochloride in spray form increases mouth comfort prior to eating, and 0.2% chlorhexidine gluconate solution, swabbed around the mouth or applied as a gel on a finger, promotes more rapid healing by keeping the area clean. Ensuring that the child has plenty of fluids is of paramount importance, as lightweight debilitated children rapidly become dehydrated.

The other area of concern to parents and carers is drooling. This can be excessive in some disabled children, although surgery to divert the submandibular flow more posteriorly may alleviate the problem. However, this is not always successful and carries the risk of increasing caries prevalence as a result of the greatly diminished salivary volume. The use of acrylic training plates, which encourage the formation of an oral seal as well as promoting a more active swallowing mechanism so that saliva does not pool in an open mouth, may be helpful (Fig. 17.20). Concurrent work with speech and language therapists will help with the necessary therapy that is fundamental to the success of such treatment. Anecdotal case reports support the use of these plates, but few studies providing objective data on their success have been published. However, one relatively non-interventional method of reducing saliva flow is the use of hyoscine hydrobromide (scopolamine), a drug which blocks parasympathetic transmission to the salivary glands. It is applied as a patch behind the ear and changed every 3 days. The use of botulinum neurotoxin type A (BoNT-A) injected into the parotid gland is now the preferred management in a number of centres, although it needs to be carried out as a day-case procedure under guided ultrasonography with a general anaesthetic.

Diet

Considerations of dietary aspects have been covered in Section 17.2.4). Because of a failure to thrive, some children will be fed through a gastrostomy site. A child fed exclusively via this route will tend to accumulate large deposits of calculus. These need to be removed, particularly from surfaces adjacent to the gingival margins. This can be difficult unless there is good cooperation from the patient; an impaired airway makes the safe removal of such deposits hazardous, with the risk of inhalation of calculus. The gastrostomy site can also be useful for sedative drugs, especially bitter intravenous sedative drugs that might not be tolerated orally. However, such sedation procedures need to be carried out in specialist units.

17.4 Physical impairment—spina bifida

Spina bifida occurs as a result of non-fusion of one or more posterior vertebral arches, with or without protrusion of some or all of the contents of the spinal canal. It may be accompanied by

hydrocephalus in up to 95% of cases. It is estimated that the defect is inherited in 50–60% of affected children and that environmental agents may be responsible for the remainder. The incidence in the

UK is 2.5 per 1000 births and, unlike other malformations, it is more common in females. A quarter of affected children will also have epilepsy and about a third will have some degree of intellectual impairment.

17.4.1 General considerations

Unless the defect is slight, children with spina bifida will spend much of their time confined to a wheelchair (Fig. 17.21) and be incontinent. Urinary tract infections are common and the child may be on frequent courses of antibiotics. Hydrocephalus, unless arrested, is treated by the insertion of a shunt (fitted with a Spitz–Holter valve) to drain fluid from the ventricles into the superior vena cava or, more usually, the peritoneum. It is important to protect the venous shunt from blockage, which may arise from a bacteraemia of oral origin, otherwise intracranial pressure will increase, causing convulsions. Although opinion is divided on the necessity of giving antibiotic cover for invasive dental procedures in children who have a venous shunt, some clinicians will err on the side of caution. However, there is no indication for antibiotic prophylaxis if a ventriculo-peritoneal shunt is used. Children with spina bifida have frequent regular exposure to latex because of catheterization for urinary infections, and they are more likely to develop type I hypersensitivity to latex. The dental team need to be aware of this potential. Such patients should be managed in a latex-screened environment and may need to be treated in a latex-free surgery.

Children who are confined to a wheelchair for much of the time will need to be either treated in their chair or transferred carefully to the dental chair. Chair adaptations to accommodate a patient in their wheelchair (Fig. 17.22) are commercially available. These are helpful if the child is too heavy to transfer easily to the dental chair or if the procedure is more easily accomplished for the operator and patient in this position. Shaped body supports, which are essentially modifications of a beanbag, are also available for use in the dental chair for any patient with a physical disability who cannot otherwise be comfortably accommodated. These supports contain a material that allows them to mould to the body shape of the patient and be remoulded for subsequent patients (Fig. 17.23).

17.4.2 Dental care

There is little in the dental literature to suggest that the oral/dental health of children with spina bifida is different from that of other children with impairments. The same principles of treatment apply to these children as to others who are impaired, namely aggressive prevention and early intervention with a radical approach if dental treatment under general anaesthesia is required.

17.4.3 Home care

The issues relevant to spina bifida have been covered in the appropriate sections under intellectual and physical impairment.

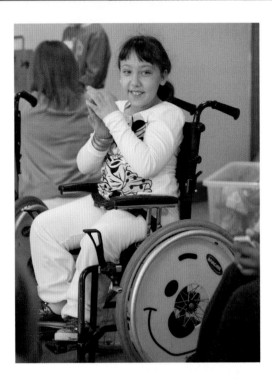

Figure 17.21 A girl with spina bifida—wheelchair-aided. (Courtesy of Shine, www.shinecharity.org.uk).

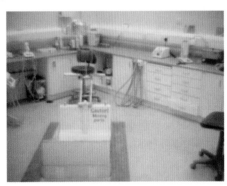

Figure 17.22 A customized floor insert to accommodate a patient's wheelchair. (Courtesy of HSE Dental Services, Dun Laoghaire, Ireland.)

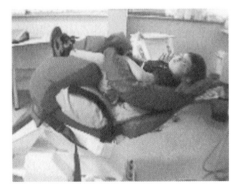

Figure 17.23 Dental chair with moulded cushion supports. (Courtesy of Dr Bitte Ahlborg, Mun-H-Center, Sweden).

17.5 Physical impairment—muscular dystrophy

Muscular dystrophy is a group of muscle diseases which present as progressive atrophy and weakness of skeletal muscles with resultant disability and deformity. The muscle fibres degenerate and are replaced by fatty and fibrous tissue. The disease is eventually fatal because of recurrent respiratory infections. Prevalence rates in children are of the order of 4 per 100 000 children.

17.5.1 General considerations

The child with muscular dystrophy will initially be mobile, but as the disease progresses, he/she will become reliant on a wheelchair to move around. A respirator will be necessary in the later stages of the disease, and patients are then confined to home or to residential care. There are a number of variants of the disease with different signs and symptoms. Males are exclusively affected in the Duchenne type, while facial musculature is always affected in the fascioscapulohumeral type but rarely in other forms.

17.5.2 Oral health

The oral/dental effects of the disease are numerous and include:

- weakness of the facial muscles;
- poor oral hygiene secondary to the general inability to provide oral self-care;
- increased dental decay;
- increased potential for periodontal disease;
- malocclusion secondary to decreased facial muscle tone while retaining tongue function;
- decreased protective reflexes and reduced ability to swallow or clear secretions from the oropharynx, thus increasing the potential for aspiration.

17.5.3 Dental care

Consideration needs to be given to wheelchair transfer techniques and padding as well as the length of appointments (see above). The use of sedation and general anaesthesia may need to be avoided because of the decreased respiratory function and the risk of post-anaesthetic complications. Frequent recall is important, with applications of topical fluorides and antiplaque agents (0.2% chlorhexidine gluconate). There are no contraindications to dental treatment, except orthodontics because of the changing muscle forces. As a consequence of tooth movement, which is seen as part of the disease, and the likely development of anterior or posterior open-bites, prosthetic appliances may become non-functional. Children with Duchenne muscular dystrophy will frequently be started on bisphosphonates early in the course of the condition. Survival is significantly enhanced by the combination of steroids and bisphosphonates but dentists need to take concurrent bisphosphonate therapy into account in their risk assessment and subsequent management.

17.5.4 Home care

Appropriate support and training needs to be given to the parent or carer so that in the later stages of the disease, when contact with dental services may be difficult, adequate plaque control can be maintained. Dental treatment may need to be provided within the home environment, although this will usually be at the stage when the patient has reached adulthood. It is important that every effort is made to optimize oral function and facial appearance and thereby encourage a positive self-image.

17.6 Other musculoskeletal impairments

A variety of other defects, some degenerative and some developmental (e.g. osteogenesis imperfecta, juvenile arthritis, and multiple sclerosis), affect children. However, these are relatively rare and are unlikely to be encountered regularly in practice. When patients present with such disabilities there may be significant oral signs; for example, in rheumatoid arthritis there is an increased incidence of Sjögren's syndrome (autoimmune) and anaemia (secondary to anti-inflammatory and steroid medication). Risk assessment and targeted preventive care are vital to prevent dental disease.

17.7 Blindness and visual impairment

Visual impairments vary from total blindness to sight limitations of size, colour, distance, and shape. The prevalence is in the order of 3 per 1000 children.

17.7.1 Oral health

The oral and dental health of children with a visual impairment is no different from that of the normal population and with good home care this can be maintained. In the UK many children are educated in residential schools and their supervision, with regard to personal hygiene and diet (restraint from between-meal snacking), often means that their oral health is good.

17.7.2 Dental care

Consideration should be given to the design and format of written material available for use by patients who may be visually impaired, for example instructions for the wearing of orthodontic appliances and diet history sheets. Highly stylized type should be avoided and a mix of upper and lower case should be used. Letters should be at least one-eighth of an inch high (about 3mm, 14 point) and be on uncoated (non-glare) paper. The best contrast for ease of reading is black type on white or off-white paper.

It is important to assist the visually impaired person according to their individual needs. Patients with a sight defect object to being forcefully guided around by a nurse or dentist who is enthusiastic to help. Many sight-impaired patients will have an increased sensitivity to bright lights and perhaps touch. Therefore the operating light should be used with caution and touch should be utilized to enhance the patient's perception of what is being done, for example being allowed to feel the instruments and the dental chair.

It is not unusual for people to shout at those with a visual impairment. Sight-impaired children are not usually deaf as well, and therefore should be addressed in a normal voice. It is important to the patient, and not only those with visual impairments, that conversation is addressed to them and not to the person with them. Because vision is impaired and the sense of touch may be heightened, it can be startling to suddenly feel a cold mirror in your mouth without warning. A 'tell–feel–then do' approach is important for these children, who may be unnerved by contact without forewarning. With these considerations in mind, there are no areas of dental treatment that are unsuitable for the child with a visual impairment, provided that they, or their parent or carer, can maintain an adequate standard of oral hygiene. Insertion of orthodontic appliances may initially be difficult and techniques like flossing take time to master.

17.8 Deafness and hearing impairment

Loss of hearing is an impairment acquired by many with increasing age. However, some children are born with either partial or total loss of hearing, and this can occur in isolation or in combination with other impairments, for example rubella syndrome (auditory, visual, intellectual, and cardiac defects). The prevalence is 3 per 1000 children.

17.8.1 General considerations

Patients who have impaired hearing may be fearful, or even hostile, because they feel that they are not going to understand what is being asked of them. The child may not hear what has been said, but pretends to have done so to avoid embarrassment. In this situation visual aids assume an even greater importance. It is important for optimizing hearing that all extraneous background noise is removed when communicating with the hearing-impaired child. Piped music in the surgery, noise from the reception area, and internal noises from aspirators and scavenging systems should be reduced or eliminated.

Many deaf or hearing-impaired children will wear aids (Fig. 17.24) to enable them to pick up more sounds, and older children may have become skilled not only in lip-reading but also in signing. However, there is now a trend towards discouraging the use of signing and to positively encourage a child to acquire some speech, utilizing any residual vocal potential.

17.8.2 Oral health

There is a paucity of data concerning the oral health of children with hearing impairment. As with visually impaired children, residence away from home in residential schools sometimes means that eating patterns are more desirable dentally, with less opportunity for between-meal snacking compared with day pupils. Supervision of oral hygiene measures can also be better in children living in residential care and is reflected in their oral hygiene scores, but this is very variable. Like many other impaired children, hearing-impaired patients are initially wary of powered toothbrushes because of the sensation they produce intra-orally. Although these brushes have not been shown to be better in terms of plaque removal than a well-manipulated manual brush, in children particularly the novelty aspect may be a motivating factor to use this type of brush to greater benefit.

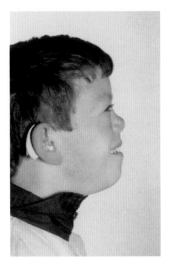

Figure 17.24 A child with Williams syndrome wearing a hearing aid.

17.8.3 Dental care

For those children who can lip-read it is necessary to sit well in front of the child, with good lighting to the operator's face. Both dentist and assistant should move their lips clearly during speech and avoid the temptation to shout. Therefore masks are to be put to one side and bearded operators should ensure that facial hair does not obscure clear visualization of lip movement! A comment as to the best hearing side should be inserted in the patient's notes so that staff are aware of this at each visit.

Children wearing hearing devices may be disturbed by the high-pitched noise produced by handpieces and ultrasonic scalers. This may make them less cooperative and less amenable to treatment. Similarly, the conduction of vibrations from the handpiece and burs via bone is more disturbing for the hearing-impaired child. After initial communications are complete, it may be advisable to suggest that the hearing device is removed or turned off and only reinserted on completion of the dental treatment in time for final instructions. Very young children often have difficulty keeping the aids in place simply because of the size of the immature pinnae. This is especially relevant when lying supine in the dental chair.

17.9 Summary

1 Children with impairments present the dental team with the challenge of adapting familiar skills to new situations.

2 To meet this challenge effectively the dental team needs to re-examine some of the stereotypes of impairment.

3 An impairment becomes a disability by virtue of other people's attitudes, the things that are done or not done, and the facilities not offered, as well as the physical barriers the environment interposes.

4 Oral and dental health are little different between children with impairments and others. What is different is the type of treatment offered, with more missing teeth and fewer filled teeth in populations with impairments.

5 Some children have specific oral conditions as a result of their impairment, for example periodontal disease in Down syndrome.

6 A degree of common sense, a willingness to be flexible, and a working familiarity with the more common medical conditions and their implications for oral and dental health are most of what a general dental practitioner requires to provide dental care for the child with impairments in his/her community.

17.10 Further reading

Carlstedt, K., Henningsson, G., and Dahllöf, G. (2007). Longitudinal study of palatal plate therapy in children with Down syndrome. Effects on oral motor function. *Journal of Disability and Oral Health*, **8**, 13–19

Faulks, D. and Hennequin, M. (2006). Defining the population requiring special care dentistry using the International Classification of Functioning, Disability and Health—a personal view. *Journal of Disability and Oral Health*, **7**, 143–52.

Nelson, L.P., Getzin, A., Graham, D., *et al.* (2011). Unmet dental needs and barriers to dental care for children with significant special health care needs. *Pediatric Dentistry*, **33**, 29–36.

Nunn, J., Foster, M., Master, S., and Greening, S. (2008). A policy document on consent and physical intervention in children. *International Journal of Paediatric Dentistry*, **18** (Suppl. 1), 39–46.

17.11 References

British Dental Association (2010). *Case mix model.* Available online at: **http://www.bda.org/dentists/representation/salaried-primary-care-dentists/cccphd/casemix/case_mix_models/index.aspx**

Department of Health (2009). *Delivering oral health: an evidence-based toolkit for prevention.* Second edition. Available online at: **http://www.dh.gov.uk/prod_consum_dh/groups/dh_digitalassets/documents/digitalasset/dh_102982.pdf**

Oral Health Services Research Centre (2010). *Oral Health Services guideline initiative.* Available online at: **http://ohsrc.ucc.ie/html/guidelines.html**

Shuman, S.K. and Bebeau, M.J. (1996). Ethical issues in nursing home care: practice guidelines for difficult situations. *Special Care in Dentistry*, **16**, 170–7.

18

Safeguarding children

J.C. Harris and R. Welbury

Chapter contents

18.1 Introduction

It is essential that everyone who provides dental care for children has an understanding of other factors that affect children's lives. This includes non-dental aspects of their health, as discussed in previous chapters, and wider issues that affect children's development and well-being. Child maltreatment is one such issue.

Abuse and neglect are forms of maltreatment of a child. Child maltreatment involves acts of commission or omission which result in harm to a child. When health professionals work with others to take action to protect children who are suffering, or are at risk of suffering, significant harm as a result of maltreatment, this is known as 'child protection'.

Child protection sits within the context of a wider agenda to 'safeguard' children. Safeguarding measures are actions taken to minimize the risks of harm to children and young people. This includes:

- protecting children from maltreatment;
- preventing impairment of children's health or development;
- ensuring that children are growing up in a safe and caring environment.

This should enable children to have optimal life chances and to enter adulthood successfully (Box 18.1). The foundation for the success of such work is an acceptance and understanding of children's internationally agreed human rights (Box 18.2). In this context the term 'child' includes children and young people up to the age of 18.

18.1.1 Historical aspects

Violence towards children has been noted between cultures and at different times within the same culture since early civilization. Infanticide has been documented in almost every culture, and ritualistic killing, maiming, and severe punishment of children in an attempt to educate them, exploit them, or rid them of evil spirits has been reported since early times. Ritualistic surgery or mutilation of children has been recorded as part of religious and ethnic traditions.

In the seventeenth century values started to change and incest was seen as a crime under church law, but until the eighteenth century society viewed children as possessions of their parents who were at liberty to treat them in any way they wished. In fact legislation to protect animals was introduced before children were afforded the same 'privilege'.

Around the turn of the twentieth century social denial of abuse continued, but the implementation of the Prevention of Cruelty to Children Act 1904 gave local authorities the power, for the first time, to remove children from their parents. In 1908 incest became a criminal offence when the Punishment of Incest Act was passed in the British Parliament. The twentieth century saw the beginnings of an acknowledgement of the problem of child abuse and recognition that children needed protection, although society was very slow to accept that carers could deliberately harm children for whom they were responsible. In 1946 Caffey, a paediatric radiologist, described bone lesions and subdural haematomas resulting from trauma, and in 1962 Kempe, a paediatrician, described 'the battered child syndrome' (Kempe *et al.* 1962).

The term 'non-accidental injury' (NAI) became the medically accepted label for this syndrome in the UK, and doctors became increasingly involved with social workers and the police in its diagnosis. In the 1980s the problem of sexual abuse began to be seriously highlighted both in society and in the medical press. However, the actual diagnosis was still based on the medical model and, to compound the problem, society's level of acknowledgement lagged behind that of professionals.

Despite the progress made on recognizing child abuse, defining what constitutes child abuse remains a matter of debate. Until recently, corporal punishment at school was deemed by society not only acceptable but also necessary. Yet nowadays previously widely accepted and almost universal practices such as caning of schoolchildren have been incorporated into the widening spectrum of child abuse. Even today the debate continues as to the appropriateness of smacking children to enforce discipline.

Today it is recognized that NAI is just one aspect of a spectrum which encompasses other types of abuse and neglect, and the current preferred term is 'child maltreatment'. The primary aim of all professionals involved in the child protection process is to ensure the safety of the child. The secondary aim is to provide help and counselling for the parents or caregivers so that the abuse stops. (See Key Points 18.1.)

Box 18.1 Five key outcomes for the well-being of children and young people

- Be healthy
- Stay safe
- Enjoy and achieve
- Make a positive contribution
- Achieve economic well-being

Every Child Matters, Department for Education and Skills, 2003. © Crown Copyright.

Box 18.2 Extracts from the United Nations Convention on the Rights of the Child

Article 19
Children should be protected from all forms of physical or mental violence, injury or abuse, neglect or negligent treatment, maltreatment or exploitation

Article 24
Children have a right to the enjoyment of the highest attainable standard of health and to facilities for the treatment of illness and rehabilitation of health

United Nations Convention on the Rights of the Child. Office of the High Commissioner for Human Rights, Geneva, 1989.

Key Points 18.1

- Children have a right to be protected from all forms of abuse and neglect.
- Child protection is the action taken to protect children who are suffering, or at risk of suffering, significant harm as a result of maltreatment.
- Safeguarding describes the wider range of measures taken to minimize the risks of harm to children.

18.2 Categories of abuse and neglect

Somebody may abuse or neglect a child by inflicting harm, or by failing to act to prevent harm. Children may be abused in a family or in an institutional or community setting, by those known to them, or, more rarely, by a stranger. They may be abused by an adult or adults, or by another child or children. There are four categories of child maltreatment.

18.2.1 Physical abuse

Physical abuse may involve hitting, shaking, throwing, poisoning, burning or scalding, drowning, suffocating, or otherwise causing physical harm to a child. Physical harm may also be caused when a parent or carer fabricates the symptoms of, or deliberately induces, illness in a child (formerly known as Munchausen syndrome by proxy or factitious illness by proxy).

18.2.2 Emotional abuse

Emotional abuse is the persistent emotional maltreatment of a child such as to cause severe and persistent adverse effects on the child's emotional development. It may involve conveying to children that they are worthless or unloved, inadequate, or valued only in so far as they meet the needs of another person. It may feature age or developmentally inappropriate expectations being imposed on children. These may include interactions that are beyond the child's developmental capability as well as overprotection and preventing participation in normal social interaction. It may involve seeing or hearing the ill-treatment of another. It may involve serious bullying, causing children frequently to feel frightened or in danger, or the exploitation or corruption of children. Some level of emotional abuse is involved in all types of maltreatment of a child, although it may occur alone.

18.2.3 Sexual abuse

Sexual abuse involves forcing or enticing a child or young person to take part in sexual activities, including prostitution, whether or not the child is aware of what is happening. The activities may involve physical contact, including penetrative acts (e.g. rape or oral sex) or non-penetrative acts (such as kissing or touching). They may include non-contact activities, such as involving children in looking at, or in the production of, sexual images, watching sexual activities, encouraging children to behave in sexually inappropriate ways, or grooming a child in preparation for abuse.

18.2.4 Neglect

Neglect is the persistent failure to meet a child's basic physical and/or psychological needs which is likely to result in the serious impairment of the child's health or development. Neglect may occur during pregnancy as a result of maternal substance abuse. Once a child is born, neglect may involve a parent or carer failing to provide adequate food, clothing, and shelter (including exclusion from home or abandonment), failing to protect a child from physical and emotional harm or danger, failing to ensure adequate supervision (including the use of inadequate caregivers), or failing to ensure access to appropriate medical care or treatment. It may also include neglect of, or unresponsiveness to, a child's basic emotional needs. (See Key Point 18.2.)

> **Key Point 18.2**
>
> There are four categories of child maltreatment: physical abuse, emotional abuse, sexual abuse, and neglect

18.3 Extent of the problem

18.3.1 Prevalence

Child maltreatment is recognized to show a spectrum of severity, with larger numbers of children subject to careless or poor parenting and a small number subject to the most severe, persistent, or malicious abuse (Fig. 18.1). The true incidence of child abuse is difficult to ascertain. For instance, there are international differences in the acceptance of physical chastisement. In addition, today's global society has led to the emergence of new aspects of child exploitation such as the international trafficking of children and internet child pornography.

Children who are recognized to be at risk of significant harm are made the subject of a 'child protection plan' (England and Wales) or placed on a 'child protection register' (Scotland). This allows us to identify at any one time the reasons for registration or being subject to a plan: an estimate of the prevalence of significant maltreatment.

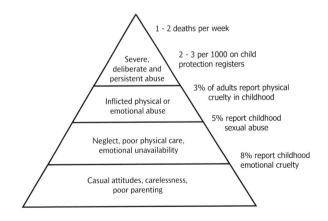

Figure 18.1 The pyramid of severity of child maltreatment (figures are UK estimates).

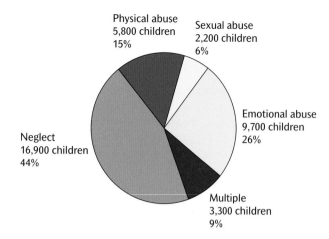

Figure 18.2 Children and young people with a child protection plan by category of abuse in England, 2009 (Department for Children, Schools and Families 2010).

Latest figures show that in England in 2010 there were 35,700 children who were the subject of a child protection plan, representing approximately 3 per 1000 of the population aged under 18. In recent years, 40–45% of cases were because of neglect, consistently the most common reason, 15–20% because of physical injury, 20–25% because of emotional abuse, 5–10% because of sexual abuse, and approximately 10% in mixed categories (Fig. 18.2). The highest rate of child protection plans is in children aged under 1 year. Young children are the most likely to be reported and registered because of the higher likelihood of very serious consequences of severe neglect and physical assault.

Children from all social, cultural, and religious backgrounds may be subject to maltreatment. Professionals need to be aware of and sensitive to differing family patterns, lifestyles, and child-rearing practices, but clear that child abuse cannot be condoned for religious or cultural reasons. Forced marriage, female genital mutilation, and 'honour'-based violence are examples of newer challenges in this field. Working in a multiracial and multicultural society requires commitment to equality in meeting the needs of all children and families.

It is now recognized that if families can be identified and supported at a stage where they are 'in need', potential crises may be averted and there may be less requirement for child protection action. 'Children in need' can be defined as 'those who require additional support or services to achieve their full potential'. In England there are currently 11–12 million children. Of these, 300 000–400 000 are recognized as being 'children in need'.

18.3.2 A shared responsibility

Child protection is the responsibility of all members of society—it is everyone's responsibility. In order to ensure that the task of protecting children is carried out effectively, different groups of professionals (Box 18.3) each have a specific role. Government guidance specifies how they should work together to fulfil this shared responsibility.

Box 18.3 A shared responsibility: agencies which work together

- Local government children's (social) services
- Health services, including dental services
- Education, including nurseries, schools, and colleges
- Criminal justice organizations, including police and probation
- Family courts and legal support
- Youth and community workers
- Sport and leisure services
- Voluntary and private sector organizations
- Faith communities

The development of legal and professional strategies and systems to safeguard children is an ongoing process. Whenever a death tragically occurs, an investigation is carried out to see what lessons can be learned. These often highlight the complexity of the process and reveal potential loopholes in a system designed to protect those who are most vulnerable. There can never be complacency in child protection. Four areas are recurrently identified where professional practice could be improved:

- recognition
- communication
- procedures
- record-keeping.

18.3.3 The role of the dental team

The dental team is well placed to take part in the shared responsibility of protecting children. The reasons for this include the following:

- Dentists are skilled at examining the head and neck and recording their findings. The head and neck is frequently a site of injury in physical abuse.
- Untreated dental disease may itself be a sign of neglect.
- Children often attend the dentist regularly, even when they may have little or no contact with other health services.
- Dentists often treat more than one family member, so may get to know about wider issues that impact on a child's well-being.

Dental professionals may observe the signs of abuse or neglect, or hear something that causes them concern about a child. Child protection concerns may also come to the attention of dental teams that only treat adults, so they also need to know about these issues and how to respond. Research has shown that dental professionals often lack confidence in this field of practice. However, it is never a task that the dental team faces alone. Advice and support are always available from experienced child protection professionals. (See Key Points 18.3.)

Key Points 18.3

- Child protection is the shared responsibility of different agencies working together.
- The dental team has a responsibility to work with other agencies to protect children and young people at risk.
- All members of the dental team can contribute to fulfilling this responsibility.
- Dental professionals can seek advice, when needed, from experienced child protection professionals.

18.4 Recognizing the signs

Abuse or neglect may present to the dental team in a number of different ways:

- through a direct allegation (sometimes termed a 'disclosure' made by the child, a parent, or some other person);
- through signs and symptoms which are suggestive of maltreatment;
- through observations of child behaviour or parent–child interaction.

However it presents, any concerns should be taken seriously and appropriate action taken. It is assumed that the dentist will be examining a child who is fully dressed, so signs and symptoms related to areas not covered by clothes will be the focus of discussion.

18.4.1 Markers of physical abuse

There are no hard-and-fast rules to make the diagnosis of physical abuse easier. The following list constitutes seven classic indicators to the diagnosis. None of them is absolute on its own, and neither does the absence of any of them preclude the diagnosis of physical abuse.

- There is a delay in seeking medical help (or medical help is not sought at all).
- The story of the 'accident' is vague and lacking in detail, and may vary with each telling and from person to person.
- The account of the accident is not compatible with the injury observed.
- The parents' mood is abnormal. Normal parents are full of creative anxiety for the child, while abusing parents tend to be more preoccupied with their own problems—for example, how they can return home as soon as possible.
- The parents' behaviour gives cause for concern—for example, they may become hostile and rebut accusations that have not been made.
- The child's appearance and interaction with the parents are abnormal. The child may look sad, withdrawn, or frightened.
- The child may say something concerning the injury that gives you cause for concern.

Orofacial trauma occurs in at least 50% of children diagnosed with physical abuse. It is always important to remember that a child with one injury may have further injuries that are not visible so, where possible, arrangements should be made for the child to have a comprehensive medical examination. Although the face often seems to be the focus of impulsive violence, facial fractures are not frequent. It is extremely important to state that there are no injuries that are pathognomonic of (i.e. only occur in or prove) child abuse. Any text that suggests so is incorrect. However, some injuries or patterns of injury will be highly suggestive of it.

The assessment of any physical injury involves three stages:

- evaluating the injury itself, its extent, site, and any particular patterns;
- taking a history with a focus on understanding how and why the injury occurred and whether the findings match the story given (Figs 18.3 and 18.4);
- exploring the broader picture, including aspects of the child's behaviour, the parent–child interaction, underlying risk factors, or markers of emotional abuse or neglect.

Bruising

Accidental falls rarely cause bruises to the soft tissues of the cheek, but instead tend to involve the skin overlying bony prominences such as the forehead or cheekbone. Inflicted bruises may occur at typical sites or fit recognizable patterns. Bruising in babies or children who are not independently mobile are a cause for concern. Multiple bruises in clusters or of uniform shape are suggestive of physical abuse and may occur with older injuries. The clinical dating of bruises according to colour is inaccurate. However, multiple bruises of different ages are suggestive of physical abuse.

Bruises on the ear may result from being pinched or pulled by the ear (Fig. 18.5) and there will often be a matching bruise on the posterior surface of the ear. Bruises or cuts on the neck may result from choking or strangling by a human hand, a cord, or some sort of collar. Accidents to this site are extremely rare and should be looked upon with suspicion.

Particular patterns of bruises may be caused by pinching (paired, oval, or round bruises) (Fig. 18.6), grabbing (a round thumb imprint on one cheek with three or four fingertip bruises on the other) (Fig. 18.7),

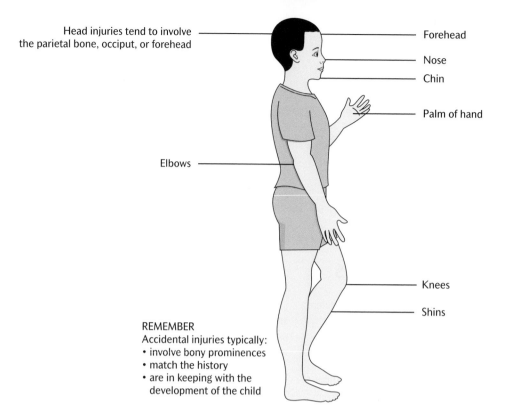

Head injuries tend to involve the parietal bone, occiput, or forehead

Forehead

Nose

Chin

Palm of hand

Elbows

Knees

Shins

REMEMBER
Accidental injuries typically:
• involve bony prominences
• match the history
• are in keeping with the development of the child

Figure 18.3 Typical sites of accidental injuries. (Reproduced from Harris, J.C. *et al.*, Child protection and the dental team. © COPDEND 2006.)

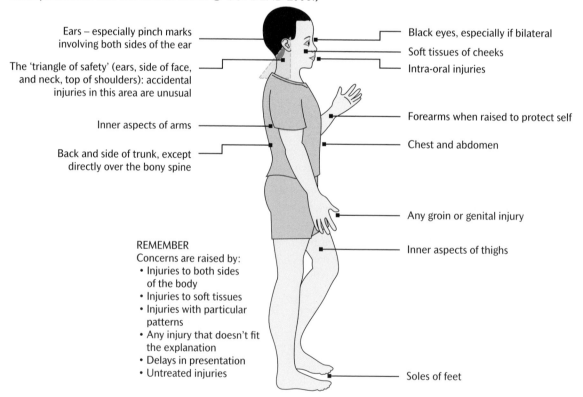

Ears – especially pinch marks involving both sides of the ear

Black eyes, especially if bilateral

Soft tissues of cheeks

The 'triangle of safety' (ears, side of face, and neck, top of shoulders): accidental injuries in this area are unusual

Intra-oral injuries

Inner aspects of arms

Forearms when raised to protect self

Chest and abdomen

Back and side of trunk, except directly over the bony spine

Any groin or genital injury

Inner aspects of thighs

REMEMBER
Concerns are raised by:
• Injuries to both sides of the body
• Injuries to soft tissues
• Injuries with particular patterns
• Any injury that doesn't fit the explanation
• Delays in presentation
• Untreated injuries

Soles of feet

Figure 18.4 Typical sites of injuries that should raise concern. (Reproduced from Harris, J.C. *et al.*, Child protection and the dental team. © COPDEND 2006.)

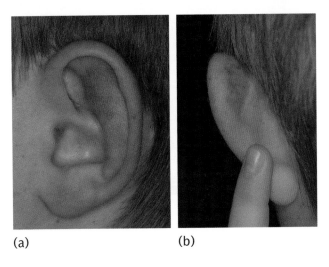

(a)　　　　　　(b)

Figure 18.5 Bruising on both the (a) inner and (b) outer surfaces of the ear in a 12-year-old child.

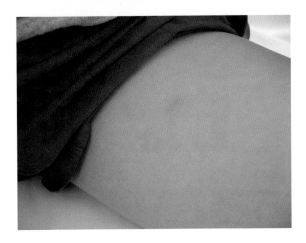

Figure 18.6 Pinch mark on the leg of a 7-year-old boy, showing the typical appearance of two small round bruises separated by a clear space.

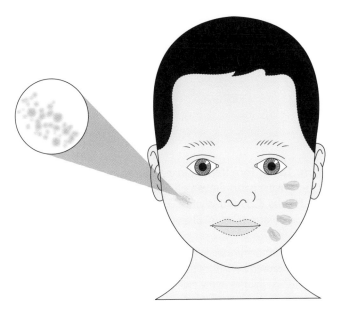

Figure 18.7 Artist's impression of grab or grip marks, showing a round bruise made with a thumb on one cheek and three or four fingertip bruises on the other cheek. (Reproduced from Harris, J.C. *et al.*, Child protection and the dental team. © COPDEND 2006.)

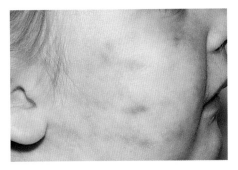

Figure 18.8 Characteristic parallel linear bruising of a slap mark on a child's cheek. (Reproduced with kind permission of Munksgaard.)

the orofacial structures. Accidental facial abrasions and lacerations are usually explained by a consistent history, such as falling off a bicycle, and are often associated with injuries at other sites, such as knees and elbows.

Burns

Approximately 10% of physical abuse cases involve burns. Burns of the oral mucosa can be the result of forced ingestion of hot or caustic fluids in young children. Burns from hot solid objects applied to the face are usually without blister formation and the shape of the burn often resembles the implement used. Intentional cigarette burns result in circular punched-out lesions of uniform size (Fig. 18.9). It is important to be aware that other medical conditions, such as bullous impetigo, may mimic the round lesions of cigarette burns.

Bite marks

Human bite marks are identified by their shape and size (Fig. 18.10). The nature and location of the bite are likely to change with increasing age of the child. They may appear only as bruising, or as a pattern of

or hand slaps (parallel linear, often petechial, marks on the cheek at finger-width spacing) (Fig. 18.8). Bizarrely shaped bruises with sharp borders are nearly always deliberately inflicted. If there is a pattern on the inflicting implement, this may be duplicated in the bruise—so-called tattoo bruising.

Abrasions and lacerations

Abrasions and lacerations on the face in abused children may be caused by a variety of objects but are most commonly due to rings or fingernails on the inflicting hand. Such injuries are rarely confined to

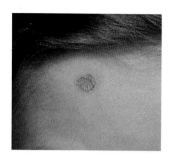

Figure 18.9 Cigarette burn on the forehead of a 7-year-old girl, showing the typical appearance of a circular lesion of diameter 0.8–1.0cm with a well-defined edge. (Reproduced from Hobbs, C.J. and Wynne, J.M., *Physical signs of child abuse: a colour atlas.* © Elsevier 2001.)

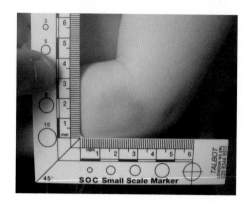

Figure 18.10 Human bite mark on a child's arm, presenting as diffuse bruising. (Reproduced with kind permission of Professor G.T. Craig.)

abrasions and lacerations. They may be caused by other children, or by adults in an assault or as an inappropriate form of punishment. Sexually orientated bite marks occur more frequently in adolescents and adults. A bite mark at any age should raise the suspicion of child sexual abuse.

The duration of a bite mark depends on the force applied and the extent of tissue damage. Tooth marks that do not break the skin can disappear within 24 hours but may persist for longer. In those cases where the skin is broken, the borders or edges will be apparent for several days, depending on the thickness of the tissue. Thinner tissues retain the marks for longer. A bite mark presents a unique opportunity to identify the perpetrator (see Section 18.7.2).

Eye injuries

Periorbital bruising in children is uncommon and should raise suspicion, particularly if bilateral. Ocular damage in child physical abuse includes acute hyphaema (bleeding in the anterior chamber of the eye), dislocated lens, traumatic cataract, and detached retina. More than half of these injuries result in permanent impairment of vision affecting one or both eyes.

Bone fractures

Fractures resulting from abuse may occur in almost any bone including the facial skeleton. They may be single or multiple, clinically obvious or occult, and detectable only by radiography. Most fractures in physically abused children occur under the age of 3. In contrast, accidental fractures occur more commonly in children of school age. Facial fractures are relatively uncommon in children.

When abuse is suspected, the presence of any fracture is an indication for a full skeletal radiographic survey. Generally the force required to produce a facial fracture in a child is greater than that required to produce fractures in long bones. A child who has suffered sustained physical abuse may show evidence of multiple fractures at different stages of healing.

Intra-oral injuries

Damage to the primary or permanent teeth can be due to blunt trauma. Such injuries are often accompanied by local soft tissue lacerations and bruising. The age of the child and the history of the incident

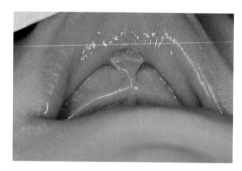

Figure 18.11 Torn frenum in a 3-month-old baby, in whom further investigation revealed fractured ribs. (Reproduced from Hobbs, C.J. and Wynne, J.M., *Physical signs of child abuse: a colour atlas.* © Elsevier 2001.)

are crucial factors in raising suspicion and determining whether the injury was caused by abusive behaviour (Maguire *et al.* 2007).

Penetrating injuries to the palate, vestibule, and floor of the mouth can occur during forceful feeding of young infants and are usually caused by the feeding utensil.

Bruising and laceration of the upper labial frenum is not uncommon in a young child who falls while learning to walk (generally between 8 and 18 months) or in older children due to accidental trauma. However, a frenum tear in a very young non-ambulatory patient (less than 1 year) should arouse suspicion (Fig. 18.11). It may be produced by a direct blow to the mouth and may remain hidden on examination unless the lip is carefully everted. Any accompanying facial bruising or abrasions should also be meticulously noted.

Fabricated or induced illness

Fabricated or induced illness may come to light because a parent or carer claims that the child has signs or symptoms, or exaggerates them, yet these are never observed by health professionals and cannot be verified. Alternatively, there may be parental interference with treatment, such as overdosing with medication or withholding medication. This may cause professionals to arrange unnecessary investigations or operations. The

Table 18.1 Differential diagnosis: conditions that may mimic physical abuse

Abusive injury	Other conditions
Unexplained, unusual, or multiple bruises	Bleeding disorder, birth marks (e.g. haemangioma, Mongolian blue spot)
Unexplained, multiple, or frequent fractures	Osteogenesis imperfecta
Burns	Photodermatitis (skin blistering caused by combined effect of a chemical, often plant oils, with sunlight), impetigo, accidental caustic burns (e.g. from leaking batteries in toys)
Skin abrasions and lacerations	Scratching due to scabies
Ocular trauma	Conjunctivitis

consequences may be physical harm to the child or emotional harm and long-term impact on the child's health and development.

Differential diagnosis

Although dental practitioners should be suspicious of all injuries to children, they should be aware that the diagnosis of child physical abuse is never made on the basis of one sign as various other conditions can be mistaken for child physical abuse (Table 18.1). The lesions of impetigo may look similar to cigarette burns, birthmarks can be mistaken for bruising, and conjunctivitis can be mistaken for trauma. All children who are said to bruise easily and extensively should be screened for bleeding disorders (see Chapter 3, Fig. 3.4). Unexplained, multiple, or frequent fractures may rarely be due to osteogenesis imperfecta; a family history, blue sclerae, and the dental changes of dentinogenesis imperfecta may all help in establishing the diagnosis (see also Section 13.7.3).

18.4.2 Markers of emotional abuse

Emotional abuse causes unhappiness and damage to the child's developing personality that may be irreversible. Such abuse often accompanies other forms of violence and neglect. It may be missed if a child appears to be well nourished and well cared for.

Clues may be found in the emotional state and behaviour of the child. For example, they may be clingy and become distressed when a parent is not present or, alternatively, they may be agitated, non-compliant, and unable to concentrate, or withdrawn, watchful, and anxious. Older children may self-harm, abuse drugs and alcohol, exhibit delinquent behaviour, run away from home, or have educational problems. Further signs of emotional abuse that may be noted in the child's presentation are shown in Box 18.4.

Alternatively, emotional abuse may come to the attention of the dental team by observation of the child's interaction with the parent. For example, the parent may ignore the child or use abusive or inappropriate language; they may threaten the child in the dental surgery or have unrealistic expectations of the child's abilities to cope with dental treatment.

Box 18.4 Signs of emotional abuse

- Poor growth
- Developmental delay
- Educational failure
- Social immaturity
- Lack of social responsiveness
- Aggression
- Attachment disorders
- Indiscriminate friendliness
- Challenging behaviour
- Attention difficulties

On occasions the dental team may become aware that a child is being exposed to the frightening and traumatic experience of witnessing domestic abuse. Perhaps it is the injured parent who is the dental patient, yet the dental team should also be concerned for any child in the family and must respond accordingly.

18.4.3 Markers of sexual abuse

Sexual abuse is an abuse of power and may be perpetrated by both men and women, or by other children. It may present to the dental team in any of the following ways:

- Intra-oral signs of sexual abuse: erythema, ulceration, or vesicle formation arising from gonorrhoea or other sexually transmitted diseases, or signs of oral trauma such as erythema and petechiae at the junction of the hard and soft palate which may indicate oral sex.

- With a 'disclosure' or allegation of abuse made by the child: children usually choose to disclose to a trusted adult, who may be a dental professional who has gained their trust.

- Pregnancy: sex with a child under 16 is illegal and pregnancy below the age of 13 is charged as rape; sexual abuse should be considered particularly where there is concern about a difference in power or mental capacity, or about exploitation.

- Emotional or behavioural signs such as delayed development, anxiety and depression, psychosomatic indicators, self-harm, soiling or wetting, inappropriate sexual behaviour or knowledge, running away, and alcohol or substance abuse.

18.4.4 Markers of neglect

Neglect is insidious and affects all aspects of a child's health and development: emotional health, social development, cognitive development, and physical health. In the long term, adults who were neglected as children are known to experience a higher incidence of adverse life events such as arrest by the police, suicide attempts, major depression, diabetes, and heart disease.

Failure of the parent to recognize or meet their child's needs and comply with professional advice is a common factor in many types of neglect (Table 18.2). Children's needs include nutrition, clothing,

Table 18.2 Neglect of a child's needs

The child's needs	Effects of neglect
Nutrition	Failure to thrive, short stature
Warmth, clothing, shelter	Inappropriate clothing (e.g. for the weather or the child's size), cold injury, sunburn
Safe environment	Frequent injuries (e.g. burns/cuts from playing with matches/knives), animal bites
Hygiene	Persistently smelly and dirty, infestation with headlice or scabies, persistently poor oral hygiene
Healthcare	Missed immunizations, compromised health including being left in ongoing pain, failure to administer essential prescribed medication, untreated dental caries
Stimulation and education	Developmental delay
Affection	Withdrawn or attention-seeking behaviour

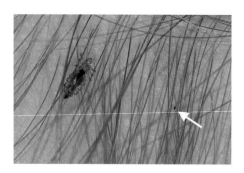

Figure 18.12 Head louse and egg (arrow). After hatching, the empty egg case or 'nit' remains attached to the hair shaft, appearing as a whitish speck. Severe and persistent infestation is cause for concern about possible neglect.

Key Points 18.4

- Child maltreatment may present to the dental team through (a) a direct allegation, (b) signs and symptoms, or (c) observations of child behaviour or parent–child interaction.
- Any injury, including oral injury, in a non-mobile baby is a cause for concern.
- Any injury with an absent or unsuitable explanation is a cause for concern.
- The dental team must be able to recognize the varied presenting features of child maltreatment.

shelter, hygiene (Fig. 18.12), and healthcare. Failure to take a child for healthcare appointments when required and for necessary dental care is neglectful. Dental neglect will be considered in more detail in Section 18.8. (See Key Points 18.4.)

18.5 Vulnerable groups

Certain individuals or groups of children may be more vulnerable to abuse or neglect because of risk factors in their family or environment, or because of the way they are perceived by their carers (Table 18.3). Recognizing these vulnerable groups may enable the dental practitioner to take steps to promote and safeguard the well-being of such children and to respond appropriately to concerns. However, it is important not to stigmatize families because of the presence of particular risk factors. Whilst the risks of maltreatment may be higher, the majority of children within these vulnerable groups are loved and cared for and do not experience abuse.

18.5.1 Parental factors

Young or single parents, parents with learning difficulties, those who themselves have experienced adverse childhoods, and those with any mental health problems, including problems of substance or alcohol abuse, are all at greater risk of abusing or neglecting their children. They may often need extra support in meeting their children's needs and may be more vulnerable to the stresses inherent in parenting.

18.5.2 Social factors

Families living in adverse social environments, for example due to poverty, social isolation, or poor housing, may find it both materially and socially harder to care for their children. Where poverty or the social environment is affecting a child's care, it may be possible to intervene to support the family at an early stage before the child suffers harm.

Children may flee from famine, war, or torture and arrive in a new country, either with their families or unaccompanied, as asylum seekers or refugees. On arrival in the host country, displaced children may face ongoing barriers to accessing healthcare, education, and social support.

Table 18.3 Vulnerable children

Parental risk factors: parents needing additional support to meet child's needs	Social risk factors: families living in adverse social environments	Child risk factors: children in need of additional help to safeguard their welfare
Young parents	Poverty	Babies and toddlers are most vulnerable
Single parents	Social isolation	Older children, particularly girls, are more vulnerable to sexual abuse
Parents with learning difficulties	Poor housing	Children with disabilities
Parental mental health problems	Family violence	Children with behavioural problems
Parental alcohol and substance abuse	Asylum seekers and refugees	Children looked after in foster or residential care
	Homeless families	Children who go missing from education

18.5.3 Child factors

Age plays an important role in the patterns of child abuse. Younger children are much more vulnerable to physical abuse and neglect, with at least 10% of all abuse involving children under the age of 1. In contrast, sexual abuse more often (though not exclusively) involves older children, particularly girls.

Children with disabilities are much more at risk of experiencing abuse of all kinds (Miller 2002). A wide variety of factors may contribute to that risk, sometimes including their greater dependence on carers (including for hygiene and intimate care), increased stress on the carers, and difficulties for the young person to communicate and express concerns. It is also well documented that people with disabilities face barriers when accessing health services. Therefore particular attention should be given to supporting the needs, including the dental needs, of children with disabilities and being alert to signs, symptoms, and behavioural indicators that may indicate abuse or neglect.

Further vulnerable groups are children who are 'looked after' in foster care or residential care and children who are 'missing from education'. They may require additional help to promote their health and well-being. (See Key Points 18.5.)

> **Key Points 18.5**
>
> - Certain groups of children may be more vulnerable to abuse or neglect because of risk factors in their family, environment, or personal circumstances.
> - Recognizing this helps dental practitioners to respond appropriately to concerns in order to safeguard and promote the well-being of these children.

18.6 Responding

In this section we describe what you should do when you have concerns about a child. The flowchart in Fig. 18.13 summarizes the process.

18.6.1 Assessing the child

As with all aspects of dentistry, assessing a child with an injury or with possible signs of abuse or neglect starts with taking a thorough history (Box 18.5). As well as getting details from the child and carer of any injury or presenting complaint, it is important to consider aspects of the past dental history, the wider medical history, and the family and social circumstances.

Particular aspects of the presentation may in themselves raise some concerns and should be carefully evaluated. These would include, for example, a delay in the presentation, discrepancies between the history and examination findings, or previous concerns about the child or siblings. A full dental examination should be carried out, noting in particular any dental, oral, or facial injuries, their site, their extent, and any

specific patterns (Box 18.5). It is also important to note the general appearance of the child, their state of hygiene, whether they appear to be growing well or are 'failing to thrive', their demeanour, and their

> **Box 18.5 Assessing the child**
>
> **History: features of concern**
> - Changing or inconsistent history
> - Developmentally inappropriate (does not fit with the age of the child)
> - Delay in presentation
> - Previous concerns, including siblings
>
> **Examination**
> - General appearance (growth, hygiene)
> - Injuries (site, extent, patterns)
> - Dental examination

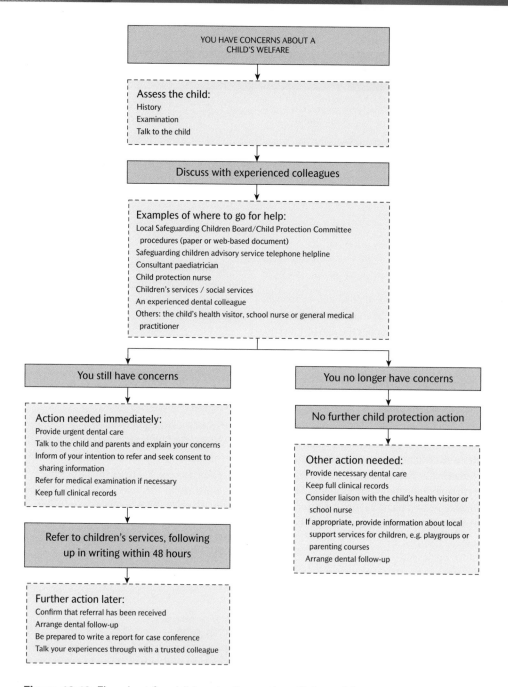

Figure 18.13 Flowchart for child protection action. (Adapted from Harris, J.C. *et al.*, Child protection and the dental team. © COPDEND 2006.)

interaction with their parents or carers and others. Look particularly for signs of 'frozen watchfulness' where the child seems to take in everything going on, but in a detached, wary, or fearful manner.

Talking to the child

It is good practice to ask the child about the cause of any injuries and to allow them to talk if they volunteer information about abuse. You should avoid asking leading questions and should respond calmly and kindly with a non-judgemental attitude. A child who makes a disclosure

of abuse should always be taken seriously. If they ask you to keep a secret, you should not do so but explain that you may have to share information, but will explain with whom and when it will be shared.

18.6.2 What to do next

Remember that you still have the responsibility for dealing with any injury or dental needs; no child should be left untreated or in pain because of underlying concerns about maltreatment. Your next step is to take action on your concerns. Research shows that most dental practitioners want to be sure that they have made the right diagnosis before they take action. In reality, the responsibility for making a diagnosis is always shared by a multi-agency team. Dentists are not required to make the diagnosis but must share any concerns appropriately. In doing so, they may contribute a vital 'piece of the jigsaw' (Fig. 18.14) and initiate the process for effective protection of the child. To delay puts that child at risk of continuing abuse. A further opportunity for someone to spot the abuse and intervene may not present for some time.

Colleagues to consult

Remember that you do not need to manage this on your own. You should discuss the case with an appropriately experienced colleague, possibly a dental colleague, or a child protection nurse advisor (safeguarding children advisor), paediatrician, or social worker. This will depend on the setting in which you are working. Hospitals may have appointed child protection liaison workers. If you work in a health centre you may have close working relationships with health visitors and school nurses, some of whom are highly experienced in child protection and may be a source of helpful advice.

Making a referral

If, having had discussions with an appropriate colleague, you remain concerned, you should make a referral to your local children's (social) services. You should already have identified in advance where and how to contact your children's services team. Referrals should be made by telephone, so that you can discuss your concerns directly, and should be followed up in writing within 48 hours. Your letter should clearly document the facts of the case and include an explicit statement of why you are concerned. The telephone discussion should be clearly recorded, documenting what was said, what decisions were made, and an unambiguous action plan.

Informing the child and parents

It is good practice to explain your concerns to the child and parents, inform them of your intention to refer, and seek their consent. Research shows that being open and honest from the start results in better outcomes for children. There are certain exceptions, and reasonable judgement must be made in each case. Usually you should *not* discuss your concerns with the parents in the following circumstances:

- where discussion might put the child at greater risk;
- where discussion would impede a police investigation or social work enquiry;
- where sexual abuse by a family member, or organized, or multiple abuse is suspected;
- where fabricated or induced illness is suspected;
- where parents or carers are being violent or abusive, and discussion would place you or others at risk;
- where it is not possible to contact parents or carers without causing undue delay in making the referral.

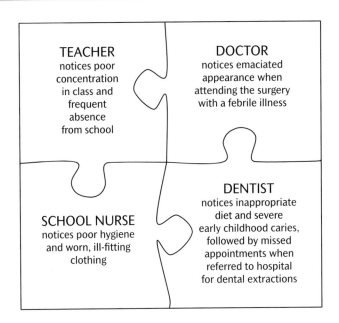

Figure 18.14 When information from different sources is shared, a more complete picture of concern emerges.

Coping with the aftermath

You should always receive feedback from children's services about the outcome of your referral and the action they intend to take. It is quite normal to have some anxiety about the consequences of making a child protection referral, including fears about potential adverse consequences for the child or family, or repercussions on your dental practice or yourself (Welbury *et al*. 2003). Talking it through or 'debriefing' with an experienced colleague may be helpful. Alternatively you may wish to seek confidential counselling through your local occupational health or child protection department.

18.6.3 What happens after referral

Many practitioners worry that by making a referral to social services, they will initiate a process that will quickly get out of hand, and end up with severe and drastic action being taken to remove the child and punish the family. This is a misperception that does not reflect current practice in the UK. Fewer than 50% of children investigated for possible abuse end up being placed on child protection registers. It is estimated that fewer than 1% of children referred to social services for possible abuse end up in judicial proceedings. Usually families are supported to make their own arrangements for safe and effective care of the child. The precise procedures followed may show regional variation or change according to prevailing government policy, but the following description illustrates the general principles.

When a child is referred to social services on suspicion of abuse, the duty social worker will note details of the child and family and the concerns that are being raised. The social work team manager will then convene a strategy discussion (often by telephone) with a senior member of the police child protection team. This happens within one working day and often involves a paediatrician or other health professional.

The purpose of this strategy discussion is to share information and decide on how best to manage the referral, taking note of the concerns that have been raised. They may decide that a social worker will visit the family to carry out an initial assessment or initiate a joint investigation with the police. If the concerns are minor, or the family is already known to other professionals, it may be appropriate for those professionals to take the lead in supporting and working with the family, rather than continuing down a child protection route. In extreme cases, where there is the risk of immediate harm to the child, legal action may be required through an emergency protection order or police powers of protection. In those cases where the initial assessment identifies ongoing concerns and risks, a multi-agency case conference may be held. Parents are normally invited to these conferences. At the conference, all those present are given an opportunity to share information about the child and family, including any concerns they may have. The conference chair then summarizes any identified risks to the child, along with any factors that may be serving to protect the child or support the family. An action plan is then agreed with the family in order to provide support and ensure the safety of the child. This plan will include a decision on whether the child's name should be placed on the child protection register—a decision that is then reviewed at a further case conference after 3 months and at any subsequent conferences that may be held until such time as the child is felt to be no longer at risk of significant harm. At any stage in this process, it may be necessary to take legal action to protect the child, but this would only be where it has been shown that the child cannot be protected without recourse to such action.

18.7 Legal aspects

18.7.1 Information sharing and confidentiality

Whenever a child dies in the UK as a result of abuse, local agencies are required to undertake a serious case review to look at the case and any lessons that might be learned from it. One consistent theme comes out in all these case reviews—a failure of communication between professionals involved with the child. If we are ever going to protect children from abuse, it is crucial that we learn to communicate with each other and share information.

You will have information about the child that no other professional will have. You may need to share it in the following circumstances:

- to refer a child about whom you have concerns, as discussed previously;
- to respond to a request for information for a child protection initial assessment or case conference regarding a child in your care.

Ethical guidance

Practitioners are often anxious about the legal or ethical restrictions on sharing information, particularly with other agencies. You should be aware of the law and should comply with the principles of current ethical guidance for the dental team. These do not provide an absolute barrier to information sharing. You should be prepared to exercise your judgement and share information proportionate to your level of concern about the child. A failure to pass on information that might prevent a tragedy could expose you to criticism in the same way as an unjustified disclosure.

Consent

In most situations, it will be appropriate to share any concerns you have identified with the family and to obtain their consent to sharing information with others. However, as discussed earlier, there may be situations where discussing your concerns with the family could put the child at greater risk or put you or your staff at risk. In practice, such situations are rare. Restrictions on sharing information are embodied in the common law duty of confidence, the Human Rights Act 1998 and the Data Protection Act 1998. Within these frameworks there is provision for sharing information in any of the following situations:

- where those likely to be affected give consent;
- the public interest in safeguarding the child's welfare overrides the need to keep the information confidential;
- disclosure is required under a court order or other legal obligation.

Therefore, if you have concerns about a child's welfare, and you consider that sharing information is important in safeguarding that child, you should share that information even if you are unable to gain parental consent to do so. Sources of further guidance include the professional defence organizations.

18.7.2 Forensic aspects of child protection practice

Any situation where a child has been harmed as a result of abuse or neglect potentially involves a criminal offence against that child. The responsibility for carrying out any criminal investigation rests with the police and will usually be carried out by the local police child protection team. All other agencies have a responsibility to cooperate with the police in carrying out such investigations. Therefore you may be required to assist the police by providing a statement, providing copies of records, or carrying out particular forensic examinations or tests where you are qualified to do so. If you are in any doubt you should seek advice from an experienced colleague. Comprehensive, contemporaneous, and accurate record-keeping is essential to this process.

Diagrams and clinical photographs

When you examine a child, you should consider whether your notes should include a diagram of your findings (such as that shown in Chapter 3, Fig. 3.10) or be supplemented by clinical photographs. Diagrams and photographs should be clearly labelled with the child's identity and the date and time marked. They should be referred to in the clinical notes. Diagrams should be annotated with descriptions and measurements of any injuries. Note the inclusion of a measurement scale in Fig. 18.10.

DNA sampling

Where a child has been assaulted, it may be possible to obtain forensic evidence, including DNA sampling. You may be asked to assist the police in obtaining such samples, for example through taking swabs of a bite mark or other injury. Strict procedures must be followed in order to ensure the validity in court of any samples. This may involve, for example, a clear documented 'chain of evidence' where a sample is passed from one person to another with no possibility of contamination.

Bite marks

Documenting and interpreting the significance of bite marks must be carried out by someone with training and experience in forensic odontology. Local police may have a preferred expert. Dental practitioners should be clear about their own limitations and only offer opinions within their level of expertise. Certain features of the injury may help to distinguish animal from human bites and adult from child bites. It may also be possible to match the impression left with the dentition of a suspected perpetrator. Assessment of these cases may involve:

- examination of the injury and provision of diagrams, documentation, and forensic photographs obtained according to a clear procedure;
- examination, photographs, and impressions of the victim's own dentition;
- examination, photographs, and impressions of any alleged perpetrator or other family members.

18.7.3 Giving evidence in court

In cases of severe child abuse or neglect, two parallel legal processes may be required: the prosecution of an alleged offender in the criminal courts and the protection of children under the Children Act in the civil courts. The two processes take different routes and rely on different levels of evidence. The decision as to whether or not criminal proceedings should be initiated is based on three main factors:

- whether or not there is sufficient evidence to prosecute;
- whether it is in the public interest that proceedings should be instigated against a particular offender;
- whether or not a criminal prosecution is in the best interests of the child.

The evidential standard required by the criminal court is proof 'beyond reasonable doubt' that the defendant committed the offence. In contrast, civil proceedings are initiated by the local authority for the protection of the child and rely on finding 'on the balance of probabilities' that a child has suffered or is likely to suffer significant harm.

As a professional involved in a case, you may be called upon to provide evidence in either court. Your responsibility to the court is to provide an accurate and unbiased account of your findings, your opinion based on those findings, and any action that you took as a consequence. In a court situation, you should never venture beyond your level of expertise or provide opinions that you are unable to back up. Those unfamiliar with court procedures should seek advice and training. (See Key Points 18.6.)

Key Points 18.6

- If you are concerned about a child, you have a duty to follow local child protection procedures and share information appropriately.
- To delay taking necessary action puts a child at risk of continuing abuse; a further opportunity for someone to spot the abuse and intervene may not present for some time.

18.8 Dental neglect

Many adults visit the dentist only for emergency treatment when they are in pain and choose not to return for treatment to restore complete oral health. They may choose to use dental services in a similar manner for their children. Dental professionals have traditionally respected this choice and not challenged this behaviour. However, children may suffer ongoing dental pain or other adverse consequences as a result and, when young, are reliant on their carers to seek treatment for them. Anecdotally, it is reported that other health professionals who work regularly with children are shocked that the dental team often fails to follow up such children rigorously.

With the rise of the safeguarding children agenda, this has become a topical issue. In the context of increasing emphasis on preventing maltreatment, improving multi-agency working, and encouraging early intervention, rather than intervening only when a crisis occurs, the dental profession has had to reconsider the diagnosis and management of child dental neglect.

18.8.1 Diagnosis of dental neglect

The British Society of Paediatric Dentistry defines dental neglect as 'the persistent failure to meet a child's basic oral health needs, likely to result in the serious impairment of a child's oral or general health or development' (Harris *et al.* 2009). It may occur in isolation or may be an indicator of a wider picture of child maltreatment. The focus of this definition is on identifying unmet need (Box 18.6), so that the family can receive the support they need, rather than on apportioning blame. Children have a right to oral health, which forms an integral part of their general health (see also Box 18.2).

When assessing a child with dental disease it is important to assess the impact of the disease on the individual. Severe untreated dental disease can cause:

- toothache;
- disturbed sleep;

Box 18.6 Children's basic oral health needs

To maintain optimal oral health, children need:

- fluoride—a regular source, usually supplied by twice daily use of fluoride toothpaste;
- diet—limited frequency of sugary snacks and drinks;
- oral hygiene—facilities, supervision, and assistance;
- dental visits—to benefit from preventive care and treatment when needed.

- difficulty with eating or change in food preferences;
- absence from school and interference with play and socialization.

It may also put a child at risk of:

- being teased because of poor dental appearance;
- needing repeated antibiotics;
- repeated exposure to the morbidity associated with general anaesthesia;
- chronic localized infection which may affect underlying developing teeth;
- severe acute infection which can cause life-threatening systemic illness.

In addition, there is a growing body of evidence indicating that untreated caries in preschool children is associated with lower body weight, slower growth, and poorer quality of life (Sheiham 2006).

However, it should be remembered that dental caries is a very common finding in children and, even when extensive, does not always indicate neglect. A 2003 survey found that by the age of 5 years, 43% of UK children had obvious decay and 5% had had teeth extracted under general anaesthesia. Therefore care should be taken to assess the child in the context of all other relevant factors. Dental caries, like any other finding in cases of suspected abuse or neglect, should never be interpreted in isolation. It must always be assessed in the context of the child's medical and social history and developmental stage (Fig. 18.15). Any previous dental treatment received by the child may be particularly relevant, for example whether a previous dentist has chosen to manage caries in primary teeth by monitoring rather than restoration or extraction. In older children and young people, whose autonomy with respect to healthcare decisions should be respected, they themselves may have made the choice to decline or delay treatment advised by the dentist. Furthermore, factors such as inequalities in dental health (e.g. regional or social class differences in caries experience) and inequalities in access to dental services (e.g. in inner city and rural areas) may need consideration.

The features that give cause for particular concern after dental problems have been pointed out to parents and appropriate and acceptable treatment offered are summarized in Box 18.7.

18.8.2 Management of dental neglect

When dental neglect is suspected and is accompanied by signs of general neglect a child protection referral should be made as already discussed. However, in cases where there is a lower level of concern and

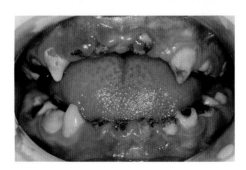

Figure 18.15 Severe untreated dental caries in a 4-year-old girl. This complex case must be interpreted in the context of her medical history (22q11 deletion syndrome resulting in congenital heart defect, learning difficulties, enamel defects, and xerostomia), previous dental history (failure to comply with preventive advice, missed appointments for extractions under general anaesthesia), social history (parental anxiety about general anaesthesia, parental mistrust of health professionals following severe illness in the neonatal period, a new baby in the family), and difficulties with access to specialist dental care (at a supra-regional centre a 3-hour journey away).

Box 18.7 Dental neglect: features of particular concern

- Severe untreated dental disease, particularly that which is obvious to a layperson or other non-dental health professional.
- Dental disease resulting in a significant impact on the child.
- Parents or carers have access to but persistently fail to obtain treatment for the child, as may be indicated by:
  - irregular attendance and repeated missed appointments
  - failure to complete planned treatment
  - returning in pain at repeated intervals
  - requiring repeated general anaesthesia for dental extractions.

---

signs of apparently isolated dental neglect, it is appropriate for the dental team to consider a tiered response. Current guidance and policy documents (Harris *et al.* 2006, 2009) advocate three stages of intervention, implemented according to the level of concern:

1. preventive dental team management
2. preventive multi-agency management
3. child protection referral

Preventive dental team management

This involves raising concerns with parents, offering support, setting targets, keeping records, and monitoring progress. The initial focus should be on relief of pain accompanied by preventive care. In order to overcome problems of poor attendance, dental treatment planning should be realistic and achievable and negotiated with the family. If concerns remain, management should progress to the next stage.

Preventive multi-agency management

This involves liaison with other professionals who are working with the family, such as the health visitor or school nurse, general medical practitioner, or social worker, to see if concerns are shared and to clarify what further steps are needed. It should be checked whether the child is subject to a child protection plan or on the child protection register. A joint plan of action should be agreed and documented, with a date specified for review.

Child protection referral

If at any point the situation is found to be too complex or deteriorating and there is concern that the child is suffering significant harm, the dental team should not delay in making a child protection referral according to local procedures.

18.9 Dental practice policy and procedures

Safeguarding children is not just about recognizing and referring when concerned about possible maltreatment, but also about changing the environment to ensure that risks to children are minimized (Fig. 18.16). The following tips for good practice are recommended to ensure that practices are well placed not only to meet their responsibilities under current legislation but also to take an active role in safeguarding children (Harris *et al*. 2006):

- Identify a staff member to take the lead on child protection.

- Adopt a child protection policy.

- Work out a step-by-step guide of what to do if you have concerns about a child (in advance, with local telephone contacts to obtain advice or to make a referral).

- Follow best practice in record-keeping.

- Undertake regular team training.

- Practice safe staff recruitment (to avoid employing someone who may pose a risk to children).

All members of the dental team have a part to play, whether dentist, dental nurse, hygienist, therapist, dental receptionist, or practice manager. In this way dentistry can make a wider contribution to the health and well-being of the local community.

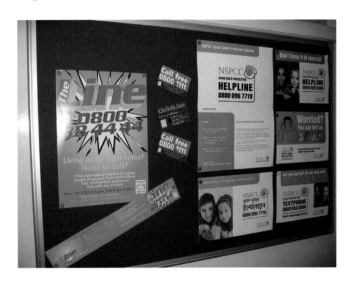

Figure 18.16 A dental practice can contribute to safeguarding children by providing information about local services and sources of help for children and families.

18.10 Summary

1 Sadly, significant numbers of children worldwide are harmed as a result of maltreatment.

2 The dental team has an important role in recognizing concerns and sharing information with child protection professionals.

3 No individual injury is diagnostic of maltreatment, but some patterns of injury make it highly likely.

4 If you recognize signs of possible maltreatment but fail to refer appropriately, a further opportunity to intervene may not present for some time, putting the child at risk of ongoing maltreatment.

In his report of the inquiry into the tragic death of an 8-year-old girl, Victoria Climbié, Lord Laming (2003) commented on how similar events might be prevented in the future saying, *'I am convinced that the answer lies in doing relatively straightforward things well. Adhering to this principle will have significant impact on the lives of vulnerable children'*. It is our belief that this can be so.

18.11 Acknowledgements

Sections of this chapter have been developed by the authors from their previous work under group authorship, *Child protection and the dental team: an introduction to safeguarding children in dental practice* (Harris *et al.* 2006). They would like to thank colleagues, particularly Dr Peter Sidebotham, and the Committee of Postgraduate Dental Deans and Directors (COPDEND UK) with whose kind permission the material is reproduced here.

18.12 Further reading

NICE (2009). *Clinical guideline 89: When to suspect child maltreatment.* Available online at: **http://guidance.nice.org.uk/CG89. (*This evidence-based guidance document is an authoritative reference for health professionals and has a useful accompanying quick reference guide.*)**

Welsh Child Protection Systematic Review Group (2010). *Core info.* Available online at: **http://www.core-info.cardiff.ac.uk. (*Website detailing systematic reviews on child protection, with extensive links and references to other published work on the topic.*)**

18.13 References

Caffey, J. (1946). Multiple fractures in the long bones of infants suffering from chronic subdural haematoma. *American Journal of Roentgenology, Radium Therapy, and Nuclear Medicine,* **56**, 162–73.

Department for Children, Schools and Families (2010). *Working together to safeguard children. A guide to inter-agency working to safeguard and promote the welfare of children.* Document DCSF-00305-2010. Available online at: **http://www.workingtogetheronline.co.uk**

Department for Education and Skills (2003). *Every child matters.* DFES, Athlone.

Harris, J., Sidebotham, P., Welbury, R., *et al.* (2006). *Child protection and the dental team: an introduction to safeguarding children in dental practice.* Committee of Postgraduate Dental Deans and Directors (COPDEND), Sheffield. Available online at: **www.cpdt.org.uk**

Harris, J.C., Balmer, R.C., and Sidebotham, P.D. (2009). British Society of Paediatric Dentistry: a policy document on dental neglect in children. *International Journal of Paediatric Dentistry,* DOI: 10.1111/j.1365-263X.2009.00996.x. Available online at: **www.bspd.co.uk**

Hobbs, C.J. and Wynne, J.M. (2001). *Physical signs of child abuses a colour atlas.* Elsevier, Amsterdam.

Kempe, C.H., Silverman, F.N., Steele, B.F., Droegemueller, W., and Silver, H.K. (1962). The battered-child syndrome. *Journal of the American Medical Association,* **181**, 105–12.

Laming, Lord (2003). *The Victoria Climbié Inquiry Report.* Publication no. CM5730, The Stationery Office, London. Available online at: **http://www.dh.gov.uk**

Maguire, S.A., Hunter, B., Hunter, L., Sibert, J.R., Mann, M., and Kemp, A.M. (2007). Diagnosing abuse: a systematic review of torn frenum and other intra-oral injuries. *Archives of Disease in Childhood,* **92**, 1113–17.

Miller, D. (2002). Disabled children and abuse. *NSPCC Information Briefings.* Available online at: **www.nspcc.org.uk/inform**

Sheiham, A. (2006). Dental caries affects body weight, growth and quality of life in pre-school children. *British Dental Journal,* **201**, 625–6.

United Nations Convention on the Rights of the Child (UNCRC) 1989. Office of the High Commissioner for Human Rights, Geneva.

Welbury, R.R., MacAskill, S.G., Murphy, J.M., *et al.* (2003). General dental practitioners' perception of their role within child protection: a qualitative study. *European Journal of Paediatric Dentistry,* **4**, 89–95.

Index